Clinical Orthopaedic Rehabilitation

Clinical Orthopaedic Rehabilitation

Second Edition

S. Brent Brotzman, M.D.

Assistant Professor
Texas A&M University System Health Science Center
College Station, Texas

Adjunct Professor
Department of Kinesiology
Texas A&M–Corpus Christi
Corpus Christi, Texas

Division I Team Physician
Department of Athletics
Texas A&M–Corpus Christi
Corpus Christi, Texas

Sports Medicine Specialist
North Austin Medical Center
Austin, Texas

Kevin E. Wilk, P.T.

Adjunct Assistant Professor
Programs in Physical Therapy
Marquette University
Milwaukee, Wisconsin

National Director
Research and Clinical Education
HealthSouth Rehabilitation Corporation

Associate Clinical Director
HealthSouth Sports Medicine and Rehabilitation Center
Birmingham, Alabama

Director of Rehabilitative Research
American Sports Medicine Institute
Birmingham, Alabama

Managing Editor:
Kay Daugherty
Memphis, Tennessee

 Mosby

An Affiliate of Elsevier

Mosby

An Affiliate of Elsevier

The Curtis Center
Independence Square West
Philadelphia, Pennsylvania 19106

NOTICE

Medicine is an ever-changing field. Standard safety precautions must be followed, but as new research and clinical experience broaden our knowledge, changes in treatment and drug therapy may become necessary or appropriate. Readers are advised to check the most current product information provided by the manufacturer of each drug to be administered to verify the recommended dose, the method and duration of administration, and the contraindications. It is the responsibility of the licensed physician, relying on experience and knowledge of the patient, to determine dosages and the best treatment for each individual patient. Neither the publisher nor the editor assumes any liability for any injury and/or damage to persons or property arising from this publication.

THE PUBLISHER

Previous edition copyrighted 1996

Library of Congress Cataloging-in-Publication Data

Clinical orthopaedic rehabilitation / editor, S. Brent Brotzman, Kevin E. Wilk.—2nd ed.
    p. ; cm.
    Includes bibliographical references.
    ISBN-13:978-0-323-01186-0   ISBN-10:0-323-01186-1
    1. People with disabilities—Rehabilitation. 2. Orthopedics. I. Brotzman, S. Brent. II. Wilk, Kevin E.
    [DNLM: 1. Orthopedics—methods. 2. Rehabilitation—standards. WE 168 C6405 2002]
RD797 .C55 2003
616.7'06515—dc21

2002025099

ISBN-13:978-0-323-01186-0

ISBN-10:0-323-01186-1

PIT/RRD

Printed in the United States of America

Last digit is the print number: 9 8 7 6

To my wife Cynthia,
whose patience, love, and understanding
throughout this long process
have provided continued inspiration
and encouragement.
To my parents,
whose love and sacrifice over the years
have opened countless opportunities.
And finally to my three beautiful children,
who make me want to be
the best surgeon, educator, and father
I can be.

S. Brent Brotzman, M.D.

Contributors

James R. Andrews, MD
Clinical Professor
Orthopaedics and Sports Medicine
University of Virginia School of Medicine
Charlottesville, Virginia
Clinical Professor of Surgery
School of Medicine, Division of Orthopaedic Surgery
University of Alabama at Birmingham
Birmingham, Alabama
Medical Director
American Sports Medicine Institute
Birmingham, Alabama
Orthopaedic Surgeon
Alabama Sports Medicine & Orthopaedic Center
Birmingham, Alabama

David W. Altchek, MD
Associate Professor of Clinical Surgery (Orthopaedics)
Weill Medical College of Cornell University
New York, New York
Associate Attending Surgeon
The Hospital for Special Surgery
New York, New York

Bernard R. Bach Jr., MD
Professor
Department of Orthopaedic Surgery
Director
Sports Medicine Section
Rush Medical College
Chicago, Illinois

Champ L. Baker Jr., MD
Orthopaedic Surgeon
Hughston Clinic
Columbus, Georgia
Clinical Assistant Professor
Department of Orthopaedics
Tulane University
New Orleans, Louisiana
Team Physician
Columbus State University
Columbus RedStixx
Columbus Cottonmouths
Columbus, Georgia

Mark Baker, PT
Hughston Sports Medicine Foundation
Columbus, Georgia

Mark Bohling, MS, ATC, LAT
Head Athletic Trainer/Instructor
Texas A&M University
Corpus Christi, Texas

Shawn Bonsell, MD
Sports Medicine Specialist
Baylor University Medical Center
Dallas, Texas

Gae Burchill, MHA, OTR/L, CHT
Clinical Specialist
Occupational Therapy—Hand and Upper Extremity Services
Massachusetts General Hospital
Boston, Massachusetts

Dann C. Byck, MD
Attending Physician
Department of Orthopaedic Surgery
McKay-Dee Hospital
Ogden, Utah

James H. Calandruccio, MD
Instructor
University of Tennessee—Campbell Clinic
Department of Orthopaedic Surgery
Memphis, Tennessee
Staff Orthopaedic Surgeon
Campbell Clinic
Memphis, Tennessee

Donna Ryan Callamaro, OTR/L, CHT
Senior Occupational Therapist
Occupational Therapy—Hand and Upper Extremity Services
Massachusetts General Hospital
Boston, Massachusetts

Hugh Cameron, MD
Associate Professor
Department of Surgery, Pathology, and Engineering
University of Toronto
Toronto, Canada

Staff Orthopaedic Surgeon
SunnyBrook Women's Hospital
Toronto, Canada

Mark M. Casillas, MD
Clinical Assistant Professor
University of Texas Health Sciences Center
San Antonio, Texas

Thomas O. Clanton, MD
Professor and Chairman
Department of Orthopaedics
University of Texas–Houston Medical School

Team Physician
Rice University Department of Athletics
Houston, Texas

Brian Cohen, MD
Attending Orthopaedic Surgeon
Center for Advanced Orthopaedics and Sports Medicine
Adena Regional Medical Center
Chillicothe, Ohio

Jenna Deacon Costella, ATC
Assistant Athletic Trainer
Instructor
Department of Kinesiology
Texas A&M University
Corpus Christi, Texas

Kevin J. Coupe, MD
Assistant Professor of Orthopaedics
Program Director
University of Texas–Houston
Houston, Texas

Michael J. D'Amato, MD
Team Physician
Shawnee State University
Portsmouth, Ohio

Adjunct Clinical Consultant
Ohio University
Athens, Ohio

Larry D. Field, MD
Partner
Mississippi Sports Medicine and Orthopaedic Center
Jackson, Mississippi

Brett Fink, MD
Foot and Ankle Specialist
Orthopaedic Surgeon
Community Hospitals
Indianapolis, Indiana

G. Kelley Fitzgerald, PT, PhD, OCS
Assistant Professor
Department of Physical Therapy
School of Health and Rehabilitation Sciences
University of Pittsburgh
Pittsburgh, Pennsylvania

Harris Gellman, MD
Professor, Co-Chief
Hand and Upper Extremity Service
Department of Orthopaedics and Plastic Surgery
University of Miami
Miami, Florida

Adjunct Clinical Professor
Department of Orthopaedic Surgery
University of Arkansas
Fayetteville, Arkansas

Robert C. Greenberg, MD
Associate Clinical Professor
Department of Orthopaedic Surgery
Berkshire Medical Center
Pittsfield, Massachusetts

James J. Irrgang, PhD, PT, ATC
Assistant Professor
Vice Chairman for Clinical Services
University of Pittsburgh
Pittsburgh, Pennsylvania

Robert W. Jackson, MD
Professor
Pulmonary and Critical Care Medicine
University of Alabama at Birmingham
Birmingham, Alabama

Margaret Jacobs, PT
Physical Therapist
Orthopaedic Store
San Antonio, Texas

Stan L. James, MD
Courtsey Professor
Department of Exercise and Movement Science
University of Oregon
Eugene, Oregon
Orthopaedic Surgeon
Orthopaedic Healthcare Northwest
Eugene, Oregon

Jesse B. Jupiter, MD
Professor
Department of Orthopaedic Surgery
Harvard Medical School
Cambridge, Massachusetts
Director
Orthopaedic Hand Service
Massachusetts General Hospital
Boston, Massachusetts

W. Ben Kibler, MD
Medical Director
Lexington Clinic Sports Medicine Center
Lexington, Kentucky

Michael L. Lee, MD
University Sports Medicine Associates
Corpus Christi, Texas

Michael Levinson, PT
Clinical Supervisor
Sports Medicine Rehabilitation Department
Hospital for Special Surgery
New York, New York

Andrew Markiewitz, MD
Clinical Assistant Professor
University of Cincinnati
Cincinnati, Ohio

Matthew J. Matava, MD
Assistant Professor
Department of Orthopaedic Surgery
Washington University School of Medicine
St. Louis, Missouri

John McMullen, MS, ATC
Manager, Sports Medicine and Physical Therapy
Sports Medicine Center
Lexington Clinic
Lexington, Kentucky

Steven J. Meyers, MD
Assistant Professor, Pediatrics
Texas A&M University Health Science Center
College Station, Texas
Team Physician
Department of Athletics
Texas A&M University—Corpus Christi
Corpus Christi, Texas

Sue Million, MHS, PT
Outpatient Program Director
Rehabilitation Institute of St. Louis
St. Louis, Missouri

Mark S. Mizel, MD
Professor
Department of Orthopaedics and Rehabilitation
University of Miami School of Medicine
Miami, Florida

Kenneth J. Mroczek, MD
Department of Orthopaedic Surgery
Assistant Professor
New York University School of Medicine
New York, New York

Kyle C. Phillips, PA-C, BHS
Clinical Instructor
Health Science
University of North Texas
Fort Worth, Texas
Physician Assistant
Allied Health
Spohn Hospital
Corpus Christi, Texas

Bruce Reider, MD
Professor of Surgery
Section of Orthopaedic Surgery and Rehabilitation Medicine
Department of Surgery
The University of Chicago
Chicago, Illinois
Director of Sports Medicine
The University of Chicago Hospitals
Chicago, Illinois

David Ring, MD
Instructor of Orthopaedics
Department of Orthopaedic Surgery
Harvard Medical School
Boston, Massachusetts

Anthony A. Romeo, MD
Associate Professor
Department of Orthopaedic Surgery
Rush Medical College
Chicago, Illinois

Melvin P. Rosenwasser, MD
Director
Orthopaedic Hand and Trauma Service
New York Presbyterian Hospital, Columbia Campus
New York, New York
Robert E. Carroll Professor of Orthopaedic Surgery
College of Physicians and Surgeons
Columbia University
New York, New York

Charles L. Saltzman, MD
Professor
Department of Orthopaedic Surgery
Department of Biomedical Engineering
University of Iowa
Iowa City, Iowa

F.H. Savoie, MD
Partner
Mississippi Sports Medicine and Orthopaedic Center
Jackson, Mississippi

K. Donald Shelbourne, MD
Associate Clinical Professor
Orthopaedic Surgery
Indiana University School of Medicine
Indianapolis, Indiana
Orthopaedic Surgeon
Methodist Sports Medicine Center
Indianapolis, Indiana

Kenneth A. Stephenson, MD
Attending Surgeon
Covenant Medical Center
Lubbock, Texas
Attending Surgeon
Northstar Surgical Center
Lubbock, Texas

Teresa Triche, M Ed
Exercise Physiologist
Certified Aquatic Specialist
Personal Trainer
San Antonio, Texas

Anna Williams, PT
Director of Physical Therapy
Crossroads Home Health
Port Lavaca, Texas

Preface

Our goal in preparing the second edition of *Clinical Orthopaedic Rehabilitation* was to widen the scope of available information for the musculoskeletal practitioner. The expanded material should prove relevant to physical therapists, orthopaedic surgeons, family practitioners, athletic trainers, chiropractors, and others who treat musculoskeletal disorders.

We have attempted to provide sound examination techniques, classification systems, differential diagnoses, treatment options, and rehabilitation protocols for common musculoskeletal problems. With this material the clinician who suspects de Quervain's tenosynovitis of the wrist, for example, may easily look up the appropriate examination, differential diagnosis, treatment options, and rehabilitation protocol.

Although the literature describing orthopaedic surgery techniques and acute fracture care is sound and comprehensive, there has been a relative paucity of information concerning nonoperative and postoperative rehabilitative care. This void exists even though rehabilitative therapy often has as much or greater an impact as the initial surgery does on the long-term results. A technically superb surgery may be compromised by improper postoperative rehabilitative techniques which allow scar formation, stiffness, rupture of incompletely healed tissue, or loss of function.

Many of the current rehabilitation protocols are empirically based. They have been shaped by years of trial and error with a large number of patients. Changes in rehabilitation protocols will be improved in the future by more clinical research and biomechanical studies. At present, however, the principles outlined in this text are those accepted by most orthopaedic surgeons and therapists.

We hope that the practitioner will find this text to be a concise, easy-to-use guide for performing precise examinations, formulating effective treatment options, and achieving successful rehabilitation of orthopaedic injuries.

Contents

Chapter 1
Hand and Wrist Injuries

*S. Brent Brotzman, MD, James H. Calandruccio, MD,
and Jesse B. Jupiter, MD*

Flexor Tendon Injuries

Important Points for Rehabilitation after Flexor Tendon Injury or Repair

- Repaired tendons subjected to *appropriate* early motion stress will increase in strength more rapidly and develop fewer adhesions than immobilized repairs.
- The **A2** and **A4** pulleys are the most important to the mechanical function of the finger. Loss of a substantial portion of either may diminish digital motion and power or lead to flexion contractures of the interphalangeal (IP) joints.
- The flexor digitorum superficialis (FDS) tendons lie on the palmar side of the flexor digitorum profundus (FDP) until they enter the A1 entrance of the digital sheath. The FDS then splits (at Champer's chiasma) and terminates into the proximal half of the middle phalanx.
- As much as 9 cm of flexor tendon excursion is required to produce composite wrist and digital flexion. Only 2.5 cm of excursion are required for full digital flexion when the wrist is stabilized in the neutral position.
- Tendons in the hand have both intrinsic and extrinsic capabilities for healing.
- Factors that influence the formation of excursion-restricting adhesions around repaired flexor tendons include
  - Amount of initial trauma to the tendon and its sheath.
  - Tendon ischemia.

- Tendon immobilization.
- Gapping at the repair site.
- Disruption of the vincula (blood supply), which decreases the recovery of tendon excursion.
- Lacerations of the palmar aspect of the finger will almost always injure the FDP before severing the FDS.
- Delayed primary repair results (within the first 10 days) are equal to or better than immediate repair of the flexor tendon.
- Immediate (primary) repair is **contraindicated** in patients with
  - Severe multiple tissue injuries to the fingers or palm.
  - Wound contamination.
  - Significant skin loss over the flexor tendons.

Rehabilitation Rationale and Basic Principles of Treatment after Flexor Tendon Repair

Timing

The timing of flexor tendon repair influences the rehabilitation and outcome of flexor tendon injuries.

- *Primary repair* is done within the first 12 to 24 hours after injury.
- *Delayed primary repair* is done within the first 10 days after injury.

If primary repair is not done, delayed primary repair should be done as soon as there is evidence of wound healing without infection.

- *Secondary repair* is done 10 and 14 days after injury.
- *Late secondary repair* is done more than 4 weeks after injury.

After 4 weeks, it is extremely difficult to deliver the flexor tendon through the digital sheath, which usually becomes extensively scarred. However, clinical situations in which the tendon repair is of secondary importance often make late repair necessary, especially for patients with massive crush injuries, inadequate soft tissue coverage, grossly contaminated or infected wounds, multiple fractures, or untreated injuries. If the sheath is not scarred or destroyed, single-stage tendon grafting, direct repair, or tendon transfer can be done. If extensive disturbance and scarring have occurred, two-stage tendon grafting with a Hunter rod should be used.

Before tendons can be secondarily repaired, these requirements must be met:

- Joints must be supple and have useful passive range of motion (ROM) (Boyes' grade 1 or 2, Table 1–1). Restoration of passive ROM is aggressively obtained with rehabilitation before secondary repair is done.
- Skin coverage must be adequate.
- The surrounding tissue in which the tendon is expected to glide must be relatively free of scar tissue.

Table 1-1

Boyes' Preoperative Classification

Grade	Preoperative Condition
1	Good: minimal scar with mobile joints and no trophic changes
2	Cicatrix: heavy skin scarring due to injury or previous surgery; deep scarring due to failed primary repair or infection
3	Joint damage: injury to the joint with restricted range of motion
4	Nerve damage: injury to the digital nerves resulting in trophic changes in the finger
5	Multiple damage: involvement of multiple fingers with a combination of the above problems

- Wound erythema and swelling must be minimal or absent.
- Fractures must have been securely fixed or healed with adequate alignment.
- Sensation in the involved digit must be undamaged or restored, or it should be possible to repair damaged nerves at the time of tendon repair directly or with nerve grafts.
- The critical A2 and A4 pulleys must be present or have been reconstructed. Secondary repair is delayed until these are reconstructed. During reconstruction, Hunter (silicone) rods are useful to maintain the lumen of the tendon sheath while the grafted pulleys are healing.

Anatomy

The anatomic zone of injury of the flexor tendons influences the outcome and rehabilitation of these injuries. The hand is divided into five distinct flexor zones (Fig. 1–1):

- *Zone 1*—from the insertion of the profundus tendon at the distal phalanx to just distal to the insertion of the sublimus.
- *Zone 2*—Bunnell's "no-man's land": the critical area of pulleys between the insertion of the sublimus and the distal palmar crease.
- *Zone 3*—"area of lumbrical origin": from the beginning of the pulleys (A1) to the distal margin of the transverse carpal ligament.
- *Zone 4*—area covered by the transverse carpal ligament.
- *Zone 5*—area proximal to the transverse carpal ligament.

As a rule, repairs to tendons injured outside the flexor sheath have much better results than repairs to tendons injured inside the sheath (zone 2).

It is essential that the A2 and A4 pulleys (Fig. 1–2) be preserved to prevent bowstringing. In the thumb, the

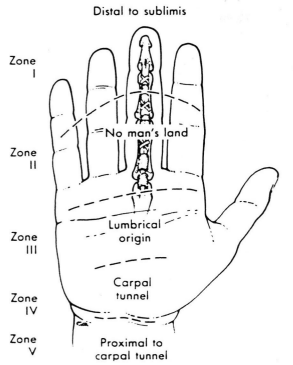

Figure 1–1. Flexor tendon zones. (From Canale ST [ed]: Campbell's Operative Orthopaedics, 9th ed. St. Louis, Mosby, 1998.)

A1 and oblique pulleys are the most important. The thumb lacks vinculum for blood supply.

Tendon Healing

The exact mechanism of tendon healing is still unknown. Healing probably occurs through a combination of extrinsic and intrinsic processes. *Extrinsic* healing depends on the formation of adhesions between the tendon and the surrounding tissue, providing a blood supply and fibroblasts, but unfortunately, it also prevents the tendon from gliding. *Intrinsic* healing relies on synovial fluid for nutrition and occurs only between the tendon ends.

Flexor tendons in the distal sheath have a dual source of nutrition via the vincular system and synovial diffusion. Diffusion appears to be more important than perfusion in the digital sheath (Green, 1993).

Several factors have been reported to affect tendon healing.

- Age—The number of vincula (blood supply) decreases with age.
- General health—Cigarettes, caffeine, and poor general health delay healing. The patient should refrain from caffeine and cigarettes during the first 4 to 6 weeks after repair.

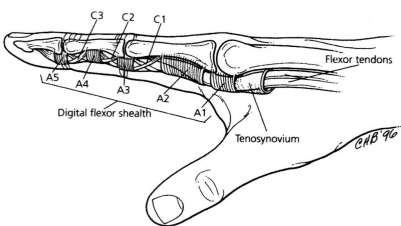

Figure 1–2. *A,* Uninvolved hand showing position of the pulleys and synovial sheaths of the fingers. *B,* Normal anatomy of the pulley system. (*A,* Modified from Idler RS: Anatomy and biomechanics of the digital flexor tendons. Hand Clin 1:6, 1985, Gary W. Schnitz, artist; *B,* from Idler RS: Helping the patient who has wrist or hand tenosynovitis. J Musculoskel Med 14[2]:21–35, 1997. Artist: Charles H. Boyter.)

A

B

- Scar formation—The remodeling phase is not as effective in patients who produce heavy keloid or scar.
- Motivation and compliance—Motivation and the ability to follow the postoperative rehabilitation regimen are critical factors in outcome.
- Level of injury—Zone 2 injuries are more apt to form limiting adhesions from the tendon to the surrounding tissue. In zone 4, where the flexor tendons lie in close proximity to each other, injuries tend to form tendon-to-tendon adhesions, limiting differential glide.
- Trauma and extent of injury—Crushing or blunt injuries promote more scar formation and cause more vascular trauma, impairing function and healing. Infection also impedes the healing process.
- Pulley integrity—Pulley repair is important in restoring mechanical advantage (especially A2 and A4) and maintaining tendon nutrition through synovial diffusion.
- Surgical technique—Improper handling of tissues (such as forceps marks on the tendon) and excessive postoperative hematoma formation trigger adhesion formation.

The two most frequent causes for failure of primary tendon repairs are formation of adhesions and rupture of the repaired tendon.

Through experimental and clinical observation, Duran and Houser (1975) determined that 3 to 5 mm of tendon glide is sufficient to prevent motion-limiting tendon adhesions. Exercises are thus designed to achieve this motion.

Treatment of Flexor Tendon Lacerations

- Partial laceration involving less than 25% of the tendon substance can be treated by beveling the cut edges.
- Lacerations between 25% and 50% can be repaired with 6-0 running nylon suture in the epitenon.
- Lacerations involving more than 50% should be considered complete and should be repaired with a core suture and an epitenon suture.
- FDP lacerations should be repaired directly or advanced and reinserted into the distal phalanx with a pull-out wire, but should not be advanced more than 1 cm to avoid the quadrigia effect (a complication of a single digit with limited motion causing limitation of excursion and, thus, the motion of the uninvolved digits).

Rehabilitation after Flexor Tendon Repair

The rehabilitation protocol chosen depends on the **timing** of the repair (delayed primary or secondary), the **location** of the injury (zones 1 through 5), and the **compliance** of the patient (early mobilization for compliant patients and delayed mobilization for noncompliant patients and children younger than 7 years of age).

Text continued on page 12

Rehabilitation Protocol
After Immediate or Delayed Primary Repair of Flexor Tendon Injury in Zones 1, 2, and 3
Modified Duran Protocol (Cannon)

Prerequisites

- Compliant patient.
- Clean or healed wound.
- Repair within 14 days of injury.

1–3 Days to 4.5 Weeks

- Remove bulky compressive dressing and apply light compressive dressing.
- Use digital-level fingersocks or Coban for edema control.
- Fit dorsal blocking splint (DBS) to wrist and digits for continual wear with the following positions:
  - Wrist—20 degrees flexion.
  - Metacarpophalangeal (MCP) joints—50 degrees flexion.
  - Distal interphalangeal (DIP) and proximal interphalangeal (PIP) joints—full extension.
- Initiate controlled passive mobilization exercises, including passive flexion/extension exercises to DIP and PIP joints individually.

- Composite passive flexion/extension exercises to MCP, PIP, DIP joints of digits (modified Duran program).

Figure 1–3. Passive flexion and extension exercises of the proximal interphalangeal (PIP) joint in a dorsal blocking splint (DBS).

Rehabilitation Protocol
After Immediate or Delayed Primary Repair of Flexor Tendon Injury in Zones 1, 2, and 3 (Continued)
Modified Duran Protocol (Cannon)

Figure 1–4. Passive flexion and extension exercises of the distal interphalangeal (DIP) joint in a DBS.

Figure 1–5. Combined passive flexion and extension exercises of the metacarpophalangeal (MCP), PIP, and DIP joints.

Active extension should be within the restraints of the DBS. If full flexion is not obtained, the patient may begin prolonged flexion stretching with Coban or taping.
- Eight repetitions each of isolated passive flexion/extension exercises of PIP, DIP, and MCP joints within the DBS (Figs. 1–3 to 1–5).

4.5 Weeks
- Continue the exercises and begin active ROM for fingers and wrist flexion, allowing active wrist extension to neutral or 0 degrees of extension only.
- Patient should perform hourly exercise with the splint removed, including composite fist, wrist flexion and extension to neutral, and composite finger flexion with the wrist immobilized (Fig. 1–6).
- Have the patient perform fist to hook fist (intrinsic minus position) exercise to extended fingers (Fig. 1–7).
- Watch for PIP joint flexion contractures. If an extension lag is present, add protected passive extension of the PIP joint with the MCP joint held in flexion. This should be done only by reliable patients or therapists. The PIP joint should be blocked to 30 degrees of flexion for 3 weeks if a concomitant distal nerve repair is done.
- Patients may reach a plateau in ROM 2 months after surgery, but maximal motion is usually achieved by 3 months after surgery.

5 Weeks
- Functional electrical stimulation (FES) can be used to improve tendon excursion. Consider the patient's quality of primary repair, the nature of the injury, and the medical history before initiating FES.

5.5 Weeks
- Add blocking exercises for PIP and DIP joints to previous home program.
- Discontinue DBS.
- Focus on gaining full passive ROM for flexion. Do not begin passive extension stretching at this time. A restraining extension splint can be used and positioned in the available range if tightness is noted.

6 Weeks
- Begin passive extension exercises of wrist and digits.
- Fit extension resting pan splint in maximal extension if extrinsic flexor tendon tightness is significant; frequently the patient may need only an extension gutter splint for night wear.

8 Weeks
- Begin resistive exercises with sponges or a Nerf ball and progress to putty and a hand-helper.
- Allow use of the hand in light work activities, but no lifting or heavy use of the hand.

A

B

Figure 1–6. Wrist is bent in flexion with a composite fist (A), then the wrist and fingers are extended (B).

continued

Rehabilitation Protocol
After Immediate or Delayed Primary Repair of Flexor Tendon Injury in Zones 1, 2, and 3 *(Continued)*
Modified Duran Protocol (Cannon)

A	B	C

Figure 1–7. Patient makes a fist (*A*), then straightens the MCP joints ("back knuckles") (*B*). Then the fingers are straightened with the wrist in neutral (*C*).

10–12 Weeks

- Allow full use of the hand in all daily activities.
- Use a work stimulator or strengthening program to improve hand strength.

The greatest achievement in total motion is seen between 12 and 14 weeks after surgery. It is not uncommon for the patient's ROM to plateau between 6 and 8 weeks.

Patients with associated digital nerve repair with some degree of tension at the nerve site should be fitted with a separate digital DBS in 30 degrees of PIP joint flexion. This splint is worn for 6 weeks and is progressively adjusted into increased extension during that time frame (see the section on Digital Nerve Repair).

[Many of the rehabilitation protocols in this chapter are taken from Diagnosis and Treatment Manual for Physicians and Therapists, 3rd ed., by Nancy Cannon, OTR, The Hand Rehabilitation Clinic of Indiana, PC. We highly recommend this manual as a detailed reference text for hand therapy.]

Rehabilitation Protocol
Early Mobilization after Immediate or Delayed Primary Repair of Flexor Tendon Injuries in Zones 4 and 5
Modified Duran Protocol (Cannon)

Prerequisites

- Compliant patient.
- Clean or healed wound.
- Repair within 14 days of injury.

7–10 Days

- Remove bulky compressive dressing and apply light compressive dressing.
- Use digital-level fingersocks or Coban for edema control.
- Fit DBS to wrist and digits for continual wear with the following positions:
  - Wrist—30 degrees palmar flexion.
  - MCP joints—50 degrees flexion.
  - DIP and PIP joints—full extension.
- Begin hourly passive ROM exercises in flexion and extension within the restraints of DBS (See Figs. 1–3 to 1–5).

3 Weeks

- Begin active ROM exercises (including blocking) 10 to 15 minutes each hour; exercises can be done within the restraints of DBS.
- FES or electrical muscle stimulation (EMS) can be initiated to improve tendon excursion within 2 days of initiation of active ROM.
- Begin scar massage, scar retraction, and scar remodeling techniques to remodel scar tissue and minimize subcutaneous adhesions.

4.5 Weeks

- Begin active ROM exercises of the wrist and digits outside of DBS. If nerve repair has been done at the wrist level, ROM exercises are done within the splint to alleviate additional stress at the nerve repair site (see digital nerve repair section).

Rehabilitation Protocol
Early Mobilization after Immediate or Delayed Primary Repair of Flexor Tendon Injuries in Zones 4 and 5 (Continued)
Modified Duran Protocol (Cannon)

6 Weeks

- Discontinue DBS.
- Begin passive ROM exercises of the wrist and digits.
- A full-extension resting pan splint or a long dorsal outrigger with a lumbrical bar can be used if extrinsic flexor tightness is present. Generally, this type of splinting is necessary with this level of repair.
- Do not allow lifting or heavy use of the hand.
- Begin gentle strengthening with a Nerf ball or putty.

7 Weeks

- May progress strengthening to include use of a hand-helper.

10–12 Weeks

- Allow full use of the injured hand.

Once active ROM exercise is begun at 3 weeks, it is important to emphasize blocking exercises along with the composite active ROM exercises. If the patient is having difficulty regaining active flexion, it is important to carefully monitor progress and request frequent patient visits to maximize flexion. *The first 3 to 7 weeks after surgery are critical for restoring tendon excursion.*

Rehabilitation Protocol
After Immediate or Delayed Primary Repair of Flexor Tendon Injuries in Zones 1, 2, and 3
Modified Early Motion Program (Cannon)

Prerequisites

- Compliant, motivated patient.
- Good repair.
- Wound healing.

1–3 Days

- Remove bulky compressive dressing and apply light compressive dressing.
- Use digital-level fingersocks or Coban for edema control.
- Fit DBS to wrist and digits for continual wear with the following positions:
  - Wrist—20 degrees palmar flexion.
  - MCP joints—50 degrees flexion.
  - DIP and PIP joints—full extension.
- Begin hourly passive ROM exercises in flexion and extension within the restraints of DBS (refer to the Modified Duran Protocol earlier in this chapter).

3 Weeks

- Begin active ROM exercises in flexion and extension within the restraints of DBS four to six times a day, in addition to the Modified Duran Protocol (earlier in this chapter).

4.5 Weeks

- Begin hourly active ROM exercises of wrist and digits outside of DBS.
- Patient should wear DBS between exercise sessions and at night.

5.5 Weeks

- Begin blocking exercises of DIP and PIP joints, as outlined in the Modified Duran Protocol (see Figs. 1–3 and 1–4).

6 Weeks

- Discontinue DBS.
- Begin passive ROM exercises in extension of wrist and digits as needed.
- Begin extension splinting if extrinsic flexor tendon tightness or PIP joint contracture is present.

8 Weeks

- Begin progressive strengthening.
- Do not allow lifting or heavy use of the hand.

10–12 Weeks

- Allow full use of the hand, including sports.

This protocol differs from the Modified Duran Protocol because the patient can begin active ROM exercises within the restraints of the DBS at 3 weeks instead of exercising out of the splint at 4.5 weeks.

Rehabilitation Protocol
Delayed Mobilization after Flexor Tendon Injury in Zones 1 through 5 in Noncompliant Patients
Cannon

Indications

- Crush injury.
- Younger than 11 years of age.
- Poor compliance and/or intelligence.
- Soft tissue loss, wound management problems.

3 Weeks

- Remove bulky compressive dressing and apply light compressive dressing.
- Fit DBS to wrist and digits for continual wear with the following positions:
  - Wrist—30 degrees palmar flexion.
  - MCP joints—50 degrees flexion.
  - DIP and PIP joints—full extension.
- Begin hourly active and passive ROM exercises within restraints of DBS; blocking exercises of PIP and DIP joints may be included.
- Active ROM is begun earlier than in other protocols because of longer (3 weeks) immobilization in DBS.

4.5 Weeks

- Begin active ROM exercises of digits and wrist outside of DBS; continue passive ROM exercises within restraints of DBS.
- Use FES or EMS to improve tendon excursion.
- If an associated nerve repair is under degree of tension, continue exercises within DBS that are appropriate for the level of nerve repair for 6 weeks.

6 Weeks

- Discontinue DBS.
- Begin passive ROM exercises in extension of wrist and digits.
- Use extension resting pan splint for extrinsic flexor tendon tightness or joint stiffness.
- Do not allow lifting or heavy use of hand.

8 Weeks

- Begin progressive strengthening with putty and hand-helper.

10–12 Weeks

- Allow full use of the hand.

This delayed mobilization program for digital-level to forearm-level flexor tendon repairs is reserved primarily for significant crush injuries, which may include severe edema or wound problems. This program is best used for patients whose primary repair may be somewhat "ragged" because of the crushing or bursting nature of the wound. It is also indicated for young children who cannot comply with an early motion protocol, such as the Modified Duran Program. *It is not indicated for patients who have a simple primary repair.*

Rehabilitation Protocol
Early Mobilization after Injury of the Flexor Pollicis Longus of Thumb
Cannon

Prerequisites

- Compliant patient.
- Clean or healed wound.

1–3 Days to 4.5 Weeks

- Remove bulky compressive dressing and apply light compressive dressing.
- Use fingersocks or Coban on thumb for edema control.
- Fit DBS to wrist and digits for continual wear with the following positions:
  - Wrist—20 degrees palmar flexion.
  - Thumb MCP and IP joints—15 degrees flexion at each joint.
  - Thumb carpometacarpal (CMC) joint—palmar abduction.

It is important to ensure that the thumb IP joint is in 15 degrees of flexion and is not extended. When the IP joint is left in a neutral position, restoration of IP joint flexion can be difficult.

- Begin hourly controlled passive mobilization program within the restraints of DBS:
  - Eight repetitions passive flexion and extension of MCP joints (Fig. 1–8).
  - Eight repetitions passive flexion and extension of IP joints (Fig. 1–9).

Rehabilitation Protocol
Early Mobilization after Injury of the Flexor Pollicis Longus of Thumb (Continued)
Cannon

Figure 1–8. Passive flexion and extension of the thumb MCP joint.

- Eight repetitions passive flexion and extension in composite manner of MCP and IP joints (Fig. 1–10).

4.5 Weeks
- Remove DBS each hour to allow performance of the following exercises:
  - Ten repetitions active flexion and extension of wrist (Fig. 1–11).
  - Ten repetitions active flexion and extension of thumb (Fig. 1–12).
- Continue passive ROM exercises.
- Patient should wear DBS between exercise sessions and at night.

5 Weeks
- Use FES or EMS within the restraints of DBS to improve tendon excursion.

Figure 1–9. Passive flexion and extension of the thumb interphalangeal (IP) joint.

Figure 1–10. Passive flexion and extension of the MCP and IP joints in the composite manner.

5.5 Weeks
- Discontinue DBS.
- Begin hourly active ROM exercises:
  - Twelve repetitions blocking of thumb IP joint (Fig. 1–13).
  - Twelve repetitions composite active flexion and extension of thumb.
- Continue passive ROM exercises as necessary.

6 Weeks
- Begin passive ROM exercises in extension of wrist and thumb.
- If needed for extrinsic flexor tendon tightness in FPL, a wrist and thumb static splint can be used to hold the wrist and thumb in extension. Often, a simple extension gutter splint in full extension can be used for night wear.

Figure 1–11. Active flexion and extension of the wrist.

continued

Rehabilitation Protocol
Early Mobilization after Injury of the Flexor Pollicis Longus of Thumb (Continued)
Cannon

Figure 1–12. Active flexion and extension of the thumb.

Figure 1–13. Blocking exercises of the thumb IP joint.

8 Weeks

- Begin progressive strengthening with a Nerf ball and progress to a hand-helper.
- Do not allow lifting or heavy use of the hand.

10–12 Weeks

- Allow full use of the hand for most activities, including sports.
- ROM generally begins to plateau at approximately 7 to 8 weeks after surgery.
- If an associated digital nerve repair is under tension, position the thumb in 30 degrees of flexion at the MCP and IP joints.
- If passive flexion is limited, taping or dynamic flexion splinting may be used.
- Scar management, including scar retraction, scar massage, and the use of Otoform or Elastomer, may be used at 2 weeks after surgery.

Rehabilitation Protocol
Delayed Mobilization after Injury of the Flexor Pollicis Longus of Thumb
Cannon

Indications

- Crush injury.
- Younger than 7 years of age.
- Poor compliance and/or intelligence.
- Soft tissue loss, wound management problems.

3 Weeks

- Remove bulky compressive dressing and apply light compressive dressing.

- Use fingersock or Coban on thumb as needed for edema control.
- Fit DBS to wrist and digits for continual wear with the following positions:
  - Wrist—30 degrees palmar flexion.
  - Thumb MCP and IP joints—15 degrees flexion at each joint.
  - Thumb CMC joint—palmar abduction.

Rehabilitation Protocol
Delayed Mobilization after Injury of the Flexor Pollicis Longus of Thumb *(Continued)*
Cannon

- Begin hourly active and passive ROM exercises within the restraints of DBS, including blocking exercises.
- If passive flexion of the thumb is limited, taping or dynamic flexion splinting may be used.
- Begin scar massage and scar management techniques.

4.5 Weeks

- Begin hourly active ROM exercises of wrist and thumb outside DBS.
- May use FES or EMS to improve tendon excursion of flexor pollicis longus (FPL).

6 Weeks

- Discontinue DBS.
- Begin passive ROM exercises in extension of wrist and thumb.
- If extrinsic flexor tendon tightness of the FPL is present, a wrist and thumb static splint may be used as needed;

the patient should wear the splint between exercise sessions and at night.
- Do not allow lifting or heavy use of the hand.

8 Weeks

- Begin progressive strengthening with a Nerf ball or putty.

10–12 Weeks

- Allow full use of the hand for most activities.
- If associated digital nerve repair is under tension, position thumb MCP and IP joints in 30 degrees flexion to minimize tension at repair site.
- Composite active flexion of the thumb tends to reach a plateau between 9 and 10 weeks after surgery.

The delayed mobilization for FPL repairs is best reserved for patients with crush injuries, soft tissue loss, wound management problems, and those in whom end-to-end repair was difficult.

Rehabilitation Protocol
After Two-stage Reconstruction for Delayed Tendon Repair
Cannon

Stage 1 (Hunter Rod)

Before Surgery
- Maximize passive ROM of digit with manual passive exercises, digital-level taping, or dynamic splinting.
- Use scar management techniques to improve suppleness of soft tissues, including scar massage, scar retraction, and use of Otoform or Elastomer silicone molds.
- Begin strengthening exercises of future donor tendon to improve postoperative strength after stage 2 procedure.
- If needed for protection or assistance with ROM, use buddy taping of the involved digit.

After Surgery

5–7 Days
- Remove bulky dressing and apply light compressive dressing; use digital-level finger socks or Coban.
- Begin active and passive ROM exercises of hand for approximately 10 minutes, six times a day.
- Fit an extension gutter splint that holds the digit in full extension to wear between exercise sessions and at night.
- If pulleys have been reconstructed during stage 1, use taping for about 8 weeks during the postoperative phase.

3–6 Weeks
- Gradually wean patient from extension gutter splint; continue buddy taping for protection.

The major goals during stage 1 are to maintain passive ROM and to obtain supple soft tissues before tendon grafting.

Stage 2 (Free Tendon Graft)

After Surgery
- Follow instructions for the early motion program for injuries in zones 1 through 3 (Modified Duran Protocol earlier in this chapter), or the delayed mobilization program for injuries in zones 1 through 5.
- For most patients, the Modified Duran Program is preferable to the delayed mobilization program because it encourages greater excursion of the graft and helps maintain passive ROM through the early mobilization exercises.
- Do not use FES before 5 to 5.5 weeks after surgery because of the initial avascularity of the tendon graft. Also consider the reasons for failure of the primary repair.

Trigger Finger (Stenosing Flexor Tenosynovitis)

Steven J. Meyers, MD, and Michael L. Lee, MD

Background

Trigger finger is a painful snapping phenomenon that occurs as the finger flexor tendons suddenly pull through a tight **A1 pulley** portion of the flexor sheath. The underlying pathophysiology of trigger finger is an inability of the two flexor tendons of the finger (FDS and FDP) to slide smoothly under the A1 pulley, resulting in a need for increased tension to force the tendon to slide and a sudden jerk as the tendon nodule suddenly pulls through the constricted pulley (triggering). The triggering can occur with flexion or extension of the finger or both. Whether this pathologic state arises primarily from the A1 pulley becoming stenotic or from a thickening of the tendon remains controversial, but both elements are usually found at surgery.

Clinical History and Examination

Trigger finger most commonly occurs in the thumb, middle, or ring fingers of postmenopausal women and is more common in patients with diabetes or rheumatoid arthritis, Dupuytren's contracture, and other tendinitis (de Quervain's tendinitis or lateral epicondylitis ["tennis elbow"]). Patients present with clicking, locking, or popping in the affected finger that is often painful, but not necessarily so.

Patients often have a **palpable nodule** in the area of the thickened A1 pulley (which is at the level of the distal palmar crease) (Fig. 1–14). This nodule can be felt to move with the tendon and is usually painful to deep palpation.

Figure 1–15. Midline palmar approach can be used for injection of corticosteroid into the flexor tendon sheath in patients with trigger finger; however, approach from the lateral base of any digit (except the thumb) is much less painful. (From Idler RS: Helping the patient who has wrist or hand tenosynovitis. Part 2. Managing trigger finger, de Quervain's disease. J Musculoskel Med 14[2]:62–75, 1997. Artist: Teri McDermott.)

To induce the triggering during examination, it is necessary to **have the patient make a full fist** and then completely extend the fingers, because the patient may avoid triggering by only partially flexing the fingers.

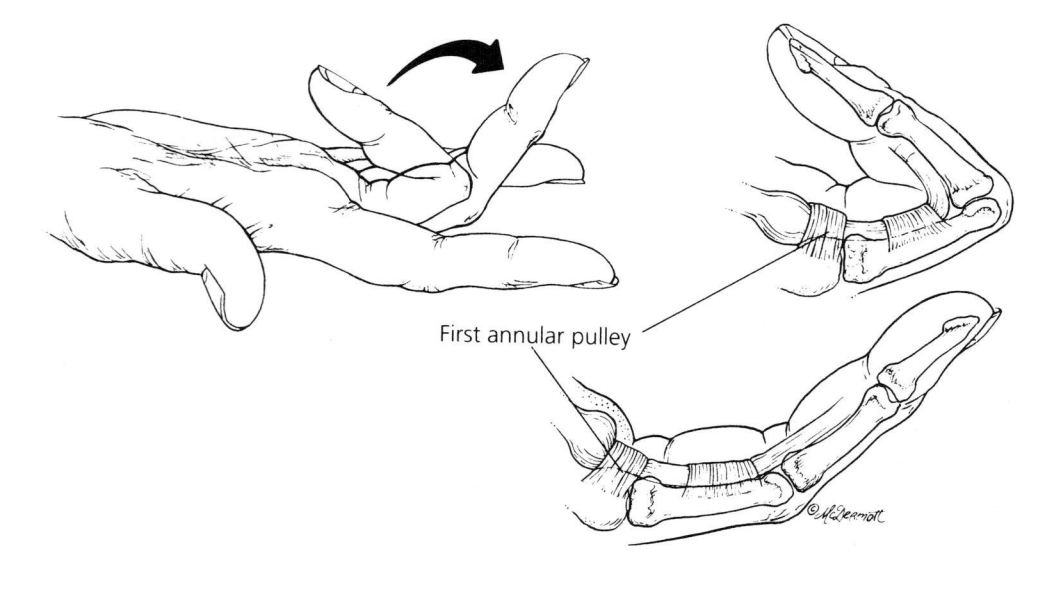

First annular pulley

Figure 1–14. Nodule or thickening in the flexor tendon, which strikes the proximal pulley, making finger extension difficult. (From Idler RS: Helping the patient who has hand tenosynovitis. J Musculoskel Med 14[2]:62–67, 1997. Artist: Teri McDermott.)

Rehabilitation Protocol
After Trigger Finger Cortisone Injection or Release

After injection

Physical therapy usually is not necessary for motion because most patients are able to regain motion once the triggering resolves.

After trigger release surgery

0–4 days	Gentle active MCP/PIP/DIP joint ROM (avoid gapping of wound).
4 days	Remove bulky dressing and cover wound with Band-Aid.
4–8 days	Continue ROM exercises. Remove sutures at 7–9 days.
8 days–3 weeks	Active/active-assisted ROM/passive ROM MCP/PIP/DIP joints.
3 weeks +	Aggressive ROM and strengthening. Return to unrestricted activities.

Treatment

Spontaneous long-term resolution of trigger finger is rare. If left untreated, the trigger finger will remain a painful nuisance; however, if the finger should become locked, the patient may develop permanent joint stiffness. Historically, conservative treatment included splinting of the finger in extension to prevent triggering, but this has been abandoned because of stiffening and poor result.

Currently, *nonoperative treatment* involves injection of corticosteroids with local anesthetic into the flexor sheath. The authors' preference is 0.5 ml lidocaine, 0.5 ml bupivicaine, and 0.5 ml methoprednisolone acetate (Depo-Medrol) (Fig. 1–15). A single injection can be expected to relieve triggering in about 66% of patients. Multiple injections can relieve triggering in 75 to 85% of patients.

About one third of patients will have lasting relief of symptoms with fewer than three injections, which means that about two thirds will require surgical intervention.

Surgery of trigger finger is a relatively simple outpatient procedure done with the patient under local anesthesia. The surgery involves a 1- to 2-cm incision in the palm to identify and completely divide the A1 pulley.

Pediatric Trigger Thumb

Pediatric trigger thumb is a congenital condition in which stenosis of the A1 pulley of the thumb in infants causes locking in flexion (inability to extend) of the IP joint. It often is bilateral. There usually is no pain or clicking, because the thumb remains locked. About 30% of children have spontaneous resolution by 1 year. The rest require surgical intervention to release the tight A1 pulley by about 2 to 3 years of age to prevent permanent joint flexion contracture. ■

Flexor Digitorum Profundus Avulsion ("Jersey Finger")

S. Brent Brotzman, MD, Michael L. Lee, MD, and Steven J. Meyers, MD

Background

Avulsion of the flexor digitorum profundus (FDP) (**"Jersey finger"**) can occur in any digit, but is most common in the ring finger. This injury usually occurs when an athlete grabs an opponent's jersey and feels sudden pain as the distal phalanx of the finger is forcibly extended as it is actively flexed (hyperextension stress applied to a flexed finger).

Lack of active flexion of the DIP joint (FDP function) must be specifically checked to make the diagnosis (Fig. 1–16). Often the swollen finger assumes a position of extension relative to the other, more flexed fingers. The level of retraction of the FDP generally denotes the force of the avulsion.

Leddy and Packer (1977) described *three types of FDP avulsions,* based on where the avulsed tendon retracts. The treatment is based on the anatomy of the injury.

Classification of Jersey Finger Injury (Flexor Digitorum Profundus Avulsion)

Type I Injury

The avulsed FDP tendon retracts into the palm (no bony fragment).

Both vincula are avulsed, disrupting the blood supply.

Early reattachment at the distal phalanx (<10 days) gives the best results. After 2 weeks, tendon elasticity decreases, preventing the tendon from reaching the distal phalanx.

continued

Classification of Jersey Finger Injury (Flexor Digitorum Profundus Avulsion) (Continued)

Type II Injury

The most common type of FDP avulsion.

The avulsed tendon retreats where the tendon is trapped by the FDS decussation and held by the vincula.

The vincula are intact.

The avulsion may or may not involve a bone fragment from the distal phalanx.

Successful surgical repair may be delayed up to 3 months, if needed, because of adequate tendon nutrition (vincula).

Early repair is the treatment of choice to avoid impaired DIP joint motion and tendon gliding.

Type III Injury

A large bony fragment (from the distal phalanx) prevents retraction past the level of the A1 pulley (middle phalanx).

The FDP blood supply remains intact, and the tendon is nourished within the sheath.

Treatment involves reduction and stabilization of the bony avulsion (suture anchors or pull-out wires).

Figure 1–16. With avulsion of the flexor digitorum profundus, the patient is unable to flex the DIP joint, shown here. (From Regional Review Course in Hand Surgery. Rosemont, Illinois, American Society of Surgery of the Hand, 1991, Fig. 7.)

Treatment

The treatment of FDP avulsion is primarily surgical. The success of the treatment depends on the acuteness of diagnosis, rapidity of surgical intervention, and level of retraction. Tendons with minimal retraction usually have significant bone fragments, which may be reattached bone-to-bone as late as 6 weeks. Tendons with a large amount of retraction often have no bone fragment and have disruption of the vascular supply (vinculum), making surgical repair greater than 10 days after injury difficult because of retraction and the longer healing time of weaker nonbone-to-bone fixation and limited blood supply to the repair.

Surgical salvage procedures for late presentation include DIP joint arthrodesis, tenodesis, and staged tendon reconstructions.

Rehabilitation Protocol
After Surgical Repair of Jersey Finger
Brotzman and Lee

With Secure Bony Repair

0–10 Days
- DBS the wrist at 30 degrees flexion, the MCP joint 70 degrees flexion, and the PIP and DIP joints in full extension.
- Gentle passive DIP and PIP joint flexion to 40 degrees within DBS.
- Suture removal at 10 days.

10 Days–3 Weeks
- Place into a removable DBS with the wrist at neutral and the MCP joint at 50 degrees flexion.
- Gentle passive DIP joint flexion to 40 degrees, PIP joint flexion to 90 degrees within DBS.
- Active MCP joint flexion to 90 degrees.
- Active finger extension of IP joints within DBS, 10 repetitions per hour.

3–5 Weeks
- Discontinue DBS (5–6 weeks).
- Active/assisted MCP/PIP/DIP joint ROM exercises.
- Begin place-and-hold exercises.

5 Weeks +
- Strengthening/power grasping.
- Progress activities.
- Begin tendon gliding exercises.
- Continue passive ROM, scar massage.
- Begin active wrist flexion/extension.
- Composite fist and flex wrist, then extend wrist and fingers.

Rehabilitation Protocol
After Surgical Repair of Jersey Finger *(Continued)*
Brotzman and Lee

With Purely Tendinous Repair or Poor Bony Repair

0–10 Days
- DBS the wrist at 30 degrees flexion and the MCP joint at 70 degrees flexion.
- Gentle passive DIP and PIP joint flexion to 40 degrees within DBS.
- Suture removal at 10 days.

10 Days–4 Weeks
- DBS the wrist at 30 degrees flexion and the MCP joint at 70 degrees flexion.
- Gentle passive DIP joint flexion to 40 degrees, PIP joint flexion to 90 degrees within DBS, passive MCP joint flexion to 90 degrees.
- Active finger extension within DBS.
- Remove pull-out wire at four weeks.

4–6 Weeks
- DBS the wrist neutral and the MCP joint at 50 degrees flexion.

- Passive DIP joint flexion to 60 degrees, PIP joint to 110 degrees, MCP joint to 90 degrees.
- Gentle place-and-hold composite flexion.
- Active finger extension within DBS.
- Active wrist ROM out of DBS.

6–8 Weeks
- Discontinue daytime splinting, night splinting only.
- Active MCP/PIP/DIP joint flexion and full extension.

8–10 Weeks
- Discontinue night splinting.
- Assisted MCP/PIP/DIP joint ROM.
- Gentle strengthening.

10 Weeks +
- More aggressive ROM.
- Strengthening/power grasping.
- Unrestricted activities.

Extensor Tendon Injuries

Anatomy

Extensor mechanism injuries are grouped into eight anatomic zones according to Kleinert and Verdan (1983). Odd-number zones overlie the joint levels so that zones

Figure 1–17. Extensor tendon zones.

1, 3, 5, and 7 correspond to the DIP, PIP, MCP, and wrist joint regions, respectively (Figs. 1–17 and 1–18; Table 1–2).

Normal extensor mechanism activity relies on concerted function between the intrinsic muscles of the hand and the extrinsic extensor tendons. Even though PIP and DIP joint extension is normally controlled by the intrinsic muscles of the hand (interossei and lumbricals), the extrinsic tendons may provide satisfactory digital extension when MCP joint hyperextension is prevented.

An injury at one zone typically produces compensatory imbalance in neighboring zones; for example, a closed mallet finger deformity may be accompanied by a more striking secondary swan-neck deformity at the PIP joint.

Disruption of the terminal slip tendon allows the extensor mechanism to migrate proximally and exert a hyperextension force to the PIP joint by the central slip attachment. Thus, extensor tendon injuries cannot be considered simply static disorders.

Extensor Tendon Injuries in Zones 1 and 2

These injuries **in children** should be considered Salter-Harris type II or III physeal injuries. Splinting of extremely small digits is difficult, and fixing the joint in full extension for 4 weeks produces satisfactory results. Open injuries are especially difficult to splint, and the DIP joint may be transfixed with a 22-gauge needle (also see Mallet Finger section).

Rehabilitation Protocol
Treatment and Rehabilitation of Chronic Extensor Tendon Injuries in Zones 1 and 2

Tenodermodesis

Tenodermodesis is a simple procedure used in relatively young patients who are unable to accept the mallet finger disability. With the use of a local anesthetic, the DIP joint is fully extended and the redundant pseudotendon is excised so that the edges of the tendon coapt. A Kirschner wire may be used temporarily to fix the DIP joint in full extension.

3–5 Days
- Remove the postoperative splint and fit the DIP joint with an extension splint. A pin protection splint may be necessary if the pin is left exposed; however, some patients have their pins buried to allow unsplinted use of the finger.
- PIP joint exercises are begun to maintain full PIP joint motion.

5 Weeks
- Remove the Kirschner wire and begin active DIP motion with interval splinting.
- Continue nightly splinting for an additional 3 weeks.

Central Slip Tenotomy (Fowler)

With the use of a local anesthetic, the insertion of the central slip is sectioned where it blends with the PIP joint dorsal capsule. The combined lateral band and the extrinsic contribution should be left undisturbed. Proximal migration of the dorsal apparatus improves the extensor force at the DIP joint. A 10- to 15-degree extensor lag at the PIP joint may occur.

0–2 Weeks
- The postoperative dressing maintains the PIP joint at 45 degrees of flexion and the DIP joint at 0 degrees.

2–4 Weeks
- Allow active DIP joint extension and flexion.
- Allow full extension of the PIP joint from 45 degrees of flexion.

4 Weeks
- Begin full finger motion exercises.

Oblique Retinacular Ligament Reconstruction

- Reconstruction of the oblique retinacular ligament is done for correction of a chronic mallet finger deformity and secondary swan-neck deformity. A free tendon graft, such as the palmaris longus tendon, is passed from the dorsal base of the distal phlanax and volar to the axis of the PIP joint. The graft is anchored to the contralateral side of the proximal phalanx at the fibro-osseous rim. Kirscher wires temporarily fix the DIP joint in full extension and the PIP joint in 10 to 15 degrees of flexion.

3 Weeks
- Remove the bulky postoperative dressing and sutures.
- Withdraw the PIP joint pin.
- Begin active flexion and extension exercises of the PIP joint.

4–5 Weeks
- With the DIP joint K-wire.
- Begin full active and passive PIP and DIP joint exercises.
- Supplement home exercises with a supervised program over the next 2 to 3 weeks to achieve full motion.
- Continue internal splinting of the DIP joint in full extension until 6 weeks after the operation.

Extensor Tendon Injuries in Zones 4, 5, and 6

Normal function is usually possible after unilateral injuries to the dorsal apparatus, and splinting and immobilization are not recommended. Complete disruptions of the dorsal expansion and central slip lacerations are repaired.

Rehabilitation Protocol
After Surgical Repair of Extensor Tendon Injuries in Zones 4, 5, and 6

0–2 Weeks
- Allow active and passive PIP joint exercises, keep the MCP joint in full extension and the wrist in 40 degrees of extension.

2 Weeks
- Remove the sutures and fit the patient with a removable splint.

Rehabilitation Protocol
After Surgical Repair of Extensor Tendon Injuries in Zones 4, 5, and 6 *(Continued)*

- Keep the MCP joints in full extension and the wrist in neutral position.
- Continue PIP joint exercises and remove the splint for scar massage and hygienic purposes only.

4–6 Weeks

- Begin MCP and wrist joint active flexion exercises with interval and night splinting with the wrist in neutral position.

- Over the next 2 weeks, begin active-assisted and gentle passive flexion exercises.

6 Weeks

- Discontinue splinting unless an extensor lag develops at the MCP joint.
- Use passive wrist flexion exercises as necessary.

Zone 5 Extensor Tendon Subluxations

Zone 5 extensor tendon subluxations rarely respond to a splinting program. The affected MCP joint can be splinted in full extension and radial deviation for 4 weeks, with the understanding that surgical intervention will probably be required. Painful popping and swelling, in addition to a problematic extensor lag with radial de-viation of the involved digit, usually require prompt re-construction.

Acute injuries can be repaired directly, and chronic injuries can be reconstructed with local tissue. Most reconstructive pro-cedures use portions of the juncturae tendinum or extensor ten-don slips anchored to the deep transverse metacarpal ligament or looped around the lumbrical tendon.

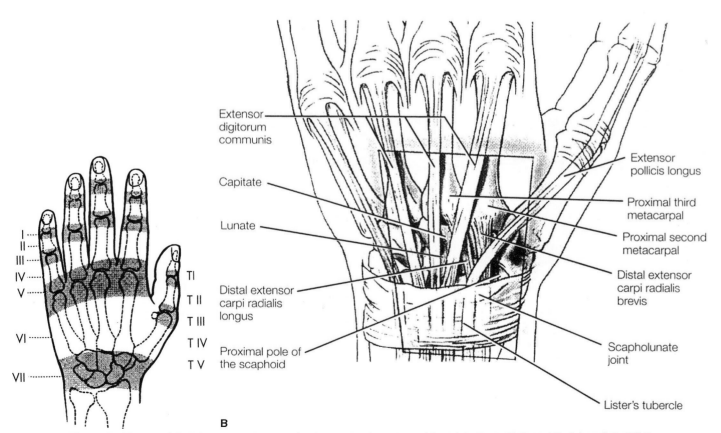

Figure 1–18. *A* and *B*, Extensor anatomy and extensor tendon zones. (*A* and *B*, From Kleinert HE, Schepel S, Gill T: Flexor tendon injuries. Surg Clin North Am 61:267, 1981.)

Rehabilitation Protocol
After Surgical Repair of Zone 5 Extensor Tendon Subluxation

2 Weeks

- Remove the postoperative dressing and sutures.
- Keep the MCP joints in full extension.
- Fashion a removable volar short arm splint to maintain the operated finger MCP joint in full extension and radial deviation.
- Allow periodic splint removal for hygienic purposes and scar massage.
- Allow full PIP and DIP joint motion.

4 Weeks

- Begin MCP joint active and active-assisted exercises hourly with interval daily and full-time night splinting.
- At week 5, begin gentle passive MCP joint motion if necessary to gain full MCP joint flexion.

6 Weeks

- Discontinue splinting during the day and allow full activity.

Table 1–2

Zones of Extensor Mechanism Injury

Zone	Finger	Thumb
1	DIP joint	IP joint
2	Middle phalanx	Proximal phalanx
3	Apex PIP joint	MCP joint
4	Proximal phalanx	Metacarpal
5	Apex MCP joint	
6	Dorsal hand	
7	Dorsal retinaculum	Dorsal retinaculum
8	Distal forearm	Distal forearm

DIP, distal interphalangeal; IP, interphalangeal; MCP, metacarpophalangeal; PIP, proximal interphalangeal.
From Kleinert HE, Verdan C: Report of the committee on tendon injuries. J Hand Surg 8:794, 1983.

Extensor Tendon Injuries in Zones 7 and 8

Extensor tendon injuries in zones 7 and 8 are usually from lacerations, but attritional ruptures secondary to remote distal radial fractures and rheumatoid synovitis may occur at the wrist level. These may require tendon transfers, free tendon grafts, or side-by-side transfers rather than direct repair. The splinting program for these, however, is identical to that for penetrating trauma.

Repairs done 3 weeks or more after the injury may weaken the extensor pollicis longus (EPL) muscle sufficiently for electrical stimulation to become necessary for tendon glide. The EPL is selectively strengthened by thumb retropulsion exercises done against resistance with the palm held on a flat surface.

Rehabilitation Protocol
After Surgical Repair of Extensor Tendon Injuries in Zones 7 and 8

0–2 Weeks

- Maintain the wrist in 30 to 40 degrees of extension with postoperative splint.
- Encourage hand elevation and full PIP and DIP joint motion to reduce swelling and edema.
- Treat any significant swelling by loosening the dressing and elevating the extremity.

2–4 Weeks

- At 2 weeks, remove the postoperative dressing and sutures.
- Fashion a volar splint to keep the wrist in 20 degrees of extension and the MCP joints of the affected finger(s) in full extension.
- Continue full PIP and DIP joint motion exercises and initiate scar massage to improve skin-tendon glide during the next 2 weeks.

4–6 Weeks

- Begin hourly wrist and MCP joint exercises, with interval and nightly splinting over the next 2 weeks.
- From week 4 to 5, hold the wrist in extension during the MCP joint flexion exercises and extend the MCP joints during the wrist flexion exercises.
- Composite wrist and flexion flexion from the fifth week forward. An MCP joint extension lag of more than 10 to 20 degrees requires interval daily splinting.
- Splinting program can be discontinued at 6 weeks.

6–7 Weeks

- Begin gentle passive ROM.
- Begin resistive extension exercises.

Rehabilitation Protocol
After Repair of Extensor Pollicis Longus Laceration (Thumb)

After repair of thumb extensor tendon lacerations, regardless of the zone of injury, apply a thumb spica splint with the wrist in 30 degrees of extension and the thumb in 40 degrees of radial abduction with full retroposition.

0–2 Weeks

- Allow activity as comfortable in the postoperative splint.
- Edema control measures include elevation and motion exercises to the uninvolved digits.

2–4 Weeks

- At 2 weeks after repair, remove the splint and sutures. Refit a thumb spica splint with the wrist and thumb positioned to minimize tension at the repair site as before.
- Fit a removable splint for reliable patients and permit scar massage.
- The vocational interests of some patients are best suited with a thumb spica cast.
- Continue edema control measures.

4–6 Weeks

- Fit a removable thumb spica splint for night use and interval daily splinting between exercises.
- During the next 2 weeks, the splint is removed for hourly wrist and thumb exercises.

- Between weeks 4 and 5, thumb IP, MCP, and CMC joint flexion and extension exercises should be done with the wrist held in extension.
- Alternately, wrist flexion and extension motion is regained with the thumb extension.
- After the fifth week, composite wrist and thumb exercises are done concomitantly.

6 Weeks

- Discontinue the splinting program unless extensor lag develops.
- Treat an extensor lag at the IP joint of more than 10 degrees with intermittent IP extension splinting in addition to nightly thumb spica splinting.
- Problematic MCP and CMC joint extension lags require intermittent thumb spica splinting during the day and night for an additional 2 weeks or until acceptable results are obtained.
- It may be necessary to continue edema control measures for 8 weeks or longer.
- Use taping to gain full composite thumb flexion.
- Use electrical stimulation for lack of extensor pull-through.

Extensor Tenolysis

Indications

- Digital active or passive motion has reached a plateau after injury.
- Restricted isolated, or composite active or passive flexion of the PIP or DIP joint.

- Otherwise passively supple digit that exhibits an extensor lag (Fig. 1–19).

Surgical intervention for extension contractures frequently follows an extensive period of presurgical therapy. Patients who have been active in their rehabilitation are more apt to appreciate that an early and postsurgical pro-

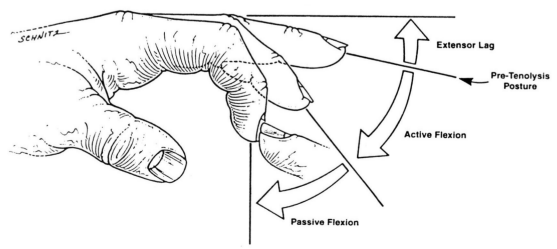

Figure 1–19. Passive supple digit with an extensor lag is an indication for possible extensor tenolysis. (From Strickland JW: The Hand: Master Techniques in Orthopaedic Surgery. Philadelphia, Lippincott-Raven, 1998.)

Rehabilitation Protocol
After Extensor Tenolysis

0–24 Hours

- Apply a light compressive postoperative dressing to allow as much digital motion as possible. Anticipate bleeding through the dressing, and implement exercises hourly in 10-minute sessions to achieve as much of the motion noted intraoperatively as possible.

1 Day–4 Weeks

- Remove the surgical dressings and drains at the first therapy visit. Apply light compressive sterile dressings.
- Edema control measures are critical at this stage.
- Continue active and passive ROM exercises hourly for 10- to 15-minute sessions. Poor IP joint flexion during the first session is an indication for flexor FES. Extensor FES should be used initially with the wrist, MCP, PIP, and DIP joints passively extended to promote maximal proximal tendon excursion. After several stimulations in this position, place the wrist, MCP, and PIP joints into more flexion and continue FES.
- Remove the sutures at 2 weeks; dynamic flexion splints and taping may be required.
- Use splints to keep the joint in question in full extension between exercises and at night for the first 4 weeks. Extensor lags of 5 to 10 degrees are acceptable and are not indications to continue splint wear after this period.

4–6 Weeks

- Continue hourly exercise sessions during the day for 10-minute sessions. Emphasis is on achieving MCP and IP joint flexion.

- Continue passive motion with greater emphasis during this period, especially for the MCP and IP joints.
- Continue extension night splinting until the sixth week.

6 Weeks

- Encourage the patient to resume normal activity.
- Edema control measures may be required. Intermittent Coban wrapping of the digits may be useful in conjunction with an oral inflammatory agent.
- Banana splints (foam cylindrical digital sheaths) can also be effective for edema control.

The therapist must have acquired some critical information regarding the patient's tenolysis. Specific therapeutic program and anticipated outcomes depend on the following:

- The quality of the tendon(s) undergoing tenolysis.
- The condition of the joint the tendon acts about.
- The stability of the joint the tendon acts about.
- The joint motions achieved during the surgical procedure. Passive motions are easily obtained; however, active motions in both extension and flexion are even more beneficial to guiding patient therapy goals.

Achieving maximal MCP and PIP joint flexion during the first 3 weeks is essential. Significant gains after this period are uncommon.

---

gram is vital to their final outcome. Presurgical patient counseling should always be attempted to delineate the immediate postsurgical tenolysis program. The quality of the extensor tendon, bone, and joint encountered at surgery may alter the intended program, and the surgeon relays this information to the therapist and the patient. Ideally, the surgical procedures are done with the patient under local anesthesia or awakened from the general anesthesia near the end of the procedure. The patient can then see the gains achieved, and the surgeon can evaluate active motion, tendon glide, and the need for additional releases. Unusual circumstances may be well served by having the therapist observe the operative procedure.

Frequently, MCP and PIP joint capsular and ligament releases are necessary to obtain the desired joint motion. Complete collateral ligament resection may be required, and special attention may be necessary in the early postoperative period for resultant instability.

Extensive tenolyses may require analgesic dosing before and during therapy sessions. Indwelling catheters also

may be needed for instillation of local anesthetics for this purpose.

Mallet Finger (Extensor Injury—Zone 1)

Background

Avulsion of the extensor tendon from its distal insertion at the dorsum of the DIP joint produces an **extensor lag** at the DIP joint. The avulsion may occur with or without a bony fragment avulsion from the dorsum of the distal phalanx. **This is termed a *mallet finger* of bony origin, or *mallet finger of tendinous origin*** (Figs. 1–20

Figure 1–20. Mallet finger of bony origin with detachment of the extensor mechanism. (From Lairmore JR, Engber WD: Serious, but often subtle, finger injuries. Physician Sports Med 26[6]:57, 1998.)

MECHANISM

Forced flexion

INJURY

A

B

C

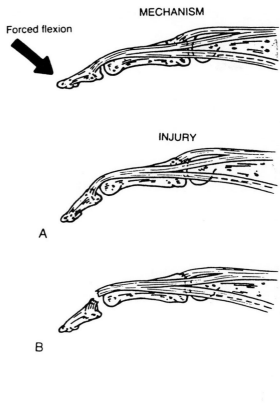

Figure 1–21. *A,* Stretching of the common extensor mechanism. *B,* Mallet finger of tendinous origin (complete disruption of the extensor tendon). *C,* Mallet finger of bony origin. (*A–C,* Delee J, Drez D [eds]: Orthopaedic Sports Medicine. Philadelphia, WB Saunders, 1994, p. 1011.)

and 1–21). The hallmark finding of a mallet finger is a flexed or dropped posture of the DIP joint (Fig. 1–22) and an inability to actively extend or straighten the DIP joint. The mechanism is typically forced flexion of the fingertip, often from the impact of a thrown ball.

Classification of Mallet Finger

Doyle (1993) described four types of mallet injury:

- Type I—extensor tendon avulsion from the distal phalanx.
- Type II—laceration of the extensor tendon.
- Type III—deep avulsion injuring the skin and tendon.
- Type IV—fracture of the distal phalanx with three subtypes:
  - Type IV A—transepiphyseal fracture in a child.
  - Type IV B—less than half of the articular surface of the joint involved with no subluxation.
  - Type IV C—more than half of the articular surface involved and may involve volar subluxation.

Treatment

Abound and Brown (1968) found that several factors are likely to lead to a **poor prognosis** after mallet finger injury:

- Age older than 60 years.
- Delay in treatment of more than 4 weeks.
- Initial extensor lag of more than 50 degrees.
- Too short a period of immobilization (<4 wk).
- Short, stubby fingers.
- Peripheral vascular disease or associated arthritis.

The results of mallet finger treatment are not universally good by any method of treatment.

Continuous extension splinting of the DIP joint, leaving the PIP free for 6 to 10 weeks (with a plastic stack splint) is the typical treatment for mallet fingers of tendinous origin (Fig. 1–23). If no extensor lag exists at 6 weeks, night splinting for 3 weeks and splinting during sports activities for an additional 6 weeks are employed.

The patient must work on active ROM of the MCP and PIP joints to avoid stiffening of these uninvolved joints. **At no point during the healing process is the DIP joint allowed to drop into flexion, or the treatment must be repeated from the beginning.** During skin care or washing, the finger must be held continuously in extension with the other hand while the splint is off.

Treatment of Mallet Finger (Fig. 1–24)

Type I: Tendinous Avulsion

Continuous extension splinting of the DIP joint (stack splint) for 4 weeks.

Bedtime splinting for another 6 weeks.

Sports splinting for another 6 weeks.

Active ROM of MCP and PIP joints.

Type II: Laceration of Extensor Tendon

Surgical repair of tendon laceration.

See type I protocol.

Type III: Deep Avulsion of Skin and Tendon

Skin grafting.

Surgical repair of tendon laceration.

See type I protocol.

Type IV: Bony Origin

Type IV A—reduction of the fracture and splinting for 6 weeks, night splinting for 6 weeks.

Type IV B—reduction and splinting for 6 weeks, night splinting for 6 weeks.

Type IV C—(controversial) Splinting versus open reduction and internal fixation (ORIF) with splinting versus percutaneous pinning with splinting for 6 weeks.

Figure 1–22. *A,* Mild mallet finger deformity (extensor lag at the DIP joint with an inability to extend the DIP joint) seen as a flexed DIP joint. It is important to treat this acute injury before further tearing of the extensor tendon and stretching of new scar tissue lead to greater deformity. *B,* No bony injury is seen on the radiograph. After 6 weeks in a splint, the finger was nearly normal. *C,* Note that the palmar fragment is concentrically reduced with the middle phalanx. In spite of a large dorsal fragment, which makes up more than one third of the articular surface, continuous splinting for 8 weeks resulted in pain-free function with only a trivial decrease in ROM. *D,* Mallet finger with a subluxated palmar fragment may need surgical reduction and internal fixation. *Arrow* points to the loss of concentricity of the joint surfaces. *E,* Intraoperative radiograph shows reduction and pinning *(arrow)* through a dorsal-ulnar approach without sectioning of the extensor tendon. Note the restored concentricity of the joint surface. *(A–E,* From Vetter WL: How I manage mallet finger. Physician Sports Med 17[3]:17–24, 1989.)

Fractures and Dislocations of the Hand

Fractures and dislocations involving the hand are classified as stable or unstable injuries to determine the appropriate treatment. **Stable** fractures are those that would not displace if some degree of early digital motion were allowed. **Unstable** fractures are those that displace to an unacceptable degree if early digital motion is allowed. Although some unstable fractures can be converted to stable fractures with closed reduction, it is very difficult to predict which of these will maintain their stability throughout the early treatment phase. For this reason, most unstable fractures should undergo closed reduction and percutaneous pinning or ORIF to allow early protected digital motion and thus prevent stiffness.

Fractures that often require surgical intervention include

- Open fractures.
- Comminuted displaced fractures.
- Fractures associated with joint dislocation or subluxation.
- Displaced spiral fractures.
- Displaced intra-articular fractures, especially around the PIP joint.
- Fractures in which there is loss of bone.
- Multiple fractures.

Because of the hand's propensity to quickly form permanently stiffening scar, unstable fractures **must** be surgically converted to stable fractures (e.g., pinning) to allow early ROM exercises. Failure to employ early ROM will result in a stiff hand with poor function regardless of bony healing.

Figure 1–23. *A,* Use of a stack splint at the DIP joint for closed treatment of mallet finger (note extension lag). The splint is held in place with paper or adhesive tape. *B,* Active ROM exercises of the PIP joint employed to keep the joint from stiffening during DIP joint immobilization. (*A* and *B,* From Regional Review Course in Hand Surgery. Memphis, American Society of Surgery of the Hand, 1991, Fig. 13.)

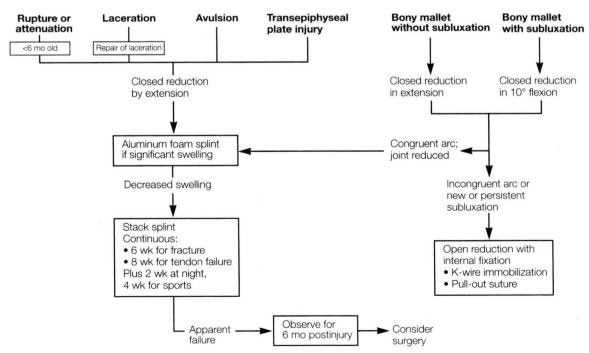

Figure 1–24. Algorithm for treatment of various mallet finger conditions. (Adapted from Damron TA, Lange RW, Engber WD: Mallet fingers: a review and treatment algorithm. Int J Orthop Trauma 1:105, 1991.)

Figure 1–25. Position of immobilization of the hand involves splinting the wrist in approximately 30 degrees of extension, the MCP joints in 60 to 80 degrees of flexion, and the IP joints in full extension. (From Delee J, Drez D [eds]: Orthopaedic Sports Medicine. Philadelphia, WB Saunders, 1994.)

Metacarpal and Phalangeal Fractures

Nondisplaced metacarpal fractures are stable injuries and are treated with application of an anterior-posterior splint in the **position of function:** the wrist in 30 to 60 degrees of extension, the MCP joints in 70 degrees of flexion, and the IP joints in 0 to 10 degrees of flexion. In this position, the important ligaments of the wrist and hand are maintained in maximal tension to prevent contractures (Fig. 1–25).

Allowing early PIP and DIP joint motion is essential. Motion prevents adhesions between the tendons and the underlying fracture and controls edema. The dorsal fiberglass splint should extend from below the elbow to the fingertips of all the **involved** digits and one adjacent digit. The anterior splint should extend from below the elbow to the distal aspect of the proximal phalanx (Fig. 1–26A), allowing the patient to resume PIP and DIP joint active flexion and extension exercises immediately (see Fig. 1–26B).

Comminuted phalangeal fractures, especially those that involve diaphyseal segments with thick cortices, may be slow to heal and may require fixation for up to 6 weeks (Fig. 1–27).

A   **B**

Figure 1–26. Anterior (*A*) and posterior fiberglass splints typically used to treat metacarpal and proximal phalangeal fractures. (*B*) PIP and DIP joint flexion and extension are allowed. The anterior splint should extend 2 cm distal to the level of the fracture.

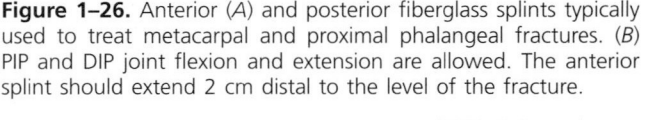

- 3-5 weeks
- 5-7 weeks
- 10-14 weeks

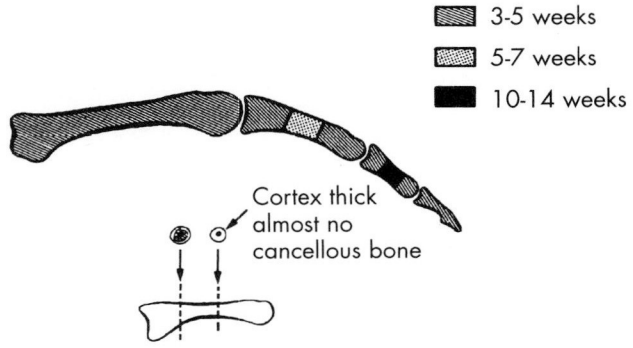

Figure 1–27. Time required for fracture healing varies, depending on the ratio of cortical to cancellous bone at the fracture site. Healing is slowest where the ratio of cortical to cancellous bone is highest. (Redrawn from Wilson RE, Carter MS: Management of hand fractures. In Hunter JM, Schneider LH, Mackin EJ, Callahan AD [eds]: Rehabilitation of the Hand. St. Louis, Mosby, 1990, p. 290.)

Rehabilitation Protocol
After Metacarpal or Phalangeal Fracture

0–4 Weeks

- Before pin removal, begin active ROM exercises while the therapist supports the fracture site.

4–6 Weeks

- Active and active-assisted intrinsic stretching exercises (i.e., simultaneous MCP joint extension and IP joint flexion) are recommended.

- Prevent PIP joint flexion contractures by ensuring that the initial splint immobilizes the PIP joint in an almost neutral position.
- When the fracture is considered solid on radiograph, a dynamic splinting program can be started. The LMB dynamic splint and the Capner splint are quite useful. They should be worn for 2-hour increments, 6 to 12

Rehabilitation Protocol
After Metacarpal or Phalangeal Fracture *(Continued)*

hours a day (Fig. 1–28) and alternated with dynamic flexion strapping (Fig. 1–29).

- Therapy may be prolonged for up to 3 to 6 months after injury.

Figure 1–28. Dynamic PIP joint extension splint (LMB, or Louise M. Barbour).

Figure 1–29. Flexion strap used to help regain PIP and DIP joint motion.

Proximal Interphalangeal (PIP) Joint Injuries (Fig. 1–30; Table 1–3)

Volar PIP joint dislocations are less common than dorsal dislocations and are often difficult to reduce by closed techniques because of entrapment of the lateral bands around the flare of the proximal phalangeal head. If not treated properly, these injuries may result in a boutonniere deformity (combined PIP joint flexion and DIP joint extension contracture). Usually, the joint is stable after closed or open reduction; however, static PIP joint extension splinting is recommended for 6 weeks to allow healing of the central slip.

Avulsion fractures involving the dorsal margin of the middle phalanx occur at the insertion of the central slip. These fractures may be treated by closed technique; however, if the fragment is displaced more than 2 mm proximally with the finger splinted in extension, ORIF of the fragment is indicated.

Rehabilitation Protocol
After Volar Proximal Interphalangeal Joint Dislocation or Avulsion Fracture

After Closed Reduction

- An extension gutter splint is fitted for continuous wear with the PIP joint in neutral position.
- The patient should perform active and passive ROM exercises of the MCP and DIP joints approximately six times a day.
- PIP joint motion is not allowed for 6 weeks.
- Begin active ROM exercises at 6 weeks in combination with intermittent daytime splinting and continuous night splinting for an additional 2 weeks.

After ORIF

- The transarticular pin is removed between 2 and 4 weeks after the wound has healed.
- Continuous splinting in an extension gutter splint is continued for a total of 6 weeks.
- The remainder of the protocol is similar to that after closed reduction.

Extension splinting is continued as long as an extensor lag is present, and passive flexion exercises are avoided as long as an extension lag of 30 degrees or more is present.

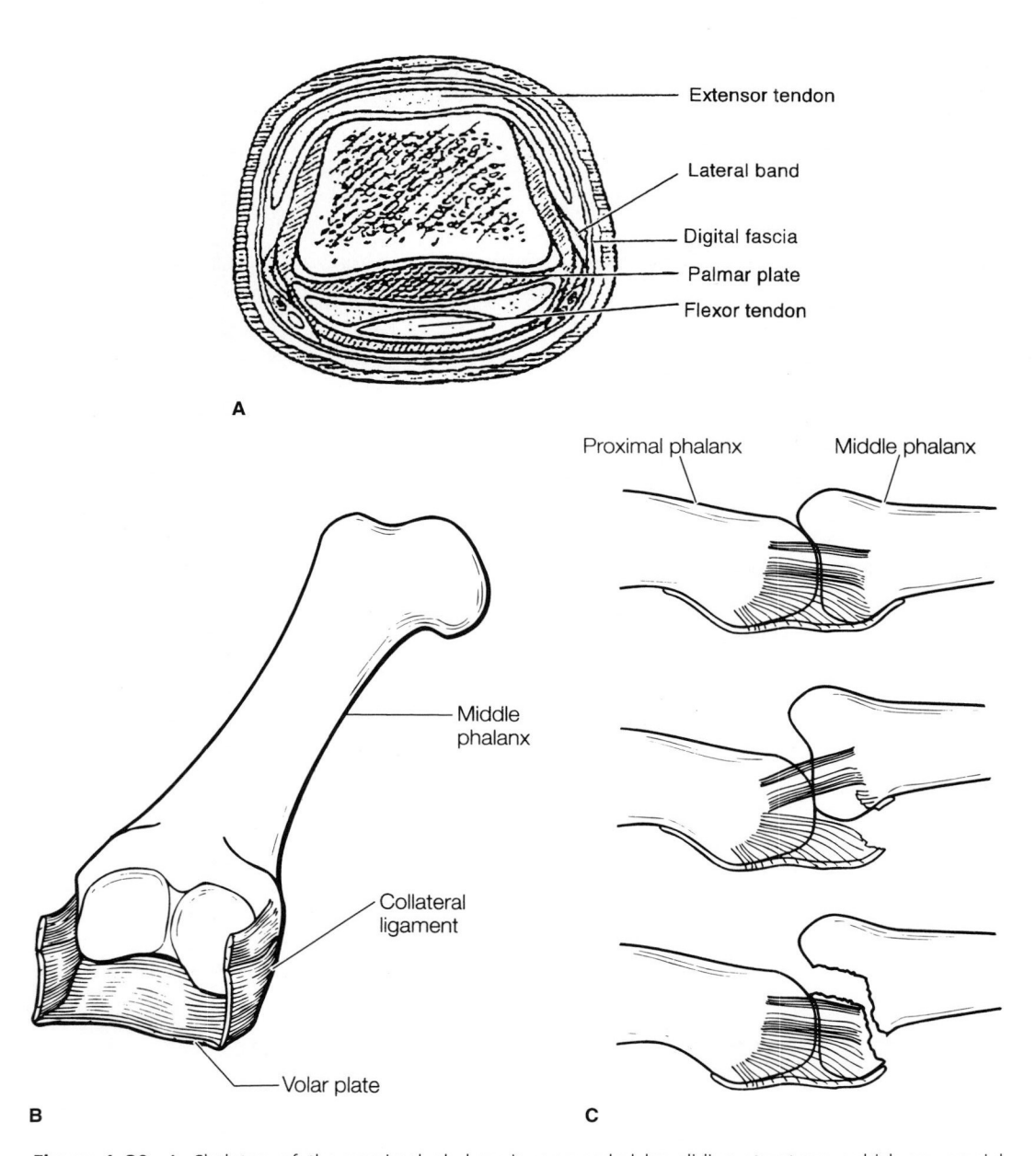

Figure 1–30. *A,* Skeleton of the proximal phalanx is surrounded by gliding structures, which are crucial for digital function. *B,* PIP joint is stabilized by a "three-dimensional ligament-box complex," consisting of collateral ligaments and a thick volar or palmar plate. *C,* PIP joint in its normal anatomy (*top*). A tear in the three-dimensional ligament-box complex (*middle*) results in a stable injury. An unstable PIP fracture-dislocation (*bottom*) occurs when stabilizers remain attached to a fragment that contains more than 40% of the articular surface. (*A,* From Jupiter JB, Axelrod TS, Belsky MR: Fractures and dislocations of the hand. In Browner B, Jupiter JB, Levine AM, Trafton PG [eds]: Skeletal Trauma, 2nd ed. Philadelphia, WB Saunders, 1998, pp. 1225–1342; *B* and *C,* from Lairmore JR, Engber WD: Serious, but often subtle, finger injuries. Physician Sports Med 26[6]:57, 1998.)

Rehabilitation Protocol
After Dorsal Fracture-Dislocation of the Proximal Interphalangeal Joint

- If the injury is believed to be stable after closed reduction, a dorsal blocking splint (DBS) is applied with the PIP joint in 30 degrees of flexion. This allows full flexion but prevents the terminal 30 degrees of extension.
- After 3 weeks, the DBS is adjusted at weekly intervals to increase PIP joint extension by about 10 degrees each week.

- The splint should be in neutral position by the sixth week, then discontinued.
- An active ROM program is begun, and dynamic extension splinting is used as needed.
- Progressive strengthening exercises are begun at 6 weeks.

Dorsal fracture-dislocations of the PIP joint are much more common than volar dislocations. If less than 50% of the articular surface is involved, these injuries usually are stable after closed reduction and protective splinting.

Dorsal fracture-dislocations involving more than 40% of the articular surface may be unstable, even with the digit in flexion, and may require surgical intervention. The Eaton volar plate advancement is probably the most common procedure used (Fig. 1–31). The fracture fragments are excised, and the volar plate is advanced into the remaining portion of the middle phalanx. The PIP joint usually is pinned in 30 degrees of flexion.

Table 1–3
Managing Proximal Interphalangeal (PIP) Joint Injuries of the Hand

Injury	Clinical Manifestations or Special Considerations	Treatment
Sprain	Stable joint with active and passive motion; negative radiographs; pain and swelling only	Buddy tape for comfort; begin early ROM exercises, ice, NSAIDs
Open dislocation	Dislocated exposed joint	Irrigation, débridement, and antibiotics; treat as any open fracture or dislocation
Dorsal PIP dislocation		
Type 1	Hyperextension, volar plate avulsion, minor collateral ligament tear	Reduction; very brief immobilization, 3–5 days, followed by ROM exercises with buddy taping and close x-ray follow-up
Type 2	Dorsal dislocation, volar plate avulsion, major collateral ligament tear	Same as type 1
Type 3	Stable fracture-dislocation: <40% of articular arc on fracture fragment	Extension block splint; *refer to hand surgeon*
	Unstable fracture dislocation: >40% of articular arc on fracture fragment	Extension block splint; *open reduction with internal fixation if closed treatment impossible; refer to hand surgeon*
Lateral dislocation	Secondary to collateral ligament injury and avulsion and/or rupture of volar plate; angulation >20 degrees indicates complete rupture	Same as dorsal dislocation types 1 and 2 above if joint is stable and congruous through active ROM
Volar PIP dislocation		
Straight volar dislocation	Proximal condyle causes significant injury to central extensor slip (may reduce easily, but extensor tendon may be seriously injured; requires careful examination)	*Refer to a hand surgeon* experienced in these rare injuries; closed reduction with traction with metatarsophalangeal and PIP flexed and extended wrist; full-extension immobilization of PIP joint if post reduction x-rays show no subluxation; if closed reduction is not achieved or subluxation persists, surgery recommended
Ulnar or radial volar displacement	Condyle often buttonholes through central slip and lateral band; reduction often extremely difficult	Same as straight volar PIP dislocation (above)

NSAIDs, nonsteroidal anti-inflammatory drugs; PIP, proximal interphalangeal; ROM, range of motion.
From Laimore JR, Engber WD: Serious, but often subtle finger injuries. Physician Sports Med 26(6):226, 1998.

Rehabilitation Protocol
After Dorsal Fracture-Dislocation of the Proximal Interphalangeal Joint Involving More Than 40% of the Articular Surface

- At 3 weeks after surgery, the pin is removed from the PIP joint and a DBS is fitted with the PIP joint in 30 degrees of flexion for continuous wear.
- Active and active-assisted ROM exercises are begun within the restraints of the DBS.

- At 5 weeks, the DBS is discontinued and active and passive extension exercises are continued.
- At 6 weeks, dynamic extension splinting may be necessary if full passive extension has not been regained.

Flexion contractures are not uncommon after this procedure. Agee (1987) described the use of an external fixation combined with rubber bands that allows early active ROM of the PIP joint in unstable fracture-dislocations while maintaining reduction. The bulky hand dressing is removed 3 to 5 days after surgery, and active ROM exercises are carried out for 10-minute sessions every 2 hours. Pins should be cleansed twice daily with cotton swabs and hydrogen peroxide, protecting the base of the pin with gauze. The external fixator can be removed between 3 and 6 weeks, at which time an unrestricted active and passive ROM exercise program is started.

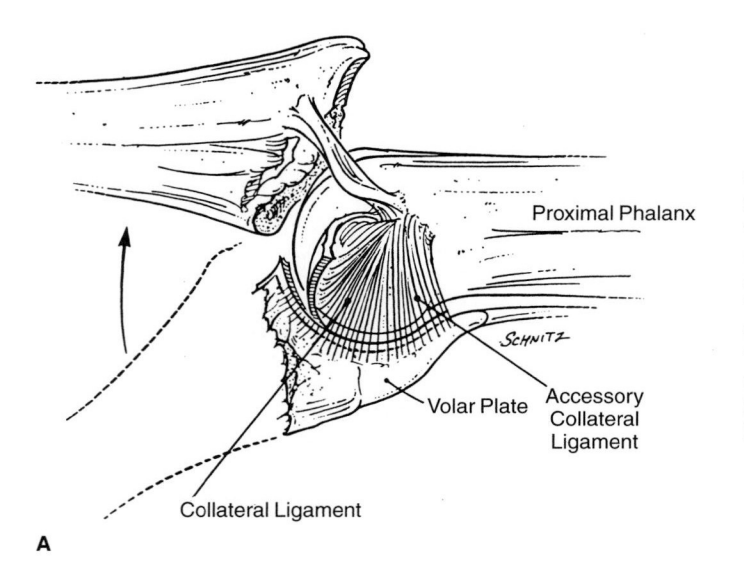

Figure 1–31. *A,* Pathology of injury demonstrating loss of collateral ligament support to the joint, producing marked instability. Eaton volar plate arthroplasty is commonly used when more than 40% comminution or impaction of the inferior aspect of the middle phalanx of the PIP joint is present. *B,* Sutures are passed through the lateral margins of the defect, exiting dorsally. The comminuted fragment has been excised, and the volar plate is being advanced. *C,* Sutures are tied over a padded button, drawing the volar plate into the defect and simultaneously reducing the PIP joint. (*A–C,* From Strickland JW: The Hand: Master Techniques in Orthopaedic Surgery. Philadelphia, Lippincott-Raven, 1999.)

Figure 1–32. Fingers are taped after dislocation, fracture, or sprain. "Buddy taping" of the injured finger to the adjacent finger provides the best support for the joint. (From Idler RS: Treatment of common hand injuries. J Musculoskel Med 17[1]:pp. 73–77, 1996.)

Dorsal dislocations of the PIP joint without associated fractures are usually stable after closed reduction. Stability is tested after reduction under digital block, and, if the joint is believed to be stable, buddy taping (Fig. 1–32; Table 1–4) for 3 to 6 weeks, early active ROM exercises, and edema control are necessary. If instability is present with passive extension of the joint, a DBS similar to that used in fracture-dislocations should be used.

Intra-articular fractures involving the base of the thumb metacarpal are classified as either *Bennett fractures* (if a single volar ulnar fragment exists) or *Rolando fractures* (if there is a T-condylar fracture pattern). These fractures often displace because of the proximal pull of the abductor pollicis longus (APL) on the base of the proximal thumb metacarpal.

Nondisplaced Bennett fractures are treated in a short arm thumb spica cast, which can be removed at 6 weeks if the fracture has healed clinically. Active and gentle passive ROM exercises are begun. At that time, the patient also is fitted with a removable thumb spica splint. This should be used between exercise sessions and at night for an additional 2 weeks. Strengthening exercises are then started,

using silicone putty. The patient generally returns to normal activity between 10 and 12 weeks. If there is persistent joint subluxation after application of a short arm cast with the thumb positioned in palmar and radial abduction, closed reduction and percutaneous pinning are carried out. After pinning, the thumb is placed in a thumb spica splint and protected for 6 weeks. After the pin is removed, therapy progresses as described for nondisplaced fractures.

Rolando fractures have a poor prognosis. The choice of treatment usually depends on the severity of comminution and the degree of displacement. If large fragments are present with displacement, ORIF with Kirschner wires or a mini-fragment plate is done. If severe comminution is present, manual molding in palmar abduction and immobilization in a thumb spica cast for 3 to 4 weeks are recommended. After stable internal fixation, motion can be started at 6 weeks in a manner similar to that for Bennett fractures.

Fifth Metacarpal Neck Fracture (Boxer's Fracture)

Steven J. Meyers, MD, and Michael L. Lee, MD

Background

Metacarpal neck fractures are among the most common fractures in the hand. Fracture of the fifth metacarpal is by far the most frequent and has been

Table 1–4
Materials for Taping the Injured Finger
1-inch white zinc oxide tape or elastic tape
Tape-adherent spray

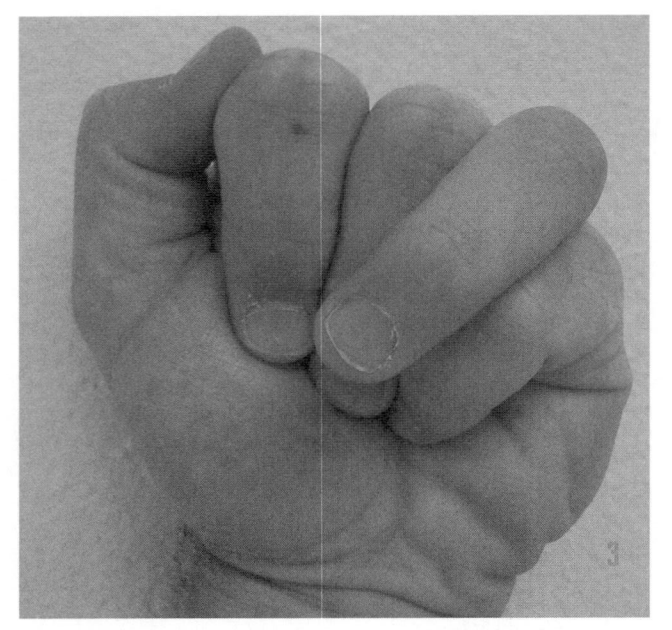

Figure 1–33. Malrotation of a fracture (and, thus, the finger).

termed a *boxer's fracture* because the usual mechanism is a glancing punch that does not land on the stronger second and third metacarpals.

Clinical History and Examination

Patients usually have pain, swelling, and loss of motion about the MCP joint. Occasionally, a rotational deformity is present. Careful examination should be performed to ensure that there is no malrotation of the finger when the patient makes a fist (Fig. 1–33), no significant prominence of the distal fragment (palmarly displaced) in the palm, and no extensor lag of the involved finger.

Radiographic Examination

On the lateral radiograph, the angle of the metacarpal fracture is determined by drawing lines down the shafts of the metacarpal and measuring the resultant angle with a goniometer.

Treatment

Treatment is based on the degree of displacement, as measured on a true lateral of the hand (Fig. 1–34). Metacarpal neck fractures are usually impacted and angulated, with the distal fragment displacing palmarly because of the intrinsic muscle pull. Excessive angulation causes loss of the MCP joint knuckle and may cause the palmar metacarpal head to be prominent during activities. *Only about 10 degrees of angulation can be accepted in second and third metacarpal neck fractures, whereas up to 30 degrees in the fourth metacarpal and 40 degrees in the fifth metacarpal can be accepted because of greater mobility in the fourth and fifth CMC joints.*

If displacement is unacceptable, closed reduction can be attempted with wrist block anesthesia using the maneuver credited to Jahss (1938), in which the proximal phalanx is flexed to 90 degrees and used to apply a dorsally directed force to the metacarpal head (Fig. 1–35). The hand is then splinted in an ulnar gutter splint for about 3 weeks with the MCP joint at 80 degrees of flex-

Angle

Figure 1–34. "Boxer's" fracture. On the lateral radiograph, a line is drawn down the middle of each fracture fragment and the angles are measured with a goniometer. More than 40 degrees of angulation of the more mobile fifth metacarpal neck fracture requires reduction (maneuver of Jahss). If the fracture is unstable, percutaneous pinning is often required.

Figure 1–36. *A,* For application of a gutter splint, the patient's elbow should be flexed 90 degrees and the wrist dorsiflexed 10 to 15 degrees. Only the fourth and fifth fingers are included in the splint. *B,* Splint should extend from the end of the fifth finger to within two to four fingerbreadths of the antecubital space. *C,* Splinting material should be wide enough to cover half the circumference of the patient's wrist. The moistened splint is molded to the patient's hand and wrist and is secured with elastic wrap. Wrapping should be done from distal to proximal so that edema can be pushed up and out of the extremity. Padding (Webril) is wrapped around the fingers, wrist, and forearm under the splint to avoid skin pressure. *D,* After the splint has been secured, the hand must be positioned properly: 10 to 15 degrees of dorsiflexion at the wrist; as close as possible to 90 degrees of dorsiflexion at the MCP joints; and 10 to 15 degrees of flexion at the PIP joints. (From Petrizzi MJ: Making an ulnar gutter splint for a boxer's fracture. Physician Sports Med 27[1]:111, 1999.)

ion, the PIP joint straight, and the DIP joint free (Fig. 1–36).

Rapid mobilization of the fingers is required to avoid scarring, adhesions, and stiffness unrelated to the fracture itself but rather to the propensity of an immobilized hand to quickly stiffen.

Operative treatment of boxer's fractures is indicated if

- Fracture alignment remains unacceptable (>40 degrees displacement).
- Late redisplacement occurs in a previously reduced fracture.
- There is any malrotation of the finger.

Operative fixation usually involves percutaneous pinning of the fracture, but ORIF may be required.

Fractures treated operatively still require about 3 weeks of immobilization. ■

Figure 1–35. Maneuver of Jahss. *A,* PIP joint is flexed 90 degrees, and the examiner stabilizes the metacarpal proximal to the neck fracture, then pushes the finger to dorsally displace the volar angulated boxer's fracture to "straight." *B,* Splint is molded in reduced position with the ulnar gutter in the position of function. (*A* and *B,* From Regional Review Course in Hand Surgery. Rosemont, Illinois, American Society for Surgery of the Hand, 1991.)

Rehabilitation Protocol
After Boxer's Fracture
Brotzman and Lee

After Closed Treatment (Nonoperative)

0–1 Week
- Elevation of hand, icing, ulnar gutter splint with the MCP joints at 80 degrees flexion, DIP joints are free.
- Active motion of nonimmobilized thumb, index, long finger.
- Radiographs at 6–8 days (three views of the hand).

1–2 Weeks
- Continue active finger ROM of nonimmobilized joints.
- Radiographs at 2 weeks.

2–3 Weeks
- Remove ulnar gutter splint at 3 weeks and x-ray.
- Apply short arm cast (that allows active motion of the fourth and fifth DIP, PIP, and MCP joints) for 3 more weeks.

3–5 Weeks
- Active/gentle assisted ROM of the fourth and fifth fingers.
- Passive extension.

5–7 Weeks
- Active/aggressive assisted/passive ROM of the fourth and fifth fingers.
- Strengthening.
- Unrestricted activities.
- Radiographs at 6 weeks.

After Operative Treatment (K-Wire, ORIF)

0–1.5 Weeks
- Elevate, ice.
- Splinted with PIP joints and DIP joints *free*.
- Gentle active ROM of the PIP and DIP joints.
- Active ROM of the uninvolved fingers and thumb.
- Remove sutures if ORIF at 10–14 days.

1.5–3 Weeks
- Continue splinting with PIP and DIP joints free.
- Gentle active ROM of the PIP and DIP joints.
- Active ROM of the uninvolved fingers and thumb.
- Remove splint at 3 weeks.
- Remove pins at 3–6 weeks.

3–5 Weeks
- Buddy taping
- Active/assisted/passive ROM of the fourth and fifth fingers.
- Passive extension of all joints.

5–7 Weeks
- Active/aggressive assisted/passive ROM of the fourth and fifth fingers.
- Strengthening.
- Unrestricted activities.

Injuries to the Ulnar Collateral Ligament of the Thumb Metacarpophalangeal Joint (Gamekeeper's Thumb)

S. Brent Brotzman, MD

Background

The classic **"gamekeeper's thumb"** was first described in Scottish gamekeepers. **"Skier's thumb"** was coined by Schultz, Brown, and Fox in 1973, with skiing being the most common cause of acute rupture (e.g., after a fall causing the ski pole to stress the UCL of the thumb).

Stability of the thumb on the ulnar side is maintained by four structures: the adductor aponeurosis, the adductor pollicis muscle, the proper and accessory ulnar collateral ligament (UCL), and the volar plate. The UCL provides resistance to radially applied forces (e.g., pinching or holding large objects). A torn UCL weakens the key pinch grip strength and allows volar subluxation of the proximal phalanx. With prolonged instability, the MCP joint frequently degenerates.

The amount of valgus laxity of normal thumbs varies widely. In full MCP joint extension, valgus laxity averages 6 degrees, and in 15 degrees of MCP joint flexion, increases to an average of 12 degrees. The adductor aponeurosis (when torn and pulled distally) occasionally entraps the UCL, preventing anatomic reduction or healing **(Stener lesion)** (Fig. 1–37). The typical **mechanism of injury** is an extreme valgus stress to the thumb (e.g., falling on an abducted thumb).

Evaluation

Patients typically have a history of a valgus injury to the thumb followed by pain, swelling, and frequently ecchymosis at the ulnar aspect of the thumb MCP joint. Palpation of the ulnar aspect of the MCP joint may reveal a small lump, which may be indicative of a Stener lesion or avulsion fracture.

Figure 1–37. *A,* In the thumb MCP joint, the adductor aponeurosis covers the ulnar collateral ligament. *B,* When thumb angulation is sufficient, the ligament can rupture and displace. *C,* If the ligament becomes trapped outside the aponeurosis, Stener lesion results. Trapped ligament that is not surgically repaired leads to chronic instability. (From Lairmore JR, Engber WD: Serious, but often subtle, finger injuries. Physician Sports Med 26[6]:57, 1998.)

In addition to plain films (three views of the thumb and carpus), valgus stress testing radiographs should be obtained. Because acutely injured patients will guard from pain, 1% lidocaine should be injected into the joint before stress testing. The integrity of the proper (ulnar collateral) ligament is **assessed by valgus stress testing with the MCP joint of the thumb in 30 degrees of flexion.** This test can be done clinically or with radiographic documentation. There is some variation in the literature as to the degree of angulation on valgus stressing that is compatible with complete rupture of the UCL. **Thirty to 35 degrees of radial deviation of the thumb on valgus stressing indicates a complete UCL rupture and is an indication for surgical correction.** With complete ruptures (>30 degrees of opening), the likelihood of an UCL ligament displacement (a Stener lesion) is greater than 80%.

Treatment of Skier's Thumb

Stable Thumb on Valgus Stressing (No Stener Lesion)

- The ligament is only partially torn, and healing will occur with nonoperative treatment.
- The thumb is immobilized for 4 weeks in a short arm spica cast or thermoplastic splint (molded), usually with the thumb IP joint free.
- Active and passive thumb motion is begun at 3 to 4 weeks, but valgus is avoided.
- If ROM is painful at 3 to 4 weeks, re-evaluation by physician is indicated.
- The thermoplastic splint is removed several times a day for active ROM exercises.
- Grip-strengthening exercises are begun at 6 weeks after injury. A brace is worn for protection in contact situations for 2 months.

Unstable Thumb on Valgus Stressing (>30 Degrees)

- Requires direct operative repair with a suture anchor (Fig. 1–38).
- Because 80% of patients with a complete rupture are found to have a Stener lesion (thus obtaining a poor healing result if treated nonoperatively), it is critical to make the correct diagnosis of stable versus unstable gamekeeper's thumb.

Rehabilitation Protocol
After Repair or Reconstruction of the Ulnar Collateral Ligament of the Thumb Metacarpophalangeal Joint

3 Weeks

- Remove bulky dressing.
- Remove MCP joint pin (K-wire) if used for joint stabilization.
- Fit with wrist and thumb static splint for continual wear.

6 Weeks

- Begin active and gentle passive ROM exercises of the thumb for 10 minutes each hour.
- *Avoid any lateral stress to the MCP joint of the thumb.*

- Begin dynamic splinting if necessary to increase passive ROM of the thumb.

8 Weeks

- Discontinue splinting. Wrist and thumb static splint or short opponens splint may be useful during sports-related activities or heavy lifting.
- Begin progressive strengthening.

12 Weeks

- Allow the patient to return to unrestricted activity.

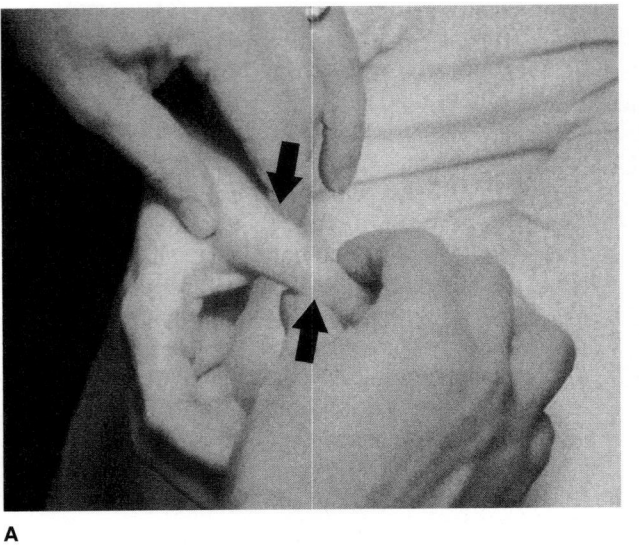

A

Figure 1–38. *A,* During stress examination of skier's thumb, the physician stabilizes the metacarpal to prevent rotation, then applies radial stress (arrows) to the distal end of the phalanx. With the thumb in 30 degrees of flexion a valgus stress is applied. Test both thumbs for symmetry, congenital laxity, etc. *B,* When complete rupture of ulnar collateral ligament occurs, the distal end of the torn ligament is usually displaced proximal and superfical to the proximal edge of the intact adductor aponeurosis. *C,* Division of the adductor aponeurosis is required for repair of the ligament. (*A,* From Wadsworth LT: How I manage skiers thumb. Physician Sports Med 20[3]:69, 1992; *B* and *C,* from Heyman P: Injuries to the ulnar collateral ligament of the thumb MCP joint. J Am Acad Orthop Surg 5:224, 1997.)

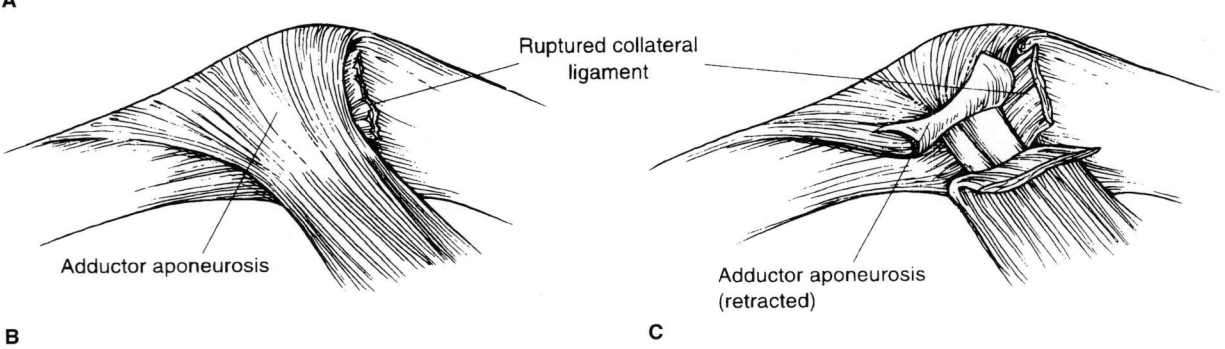

B   **C**

Nerve Compression Syndromes

Carpal Tunnel Syndrome

S. Brent Brotzman, MD

Background

Carpal tunnel syndrome (CTS) is relatively common (the most common peripheral neuropathy), affecting 1% of the general population. It occurs most frequently during middle or advanced age, with 83% of 1215 study patients older than 40 years with a mean age of 54 years. Women are affected twice as frequently as men.

The carpal tunnel is a rigid, confined fibro-osseous space that physiologically acts as a "closed compartment." CTS is caused by compression of the median nerve at the wrist. The clinical syndrome is characterized by pain, numbness, or tingling in the distribution of the median nerve (the palmar aspect of the thumb, index, and long finger). These symptoms may affect all or a combination of the thumb, index, long, and ring fingers. Pain and **paresthesias at night** in the palmar aspect of the hand (median nerve distribution) are common symptoms.

The prolonged flexion or extension of the wrists under the patient's head or pillow during sleep is be-lieved to contribute to the prevalence of nocturnal symptoms. Conditions that alter fluid balance (pregnancy, use of oral contraceptives, hemodialysis) may predispose to CTS. CTS associated with **pregnancy** is transitory and typically resolves spontaneously. Therefore surgery should be avoided during pregnancy.

Types of Carpal Tunnel Syndrome

Acute Etiology

Sudden trauma

Wrist fracture

Crush injury

Burns

Gunshot wound

Chronic Etiology (Usually Idiopathic; Other Causes Include:)

Extrinsic causes

    Constrictive casts (must be released quickly and wrist taken out of flexion and placed into neutral)

Types of Carpal Tunnel Syndrome (*Continued*)

Handcuffs

Tight gloves

Repetitive and forceful gripping and/or power vibrating tools

Intrinsic causes

Anatomic anomalies such as hypertrophy or proximal
location of lumbricals, palmaris longus, or palmaris
profundus

Inflammatory proliferative tenosynovium

Perineural scarring from previous carpal tunnel release

Occupational Etiology (Controversial and Inconclusive)

Repetitive wrist flexion/extension

Intense gripping

Awkward (poor ergonomics) wrist flexion

Computer keyboards

Power vibratory tools

Typical Clinical Presentation

Paresthesias, pain, and numbness or tingling in the palmar surface of the hand in the distribution of the median nerve (Fig. 1–39) (i.e., the palmar aspect of the three and one-half radial digits) are the most common symptoms. Nocturnal pain is also common. Activities of daily living (such as driving a car, holding a cup, and typing) of-ten aggravate pain. Pain and paresthesias are sometimes relieved by the patient massaging or shaking the hand.

Provocative Testing Maneuvers (Table 1–5)

Phalen Maneuver (Fig. 1–40)

- The patient's wrists are placed in complete (but not forced) flexion.
- If paresthesias in the median nerve distribution occur within the 60-second test, the test is positive for CTS.
- Gellman and associates (1986) found this to be the most sensitive (sensitivity, 75%) of the provocative maneuvers in their study of CTS.

Tinel Sign (Median Nerve Percussion)

- Tinel sign may be elicited by lightly tapping the patient's median nerve at the wrist, moving from proximal to distal.
- The sign is positive if the patient complains of tingling or electric shock–like sensation in the distribution of the median nerve.

Sensory Testing of the Median Nerve Distribution

Decreased sensation may be tested by:

- *Threshold tests:* Semmes-Weinstein monofilament; vibrometry perception of a 256-cps tuning fork.
- *Innervation density tests:* two-point discrimination.

Sensory loss and thenar muscle weakness often are *late findings.*

Electrodiagnostic Tests

- Electrodiagnostic studies are a useful adjunct to clinical evaluation, but do not supplant the need for a careful history and physical examination.
- These tests are indicated when the clinical picture is ambiguous or there is suspicion of other neuropathies.

The criterion for a positive electrodiagnostic test is a motor latency greater than 4.0 M/sec and a sensory latency of greater than 3.5 M/sec.

The interpretation of findings in patients with CTS is classified in Table 1–6.

Special Tests for Evaluation

- Phalen maneuver (60 seconds).
- Tinel sign at carpal tunnel (percussion test).
- Carpal tunnel direct compression (60 seconds).
- Semmes-Weinstein monofilament sensory testing.
- Palpation of pronator teres/Tinel's (rule out pronator syndrome).
- Spurling's test of the neck (rule out cervical radiculopathy). (See Chapter 3, Shoulder Injuries.)
- Radicular testing (motor, sensory, reflexes) of involved extremity (rule out radiculopathy).

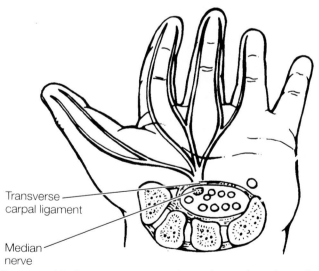

Transverse carpal ligament

Median nerve

Figure 1–39. Sensory symptoms of carpal tunnel syndrome localize to the sensory distribution of the median nerve. They most commonly consist of pain, numbness, and burning or tingling of the palmar surfaces of the thumb, index finger, middle finger, and radial half of the ring finger (*shaded area*). (From Steyers CM, Schelkuns PH: Practical management of carpal tunnel. Physician Sports Med 23[1]:83, 1995.)

Table 1–5

Available Tests used to Diagnose Carpal Tunnel Syndrome

N	Test	Method	Condition Measured	Positive Result	Interpretation of Positive Result
1*	Phalen maneuver	Patient holds wrist in marked flexion for 30–60 sec	Paresthesias in response to position	Numbness or tingling on radial side digits	Probable CTS (sensitivity, 0.75; specificity, 0.47) Gellman found best sensitivity of provocative tests.
2*	Percussion test (Tinel sign)	Examiner lightly taps along median nerve at the wrist, proximal to distal	Site of nerve lesion	Tingling response in fingers	Probable CTS if response is at the wrist (sensitivity, 0.60; specificity, 0.67).
3*	Carpal tunnel compression	Direct compression of median nerve by examiner	Paresthesias in response to pressure	Paresthesias within 30 sec	Probable CTS (sensitivity, 0.87; specificity, 0.90)
4	Hand diagram	Patient marks sites of pain or altered sensation on outline.	Patient's perception of site of nerve deficit	Pain depiction on palmar side of radial digits without depiction of the palm	Probable CTS (sensitivity, 0.96; specificity, 0.73), negative predictive value of a negative test, 0.91
5	Hand volume stress test	Measure hand volume by water displacement; repeat after 7-min stress test and 10-min rest.	Hand volume	Hand volume increased by ≥10 ml	Probable dynamic CTS
6	Static two-point discrimination	Determine minimum separation of two points perceived as distinct when lightly touched on palmar surface of digit.	Innervation density of slowly adapting fibers	Failure to discriminate points <6 mm apart	Advanced nerve dysfunction (late finding)
7	Moving two-point discrimination	As above, but with points moving	Innervation density of slowly adapting fibers	Failure to discriminate points <5 mm apart	Advanced nerve dysfunction (late finding)
8	Vibrometry	Vibrometer head is placed on palmar side of digit; amplitude at 120 Hz increased to threshold of perception; compare median and ulnar nerves in both hands.	Threshold of quickly adapting fibers	Asymmetry in contralateral hand or between radial and ulnar digits	Probable CTS (sensitivity, 0.87)
9*	Semmes-Weinstein monofilament test	Monofilaments of increasing diameter touched to palmar side of digit until patient can tell which digit is untouched	Threshold of slowly adapting fibers	Value >2.83 in radial digits	Median nerve impairment (sensitivity, 0.83)
10*	Distal sensory latency and conduction velocity	Orthodromic stimulus and recording across wrist	Latency and conduction velocity of sensory fibers	Latency >3.5 ms or asymmetry >0.5 ms compared with contralateral hand	Probable CTS
11*	Distal motor latency conduction	Orthodromic stimulus and recording across wrist	Latency and conduction velocity of motor fibers of median nerve	Latency >4.5 ms or asymmetry >1 ms	Probable CTS
12	Electromyography	Needle electrodes placed in muscle	Denervation of thenar muscles	Fibrillation potentials, sharp waves, increased insertional activity	Very advanced motor median nerve compression

CTS, carpal tunnel syndrome.
*Most common tests/methods utilized in our practice.
Adapted from Szabo RM, Madison M: Carpal tunnel syndrome. Orthop Clin North Am 1:103, 1992.

Figure 1-40. Phalen test. When the patient holds the wrists flexed for 60 seconds, numbness and tingling along the distribution of the median nerve indicate carpal tunnel syndrome. (From Slade JF, Mahoney JD, Dailinger JE, Boxamsa TH: Wrist injuries in musicians. J Musculoskel Med 16:548, 1999. Artist: Amy Collins [Art and Science].)

- Inspection for weakness or atrophy of thenar eminence (a *late* finding of CTS).
- Exploration for possible global neuropathy on history and examination (e.g., diabetic).
- If gray area, electromyographic/nerve conduction velocity (EMG/NCV) testing of *entire* involved upper extremity to exclude cervical radiculopathy versus CTS versus pronator syndrome.

Evaluation

- Patients with **systemic peripheral neuropathies** (e.g., diabetes, alcoholism, hypothyroidism) typically have sensory abnormality distribution that is not solely isolated to the median nerve distribution.
- More proximal compressive neuropathies (e.g., C6 **cervical radiculopathy**) will produce sensory deficits in the C6 distribution (well beyond median nerve distribution); plus weakness in the C6 innervated muscles (biceps) and an abnormal biceps reflex.
- Electrodiagnostic tests are helpful in distinguishing local compressive neuropathies (such as CTS) from peripheral systemic neuropathies (such as diabetic neuropathy).

Differential Diagnosis of Carpal Tunnel Syndrome

Thoracic outlet syndrome (TOS)
   TOS exhibits positive Adson test (see Chapter 3, Shoulder Injuries), costoclavicular maneuver, Roos test, etc.

Cervical radiculopathy (CR)
   CR has a positive Spurling test of the neck (see Chapter 3, Shoulder Injuries), *proximal* arm/neck symptoms, dermatomal distribution, occasional neck pain.

Brachial plexopathy

Pronator teres syndrome (PTS)
   Median nerve compression in the *proximal* forearm (PTS) rather than the wrist (CTS) has similar median nerve symptoms.
   PTS is usually associated with activity-induced *daytime* paresthesias rather than nighttime (CTS).
   Tenderness and Tinel palpable at pronator teres in the forearm, not at the carpal tunnel.
   PTS (more proximal) involves the median nerve innervated extrinsic forearm motors *and* the palmar cutaneous nerve branch of the median nerve (unlike CTS).
   Employ the provocation test for PTS (see Figure 1-43 on p. 40).

Digital nerve compression (bowler's thumb)
   Caused by direct pressure applied to the palm or digits (base of the thumb in bowler's thumb)
   Tenderness and Tinel sign localized to the thumb digit rather than carpal tunnel.

Neuropathy (systemic)
   Alcohol, diabetes, hypothyroidism—more diffuse neuropathy findings noted

Tenosynovitis (RA)

Reflex sympathetic dystrophy (RSD) (see Chapter 8)
   RSDS has skin color, temperature changes, hyperesthesias, etc.

Table 1-6

Interpreting Findings in Patients with Carpal Tunnel Syndrome

Degree of CTS	Findings
Dynamic	Symptoms primarily activity-induced; patient otherwise asymptomatic; no detectable physical findings.
Mild	Patient has intermittent symptoms; decreased light-touch sensibility; digital compression test usually positive but Tinel sign, as well as positive result on Phalen maneuver, may or may not be present.
Moderate	Frequent symptoms; decreased vibratory perception in median nerve distribution; positive Phalen maneuver and digital compression test; Tinel sign present; increased two-point discrimination; weakness of thenar muscles.
Severe	Symptoms are persistent; marked increase in or absence of two-point discrimination; thenar muscle atrophy.

CTS, carpal tunnel syndrome.

Treatment

- All patients should undergo **initial conservative management,** unless the presentation is acute and associated with trauma (such as CTS associated with acute distal radius fracture).
- All patients with **acute CTS** should have the wrist taken out of flexion in the cast and placed in neutral (see section on distal radius fractures).
- Circumferential casts should be removed or bivalved, and icing and elevation above the heart should be initiated.

- Close serial observation should check for possible "emergent" carpal tunnel release if symptoms do not improve.
- Some authors recommend measurement of wrist compartment pressure.

Nonoperative Management

- Pregnant women are all treated nonoperatively because of spontaneous resolution after delivery of the baby.
- Nonoperative treatment may include:
  - The use of a **prefabricated wrist splint,** placing the wrist in a neutral position, worn at night; daytime splinting if patient's job allows.
  - **Activity modification** (discontinuing vibratory machinery or placing a support under unsupported arms at the computer).
  - **Cortisone injection** of the carpal tunnel (Fig. 1–41) (**not** the actual median nerve). Studies have shown that fewer than 25% of patients who had cortisone injection into the carpal tunnel were symptom free at 18 months after injection. As many as 80% of patients do have *temporary relief* with cortisone injection and splinting. Green found that symptoms typically recurred 2 to 4 months after cortisone injection, leading to operative treatment in 46% of patients.
- The technique for injection is shown in Figure 1–41. If injection creates paresthesias in the hand, the needle should be immediately withdrawn and redirected; injection **should not** be into the median nerve.
- Vitamin B_6 has not been shown in clinical trials to have any therapeutic effect on CTS, but may help "missed" neuropathies (pyridoxine deficiency).

Rehabilitation Protocol
After Open Release of Carpal Tunnel Syndrome

0-7 Days
- Encourage gentle wrist extension and flexion exercises and full finger flexion and extension exercises immediately after surgery in the postsurgical dressing.

7 Days
- Remove the dressing.
- Prohibit the patient from submerging the hand in liquids, but permit showering.
- Discontinue the wrist splint if the patient is comfortable.

7-14 Days
- Permit the patient to use the hand in activities of daily living as pain allows.

2 Weeks
- Remove the sutures and begin ROM and gradual strengthening exercises.

- Achieve initial scar remodeling by using Elastomer or silicon gel-sheet scar pad at night and deep scar massage.
- If scar tenderness is intense, use desensitization techniques such as applying various textures to the area using light pressure and progressing to deep pressure. Textures include cotton, velour, wool, and Velcro.
- Control pain and edema with the use of Isotoner gloves or electrical stimulation.

2-4 Weeks
- Advance the patient to more rigorous activities; allow the patient to return to work if pain permits. The patient can use a padded glove for tasks that require pressure to be applied over the tender palmar scars.
- Begin pinch/grip strengthening with Baltimore Therapeutic Equipment work-simulator activities.

- Nonsteroidal anti-inflammatory drugs (NSAIDs) can be used for control of inflammation.
- Any underlying systemic disease (such as diabetes, rheumatoid arthritis, or hypothyroidism) must be controlled.

Surgical Treatment

Indications for surgical treatment of CTS include:

- Thenar atrophy or weakness.
- Sensation loss on objective measures.
- Fibrillation potentials on electromyelograms.
- Symptoms that persist more than a year despite appropriate conservative measures.

The goals of carpal tunnel release are:

- Decompression of the nerve.
- Improvement of excursion.
- Prevention of progressive nerve damage.

Our recommendation is **open carpal tunnel release** (complication rate of 10 to 18%) rather than endoscopic release (complication rate up to 35% in some studies). In our experience, the times to return to work and sporting activities have not been different enough between the two procedures to warrant the differences in complication rate (dramatically increased frequency of digital nerve lacerations with endoscopic technique).

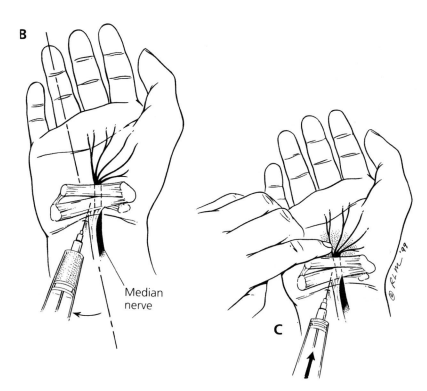

Figure 1–41. *A,* During carpal tunnel injection, a 25- or 27-gauge needle is used to introduce a mixture of dexamethasone and lidocaine into the carpal canal. *B,* Needle is aligned with the ring finger and directed 45 degrees dorsally and 30 degrees radially as it is advanced slowly beneath the transverse carpal ligament into the tunnel. *C,* After injection, lidocaine is dispersed. Injection into the nerve should be avoided. If any paresthesias occur during injection, the needle is immediately withdrawn and redirected. (From Royan GM: Understanding and managing carpal tunnel syndrome. J Musculoskel Med 16:661, 1999. Artist: Robert Marguiles.)

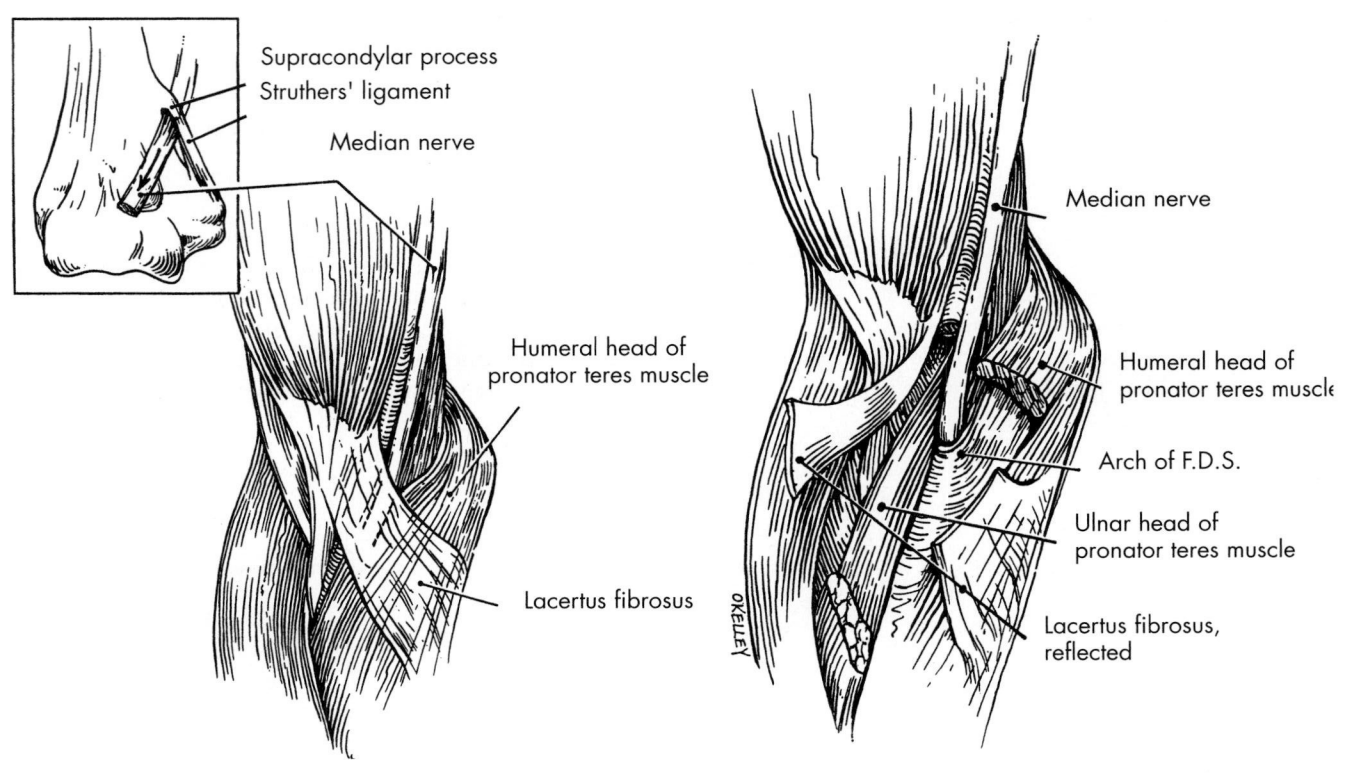

Figure 1–42. Anatomy of the antecubital fossa and structures overlying the course of the median nerve. *Inset* shows the supracondylar process that is occasionally present. F.D.S., flexor digitorum superficialis. (From Idler RS, Strickland JW, Creighton JJ Jr: Hand clinic: pronator syndrome. Indiana Med 84:124, 1991.)

Pronator Syndrome

A less common cause of median nerve entrapment occurs in the proximal forearm where the median nerve is compressed by either the pronator teres, the flexor superficialis arch, or the lacertus fibrosus in a condition referred to as *pronator syndrome* (Fig. 1–42). In addition to dysesthesias in the thumb and in the index, middle, and ring fingers, there may be a sensory disturbance of the volar base of the thenar eminence because of involvement of the palmar cutaneous branch of the medial nerve.

Physical findings include marked proximal forearm tenderness; a proximal median nerve compression test will reproduce the symptoms. The most common cause of this disorder is entrapment of the median nerve by the fascia of the pronator teres proximally, which can be tested by resisted pronation with gradual extension of the elbow (Fig. 1–43). A positive resisted middle finger flexion test may suggest median nerve entrapment by the FDS arch, and resisted supination with the elbow flexed may suggest entrapment by the lacertus fibrosus, a fascial extension of the biceps tendon.

Treatment

Nonoperative management of this disorder includes minimizing resisted pronation activities and repetitive gripping and squeezing. Long-arm splinting with the elbow at 90 degrees and the forearm in neutral rotation, in addition to anti-inflammatory medications and vitamin B, may be beneficial. Conservative management of this disorder often is ineffective, and surgery is usually required.

Figure 1–43. Provocative tests for pronator syndrome. *A*, Pronator teres: resisted forearm pronation with the elbow relatively extended. *B*, Lacertus fibrosus: resisted elbow flexion with the forearm supinated. *C*, FDS: resisted middle finger extension. (From Idler RS, Strickland JW, Creighton JJ Jr: Hand clinic: pronator syndrome. Indiana Med 84:124, 1991.)

Rehabilitation Protocol
After Surgical Decompression for Pronator Teres Syndrome

0–7 Days
- Keep a soft, light compressive dressing in place to allow full elbow, forearm, and wrist motion.

7 Days
- Remove the dressing and encourage activities as tolerated, including light manual labor.
- Begin ROM to the wrist and elbow, including gripping in extension with putty.

2 Weeks
- Remove the sutures and encourage progressive strengthening and use of the upper extremity.

4 Weeks
- Allow moderate to heavy work.

6 Weeks
- Allow full, unprotected use of the arm.

Discomfort after surgical decompression of the median nerve in the proximal forearm is less than after decompression of the median nerve at the wrist level, and desensitization techniques are unnecessary.

Ulnar Tunnel Syndrome

Compression of the ulnar nerve **at the wrist** level may result from a pathologic condition within Guyon's canal, such as an ulnar artery aneurysm, thrombosis, ganglia, anomalous muscle bellies, or anomalous ligaments. External compression of the nerve can be caused by idiopathic fascial thickening, repetitive trauma, palmaris brevis hypertrophy, and other muscle anomalies or hypertrophies. Conservative management for this disorder is similar to that for CTS, although injections should be done with caution because of the proximity of the ulnar nerve to the ulnar artery.

Radial Tunnel Syndrome, Posterior Interosseous Nerve Syndrome

Entrapment of the posterior interosseous nerve may be associated with pain and tenderness in the proximal forearm without weakness **(radial tunnel syndrome)** or with motor loss **(posterior interosseous nerve syndrome).** Sites of compression include fibrous bands over the radiocapitellar joint, synovitis of the radiocapitellar joint (as in rheumatoid arthritis), the vascular leash of Henry, the proximal fascial edge of the extensor carpi radialis brevis muscle, the arcade of Frohse (proximal edge of the super-

---

Rehabilitation Protocol
After Surgical Decompression of Ulnar Tunnel Syndrome at the Wrist

0–7 Days
- Fit the patient with a soft splint and encourage wrist flexion and extension exercises.

7 Days
- Remove the splint and increase wrist extension and flexion exercises to full motion.

7–14 Days
- Emphasize light grip activities and finger motion (marble hunt in corn or rice or soft putty exercises).
- Remove sutures at 2 weeks.

2–4 Weeks
- Treat the scar with deep friction massage using a silicone-based scar pad.
- Begin resistive exercises (hand-helper, clothes-pin pinch, forearm and wrist curls).

4–6 Weeks
- Encourage normal activity.
- Allow work-related activities.
- Desensitization techniques may be necessary for palmar scar tenderness, and a padded glove may allow the patient an early return to moderate to heavy work activities.

Rehabilitation Protocol
After Surgical Decompression of Radial Tunnel/Posterior Interosseous Syndrome

0–7 Days

- Remove light compressive surgical dressing at 3–5 days.
- Initiate full active forearm and elbow flexion and extension exercises.

7–14 Days

- Remove the dressing at 7 days.
- Begin active and active-assisted wrist, forearm, and elbow exercises.

- Continue edema control with compressive sleeve and high-voltage galvanic stimulation.

2–4 Weeks

- Begin resistive exercises for wrist and forearm supination.

6 Weeks

- Allow unrestricted activity.

---

ficial head of the supinator muscle), and the distal edge of the supinator. Although often associated with tennis elbow, this syndrome may exist as an isolated compression neuropathy. Patients with distal posterior interosseous syndrome typically present with chronic dorsal wrist pain that is exacerbated by forced dorsiflexion of the wrist.

Treatment

Conservative management of entrapment of the posterior interosseous nerve includes a trial of long arm splinting with the elbow at 90 degrees and the forearm in neutral, refraining from resisted supination and wrist extension types of activities. Anti-inflammatory medications and vitamin B_6 may be prescribed.

Rehabilitation after posterior interosseous nerve decompression may vary, depending on the surgical approach. The interval between the brachioradialis and the extensor carpi radialis longus gives excellent exposure of the posterior interosseous nerve from the radiocapitellar articulation through the proximal half of the supinator. Subsequent rehabilitation may be easier because the muscle fibers of the brachioradialis are not violated.

Nerve Injuries

Nerve injuries are most commonly caused by direct trauma, laceration, traction or stretching, entrapment, or compression. Obtaining optimal hand function after nerve injury depends on preservation of passive ROM of the hand and prevention of secondary damage from attenuation or stretching of involved structures owing to poor positioning or substitution patterns. Combined with the appropriate exercise regimens, splinting techniques can be effective for attaining these goals.

Evaluation

The status of tendon and nerve function should be documented at initial examination:

- Motor and sensory examination for radial, median, and ulnar nerves.
- Flexors and extensors to digits and wrist.

Tendon and nerve function can be difficult to evaluate initially in patients with extensive upper extremity trauma because of pain and skeletal instability. If the examination is equivocal, this should be documented.

Median nerve lesions result in a loss of coordination, decreased strength, and a decrease in or loss of sensory input from the thumb, index, long, and ring fingers. Distal lesions primarily impair opposition and adduction, and splinting is aimed primarily at preventing first web contracture and maintaining passive motion of the thumb CMC joint.

Ulnar nerve lesions compromise coordination, pinch and grip strength, and thumb stability and frequently cause "clawing" of the ring and small fingers. Splinting is aimed at prevention of this clawing, while allowing full digital flexion and IP joint extension.

Radial nerve lesions result in loss of active extension of the wrist, thumb, and fingers, weakness of thumb abduction, decreased grip strength, and diminished coordination. The emphasis of splinting is on providing wrist stability and maintaining thumb position.

Classification of Nerve Injuries

Seddon and Sunderland

Neurapraxia (first-degree injury)	Local conduction block with segmental demyelination. No axonal abnormality. Excellent recovery.
Axonotmesis (second-degree injury)	Axonal injury such that wallerian degeneration will occur distally. Axonal sprouting within the appropriate endoneurial tube. Excellent recovery anticipated.
Third-degree injury	Axonal injury and varying degrees of scarring with the endoneurium. Recovery is not complete but varies from almost complete recovery to almost no recovery, depending on the degree of endoneurial scarring and the degree of mismatching of regenerating sensory and motor fibers within the injured fascicle.
Fourth-degree injury	Nerve physically in continuity but scar tissue prevents nerve regeneration across the area of injury.
Neurotmesis (fifth-degree injury)	Transection of the nerve. No functional recovery.
Mixed injury (sixth-degree injury, neuroma incontinuity)	Combines various patterns of injury from fascicle to fascicle. Injury pattern may vary along length of nerve as well.

Treatment (Table 1–7)

Eight Principles of Nerve Repair

1. Quantitative preoperative and postoperative clinical assessment of both the motor and the sensory systems:
   - Pinch and grip measurements.
   - Static and moving two-point discrimination (innervation density test).
   - Vibration or pressure stimulus measurements (measurement of threshold).
2. Microsurgical technique.
   - Magnification.
   - Microsurgical instruments.
   - Sutures.
3. Tension-free repair.
4. Use of an interposition nerve graft when a tension-free repair is not possible.
5. Nerve repair and nerve graft with:
   - Extremity in neutral position.
   - No tension at the repair site.
6. Primary repair when clinical and surgical conditions permit.
7. Epineural repair when function of the fascicles is mixed sensory and motor without well-defined groups of fascicles. A group fascicular repair can be done when a particular fascicle(s) is recognized as mediating a specific function.
8. Postoperative motor and sensory re-education to maximize the potential surgical result.

Table 1-7

Treatment of Nerve Injuries

Degree of Injury	Tinel Sign Present/ Progresses Disability	Recovery Pattern	Rate of Recovery	Surgical Procedure
I. Neurapraxia	− / −	Complete	Fast, days to 12 wk	None
II. Axonotmesis	+ / +	Complete	Slow (1 inch/mo)	None
III. Third degree injury	+ / +	Great variation*	Slow (1 inch/mo)	None or neurolysis
IV. Neuroma incontinuity	+ / −	None	No recovery	Nerve repair or nerve graft
V. Neurotmesis	+ / −	None	No recovery	Nerve repair or nerve graft
VI. Mixed injury—varies with each fascicle, depending on the combination of injury pattern as noted above.				

*Recovery is at least as good as a nerve repair, but can vary from excellent to poor, depending on the degree of endoneurial scarring and the amount of sensory and motor axonal misdirection that occurs with the injured fascicle.

Epineural versus Fascicular Repair

The superiority of one technique over another has not been demonstrated, possibly because the theoretical benefits of fascicular alignment are lost clinically because of increased surgical manipulation. A repair of an inappropriate fascicle (e.g., motor sensory) would ensure a poor result.

Timing of the Nerve Repair

- Primary repair—variable: sharp laceration + skilled surgeon + appropriate instrumentation available.
- Delayed repair (nerve graft)—variable: avulsive injury + questionable proximal and distal extent of injury (at the earliest, three weeks after injury).
- With a closed injury:
  - Expectant treatment until 3 months, then explored if no clinical or EMG recovery.
  - If closed injury localizes to an area of nerve entrapment (such as the carpal tunnel), early decompression of the nerve is recommended so that the nerve is allowed to recover without an added superimposed element of nerve compression.
- General guidelines:
  - Nerve deficit due to sharp injury—assume nerve is cut.
  - Nerve deficit due to closed injury—generally nerve is in continuity; EMG/NCS after 4 weeks should clarify.

Nerve Gap versus Nerve Defect

Nerve defect: the actual amount of neural tissue lost; constant for any given injury.

Nerve gap: the distance between the proximal and the distal ends of the nerve; can vary (e.g., joint movement or soft tissue contracture). The *neuroma incontinuity* is evaluated with clinical examination and electrodiagnostic testing to determine which fascicles have first-, second-, or third-degree injuries with likelihood of spontaneous recovery as opposed to fourth- or fifth-degree injuries that require surgical reconstruction. Microsurgical exploration of the nerve with neurolysis will assist in making the surgical decision. Occasionally, intraoperative nerve conduction studies are useful.

Nerve grafting is done when an end-to-end repair cannot be done without tension. Donor nerves include the sural nerve, the anterior branch of the medial antebrachial cutaneous nerve, and the lateral antebrachial cutaneous nerve. The clinical role of *vascularized nerve grafts* is not established. Potential indications include reconstruction of large nerve gaps, proximal injuries, reconstruction in compro-

mised beds, and the use of large-caliber donor nerve grafts. ■

Splinting for Nerve Palsies

Nancy Cannon, OTR

Median Nerve: Splint Recommendation—Web Spacer
Purpose

- Maintain width of the first web space, preventing first web contracture. This is necessary because of the paralysis of the thenar musculature.

Warning/Precautions

- When fabricating the splint, avoid hyperextension of the thumb MCP joint or stress to the UCL of the MCP joint.

Wearing Time

- Night only.
- If any first web space contracture is noted, periodic daywear is added.

Ulnar Nerve: Splint Recommendation—Single Wynn-Parry Splint or Static Metacarpophalangeal Joint Extension Block Splint
Purpose

- Prevent clawing of the ring and small fingers while allowing full digital flexion and IP joint extension.
- The splint is required because of paralysis of the ulnar innervated intrinsics.

Warning/Precautions

- Monitor carefully to prevent pressure sores in patients who do not have sensory return.

Wearing Time

- Continuous wear until the MCP volar plates tighten so that hyper extension is no longer present, the intrinsics return, or tendon transfers are done to replace the function of the intrinsics.

Radial Nerve: Splint Recommendation—Wrist Immobilization Splint or Possibly a Long Dorsal Outrigger Splint
Purpose

- Positioning the wrist in approximately 15 to 20 degrees of dorsiflexion allows improved functional use of the hand and prevents wrist drop.

Rehabilitation Protocol
After Repair of Digital Nerve

2 Weeks

- Remove bulky dressing and initiate edema control with Coban or fingersocks.
- Fit DBS in 30 degrees of flexion at the PIP joint for continual wear, assuming the repair is near the PIP joint level or slightly distal to this point. The DBS may be fitted in more flexion at the MCP or PIP joint level if the digital nerve repair is under more tension.
  Note: if nerve repair is near the MCP joint, the DBS should include the MCP joint only, with approximately 30 degrees of flexion at the MCP joint.
- Begin active and passive ROM exercises six times a day within the restraints of the DBS.
- Begin scar massage with lotion and/or the use of Otoform or Elastomer within 24 hours after suture removal.

3–6 Weeks

- Adjust the DBS into extension 10 degrees each week until neutral position is achieved at 6 weeks.

6 Weeks

- Discontinue the DBS.
- Initiate passive extension at the MCP joint.
- Begin extension splinting if passive extension is limited, but generally patients regain extension and extension splints are not necessary.
- Begin progressive strengthening.

8–10 Weeks

- Begin sensory re-education when some sign of sensory return (protective sensation) is present.

- Incorporation of the outrigger component of the splint allows assistance with extension at the MCP level of the digits.

Wearing Time

- The patient wears the splint until there is return of the radial nerve innervated muscles or tendon transfers are done to improve wrist and/or finger extension.

Digital Nerve Repair

Most lacerations of digital nerves should be repaired as soon as possible (within 5 to 7 days of injury) if the wound is clean and sharp. The condition of the patient, the presence of other injuries that may take precedence over nerve repair, skin conditions such as extensive soft tissue loss, wound contamination, and the availability of personnel and equipment also must be considered in the timing of digital nerve repair.

Bowler's Thumb (Digital Nerve Injury)

- Digital nerve compression, or bowler's thumb, is a compression neuropathy of the ulnar digital nerve of the thumb.
- Repetitive pressure of the thumbhole of the bowling ball to this area results in formation of a perineural fibrosis or neuroma-type formation of the ulnar digital nerve.

- Patients present with a painful mass at the base of the thumb and paresthesias.
- A Tinel sign is usually elicited; and the mass is tender to palpation.
- Differential diagnoses include ganglion, inclusion cyst, and painful callous.
- Treatment includes:
  - A protective thumb shell.
  - Backsetting the thumbhole of the bowling ball to increase thumb extension and abduction.
  - Avoiding full insertion of the thumb into the thumbhole.
- If conservative measures fail, decompression and internal neurolysis or neuroma resection with primary repair should be considered.

Replantation

Replantation of amputated parts and revascularization for salvaging mangled extremities require intense commitment from both the patient and the surgeon. Emotional and financial investments are enormous, and successful replantation and revascularization require long postsurgical rehabilitation programs that are frequently interrupted and prolonged by multiple reconstructive surgical procedures.

Proper candidate selection is critical to the success of replantation and revascularization of amputated parts.

Contraindications

Absolute contraindications for replantation and revascularization include multiple-trauma victims with significant associated injuries in whom treatment of other organ systems takes precedence over extremity salvage. Digits have been refrigerated and replanted up to 3 days after injury. Extensive injury to the affected limb, chronic illness, previously nonfunctioning parts, and psychiatric illness also prohibit salvage procedures.

Relative contraindications include avulsion injuries, lengthy ischemia time, and patients older than 50 years. Major limbs are defined as those with significant skeletal muscle content. These may be salvaged if appropriately cooled 12 hours after the injury; up to 6 hours of warm ischemia time can be tolerated. Only under unusual circumstances should single digits be replanted, especially those proximal to the FDS insertion.

Indications

The ideal candidate for replantation is a young patient with a narrow zone of injury. Power saws and punch presses often result in replantable parts. Indications for replantation include any upper or lower extremity in a child, as well as thumbs, multiple digits, hands, and wrist-level and some more proximal-level amputations in adults.

Postsurgical Considerations

Postsurgical care typically begins in the operating room, where brachial plexus blocks are given before the patient leaves. A bulky, noncompressive dressing reinforced with plaster splints is applied in the operating room and usually is kept in place for 3 weeks. When the likelihood of thrombosis is increased, such as in wide-zone injuries, heparin may be used. Postsurgical orders include keeping the patient nil per os (NPO) for 12 to 24 hours after surgery, because vascular compromise may necessitate emergency surgical intervention. The replanted part is kept warm either with a thermal blanket or by elevating the room temperature to 78°F to 80°F. Caffeine-containing products, such as coffee, tea, colas, and chocolate, are prohibited, as is smoking and the use of tobacco products by both the patient and the visitors. Ice and iced drinks are not allowed, and visitation is limited to one to two visitors at a time to try to prevent emotional disturbance. The patient is restricted to bed rest for approximately 3 days, and the replanted part is kept at or slightly above heart level.

Rehabilitation Protocol
Replantation and Revascularization in Adults

1 Day

- Appropriate and liberal use of analgesics is recommended, although postoperative discomfort is usually minimal with replantations. Revascularization procedures typically require more postoperative pain management, especially when neural connections remain.
- Low-molecular-weight dextran 40 in 500 ml of 5% dextrose in water (D_5W) is given over 6–24 hours. In patients with pulmonary problems, continuous intravenous infusion at a lower rate is recommended.
- Aspirin (325 mg, one by mouth two times a day).
- Thorazine (25 mg by mouth three times a day).
- Antibiotics—cefazolin or a similar antibiotic for 3–5 days.
- Administer low-molecular-weight dextran 40 and 500 ml D_5W at a rate of 10 ml/kg/day for 3 days to the pediatric patient.
- Automated monitors with alarms provide continuous feedback, although hourly visual inspection for the first 12 hours provides important information, including color, capillary refill, turgor, and bleeding of the replanted part.

Management of Early Complications

- Five to 10 days of hospitalization are necessary after replantation. After that time, replantation failure from vascular compromise occurs infrequently. Arterial insufficiency from thrombosis or vasoconstriction usually requires immediate return to the operating room. Give a plexus block, explore the arterial anastomosis, excise the damaged segment, and perform vein grafting if necessary. Administer heparin in savage procedures of this sort and attempt to keep the partial thromboplastin time 1.5 to 2.0 times normal.
- Venous congestion indicates either insufficient venous outflow, or venous thrombosis. At the first sign of venous congestion, loosen all postoperative dressings to eliminate external construction. Digital replantations with venous congestion may benefit from a longitudinal laceration through the digital pulp or removal of the nail plate. Heparinized-saline drops applied to the nailbed and pulp may promote venous drainage. If the venous outflow from the nailbed or drainage site is inadequate but present, leech therapy may be indicated.

Rehabilitation Protocol
Replantation and Revascularization in Adults *(Continued)*

Apply a medical leech to the finger or area of congestion with the remaining sites shielded by plastic sheathing. A leech cage may be fashioned from the plastic bag in which intravenous bags are stored. Tape the open end of the plastic bag around the bulky postoperative dressing, introduce a leech through a vertical slit in the bag, then tape the vertical slit. Adequate oxygenization occurs through the porous surgical dressing. Leeches have a long-lasting anticoagulant and vasodilating effect in addition to withdrawing approximately 5 ml of blood. However, arterial inflow must be present for the leech to attach. If the leech does not attach, the digit may have arterial as well as venous insufficiency, and further salvage requires immediate surgical exploration of the artery and venous anastomoses.

5–10 Days

- The patient may be discharged from the hospital if the appearance of the replanted part is acceptable.
- Dietary and environmental restrictions remain the same, and the patient receives aspirin (325 mg) twice daily for an additional 2 weeks.

3 Weeks

- Remove the dressing and assess the wound. Replanted digits are usually markedly edematous with granulating wounds.
- Wound care management consists of hydrogen peroxide wound cleansing and silver nitrate cauterization of redundant granulation tissue.

- Apply soft, nonadherent dressings and fit the wrist with a splint in slight wrist flexion and MCP joint flexion to about 50 to 60 degrees.
- Begin passive wrist flexion and MCP joint flexion exercises, with emphasis on flexor tendon glide.

6 Weeks

- Begin active and active-assisted ROM and flexion and extension with interval splinting.
- Continue edema control measures.

8 Weeks

- Accelerate active and active-assisted flexion and extension exercises of all joints and use electrical stimulation if necessary.
- Remove temporary bony fixation.

4 Months

- Perform soft tissue and bony reconstruction procedures.
- PIP joint injuries are commonly treated by fusion. Active digital extension and flexion are often inhibited by tendon adhesions.
- Motion is best achieved through a two-stage tenolysis program. Perform extensor tenolysis first, followed by a flexor tenolysis approximately 2 to 3 months after the initial procedure.

Major Limb Replantation

Major limb replantation requires the wrist and hand to be splinted in a functional position. Full passive motion of each joint at the more proximal soft tissue and neurologic injury is allowed. Motion exercises are continued until proximal neuromuscular function returns. The results of replantation depend primarily on the outcome of the nerve repairs. The age of the patient, mechanism of injury, level of injury, and the quality of the replantation procedure, especially the extent of revascularization, are also important factors.

Dupuytren's Contracture

The manifestations of Dupuytren's disease are variable and may be confined to a single digit, but palmar and digital involvement of the ring and small fingers is more common. Diffuse involvement of the first web space and thumb in addition to the fingers is less common.

No exact criteria exist for surgical intervention in Dupuytren's disease. Some patients who have severe MCP and PIP joint contractures have surprisingly few complaints of functional disability, whereas some patients with pretendinous cords and nodules without contractures desire surgical intervention.

Guidelines for surgical intervention include:

- 30 degrees of MCP joint contracture.
- 15 degrees of PIP joint contracture.
- Inability to place the hand into a pocket, lay it flat on a table, or bring it together with the opposite hand (as in prayer).

Regardless of the criteria used for surgical intervention, the PIP joint contracture is the most difficult to correct and warrants early intervention.

Surgical procedures used in the treatment of Dupuytren's contracture include subcutaneous fasciotomy, partial selective fasciectomy, complete fasciectomy, fasciectomy with skin grafting, and amputation.

Rehabilitation Protocol
Dupuytren's Contracture, Subcutaneous Fasciotomy

0–7 Days

- Encourage the patient to work on stretching exercises immediately after the surgery. Maintain digital extension with a resting pan splint with Velcro straps.

- Have the patient wear the splint during the day between exercises and at night for the first week.
- Continue night splints for 6 weeks after surgery.

Subcutaneous Fasciotomy

In elderly patients with MCP joint contracture, subcutaneous fasciotomy is ideal, regardless of whether one or two digits are involved. This procedure may be done in the office with local anesthesia.

Technique of Subcutaneous Fasciotomy

With the palm anesthetized, a No. 15 blade is introduced across the palm between the skin and the pretendinous cord. The finger is extended and the knife blade is gently pressed onto the taut cord. An abrupt release of the MCP joint contracture follows when the cord transection is complete. Manipulation of the fingers may result in some tearing of the palmar skin; however, this is usually minor, and the wound can be left open and covered with a sterile dressing.

Surgical procedures other than cordotomy for Dupuytren's disease require considerable dissection, and subsequent palmar and finger hematomas become more likely. Small suction drain systems may be in corporated to prevent these hematomas.

Arthroplasty

Proximal Interphalangeal Joint Arthroplasty

PIP joint arthroplasty is primarily indicated for patients who are relatively free of disease at the MCP joints. This usually precludes patients with rheumatoid arthritis with significant MCP joint involvement. The best treatment option for these patients is MCP joint arthroplasty and either soft tissue procedures for correction of the soft tissue deformities or PIP joint fusion. Patients with osteoarthritis may benefit from isolated PIP joint arthroplasty, other than the index finger.

A volar approach for placement of the implant may be used when the extensor mechanism does not require repair or corrective surgery. Active flexion and extension exercises may be started immediately after surgery.

Rehabilitation after PIP joint arthroplasty depends on whether the arthroplasty is done for a stiff IP joint, for reconstruction with lateral deviation, or to correct a boutonnière deformity.

Rehabilitation Protocol
Proximal Interphalangeal Joint Arthroplasty for Joint Stiffness

0–3 Weeks

- Begin active flexion and extension exercises at 3–5 days after surgery.
- Have the patient use a padded aluminum splint between hourly exercises to maintain full PIP joint extension.

3–6 Weeks

- Continue interval PIP joint splinting during the day for 6 weeks.

6 Weeks

- Begin resistive exercises.
- Continue interval splinting to correct any angular deviation and extensor lag of more than 20 degrees.
- Have the patient wear protective splint at night for 3 months after surgery.

The ideal ROMs obtained are 0–70 degrees of flexion in the ring and small fingers, 60 degrees of flexion in the middle finger, and 45 degrees of flexion in the index finger.

Rehabilitation Protocol
Metacarpophalangeal Joint Arthroplasty

0–7 Days

- Remove drains 2 days after surgery.
- Use postoperative splint to maintain MCP joints in full extension and neutral to slight radial deviation.

7 Days

- Fashion dynamic extension outrigger splint and resting hand splints.
- Begin active MCP joint exercises.
- Apply a supinator tab to index finger.

2–4 Weeks

- Remove the sutures. Continue the night resting pan splint.
- Continue dynamic extension outrigger splint for daily use.

4 Weeks

- Allow light hand use and activities of daily living.
- Continue night splinting for 4 months to help reduce extensor lag.

Note: If MCP joint motion is not obtained in 2 weeks, the PIP joint should be splinted in full extension and flexion force concentrated at the MCP joint level. Careful follow-up is necessary during the first 3 weeks, when the desired motion should be achieved. At 3 weeks, the capsular structures are significantly tight, and no further ROM should be expected. Dynamic flexion may be necessary to regain early MCP joint flexion.

Rehabilitation Protocol
Proximal Interphalangeal Joint Arthroplasty for Lateral Deviation

The central slip and collateral ligaments are reconstructed in this deformity.

2–3 Weeks

- Use an extension splint and gutter splints to correct residual angular deformities.
- Perform active exercises three to five times a day with taping or radial outriggers.

- Have the patient wear splints for 6–8 weeks after surgery.

6–8 Weeks

- Continue night splinting for 3–6 months.

Metacarpophalangeal Joint Arthroplasty

MCP joint arthroplasty is indicated primarily for patients with rheumatoid arthritis, although unusual post-traumatic or osteoarthritic conditions may require implant arthroplasty. Correction of radial deviation of the metacarpals as well as intrinsic imbalance is necessary for acceptable results. The procedure increases the range of functional motion of the fingers, although grip and pinch strength do not improve significantly.

Thumb Carpometacarpal Joint Arthroplasty

The arthritic basilar joint of the thumb offers another clear example that radiographic appearance has no correlation with the severity of clinical symptoms. Radiographic evidence of advanced arthritic change may be an incidental finding, whereas a radiographically normal thumb may have significant disability. Treatment regimens with steroid injection splinting, and NSAIDs should be exhausted before surgical intervention.

Total joint arthroplasty, implant arthroplasty, inter position arthroplasty, suspension arthroplasties, and CMC joint fusion have been used to alleviate pain and restore function in the diseased basilar joint of the thumb.

Interposition and Sling Suspension Arthroplasties

Trapezial excision techniques combined with soft tissue interposition or sling suspension arthroplasties have similar postsurgical protocols. Sling suspension arthroplasties are designed to prevent thumb osteoarticular column shortening and provide stability beyond that afforded by simple trapezial excision.

Rehabilitation Protocol
Interposition and Sling Suspension Arthroplasties

2 Weeks

- Remove the surgical thumb spica splint and sutures. Apply a short arm thumb spica cast for an additional 2 weeks.

4 Weeks

- Begin active, active-assisted, and passive ROM exercises with interval splinting.
- Ideally the splint or cast should include only CMC joint, leaving the MP or IP joint free for ROM.

6 Weeks

- Begin gentle strengthening exercises.

8 Weeks

- Encourage light to moderate activity.
- The wrist and thumb static splint may be discontinued in the presence of a pain-free and stable joint.

3 Months

- Allow normal activity.

Discomfort frequently lasts for 6 months after surgery. The function and strength of the thumb will improve over a 6- to 12-month period.

Wrist Disorders

Scaphoid Fractures

S. Brent Brotzman, MD, Steven J. Meyers, MD, and Michael L. Lee, MD

Background

The scaphoid (carpal navicular) is the most commonly fractured of the carpal bones and is often difficult to diagnose and treat. Complications include nonunion and malunion, which alter wrist kinematics and can lead to pain, decreased ROM, decrease in strength, and early radiocarpal arthrosis.

The **scaphoid blood supply is precarious.** The radial artery branches enter the scaphoid on the dorsum, distal third, and lateral-volar surfaces. The **proximal third** of the scaphoid receives its blood supply from interosseous- only circulation in about one third of scaphoids, and thus is **at high risk of avascular necrosis (AVN).**

Scaphoid fractures usually are **classified by location of fracture: proximal third, middle third (or waist), distal third, or tuberosity** (Fig. 1–44). Fractures of the middle third are most common, and distal third fractures are very rare.

Clinical History and Examination

Scaphoid fractures usually occur with hyperextension and radial flexion of the wrist, most often in young active male patients. Patients usually have **tenderness in the anatomic snuffbox** (Fig. 1–45) (between the first and the third dorsal compartments), less commonly on the distal scaphoid tuberosity volarly, and

may have increased pain with axial compression of the thumb metacarpal. *Scaphoid* is derived from the Greek word for boat, and it is often difficult to evaluate radiographically because of its oblique orientation in the wrist.

Initial radiographs should include posteroanterior (PA), oblique, lateral, and ulnar flexion PA. If there is any question clinically, an MRI is extremely sensitive in detecting scaphoid fractures as early as 2 days after injury.

Figure 1–44. A dorsal view of the scaphoid bone demonstrates various fracture orientations. Determining the orientation on radiographs is important because the orientation helps guide treatment decisions. (From Gutierrez G: Office management of scaphoid fractures. Physician Sports Med 24[8]:60, 1996).

Figure 1–45. Evaluation of scaphoid fractures. *A,* Scaphoid tenderness can be identified by palpation dorsally within the anatomic snuffbox. *B,* Tenderness may also be identified palmarly at the scaphoid tuberosity radial to the flexor carpi radialis tendon and the proximal wrist crease (the wrist should be extended). (From Zabinski SJ: Investigating carpal injuries. Sports Med Update, 1999.)

If an MRI is unavailable, patients with snuffbox tenderness should be immobilized for 10 to 14 days and then return for repeat radiographs out of the splint. If the diagnosis is still questionable, a bone scan is indicated.

Assessment of scaphoid fracture displacement is crucial for treatment and is often best assessed with **thin section** (1-mm) CT scans (Fig. 1–46). Displacement is defined as a fracture gap of more than 1 mm,

Figure 1–46. CT of the scaphoid is easier to interpret if the images are obtained in planes defined by the long axis of the scaphoid. To achieve this, the patient lies prone on the table with the arm overhead. *A,* For sagittal plane images, the forearm is held pronated (palm down) and the hand lies flat on the table. The forearm crosses the gantry at an angle of approximately 45 degrees (roughly in line with the abducted thumb metacarpal). *B,* Scout images are obtained to confirm the appropriate orientation and ensure that the entire scaphoid is imaged. Sections are obtained at 1-mm intervals. *C,* Images obtained in the sagittal plane are best for measuring the intrascaphoid angle. *D,* For coronal plane images, the forearm is in neutral position. *E,* Scout images demonstrate alignment of the wrist through the gantry of the scanner. *F,* Interpretation of the images obtained in the coronal plane is straightforward. (From Ring D, Jupiter JB, Herndon JH: Acute fractures of the scaphoid. J Am Acad Orthop Surg 8[4]:225–231, 2000.)

Figure 1–47. *A,* Lateral radiograph shows the normal colinear relationship of the radius, lunate, capitate, and third metacarpal. With normal carpal alignment, the scapholunate angle is between 30 and 60 degrees (*B*) and the capitolunate angle is less than 30 degrees (*C*). Note that the scaphoid axis can be drawn through the center of the scaphoid, but it is also adequate and may be easier to draw a line along the inferior pole as shown in *C. D,* Dorsiflexion instability—dorsal intercalary segment instability (DISI)—is suspected when dorsal tilting of the lunate and volar tilting of the scaphoid are present with a resulting increase in the scapholunate angle to more than 60 degrees. *E,* Palmar flexion instability—volar intercalary segment instability (VISI)—is suspected with volar tilting of the lunate, resulting in a scapholunate angle of less than 30 degrees and/or a capitolunate angle of more than 30 degrees. *F,* DISI parameters for radioscaphoid, radiolunate, and scapholunate angles. (*A,* From Honing EW: Wrist injuries. Part 2: Spotting and treating troublemakers. Physician Sports Med 26[10]:62, 1996; *B–E,* from Mann FA, Gilula LA: Posttraumatic wrist pain and instability: a radiographic approach to diagnosis. In Lichtman DM, Alexander AH [eds]: The Wrist and Its Disorders, 2nd ed. Philadelphia, WB Saunders, 1997, p. 105; *F,* from Regional Review Course in Hand Surgery. Rosemont, Illinois, American Society for Surgery of the Hand, 1991, p. 12–21.)

Figure continues

a lateral scapholunate angle greater than 60 degrees (Fig. 1–47), lateral radiolunate angle greater than 15 degrees, or intrascaphoid angle greater than 35 degrees.

Treatment

- Truly nondisplaced fractures can be treated closed and nearly always heal with thumb spica cast immobilization.
- Above- or below-elbow casting is still the subject of controversy. The authors prefer 6 weeks of sugar tong (long arm) thumb spica casting, followed by a minimum of 6 weeks of short arm thumb spica casting.

- Scaphoid union is verified with thin-section CT scan.
- **Surgical treatment is indicated for** nondisplaced fractures in which the complications of prolonged immobilization (wrist stiffness, thenar atrophy, and delayed return to heavy labor or sports) would be intolerable, scaphoid fractures previously unrecognized or untreated, all displaced scaphoid fractures (see above for criteria for displacement), and scaphoid nonunions.
- For nondisplaced fractures, percutaneous fixation with cannulated screws has recently become accepted treatment.
- For fractures with displacement, ORIF is mandatory.

RADIO-SCAPHOID ANGLE

47°   >60°

A   B

NORMAL   DORSI FLEXION INSTABILITY

RADIO-LUNATE ANGLE

>15°

A   B

NORMAL   DORSI FLEXION INSTABILITY

SCAPHO-LUNATE ANGLE

47°   >75°

A   B

NORMAL   DORSI FLEXION INSTABILITY

F

Figure 1–47. *Continued*

Rehabilitation Protocol
Treatment and Rehabilitation for Scaphoid Fractures

For Fractures Treated Closed (Nonoperative), Treatment in Thumb Spica Cast

0–6 Weeks
- Sugar-tong thumb spica cast
- Active shoulder ROM
- Active second through fifth MCP/PIP/DIP joint ROM

6–12 Weeks (Bony Union)
- Nontender to palpation, painless ROM with cast off
- Short arm thumb spica cast
- Continue shoulder and finger exercises
- Begin active elbow flexion/extension/supination/pronation

12 Weeks
- CT scan to confirm union. If ununited, continue short arm thumb spica cast (Fig. 1–48)

Figure 1–48. Thumb spica cast. (From Zabinski JJ: Investigating carpal tunnel. Sports Med Update, 1999.)

12–14 Weeks
- Assuming union at 12 weeks, removable thumb spica splint
- Begin home exercise program
    - Active/gentle-assisted wrist flexion/extension ROM
    - Active/gentle-assisted wrist radial/ulnar flexion ROM
    - Active/gentle-assisted thumb MCP/IP joint ROM
    - Active/gentle-assisted thenar cone exercise

14–18 Weeks
- Discontinue all splinting
- Formalized occupational therapy
    - Active/aggressive-assisted wrist flexion/extension ROM
    - Active/aggressive-assisted wrist radial/ulnar flexion ROM
    - Active/aggressive-assisted thumb MCP/IP joint ROM
    - Active/aggressive-assisted thenar cone exercise

18 Weeks +
- Grip strengthening, aggressive ROM
- Unrestricted activities

For Scaphoid Fractures Treated with ORIF

0–10 Days
- Elevate sugar-tong thumb spica splint, ice
- Shoulder ROM
- MCP/PIP/DIP joint active ROM exercises

10 Days–4 Weeks
- Suture removal
- Sugar-tong thumb spica cast (immobilizing elbow)
- Continue hand/shoulder ROM

4–8 Weeks
- Short arm thumb spica cast
- Elbow active/assisted extension, flexion/supination/pronation; continue fingers 2 through 5 active ROM and shoulder active ROM

8 Weeks
- CT scan to verify union of fracture

8–10 Weeks (Assuming Union) (Fig. 1–49)
- Removable thumb spica splint
- Begin home exercise program
    - Active/gentle-assisted wrist flexion and extension ROM
    - Active/gentle-assisted wrist radial/ulnar flexion ROM
    - Active/gentle-assisted thumb MCP/IP joint ROM
    - Active/gentle-assisted thenar cone exercise

Figure 1–49. CT scan identified union without avascular necrosis or loss of anatomic reduction. (From Zabinski JJ: Investigating carpal tunnel. Sports Med Update, 1999.)

10–14 Weeks
- Discontinue all splinting
- Formalized occupational therapy
    - Active/aggressive-assisted wrist flexion/extension ROM

Rehabilitation Protocol
Treatment and Rehabilitation for Scaphoid Fractures *(Continued)*

- Active/aggressive-assisted wrist radial/ulnar flexion ROM
- Active/aggressive-assisted thumb MCP/IP joint ROM
- Active/aggressive-assisted thenar cone exercise

14 Weeks +
- Grip strengthening
- Aggressive ROM
- Unrestricted activities

Fracture of the Distal Radius

David Ring, MD, Gae Burchill, OT, Donna Ryan Callamaro, OT, Jesse B. Jupiter, MD

Background

Successful treatment of a fracture of the distal radius must respect the soft tissues while restoring anatomic alignment of the bones (Fig. 1–50). The surgeon must choose a treatment method that maintains bony alignment without relying on tight casts or restricting the gliding structures that control the hand. **MCP joint motion must remain free. The wrist should not be distracted or placed in a flexed position,** because these abnormal positions diminish the mechanical advantage of the extrinsic tendons, increase pressure in the carpal canal, exacerbate carpal ligament injury, and contribute to stiffness. Recognition and prompt treatment of median nerve dysfunction and the avoidance of injury to branches of the radial sensory nerve are also important. **Special attention should be given to limiting swelling of the hand. Swelling can contribute to stiffness and even contracture of the intrinsic muscles of the hand.** Mobilization and functional use of the hand, wrist, and forearm complete the rehabilitation of the fractured wrist.

The keys to successful treatment of distal radial fractures include restoration of articular congruity, radial length, proper volar inclination, avoidance of stiffness, and early motion of a stable construct.

Clinical Background

Fractures of the distal radius are common in older persons, particularly women, because they have weaker bones and are more susceptible to falls. Older persons are healthier, more active, and more numerous than ever, and treatment decisions cannot be based upon patient age alone, but must consider the possibility of poor bone quality.

Considerable energy is required to fracture the distal radius of a younger adult, and most such fractures occur in motor vehicle accidents, falls from heights, or sports. Displaced fractures in younger adults are more likely to be associated with concomitant carpal fractures and ligament injuries, acute compartment syndrome, and multitrauma. ***The distal end of the radius has two important functions: it is both the primary support of the carpus and part of the forearm articulation.*** When a fracture of the distal radius heals with malalignment, the surface pressures on the articular cartilage may be elevated and uneven, the carpus may become malaligned, the ulna may impact with the carpus, or the distal radioulnar joint (DRUJ) may be incongruent. These conditions can produce pain, loss of motion, and arthrosis.

The alignment of the distal radius is monitored using radiographic measurements to define alignment in three planes. Shortening of the distal radius is measured best as the offset between the ulnar head and the lunate facet of the distal radius on the PA view—**the ulnar variance.** The alignment of the distal radius in the sagittal plane is evaluated by measuring the inclination of the distal radial articular surface on the PA radiograph—**the ulnar inclination.** The alignment of the distal radius in the coronal plane is evaluated by measuring the inclination of the distal radial articular surface on the lateral radiograph. Studies of normal volunteers have determined that the articular surface of the distal radius is usually oriented about 11 degrees palmar and 22 degrees ulnar, and has neutral ulnar variance.

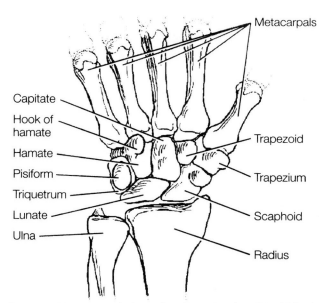

Figure 1–50. Bones of the wrist. (From Honing EW: Wrist injuries. Part 2: Spotting and treating troublemakers. Physician Sports Med 26[10]:62, 1998.)

-2 to +2mm

Figure 1–51. Impaction (loss of length). *A,* Normal radius is usually level with or within 1 to 2 mm distal or proximal to the distal ulnar articular surface. *B,* With a Colles fracture, significant loss of radial length causes loss of congruency with the distal radioulnar joint. (From Newport ML: Colles fractures. J Musculoskel Med 17[1]:292, 2000. Artist: Charles H. Boyter.)

Impaction of Distal Radius (Loss of Radial Length)

This involves the loss of radial length or height. Normally, the radial articular surface is level with or within 1 to 2 mm distal (ulnar positive) or proximal (ulnar negative) to the distal ulnar articular surface (Fig. 1–51). Colles fractures tend to lose significant height, which causes loss of congruency with the distal radioulnar joint (DRUJ) and difficulties with wrist rotation.

Dorsal Angulation (Loss of Volar Inclination)

Normally, the distal radius has a volar inclination of 11 degrees on the lateral view (Fig. 1–52). A Colles fracture often reverses that volar inclination. Dorsal inclination of **20 degrees or more** significantly affects the congruency of the DRUJ and may cause compensatory changes in the carpal bone alignment.

Dorsal Displacement

Dorsal displacement contributes significantly to the increased instability of the distal fragment by decreasing the contact area between fragments (Fig. 1–53).

Radial Displacement (Lateral Displacement)

Radial displacement occurs when the distal radial fragment displaces away from the ulna (Fig. 1–54).

Loss of Radial Inclination

The radius normally has a radial-to-ulnar inclination of approximately 22 degrees, measured from the tip of the radial styloid to the ulnar corner of the radius and compared with the longitudinal line along the length of the radius (Fig. 1–55). Loss of inclination can cause hand weakness and fatigability following the fracture.

Unrecognized supination of the distal radial fragment also creates fracture instability (Fig. 1–56).

Classification

Successful treatment of fractures of the distal radius requires accurate identification of certain injury characteristics and an understanding of their importance (Table 1–8). Whereas a number of classification systems have been described, most of the important injury elements are captured in the **system of Fernandez** (Fig. 1–57), **which**

90°

11 - 12°

Dorsal

Volar

Figure 1–52. Dorsal angulation. *A,* In the normal radius, volar inclination averages 11 degrees. *B,* Colles fracture can reverse inclination. Dorsal inclination of 20 degrees or more significantly affects congruency of the distal radioulnar joint and may alter carpal alignment. (From Newport ML: Colles fracture. J Musculoskel Med 17[1]:292, 2000. Artist: Charles H. Boyter.)

Figure 1–53. Dorsal displacement in Colles fracture contributes to instability of the distal fragment. (From Newport ML: Colles fracture. J Musculoskel Med 17[1]:296, 2000. Artist: Charles H. Boyter.)

distinguishes bending fractures (type 1), shearing fractures (type 2), compression fractures (type 3), fracture-dislocations (type 4), and high-energy fractures combining multiple types (type 5). **Type 1,** or bending-type fractures, are extra-articular, metaphyseal fractures. Dorsally displaced fractures are commonly referred to by the eponym *Colles fracture.* Volarly displaced bending fractures are often called *Smith's fractures.* **Type 2,** or articular shearing fractures, comprise volar and dorsal Barton's fractures, shearing fracture of the radial styloid (the so-called chauffeur's fracture), and shearing fractures of the lunate facet. **Type 3,** or compression fractures, include fractures that split the articular surface of the distal radius. There is a progression of injury with greater injury force—separation of the scaphoid and lunate facets occuring first, with progression to coronal splitting of the lunate or scaphoid facets and then further fragmentation. **Type 4,** radiocarpal fracture-dislocations, feature dislocation of the radiocarpal joint with small ligamentous avulsion fractures. **Type 5** fractures may combine features of all the other types and may also involve forearm compartment syndrome, open wound, or associated injury to the carpus, forearm, or elbow.

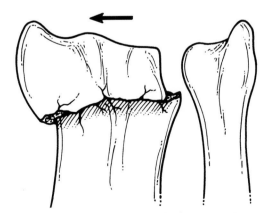

Figure 1–54. Radial (or lateral) displacement. In a displaced Colles fracture, it is possible for the distal fragment to slide away from the ulna. (From Newport ML: Colles fracture. J Musculoskel Med 17[1]:294, 2000. Artist: Charles H. Boyter.)

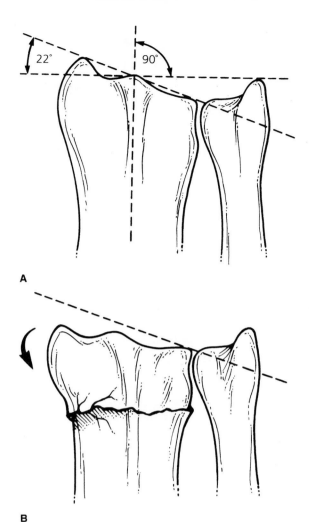

Figure 1–55. Loss of radial inclination. *A,* In a normal radius, the radial-to-ulnar inclination averages 22 degrees as measured from tip of the radial styloid to the ulnar corner of the radius compared with a vertical line along the midline of the radius. *B,* With a Colles fracture, radial inclination is lost because of imbalances in force on the radial versus the ulnar side of the wrist. (From Newport ML: Colles fracture. J Musculoskel Med 17[1]:296, 2000. Artist: Charles H. Boyter.)

Another classification used by orthopaedic surgeons is the universal classification system (Fig. 1–58).

Diagnosis and Treatment

The wrist often appears deformed with the hand dorsally displaced. This is called a "silver fork" deformity because of the semblance to a dinner fork when viewed from the side. The distal ulna also may be prominent. The wrist is swollen and tender, and palpation may elicit crepitus.

Patients with substantially displaced fractures should have rapid closed manipulation under anesthesia to reduce pressure on the soft tissues including nerves and skin and to help define the pattern of injury. Closed manipulation and sugar-tong splints provide definitive treatment in many patients. This is most often accomplished

Figure 1–56. Supination of the distal fragment of a Colles fracture creates instability. Supination deformity is usually not visible on a radiograph and is best appreciated during open reduction of the fracture. (From Newport ML: Colles fracture. J Musculoskel Med 17[1]:298, 2000. Artist: Charles H. Boyter.)

with a so-called hematoma block anesthetic. Five to 10 ml of 1% lidocaine anesthetic without epinephrine is injected into the fracture site. Consideration should be given to injecting the DRUJ and an ulnar styloid fracture in some patients. Injection of the fracture site is easiest from the volar-radial aspect of the wrist in the more common dorsally displaced fractures. Manipulation is performed manually. The use of finger traps is cumbersome, limits the surgeon's ability to correct all three dimensions of the deformity, and will not help to maintain length in metaphyseal impaction or fragmentation.

Radiographs taken after closed reduction may need to be supplemented by CT scanning to precisely define the pattern of injury. In particular, it can be difficult to tell whether the lunate facet of the distal radial articular surface is split in the coronal plane.

Bending fractures are extra-articular (metaphyseal) fractures. They may displace in either a dorsal or a volar direction. Dorsal displacement—known eponymically as **Colles** fracture—is much more common. Many dorsally displaced bending fractures can be held reduced in a cast or splint. **In older patients, more than 20 degrees of dorsal angulation of the distal radial articular surface on a lateral radiograph taken before manipulative reduction usually indicates substantial fragmentation and impaction of dorsal metaphyseal bone. Many such fractures require operative fixation to maintain reduction.** Dorsally displaced fractures are reduced under hematoma block and splinted with either a sugar-tong or a Charnley type of splint. The reduction maneuver consists of traction, flexion, ulnar deviation, and pronation. **The wrist should be splinted in an ulnar deviated position, but without wrist flexion.** Circumferential casts and tight wraps should not be used (Fig. 1–59). **Great care must be taken to ensure that motion of the MCP joints is not restricted.**

Options for the treatment of **unstable dorsal bending fractures** include external fixation that crosses the wrist, so-called nonbridging external fixation that gains hold of the distal fracture fragment and does not cross the wrist, percutaneous Kirschner wire fixation, and internal plate fixation. External fixation that crosses the wrist should be used with great care. **The wrist should not be left in a flexed position, and there should be no distraction across the wrist.** Usually, this means that Kirschner wires are needed in combination with the external fixator.

Table 1–8

Treatment-Based Classification of Distal Radius Fractures

Type	Description	Management
I	Undisplaced, extra-articular	Splinting or casting with the wrist in a neutral position for 4–6 wk. The splint chosen depends on the patient and his or her condition and compliance, as well as on physician preference.
II	Displaced, extra-articular	Fracture reduced under local or regional anesthesia
A	Stable	Splint, then cast
B	Unstable, reducible*	Remanipulation, with possible percutaneous pinning for improved stability
C	Unreducible	Open reduction and internal fixation
III	Intra-articular, undisplaced	Immobilization and possible percutaneous pinning for stability
IV	Intra-articular, displaced	
A	Stable, reducible	Adjunctive fixation with percutaneous pinning and, sometimes, external fixation
B	Unstable, reducible	Percutaneous pinning and, probably, external fixation to improve rigidity and immobilization. Dorsal comminution contribute to instability, so bone graft may be necessary.
C	Unreducible	Open reduction and internal fixation, often external fixation
D	Complex, significant soft tissue injury, carpal injury, distal ulnar fracture, or comminuted metaphyseal-diaphyseal area of the radius	Open reduction and pin or plate fixation, often supplemented with external fixation

*Instability becomes evident when radiographs show a change in position of the fracture fragments. Patients should be seen at 3, 10, and 21 days after injury to check for any change in fracture position.
From Cooney WP: Fractures of the distal radius: a modern treatment-based classification. Orthop Clin North Am 24(2):211, 1993.

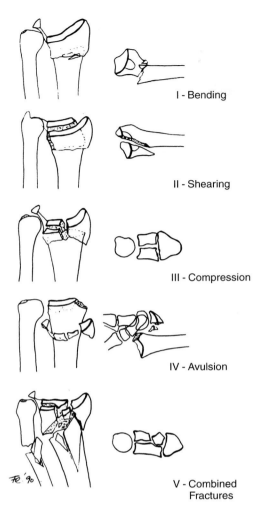

Figure 1–57. Classification of distal radius fractures based on the mechanism of injury (Fernandez): bending (I), shearing (II), compression (III), avulsion (IV), and combined (V) mechanisms. This classification is useful because the mechanism of injury influences the management of injury. (From Fernandez DL: Fractures of the distal radius: operative treatment. In Heckman JD [ed]: Instructional Course Lectures 42. Rosemont, III, American Academy of Orthopaedic Surgeons, 1993, pp. 74–75.)

Plate fixation is usually reserved for fractures with incipient callus formation that are resistant to closed manipulation (this can occur as early as 2 weeks after injury) and fractures with fragmentation of the volar as well as the dorsal metaphysis. All of these methods place the radial sensory nerve at risk. Great care must be taken to protect this nerve and its branches.

Volarly displaced bending fractures (or **Smith's fractures**) are subclassified as *transverse, oblique,* or *fragmented.* Oblique and fragmented fractures will not be stable in a cast and require operative fixation. Fixation of the distal radius with a plate applied to its volar surface is straightforward and associated with few problems. Therefore, unstable volar bending fractures are best treated with internal plate fixation.

Shearing fractures may involve the volar or dorsal articular margin (so-called **Barton's fractures**), the radial styloid, or the lunate facet of the distal radius. These partial articular fractures are inherently unstable. Failure to securely realign the fragment risks subluxation of the carpus. For this reason, shearing fractures are most predictably treated with open reduction and plate and screw fixation.

Many simple **compression articular fractures** can be treated with closed manipulation, external fixation, and percutaneous Kirschner wire fixation. When the lunate facet is split in the coronal plane, the volar lunate facet fragment is usually unstable and can be held only by a plate or tension band wire applied through a small volar-ulnar incision.

Radiocarpal fracture-dislocations and high-energy fractures require ORIF, in some cases supplemented by external fixation. One must also be extra vigilant regarding the potential for forearm compartment syndrome and acute CTS with these fractures.

Figure 1–58. Universal classification of distal radial fractures. *A,* Type I, nonarticular, undisplaced. *B,* Type II, nonarticular, displaced. *C,* Type III, intra-articular, undisplaced. *D,* Type IV, intra-articular, displaced. (From Cooney WP, Agee JM, Hastings H, et al: Symposium: management of intra-articular fractures of the distal radius. Contemp Orthop 21:71–104, 1990.)

Figure 1–59. *A,* Sugar-tong splint is made from approximately 10 thicknesses of 4-inch-wide plaster. Four layers of cast padding are used over the splint on the skin side. The splint goes from the palm, reaches around the elbow, and ends on the dorsum of the hand. The fingers are free to actively exercise. *B,* MCP joints must not be restricted. (*A,* From Newport ML: Colles fractures. J Musculoskel Med 17[1]:300, 2000. Artist: Charles H. Boyter; *B,* from Ring *D,* Jupiter JB: Managing fractures of the distal radius. J Musculoskel Med 12[10]:66, 1995. Artist: Robert Marguiles.)

For all of these fracture types, the stability of the DRUJ should be evaluated after the distal radius has been fixed. Instability of the distal ulna merits treatment of the ulnar side of the wrist. A large ulnar styloid fracture contains the origin of the triangular fibrocartilage complex (TFCC), and ORIF of such a fragment will restore stability. Similarly, unstable ulnar head and neck fractures may benefit from internal fixation. If the DRUJ is unstable in the absence of ulnar fracture, the radius should be pinned or casted in midsupination (45 degrees supination) for 4 to 6 weeks to enhance stability of the DRUJ.

Indications for operative treatment of distal radial fractures include an unstable fracture, irreducible fracture, more than 20 degrees of dorsal angulation of the distal fragment, intra-articular displacement or incongruity of 2 mm or more of articular (joint) fragments, and radial (lateral) displacement (Table 1–9).

Rehabilitation after Distal Radial Fractures

The rehabilitation after fracture of the distal radius is nearly uniform among various fracture types, provided that the pattern of injury has been identified and appropriately treated. The stages of rehabilitation can be divided into early, middle, and late.

Text continued on page 67

Rehabilitation Protocol
After Distal Radial Fracture
Ring, Jupiter, Burchill, and Calamaro

Early Phase (0–6 Weeks)

The critical part of the early phase of rehabilitation is limitation of swelling and stiffness in the hand.

- Swelling can be limited and reduced by encouraging elevation of the hand above the level of the heart, by encouraging frequent active mobilization, and by wrapping the digits and hand with self-adhesive elastic tapes (e.g., Coban, 3M, St. Paul, Minn), and applying a compressive stocking to the hand and wrist (Fig. 1–60).

- Stiffness can be limited by teaching the patient an aggressive program of active and passive digit ROM exercises (Fig. 1–61).
- The use of an external fixator as a splint to protect percutaneous or internal fixation is useful to avoid the use of restrictive circumferential dressings in the early postoperative period.
- Stable fractures and fractures with internal fixation can be supported with a light, removable thermoplastic

Rehabilitation Protocol
After Distal Radial Fracture *(Continued)*
Ring, Jupiter, Burchill, and Calamaro

Figure 1–60. Compressive dressings can help eliminate swelling of the fingers, hand, and wrist. *A,* Self-adhesive elastic tape should be applied by rolling the tape out and laying it on, applying a safe and limited amount of compression. *B,* Hand and wrist are compressed by an elastic stocking.

splint. We use a Corpus wrist splint, which is a well-padded thermoplastic brace that comes "off the shelf" but is custom moldable to each patient.
- A well-padded sugar-tong is used initially for stable, nonoperatively treated distal radial fractures. Eventually the elbow is "freed" from the sugar-tong (to avoid elbow stiffness) when the fracture looks sticky (approximately 3–4 weeks).

Another critical part of the early rehabilitation phase is functional use of the hand. Many of these patients are older and have a diminished capacity to adapt to their wrist injury.

- Appropriate treatment should be sufficiently stable to allow functional use of the hand for light activities (i.e., <5 pounds of force).
- When the hand is used to assist with daily activities such as dressing, feeding, and toileting, it will be more quickly incorporated back into the patient's physical role and may be less prone to becoming dystrophic.
- Functional use also helps restore mobility and reduce swelling.
- Most fractures are stable with forearm rotation. Supination, in particular, can be very difficult to regain after fracture of the distal radius. Initiation of active and gentle assisted forearm rotation exercises in the early phase of rehabilitation may speed and enhance the recovery of supination (Fig. 1–62).
- Some methods of treatment (e.g., nonbridging external fixation and plate fixation) offer the potential to initiate wrist flexion/extension and radial/ulnar deviation during the early phase of healing. Provided that fixation of the fragments is secure, we usually allow wrist mobilization at the time of suture removal (10–14 days after the operation) (Fig. 1–63).
- Scar massage may help limit adhesions in the area of incisions. In some patients with raised or hypertrophic scars, we recommend Otoform (Dreve-Otoplastik GMBH, Unna, Germany) application to help flatten and diminish the scar (Fig. 1–64).
- Active motion of the ipsilateral shoulder and elbow are used to avoid a frozen shoulder or elbow throughout the postoperative rehabilitation.

Middle Phase (6–8 Weeks)
- Once early healing of the fracture is established (between 6 and 8 weeks after the injury or operation), the pins and external fixation can be removed and the patient weaned from external support.
- Radiographs should guide this transition because some very fragmented fractures may require support for longer than 8 weeks.
- Active-assisted forearm and wrist mobilization exercises are used to maximize mobility (see Figs. 1–65 and 1–66). *There is no role for passive manipulation in the rehabilitation of fractures of the distal radius.*
- Dynamic splinting may help to improve motion. In particular, if supination is slow to return, a dynamic supination splint can be used intermittently (Fig. 1–65).

Late Phase (8–12 Weeks)
- Once healing is well established (between 6 and 12 weeks from the injury or operation), strengthening exercises can be initiated while active-assisted mobilization is continued.

continued

Rehabilitation Protocol
After Distal Radial Fracture *(Continued)*
Ring, Jupiter, Burchill, and Calamaro

Figure 1–61. Restoration of digit mobility in the first and most important element of rehabilitation after fracture of the distal radius. Varied exercises are done by the patient. *A,* Mobilization of the MCP joints. *B,* Hook fist to mobilize the IP joints. *C,* Opposition of each finger to the thumb. *D,* Tight fist posture, to hook fist, to straight. *E,* Digit abduction and adduction.

• The wrist and hand have been rested for a number of months from the time of the injury and will benefit from focused strengthening exercises, including digit strength-ening with Theraputty (Smith and Nephew, Memphis, Tennessee) (Fig. 1–66), the use of small weights (Fig. 1–67), and the use of various machines (Fig. 1–68).

Rehabilitation Protocol
After Distal Radial Fracture (Continued)
Ring, Jupiter, Burchill, and Calamaro

Figure 1–62. Forearm ROM is part of the early phase of rehabilitation of most distal radial fractures. *A,* Active forearm ROM is done with the elbow stabilized at the side to avoid "cheating" by moving the shoulder instead. *B,* Gentle assistive stretch can be provided by either the other hand or using the weight of a mallet grasped in the hand. *C,* Mallet can be used assist pronation.

continued

Rehabilitation Protocol
After Distal Radial Fracture (*Continued*)
Ring, Jupiter, Burchill, and Calamaro

Figure 1–63. *A,* Wrist mobilization is usually delayed for 6 to 8 weeks, but it can be begun as early as the second week when stable plate fixation is obtained. *B,* Gravity-assisted wrist flexion—hanging the hand off a towel. *C,* Wrist extension exercises. *D,* Radial and ulnar deviation. *E,* Wrist and ulnar deviation.

Rehabilitation Protocol
After Distal Radial Fracture *(Continued)*
Ring, Jupiter, Burchill, and Calamaro

Figure 1–64. Conforming plastics can be applied with pressure (such as under a Coban wrap) to help diminish the prominence of the scar.

Figure 1–65. Supination splint provides a constant stretching force that is useful when stiffness is resistant to simple active-assisted exercises.

A   B

Figure 1–66. Digit strengthening can be accomplished by exercises incorporating the manipulation of putty. Separate exercises emphasize manipulation with the fingertips (*A*) and in the clenched fist (*B*).

continued

Rehabilitation Protocol
After Distal Radial Fracture (Continued)
Ring, Jupiter, Burchill, and Calamaro

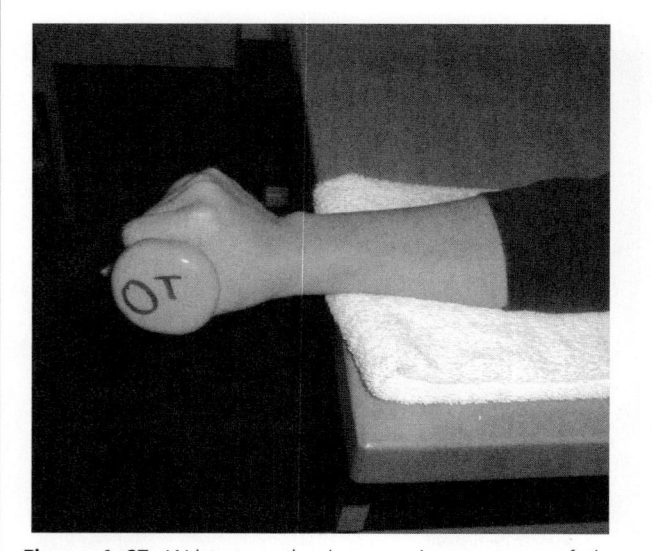

Figure 1–67. Wrist-strengthening exercises are part of the final phase of rehabilitation. Small weights can be used.

Figure 1–68. More sophisticated machines, such as this one made by Baltimore Therapeutic Equipment (Baltimore, Md), can provide more controlled and quantifiable methods of strengthening.

Table 1–9

Palmar Treatment Algorithm for Distal Radius Fractures

Fracture Type	Treatment Protocol	
	Group 1 (physiologically young and/or active)	Group 2 (physiologically old and/or inactive)
Nondisplaced fracture	STS—3 wk SAC—3 wk Splint (R)—3 wk	STS—2 wk SAC—2 wk Splint (R)—3 wk
Displaced fracture	Closed reduction X-ray findings	Closed reduction 1. STS—2 wk 2. SAC—3 wk Splint (R)—3 wk 3. Late-distal ulna resection

Acceptable reduction ⟶ / Unacceptable reduction
(> 2 mm radial shortening)
(> 2 mm displacement of articular fragment)
(> 15° dorsiflexion of radius)

Stable fracture
STS—3 wk
LAC—3 wk
Splint (R)—3 wk

Unstable fracture
1. External fixation with supplemental percutaneous pins
   Ex. fix—6 wk
   Pins—8 wk
   Splint (R)—3 wk
2. ORIF (plate)
   SAS—10 days
   Splint (R)—5 wk
3. Percutaneous pins
   STS—3 wk
   SAC—3 wk
   Pins—6 wk
   Splint (R)—3 wk

1. External fixation with fragment elevation (pins optional) and iliac crest bone graft—5 wk

2. ORIF (K-wire) with iliac crest bone graft
   Ex. fix—6 wk
   Pins—6 wk
   SAS—6 wk
   Splint (R)—4 wk

Table 1–9 (Continued)

Palmar Treatment Algorithm for Distal Radius Fractures

Ex., external; LAC, long arm cast; ORIF, open reduction and internal fixation; R, removable; SAC, short arm cast; SAS, short arm splint; STS, sugar-tong splint. From Palmar AK: Fractures of the distal radius. In Green D (ed): Operative Hand Surgery, 3rd ed. New York, Churchill Livingstone, 1993. Our protocol of the treatment of nondisplaced and displaced distal radial fractures in the physiologically young and/or active (group 1) and the physiologically old and/or inactive (group 2). Nondisplaced fractures are easily treated with immobilization alone in both groups. Displaced fractures require reduction in both groups, but only in group 1 do we recommend further treatment. Based on the reduction and whether the fracture is stable or not, immobilization is recommended with or without operative treatment. Fractures in which the reduction is unacceptable require reduction of the fragments with external fixation and/or internal fixation and bone grafting.

Conclusions

Rehabilitation after fracture of the distal radius focuses first on preventing a problem with the wrist from creating a problem with the hand; second, on restoring functional mobility quickly; and finally, on optimizing the function of the wrist after injury. Any method of treatment that contributes to excessive swelling or restriction of digit motion or tendon gliding should be abandoned. For instance, if a cast that is molded tightly to maintain fracture reduction increases edema, the surgeon should consider changing to percutaneous pinning and external fixation to avoid a constrictive dressing. Once effective treatment is administered, the rehabilitation program is straightforward. ■

Triangular Fibrocartilage Complex Injury

Dan C. Byck, MD, Felix H. Savoie III, MD, and Larry D. Field, MD

Clinical Background

The triangular fibrocartilage complex (TFCC) is an arrangement of several structures. **The primary structure is the triangular fibrocartilage or meniscal disc that is a relatively avascular disc-like structure that provides a cushion effect between the distal articular surface of the ulna and the proximal carpal row, primarily the triquetrum.** Much like the menisci in the knee, vascular studies have demonstrated poor central vascularity, whereas the peripheral 15 to 20% has the arterial inflow required for healing. In addition, there is no vascular contribution from the radial base of the TFCC. **Thus, central defects or tears tend to have difficulty healing and more peripheral injuries heal at a much higher rate.**

The disc is a biconcave structure with a radial attachment that blends with the articular cartilage of the radius. The ulnar attachment lies at the base of the ulnar styloid. There are superficial and deep layers of the TFCC, which attach separately at the base of the ulna styloid (Fig. 1–69). The anterior and posterior thickenings of the TFCC are confluent with the anterior and posterior radioulnar capsule and are called the *palmar* and *dorsal radioulnar ligaments*. These structures develop tension as the forearm is pronated and supinated and provide the primary stabilization to the DRUJ (Fig. 1–70). The TFCC itself is under maximal tension in neutral rotation. Additional attachments to the lunate, triquetrum, hamate, and the base of the fifth metacarpal have been de-

Figure 1–69. Scaphoid (S) and lunate (L) articulate with the distal articular surface of the radius, and the ulnar head articulates with the sigmoid notch. The triangular fibrocartilage complex (TFCC) is interposed between the ulnar carpus and the ulnar head.

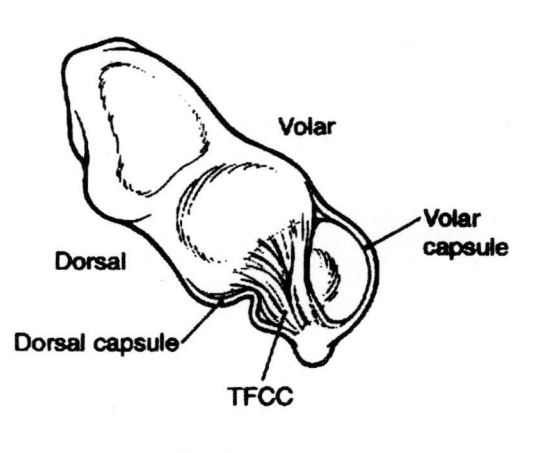

Figure 1–70. *A,* Right wrist in pronation. The dorsal capsule is tight, and the volar margin of the triangular fibrocartilage complex (TFCC; the volar radioulnar ligament) is tight. *B,* Right wrist in supination. The volar distal radioulnar joint capsule is tight, and the dorsal margin of the TFCC (dorsal radioulnar ligament) is tight as the dorsal margin of the radius moves farther away from the base of the ulnar styloid.

Differential Diagnosis of Ulnar-sided Wrist Pain

Radial shortening (e.g., comminuted distal
    radial fracture)

TFCC tear (central versus peripheral)

Degenerative joint disease

Lunotriquetral arthritis

Extensor carpi ulnaris (ECU) instability or tendinitis

Fracture of the hook of the hamate

Flexor carpi ulnaris (FCU) calcific tendinitis

Pisotriquetral arthritis

Ulnar artery stenosis

Guyon's canal syndrome

Ulnar styloid fracture

Congenital positive ulnar variance

Ulnar nerve disease

---

scribed. These structures, combined with the extensor carpi ulnaris subsheath, make up the TFCC. Normal function of the DRUJ requires the normal relationship of these anatomic structures. Tear, injury, or degeneration of any one structure leads to pathophysiology of the DRUJ and abnormal kinesis of the wrist and forearm. When evaluating **ulnar-sided wrist pain** or painful forearm rotation, several entities should be considered.

Classification

The most widely accepted classification system of TFCC injuries is that developed by Palmer (1989). **TFCC tears are divided into two categories: traumatic**

and degenerative. The system uses clinical, radiographic, anatomic, and biomechanical data to define each tear. Rehabilitation of these lesions is based on the type of procedure performed. In **Class 1A or 2A lesions,** the central portion of the disc is débrided, and in this case, the rehabilitation is a return to activities as tolerated after wound healing has taken place. For most other TFCC lesions, a more extensive immobilization period followed by aggressive physical therapy is required.

Classification of Triangular Fibrocartilage Complex Lesions (Palmer)

Class 1: Traumatic

  A. Central perforation
  B. Ulnar avulsion
     With ulnar styloid fracture
     Without ulnar styloid fracture
  C. Distal avulsion
  D. Radial avulsion
     With sigmoid notch fracture
     Without sigmoid notch fracture

Class 2: Degenerative (Ulnocarpal Abutment Syndrome)

  A. TFCC wear
  B. TFCC wear
     With lunate or ulnar chondromalacia
  C. TFCC perforation
     With lunate or ulnar chondromalacia
  D. TFCC perforation
     With lunate or ulnar chondromalacia
     With lunotriquetral ligament perforation
  E. TFCC perforation
     With lunate or ulnar chondromalacia
     With lunotriquetral ligament perforation
     With ulnocarpal arthritis

Diagnosis

A thorough history is critical to the diagnosis of TFCC lesions. Factors such as onset and duration of symptoms, type and force of trauma, eliciting activities, recent changes in symptoms, and past treatment attempts should be noted. Most TFCC injuries are caused by a fall on an outstretched hand, rotational injuries, or repetitive axial loading. *Patients complain of ulnar-sided wrist pain and clicking and often crepitation with forearm rotation, gripping, or ulnar deviation of the wrist.* Tenderness often is present on either the dorsal or the palmar side of the TFCC. Instability of the DRUJ or clicking may or may not be elicited. Care should be taken to rule out ECU tendon subluxation and radial-sided wrist injuries as well.

Provocative maneuvers are often helpful in differentiating TFCC injuries from lunotriquetral pathology. First, however, the pisotriquetral joint should be tested to rule out disease at this joint. With the wrist in neutral rotation, the triquetrum is firmly compressed against the lunate. The **"shuck test"** described by Reagan and coworkers (1984) is a more sensitive test of the lunotriquetral joint. The lunotriquetral joint is grasped between the thumb and the index finger while the wrist is stabilized with the other hand and the lunotriquetral joint is "shucked" in a dorsal-to-palmar direction. Kleinman and Graham (1996) suggested that the most sensitive test to elicit lunotriquetral pathology is the **shear test.** In this test, one thumb is placed against the pisiform and the other thumb stabilizes the lunate on its dorsal surface. As the examiner's thumbs are forced toward the carpus, a shear force is created in the lunotriquetral joint. Lester and colleagues (1995) described a **press test** to diagnose TFCC tears. They did not differentiate the region of the tear, but stated that the test was 100% sensitive for tears. In the press test, the patient grasps both sides of a chair seat while sitting in the chair. The patient then presses the body weight directly upward, and if the pain replicates the ulnar-sided pain, the test is considered positive.

Once a normal lunotriquetral joint is established, the TFCC is then evaluated. The **TFCC grind test** is very sensitive in eliciting tears in the TFCC and DRUJ instability. With the wrist in neutral rotation and ulnarly deviated, it is then rolled palmarly then dorsally. Pain or a click suggests a TFCC tear. When done with the forearm fully pronated, the dorsal radioulnar ligaments are tested. With the forearm fully supinated, the volar radioulnar ligaments are assessed.

The **piano key test** evaluates DRUJ stability. With the forearm fully pronated, the distal ulna is balloted from dorsal to volar. This test correlates with the "piano key sign" seen on lateral wrist radiographs.

Diagnostic Studies

Radiographs of the wrist include PA, lateral, and oblique views taken with the shoulder abducted to 90 degrees, the elbow flexed to 90 degrees, and the forearm flat on the table. *When indicated, specialty views such as a supination-pronation, a clenched-fist PA, and a 30-degree supination view to assess the pisotriquetral joint may be obtained.*

Arthrography may be used as a confirmatory test. Radiopaque contrast material is injected directly into the radiocarpal joint. If a tear is present, the dye will extravasate into the region of the tear. More recent reports suggest that three-compartment (radiocarpal, DRUJ, and midcarpal) injections are a more accurate method of assessing TFCC lesions. Care must be taken when interpreting wrist arthrograms because a high occurrence of false-negative readings has been reported. Asymptomatic TFCC, interosseous ligament tears, and details of the exact tear location may also appear on wrist arthrography, although adjacent soft tissue structures or articular surfaces are not well delineated.

MRI of the wrist has evolved into a useful resource in diagnosing TFCC lesions. Although an experienced radiologist is imperative, the coils and techniques are now approaching arthroscopy in sensitivity and predictive value of TFCC tears. *Potter and associates (1997) reported that MRI had a sensitivity of 100%, specificity of 90%, and accuracy of 97% in 57 wrists with arthroscopically verified TFCC lesions.* The advantage of MRI over arthrography lies in the ability to identify the location of the lesion. Potter and associates reported sensitivity of 100%, specificity of 75%, and accuracy of 92% in locating the structure injured. Gadolinium MRI arthrograms are no longer necessary to produce significant results.

The "gold standard" in diagnosing wrist injuries is arthroscopy. No other technique is as accurate or reliable in locating the lesion. In addition, arthroscopy allows the surgeon to palpate and observe every structure in the wrist, making it easier to treat all possible components of the injury. Arthroscopy also avoids the complications associated with open wrist surgery and allows a speedier rehabilitation after immobilization.

Treatment

Surgical intervention for TFCC injuries is indicated only after a full course of nonoperative measures.

Initially, the wrist is **braced** for 4 to 6 weeks. NSAIDs are used and occasionally a **corticosteroid injection** may be beneficial. After **immobilization, physical therapy** is initiated. First, active-assisted and passive ROM exercises are begun. Then, aggressive motion exercises and resisted strengthening rehabilitation are added, followed by plyometric and sports-specific therapy. Most patients with TFCC tears respond well to bracing and therapy.

If nonoperative care fails and symptoms persist, surgery is indicated. In athletes, surgery may be done earlier because of competitive and seasonal considerations. Although a controversial issue, delaying surgical treatment of TFCC tears may adversely affect the outcome.

Surgical intervention is predicated on the type of TFCC tear. Treatment of some tears remains controversial, whereas treatment of others is more widely accepted.

For **type 1A** tears, débridement of the central tear is usually preferred if there is no DRUJ instability. Up to two thirds of the central disc can be removed without significantly altering the biomechanics of the wrist. Care must be taken to avoid violating the volar or dorsal radioulnar ligaments to prevent DRUJ instability.

Type 1B tears affect the periphery of the TFCC. This is recognized by the loss of the "trampoline" effect of the central disc. Repairs of these tears usually heal because of the adequate blood supply.

Type 1D tears fall in the controversial category. Traditional treatment has been débridement of the tear, followed by early motion. Several authors, however, have reported improved results with surgical repair of these tears. In our clinic, repair of radial-sided tears to the sigmoid notch of the radius is preferred.

Type 2 tears are degenerative by definition and often occur in athletes who stress their wrists (gymnastics, throwing and racquet sports, wheelchair sports). Nonoperative treatment should be continued for at least 3 months before arthroscopy. Most of these lesions are in patients with an ulna neutral or positive wrist. In these patients, débridement of the central degenerative disc tear is followed by an extra-articular ulnar shortening procedure such as the wafer procedure.

Rehabilitation Protocol
After TFCC Débridement
Byrk, Savoie, and Field

The protocol initially focuses on tissue healing and early immobilization. **When TFCC *repair* is performed, the wrist is immobilized for 6–8 weeks and forearm pronation/supination is prevented for the same period of time with the use of a Münster cast.**

Phase 1: 0–7 Days

- Soft dressing to encourage wound healing and decrease soft tissue edema.

Phase 2: 7 Days–Variable

- ROM exercises are encouraged.
- Return to normal activities as tolerated.

Phase 3: When Pain Free

- Resisted strengthening exercises, plyometrics and sports-specific rehabilitation (see later).

Rehabilitation Protocol
After Repair of TFCC Tear (with or without Lunotriquetral Pinning)
Byrk, Savoie, and Field

Phase 1

0–7 Days

- The immediate postoperative period focuses on decreasing the soft tissue edema and the joint effusion. Maintaining an immobilized wrist and elbow is important, and a combination of ice or cold therapy and elevation are desired. The upper extremity is placed in a sling.
- Finger flexion/extension exercises are initiated to prevent possible tenodesis and decrease soft tissue edema.

- Active-assisted and passive shoulder ROM exercises are instituted to prevent loss of motion in the glenohumeral joint. These are performed at home.

7 Days–2 Weeks

- During the first office visit, the sutures are removed and a Münster cast is applied. Once again, the wrist is completely immobilized and elbow flexion/extension is encouraged.
- Hand and shoulder ROM exercises are continued.
- Sling is removed.

Rehabilitation Protocol
After Repair of TFCC Tear (with or without Lunotriquetral Pinning) *(Continued)*
Byrk, Savoie, and Field

Phase 2

4–8 Weeks

- The Münster cast is removed and a removable Münster cast is applied. Elbow flexion and extension are continued, but forearm rotation is avoided.
- Gentle wrist flexion/extension exercises are initiated.
- Progression to a squeeze ball is begun.
- Hand and shoulder exercises are continued.

Phase 3

8 Weeks

- The Münster cast is removed and a neutral wrist splint is used as needed.
- Lunotriquetral wires are removed in the office.

3 Months

- Progressive active and passive ROM exercises are instituted in the six planes of wrist motion (see section on distal radial fractures).
- Once pain-free ROM exercises are accomplished, strengthening exercises are begun.
  1. Weighted wrist curls in six planes of wrist motion using small dumbbells or elastic tubing. This includes the volar, dorsal, ulnar, radial, pronation, and supination directions. Once strength returns, the Cybex machine may be used to further develop pronation-supination strength.
  2. Four-way diagonal upper extremity patterns utilizing dumbbells, cable weights, or elastic tubing.
  3. Flexor-pronator forearm exercises. Wrist begins in extension, supination, and radial deviation, and utilizing a dumbbell as resistance, the wrist is brought into flexion, pronation, and ulnar deviation.
  4. Resisted finger extension/flexion exercise with hand grips and elastic tubing.
  5. Upper extremity plyometrics are instituted. Once wall-falling/push-off is accomplished (see 6A, below), weighted medicine ball exercises are begun. Initially, a one-pound ball is used; then the weight of the ball is progressed as indicated.
  6. The plyometric exercises are tailored to the patient's activity interests. If the patient is an athlete, sports-specific exercises are added.

    Wall-falling in which a patient stands 3–4 feet from a wall. Patient falls into the wall, catching on hands, and rebounds to starting position.
    Medicine ball throw in which a medicine ball is grasped with both hands in overhead position. Ball is thrown to a partner or trampoline. On return, the ball is taken into the overhead position.
    Medicine ball throw in which a medicine ball is grasped with both hands in chest position.
    Ball is push-passed to a partner or trampoline. On return, the ball is taken into the chest position.
    Medicine ball throw in which a medicine ball is push-passed off a wall and rebounded in the chest position.
    Medicine ball throw in which the ball is grasped in one hand in the diagonal position and thrown to a partner or trampoline. Rebound is taken in the diagonal position over the shoulder. This may be performed across body or with both hands.
    Medicine ball throw in which the patient is lying supine with upper extremity unsupported abducted to 90 degrees and externally rotated to 90 degrees. A medicine ball weighing 8 ounces–2 pounds is dropped by a partner from a height of 2–3 feet. When the ball is caught, it is returned to partner in a throwing motion as rapidly as possible.
    Medicine ball push-up with wrist in palmar flexion, dorsiflexion, radial deviation, and ulna deviation. This may be performed with the knees on the ground to begin with and progress to weight on toes as strength returns.
- Sports-specific exercises are designed to emulate the biomechanical activity encountered during play. With overhead and throwing athletes, the following program should be instituted:
  - Initially, ROM exercises establish pain-free motion. All aforementioned exercises are instituted and developed.
  - Weighted baton is used to re-create the motion of throwing, shooting, or racquet sport. This is progressed to elastic resistance. Ball-free batting practice is likewise begun.
  - Finally, actual throwing, shooting, or overhead racquet activities are begun.
  - Contact athletes, such as football linemen, will begin bench presses and bench flies. Initially, the bars are unweighted. Painless weight progression and repetition progression as tolerated is performed.
- Work-hardening tasks such as using a wrench and pliers to tighten nuts and bolts. A screwdriver may be used to tighten/loosen screws.

Phase 4

3 Months

- Minimum time for splint-free return to sports.

De Quervain's Tenosynovitis

S. Brent Brotzman, MD, Steven J. Meyers, MD, and Kyle Phillips, PA

Background

This disorder is the most common overuse injury involving the wrist and often occurs in individuals who regularly use a forceful grasp coupled with ulnar deviation of the wrist (such as in a tennis serve).

Injury occurs because of inflammation around the tendon sheath of the abductor pollicis longus (APL) and extensor pollicis brevis (EPB) in the **first dorsal compartment** (Fig. 1–71A). Pain and tenderness localized over the radial aspect of the wrist (over the first dorsal compartment) are the typical presenting symptoms.

Finklestein test is diagnostic for de Quervain's tenosynovitis (Fig. 1–71B). This test places stress on the APL and EPB by placing the thumb into the palm of a "fist," then ulnarly deviating the wrist. Mild de Quervain's may present with pain only on resisted thumb MCP joint extension.

The **other possible causes of pain in the "radial dorsal pain" category** include:

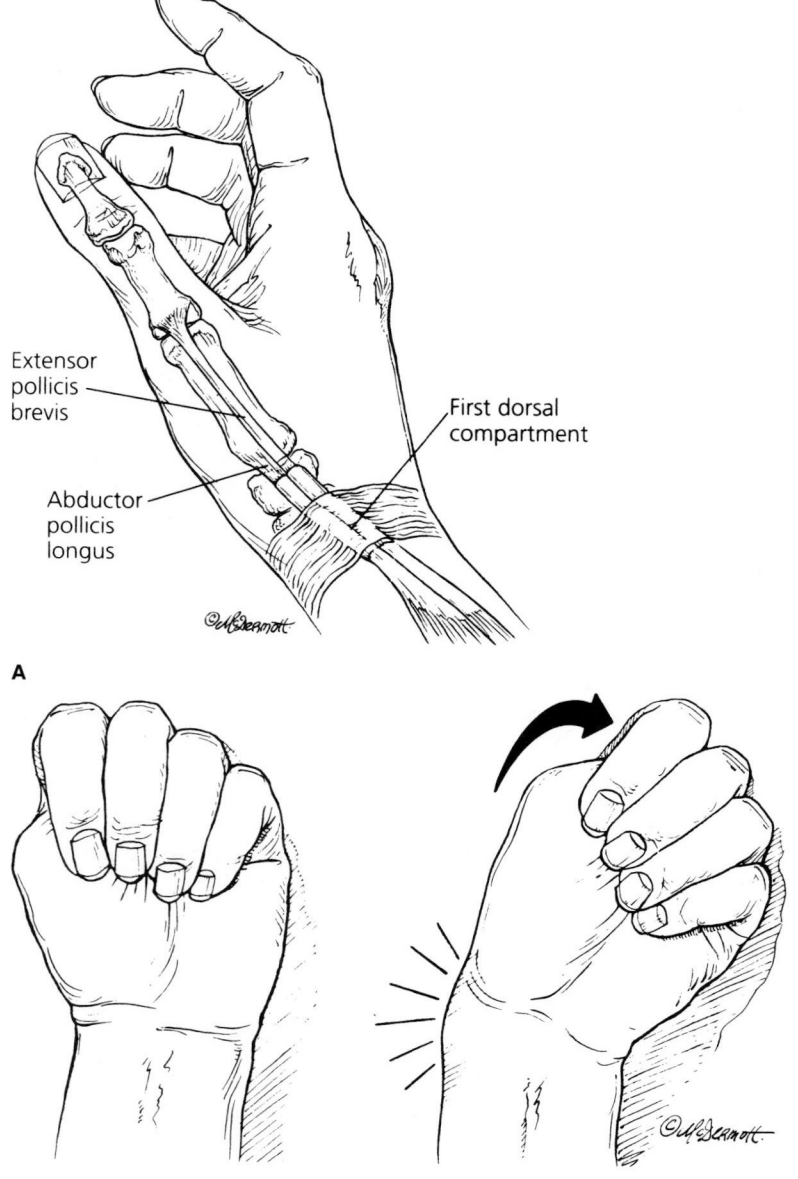

Extensor pollicis brevis

First dorsal compartment

Abductor pollicis longus

A

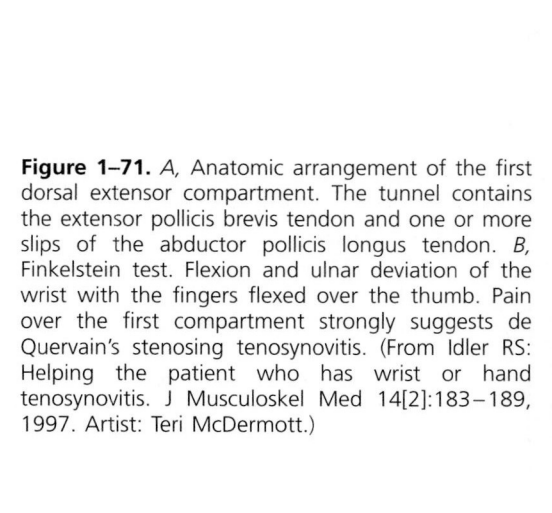

Figure 1–71. *A,* Anatomic arrangement of the first dorsal extensor compartment. The tunnel contains the extensor pollicis brevis tendon and one or more slips of the abductor pollicis longus tendon. *B,* Finkelstein test. Flexion and ulnar deviation of the wrist with the fingers flexed over the thumb. Pain over the first compartment strongly suggests de Quervain's stenosing tenosynovitis. (From Idler RS: Helping the patient who has wrist or hand tenosynovitis. J Musculoskel Med 14[2]:183–189, 1997. Artist: Teri McDermott.)

B

- CMC arthritis of the thumb—pain and crepitance are present with the thumb "crank and grind test." This test is done by applying axial pressure to the thumb while palpating the first CMC joint. (The crank and grind test is positive only with CMC arthritis of the thumb. Both de Quervain's and CMC arthritis may have a "positive" Finklesteins test and pain on thumb motion; however, the crank and grind test will be positive *only* in arthritis of the basal joint [CMC] of the thumb.)
- Scaphoid fracture—tender in the anatomic snuff box.
- Chauffeur's fracture—radial styloid fracture.
- Intersection syndrome—more proximal pain and tenderness (see later in this chapter).

Conservative Management

A thumb spica splint is used to immobilize the first dorsal compartment tendons with a commercially available splint or, depending on the patient's comfort, a custom-molded Orthoplast device. The splint maintains the wrist in 15 to 20 degrees of extension and the thumb in 30 degrees of radial and palmar abduction. The IP joint is left free, and motion at this joint is encouraged. The patient wears the splint during the day for the first 2 weeks and at night until the next office visit, generally at 6 to 8 weeks. Splinting may continue longer, depending on the response to treatment. The splint can be discontinued during the day if symptoms permit and if daily activities are gradually resumed. Workplace activities are advanced accordingly. Other considerations include:

- **A corticosteroid sheath injection** can be offered to patients with moderate to marked pain or with symptoms lasting more than 3 weeks. The injection should individually distend the APL and EPB sheaths. Discomfort after injection is variable, and

a 2- to 3-day supply of mild analgesic is recommended.
- A systemic **NSAID** is commonly prescribed for the initial 6 to 8 weeks of treatment.
- Thumb use is restricted so that the first dorsal compartment tendons are at relative rest. Activities that require prolonged thumb IP joint flexion, pinch, or repetitive motions are avoided.
- Distal-to-proximal thumb Coban wrapping, retrograde lotion, or ice massage over the radial styloid.
- Phonophoresis with 10% hydrocortisone can be used for edema control.
- Gentle active and passive thumb and wrist motion are encouraged 5 minutes every hour to prevent joint contracture and tendon adhesions.

Operative Management

Symptoms are often temporarily relieved and the patient elects to repeat the management outlined previously. Unsatisfactory symptom reduction or symptom persistence requires surgical decompression.

Multiple separate compartments for the APL (which typically has two to four slips) and the EPB require decompression. Extreme caution in the approach will spare sensory branches of the lateral antebrachial cutaneous nerve and dorsal sensory branches of the radial nerve. Before decompression, the encasing circular retinacular fibers that arc across the radial styloid should be exposed. The floor of this compartment is the tendinous insertion of the brachioradialis tendon, which sends limbs to the volar and dorsal margins of the compartment. The APL and EPB tendons may be difficult to differentiate, especially in the absence of septation. When this Y tendinous floor is identified, it can serve as a landmark to indicate decompression of the first dorsal compartment. ∎

Rehabilitation Protocol
After Decompression for de Quervain's Tenosynovitis

0–2 Days
- Leave the IP joint free and encourage motion as allowed by the soft tissue compressive surgical dressing.
- Remove the dressing 2 days after surgery.
- Begin gentle active motion of the wrist and thumb.

2–14 Days
- The presurgical splint is worn for comfort and motion exercises are continued.
- At the 10th–14th day, sutures are removed.
- Patients commonly complain of some hypersensitivity

and numbness at and distal to the incision site. Desensitization may be necessary. Digital massage of the area is usually sufficient, and the complaint almost always resolves.

1–6 Weeks
- Strengthening program is advanced and scar desensitization is continued as necessary.
- Unrestricted activity generally should not be allowed until about 6 weeks after surgery.

Intersection Syndrome of the Wrist

S. Brent Brotzman, MD

Background

Intersection syndrome is tendinitis or tenosynovitis of the first and second dorsal compartments of the wrist (Fig. 1–72). The muscle and tendons of these two compartments traverse each other at a 60-degree angle, three fingerbreadths proximal to the wrist joint on the dorsal aspect (several centimeters proximal to Lister's tubercle). This is *proximal* to the location of de Quervain's tenosynovitis.

This overuse syndrome most often occurs in rowing, skiing, racquet sports, canoeing, and weightlifting. In skiers, the mechanism of injury is repetitive dorsiflexion and radial deviation of the wrist as the skier withdraws the planted ski pole from resistance of deep snow. Weightlifters who overuse their radial extensors of the wrist and perform excessive curling get intersection syndrome.

Physical Examination

- Examination reveals point tenderness to palpation on the dorsum of the wrist, three fingerbreadths proximal to the wrist joint.
- Crepitation or "squeaking" may be noted with passive or active motion of the involved tendons, and swelling (tenosynovitis) may be visible along the two compartments.
- Pain is present on wrist flexion or extension (dorsally), rather than on radial and ulnar deviation as in de Quervain's tenosynovitis (e.g., Finklestein test is positive in de Quervain's; Table 1–10).

Prevention

Skiers should be instructed in proper powder skiing pole techniques, such as avoiding deep pole planting and pole dragging. Decreasing ski pole length by 2 inches and

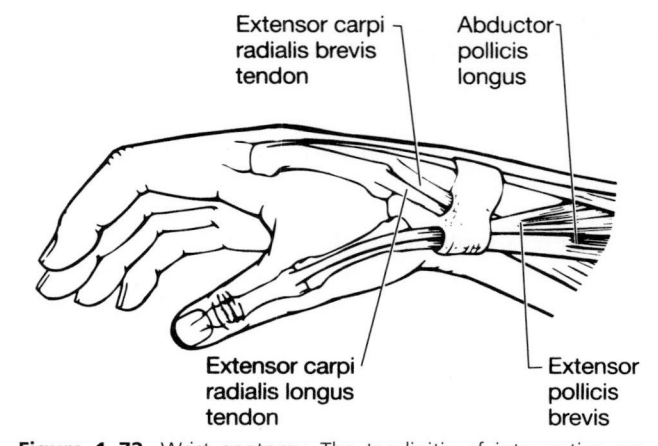

Figure 1–72. Wrist anatomy. The tendinitis of intersection syndrome occurs in the area shown. (From Servi JT: Wrist pain from overuse. Physician Sports Med 25[12]:41, 1997.)

decreasing the basket diameter to 2 inches may help prevent intersection syndrome.

Treatment

- Exacerbating activities (e.g., rowing) are avoided for several weeks.
- A removable commercial thumb spica splint (wrist in 15 degrees of extension) is used to immobilize and support the thumb for 3 to 6 weeks.
- Training modifications are made on resumption of activity (e.g., avoid excessive weight curling).
- Cryotherapy is used several times a day (ice massage with frozen water from a peeled-away Styrofoam cup).
- NSAIDs are given, and a corticosteroid injection of the compartment may be effective (avoid injection of the actual tendon).
- Gentle ROM exercises of the wrist and hand are begun, and wrist extensor strengthening is begun after the patient is asymptomatic for 2 to 3 weeks to avoid repetitive "overuse" of relatively "weak" musculotendinous units. ■

Rehabilitation Protocol
After Surgical Decompression of Intersection Syndrome

0–14 Days

- Keep the wrist in neutral position within the surgical plaster splint.
- Encourage digital, thumb, and elbow motion as comfort allows.
- Remove the sutures at 10–14 days after surgery.

2–4 Weeks

- Maintain the presurgical splint until the patient can perform the activities of daily living with little pain.
- Active and active-assisted wrist extension and flexion exercises should attain full preoperative values by 4 weeks after surgery.

4–6 Weeks

- Advance the strengthening program.
- Anticipate full activities at the end of the sixth week after surgery.
- Use the splint as needed.
- Scar desensitization techniques may be necessary, including the use of a transcutaneous electric nerve stimulation (TENS) unit if the scar region is still tender 6 weeks after surgery.

Table 1–10

Distinctive Clinical Findings in Common Forms of Tenosynovitis

Tenosynovitis	Findings	Differential Diagnosis
Intersection syndrome	Edema, swelling, and crepitation in the intersection area; pain over the **dorsum** of the wrist that is exacerbated by wrist flexion and extension, unlike the pain of de Quervain's tenosynovitis, which is exacerbated by radial and ulnar deviation; pain extends less radially than it does in de Quervain's tenosynovitis.	Wartenberg's syndrome, de Quervain's tenosynovitis
de Quervain's	Pain along the radial aspect of the wrist that worsens with radial and ulnar wrist deviation; pain on performing Finkelstein maneuver is pathognomonic	Arthritis of the first carpometacarpal joint; scaphoid fracture and nonunion; radiocarpal arthritis; Wartenberg's syndrome; intersection syndrome
Sixth dorsal compartment	Pain over the ulnar dorsum of the wrist that is worsened by ulnar deviation and wrist extension; other planes of motion may also be painful; tenderness over the sixth dorsal compartment; instability of the extensor carpi ulnaris is shown by having the patient circumduct the wrist while rotating the forearm from pronation to supination.	Extensor carpi ulnaris instability; triangular fibrocartilage complex tears; lunotriquetral ligament tears; ulnocarpal abutment syndrome; distal radioulnar joint arthritis; traumatic rupture of the subsheath that normally stabilizes this tendon to the distal ulna
Flexor carpi radialis tunnel syndrome	Pain, swelling, and erythema around the *palmar* radial aspect of the wrist at the flexor carpi radialis tunnel; pain exacerbated by resisted wrist flexion	Retinacular ganglion; scaphotrapezial arthritis, first carpometacarpal arthritis; scaphoid fracture/nonunion; radial carpal arthritis; injury to the palmar cutaneous branch of the median nerve; Lindberg's syndrome (tendon adhesions between the flexor pollicis longus and the flexor digitorum profundus)
Trigger finger	Pain on digital motion, with or without associated triggering or locking at the interphalangeal joint of the thumb or proximal interphalangeal joint of other fingers; may be crepitus or a nodular mass near the first annular pulley that moves with finger excursion.	Connective tissue disease; partial tendon laceration; retained foreign body; retinacular ganglion; infection; extensor tendon subluxation

From Idler RS: Helping the patient who has wrist or hand tenosynovitis. J Musculoskel Med 14(2):62, 1997.

Dorsal and Volar Carpal Ganglion Cysts

S. Brent Brotzman, MD, and Anna Williams, PT

Background

Dorsal carpal ganglion cysts rarely originate from sites other than near the scapholunate interval. These cysts may decompress into the EPL or common extensor tendon sheaths and may appear to arise from sites remote from their origin (Fig. 1–73).

A dorsal transverse incision in a Langer line over the scapholunate interval clearly exposes the pathology through a window bounded by the second and third dorsal compartments radially, the fourth compartment ulnarly, the dorsal intercarpal ligament distally, and the dorsal radiocarpal ligament proximally.

Volar carpal ganglion cysts originate from the flexor carpal radialis tendon sheath or from the articulations between the radius and the scaphoid, the scaphoid and the trapezium, or the scaphoid and the lunate. Excision of these cysts, as with dorsal carpal ganglion cysts, should include a generous capsulectomy at the site of the cyst origin.

Differential Diagnosis of Wrist Ganglia

Non-neoplastic Masses	Neoplastic Masses
Extraskeletal	Soft Tissue
Aneurysm/arteriovenous malformation	Benign tumor (chondroma, fibroma, giant cell tumor of tendon sheath, hemangioma, lipoma, neuroma)
Anomalous muscle and other anomalous structure	
Bursa	Malignant tumor (epithelioid sarcoma, malignant fibrous histiocytoma, metastasis, synovial sarcoma)
Displaced tendon	

continued

Differential Diagnosis of Wrist Ganglia (*Continued*)

Non-neoplastic Masses	Neoplastic Masses
Extraskeletal	**Soft Tissue**
Foreign body granulomas	Skeletal
Hypertrophic structure	Benign tumor (cyst, chondroma, giant cell tumor, collagen
Nerve entrapment	osteochondroma, osteoid osteoma)
Nerve ganglion	Malignant tumor (chondrosarcoma, metastasis, osteosarcoma)
Periarticular calcaneal	Infectious
Post-traumatic (neuroma, tendon remnant)	Fungus, mycobacteria, pyogen, tuberculosis
Repetitive use fibrosis	Disease/Metabolic
Scar	Rheumatoid arthritis and disease, rheumatoid nodule, synovial
Tendon entrapment	cyst, tenosynovitis
Tuberous sclerosis	Gout and pseudogout
Skeletal	Neuritis (PIN), vasculitis, amyloidosis
Arthritic residuum	
Pigmented villonodular synovitis	
Post-traumatic residuum: subluxed scaphoid	

From Kozin SH, Urban MA, Bishop AT, Dobyns JH: Wrist ganglia: diagnosis and treatment. J Musculo Med 10(1):21, 1993.

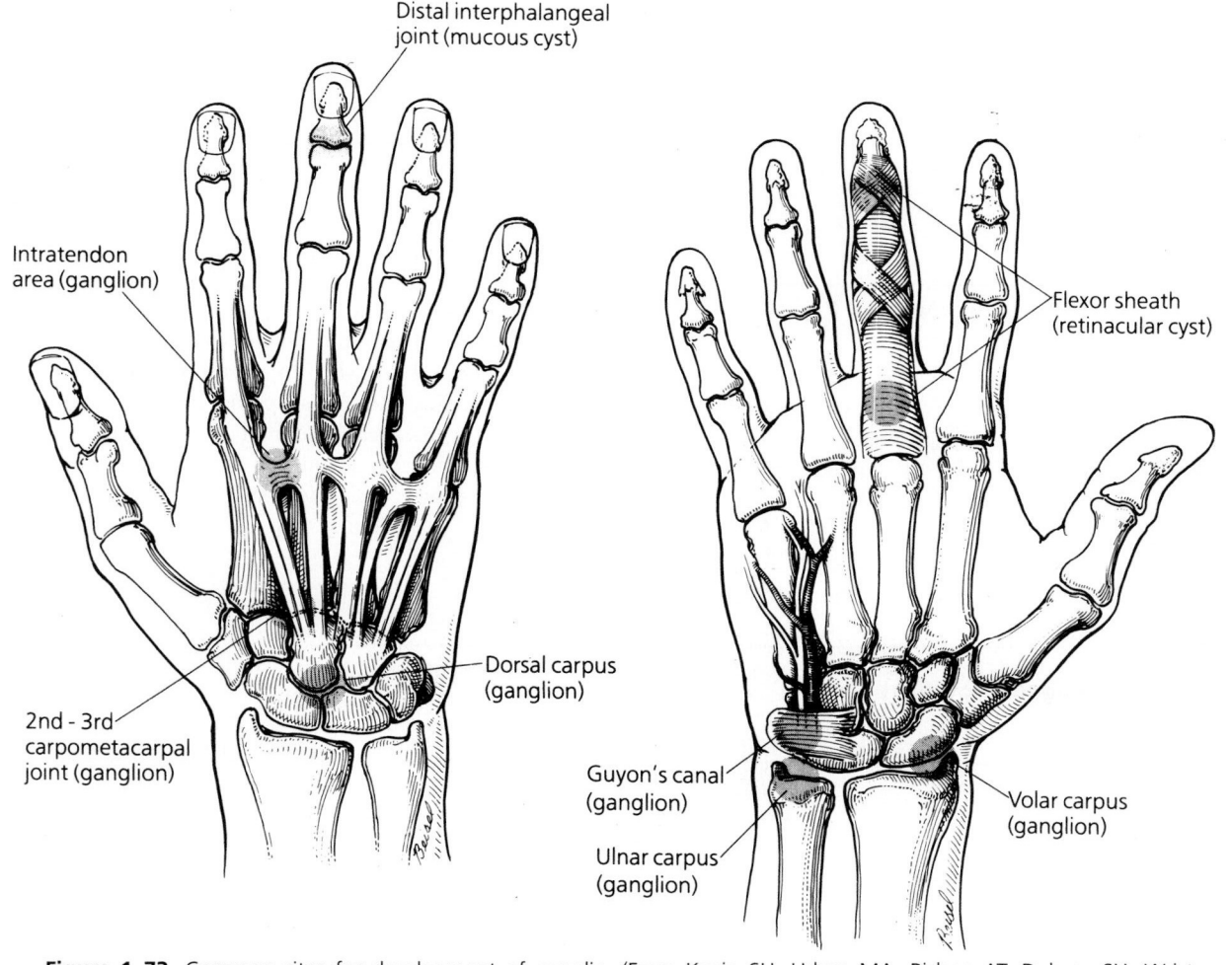

Figure 1–73. Common sites for development of ganglia. (From Kozin SH, Urban MA, Bishop AT, Dobyns SH: Wrist ganglia: diagnosis and treatment. J Musculoskel Med 10[1]:21, 1993. Artist: Dan Beisiel.)

Physical Examination (Fig. 1–74)

- Dorsal ganglion cysts are most visible with the wrist flexed.
- Palpation may produce mild discomfort, and provocation motion (extremes of wrist flexion and wrist extension) often increases pain.
- For volar wrist ganglion, differential diagnosis includes vascular lesions, and an Allen test should be performed for vascular patency.

Treatment

- Conservative treatment, which may include corticosteroid injection, is tried first.
- If symptoms persist, excision of the ganglion may be indicated.
- Postoperative resolution is usual for both volar and dorsal ganglia (more than 90% with ideal technique), but recurrence or even new formation of ganglion or pain is possible.

Rehabilitation Protocol
After Excision of Wrist Ganglion

2 Weeks

- Remove the short arm splint and sutures.
- Initiate active and active-assisted wrist extension and flexion.
- Continue interval splint wear during the day between exercises and at night.

2–4 Weeks

- Advance ROM exercises to resistive and gradual strengthening exercises.
- Discontinue the splint at 4 weeks.

4–6 Weeks

- Allow normal activities to tolerance.

6 Weeks

- Allow full activity.

Findings in Common Conditions of the Hand and Wrist

Degenerative Arthritis of the Fingers

- Heberden's nodes (most common).
- Bouchard's nodes (common).
- Mucous cysts (occasional).
- Decreased motion at involved IP joints.
- Instability of involved joints (occasional).

Basilar Joint Arthritis of the Thumb

- Swelling and tenderness of the basilar joint.
- Subluxation of the basilar joint (shuck test) (more severe cases).
- Reduced motion at the basilar joint (palmar abduction, opposition).
- Weakened opposition and grip strength.
- Abnormal compression grind test.
- Hyperextension of the first MCP joint (more severe cases).

Carpal Tunnel Syndrome

- Median nerve compression and Phalen test abnormal (most sensitive tests).
- Tinel sign over the median nerve (frequent).
- Abnormal sensation (two-point discrimination) in the median nerve distribution (more severe cases).
- Thenar eminence softened and atrophied (more severe cases).
- Weakened or absent thumb opposition (more severe cases).

continued

Findings in Common Conditions of the Hand and Wrist *(Continued)*

de Quervain's Stenosing Tenosynovitis

- Tenderness and swelling over the first dorsal compartment at the radial styloid.
- Finkelstein's test aggravates pain.

Ganglion

- Palpable mass (may be firm or soft).
- Most common locations: the volar hand at the web flexion crease of the digits or the transverse palmar crease, the dorsal wrist near the ECRL and ECRB tendons, the volar wrist near the radial artery.
- Mass transilluminates (larger ganglia).

Dupuytren's Disease

- Palpable nodules and pretendinous cords in palmar aponeurosis, most commonly affecting the ring or the little finger.
- Secondary flexion contracture of the MCP and, occasionally, PIP joints.

Rheumatoid Arthritis

- Boggy swelling of multiple joints (MCP joints and wrist joint most commonly involved).
- Boggy swelling of the tenosynovium of the extensor tendons over the dorsum of the wrist and the hand (common).
- Boggy swelling of the tenosynovium and the flexor tendons on the volar surface of the wrist (common).
- Secondary deformities in more severe cases, such as ulnar deviation of the MCP joints and swan-neck and boutonnière deformities.
- Secondary rupture of extensor or flexor tendons (variable).

Flexor Tendon Sheath Infection

- Cardinal signs of Kanavel present.
- Finger held in flexed position at rest.
- Swelling along the volar surface of the finger.
- Tenderness on the volar surface of the finger along the course of the flexor tendon sheath.
- Pain exacerbated by passive extension of the involved finger.

Injury to the Ulnar Collateral Ligament of the Metacarpophalangeal Joint of the Thumb (Skier's or gamekeeper's thumb)

- Swelling and tenderness over the ulnar aspect of the thumb MCP joint.
- Pain exacerbated by stress of the UCL.
- Increased laxity of the thumb UCL (more severe injuries)

Ulnar Nerve Entrapment at the Wrist

- Compression of the ulnar nerve at Guyon's canal reproduces symptoms (most sensitive test).
- Abnormal Tinel sign over Guyon's canal (variable).
- Weakness of intrinsic muscles (finger abduction or adduction) (most severe cases).
- Atrophy of the interossei and the hypothenar eminence (most severe cases).
- Abnormal sensation in the little finger and the ulnar aspect of the ring finger (variable).
- Abnormal Froment sign (variable).

Scapholunate Instability

- Swelling over the radial wrist. X-rays show increased scapholunate gap on clenched fist view (> 1 mm).
- Tenderness over the dorsal wrist over the scapholunate ligament.
- Scaphoid shift test produces abnormal popping and reproduces the patient's pain.

Mallet Finger

- Flexed or dropped posture of the finger at the DIP joint.
- History of jamming injury (impact of a thrown ball).
- Inability to actively extend or straighten the DIP joint.

Jersey Finger (FDP Avulsion)

- Mechanism is hyperextension stress applied to a flexed finger (e.g., grabbing a player's jersey).
- Patient lacks active flexion at the DIP joint (FDP function lost).
- Swollen finger often assumes a position of relative extension compared to the other more flexed fingers.

Modified from Reider B: The Orthopaedic Physical Examination, Philadelphia, WB Saunders, 1999.

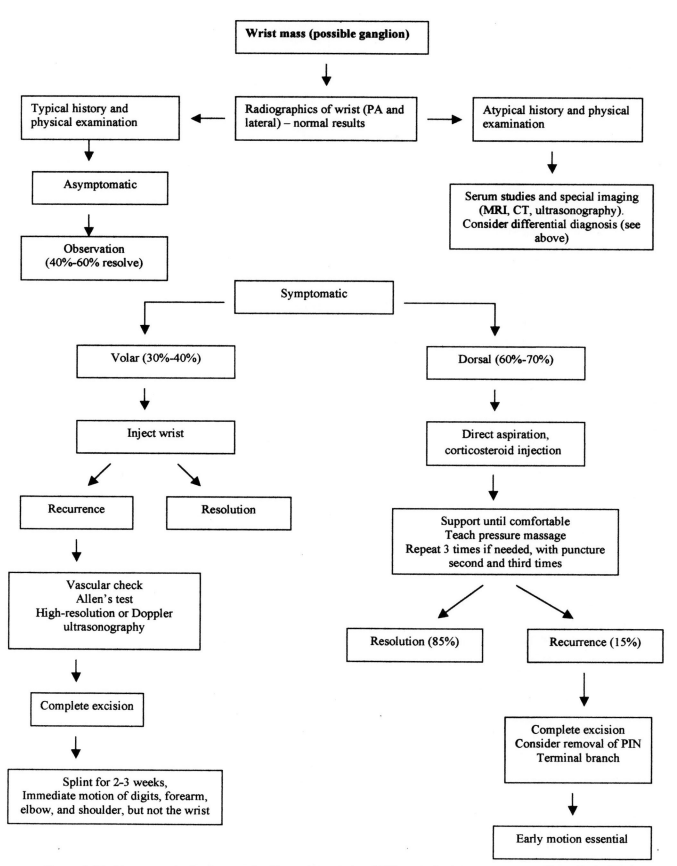

Figure 1–74. Management of wrist ganglia. PA, posteroanterior; POIN, posterior interosseus nerve. (From Kozin SH, Urban MA, Bishop AT, Dobyns SH: Wrist ganglia: diagnosis and treatment. J Musculoskel Med 10[1]:21, 1993.)

Bibliography—Chapter 1

Flexor Tendon Injuries

Trigger Digits

Boyes JH: Flexor tendon grafts in the fingers and thumb: an evaluation of end results. J Bone Joint Surg 32A:489, 1950.

Bunnell S: Surgery of the Hand, 3rd ed. Philadelphia, JB Lippincott, 1956.

Cannon NM: Diagnosis and Treatment Manual for Physicians and Therapists, 3rd ed. Indianapolis, The Hand Rehabilitation Center of Indiana, PC, 1991.

Creighton JJ, Idler RS, Strickland JW: Hand clinic, trigger finger and thumb. Indiana Med 83(4):260, 1990.

Dinham JM, Meggitt BF: Trigger thumbs in children: a review of the natural history and indications for treatment in 105 patients. J Bone Joint Surg 56B:153, 1974.

Duran RJ, Houser RG: Controlled passive motion following flexor tendon repair in zones 2 and 3. AAOS Symposium on Tendon Surgery in the Hand. St. Louis, Mosby–Year Book, 1975, pp 105–114.

Fahey JJ, Bollinger JA: Trigger finger in adults and children. J Bone Joint Surg 36A:1200, 1954.

Green D: Operative Hand Surgery, 3rd ed. New York, Churchill Livingstone, 1993.

Hunter JH: Rehabilitation of the Hand, 3rd ed. St. Louis, Mosby, 1992.

Idler RS: Anatomy and biomechanics of the digital flexor tendons. Hand Clin 1:3, 1985.

Leddy JP, Packer JW: Avulsion of the profundus tendon insertion in athletes. J Hand Surg 1:66, 1977.

Rhoades CE, Gelberman RH, Manjarris JF: Stenosing tenosynovitis of the fingers and thumbs. Clin Orthop 190:236, 1984.

Extensor Tendon Injuries

Mallet Finger

Abound JM, Brown H: The treatment of mallet finger: the results in a series of consecutive cases and a review of the literature. Br J Surg 9:653, 1968.

Bowers WH, Hurst LC: Chronic mallet finger: the use of Fowler's central slip release. J Hand Surg 3:373, 1978.

Doyle JR: Extensor tendons—acute injuries. In Green, D (ed): Operative Hand Surgery, 3rd ed. New York, Churchill Livingstone, 1993.

Fess EE, Gettle KS, Strickland JW: Hand Splinting Principles and Methods. St. Louis, Mosby, 1981.

Hillman FE: New technique for treatment of mallet fingers and fractures of the distal phalanx. JAMA 161:1135, 1956.

Iselin F, Levame J, Godoy J: A simplified technique for treating mallet fingers: tenodermodesis. J Hand Surg 2:118, 1977.

Kleinert HE, Verdan C: Report of the committee on tendon injuries. J Hand Surg 5(2):794, 1983.

Kleinman WB, Peterson DP: Oblique retinacular ligament reconstruction for chronic mallet finger deformity. J Hand Surg 9A:399, 1984.

McCoy FJ, Winsky AJ: Lumbrical loop for luxation of the extensor tendons of the hand. Plast Reconstr Surg 44(2):142, 1969.

Stark HH, Gainor BJ, Ashworth CR et al: Operative treatment of intraarticular fractures of the dorsal aspect of the distal phalanx of digits. J Bone Joint Surg 69A:892, 1987.

Stern PJ, Kastrup JJ: Complications and prognosis of treatment of mallet finger. J Hand Surg 13A:329, 1988.

Wehbe MA, Schneider LH: Mallet fractures. J Bone Joint Surg 66A:658, 1984.

Wood VE: Fractures of the hand in children. Orthop Clin North Am 7:527, 1976.

Fractures and Dislocations

Agee JM: Unstable fracture-dislocations of the proximal interphalangeal joint: treatment with the force couple splint. Clin Orthop 214:101, 1987.

Cannon NM: Diagnosis and Treatment Manual for Physicians and Therapists, 3rd ed. Indianapolis, The Hand Center of Indiana, 1991.

Crenshaw AH: Campbell's Operative Orthopaedics, 8th ed. St. Louis, Mosby, 1992.

Greene D: Operative Hand Surgery, 3rd ed. New York, Churchill Livingstone, 1993.

Hunter JM, et al: Rehabilitation of the Hand: Surgery and Therapy, 3rd ed. St. Louis, Mosby, 1990.

Jahss SA: Fractures of the metacarpals: a new method of reduction and immobilization. J Bone Joint Surg 20:278, 1938.

Jobe MT: Fractures and dislocations of the hand. In Gustilo RB, Kyle RK, Templeman D (eds): Fractures and Dislocations. St. Louis, Mosby, 1993.

Kaukonen JP, Porras M, Karaharju E: Anatomical results after distal forearm fractures. Ann Chir Gynaecol 77:21, 1988.

Knirk JL, Jupiter JB: Intra-articular fractures of the distal end of the radius in young adults. J Bone Joint Surg 63A:647, 1986.

Moberg E: Emergency Surgery of the Hand. Edinburgh, Churchill Livingstone, 1968.

Putnam MD: Fractures and dislocations of the carpus including the distal radius. In Gustillo RB, Kyle RF, Templeman D (eds): Fractures and Dislocations. St. Louis, Mosby, 1993.

Ryu J, Watson HK, Burgess RC: Rheumatoid wrist reconstruction utilizing a fibrous nonunion and radiocarpal arthrodesis. J Hand Surg 10A:830, 1985.

Schultz RJ, Brown V, Fox JM: Gamekeeper's thumb: results of skiing injuries. NY State J Med 73:2329, 1973.

Nerve Compression Syndromes

Carpal Tunnel Syndrome

Gellman H, Gelberman RH, Tan AM, Botte MJ: Carpal tunnel syndrome: an evaluation of provocative diagnostic tests. J Bone Joint Surg 5:735, 1986.

Green D: Operative Hand Surgery, 3rd ed. New York, Churchill Livingstone, 1993.

Szabo RM, Madison M: Carpal tunnel syndrome. Orthop Clin North Am 1:103, 1992.

Pronator Syndrome

Gainor BJ: The pronator compression test revisited. Orthop Rev 19:888, 1990.

Hartz CR, Linscheid RL, Gramse RR, Daube JR: The pronator teres syndrome; compressive neuropathy of the median nerve. J Bone Joint Surg 63(6):885, 1981.

Idler RS, Strickland JW, Creighton JJ: Pronator syndrome. Indianapolis Hand Clinic, Indiana Center for Surgery and Rehabilitation of the Hand and Upper Extremity.

Ulnar Tunnel Syndrome

Amadio PC, Beckenbaugh RD: Entrapment of the ulnar nerve by the deep flexor-pronator aponeurosis. J Hand Surg 11:83, 1986.

Dupont C: Ulnar-tunnel syndrome at the wrist. J Bone Joint Surg 47A:757, 1965.

Johnson RK, Spinner M, Shrewsbury MM: Median nerve entrapment syndrome in the proximal forearm. J Hand Surg 4:48, 1979.

Kleinert HE, Hayes JE: The ulnar tunnel syndrome. Plast Reconstr Surg 47:21, 1971.

Kleinman WB: Anterior intramuscular transposition of the ulnar nerve. J Hand Surg 14A:972, 1989.

Kuschner SH, Gelberman RH, Jennings C: Ulnar nerve compression at the wrist. J Hand Surg 13A:577, 1988.

Leffert RD: Anterior submuscular transposition of the ulnar nerves by the Learmonth technique. J Hand Surg 7:147, 1982.

Magassy CL, Ferris PJ: Ulnar tunnel syndrome. Orthop Rev 11:21, 1973.

Roles NC, Maudsley RH: Radial tunnel syndrome: resistant tennis elbow as a nerve entrapment. J Bone Joint Surg 54B:499, 1972.

Shea JD, McClain EJ: Ulnar nerve compression syndromes at and below the wrist. J Bone Joint Surg 51A:1095, 1969.

Szabo RM, Steinberg DR: Nerve entrapment syndromes of the wrist. J Am Acad Orthop Surg 3:115, 1994.

Radial Tunnel Syndrome

Lister GD, Belsole RB, Kleinert HE: The radial tunnel syndrome. J Hand Surg 4:52, 1979.

Spinner M: The arcade of Frohse and its relationship to posterior interosseous nerve paralysis. J Bone Joint Surg 50B:809, 1968.

Sponseller PD, Engber WD: Double-entrapment radial tunnel syndrome. J Hand Surg 8:420, 1983.

Nerve Injuries

Seddon PC, Sunderland D, Flores AJ, Lavernia CJ, Owens PW: Anatomy and physiology of peripheral nerve injury and repair. Am J Orthop 3:167, 2000.

Replantation

Entin MA: Crushing and avulsing injuries of the hand. Surg Clin North Am 44:1009, 1964.

Kleinder HE, Kasdan ML: Salvage of devascularized upper extremities, including studies on small vessel anastomosis. Clin Orthop 29:29, 1963.

Moberg E: The treatment of mutilating injuries of the upper limb. Surg Clin North Am 44:1107, 1964.

Arthroplasty

Finger Arthroplasty

Bieber EJ, Weiland AJ, Volenec-Dowling S: Silicone-rubber implant arthroplasty of the metacarpophalangeal joints for rheumatoid arthritis. J Bone Joint Surg 68A:206, 1986.

Blair WF, Shurr DG, Buckwalter JA: Metacarpophalangeal joint implant arthroplasty with a Silastic spacer. J Bone Joint Surg 66A:365, 1984.

Cannon NM: Diagnosis and Treatment Manual for Physicians and Therapists, 3rd ed. Indianapolis, The Hand Rehabilitation Center of Indiana, PC, 1991.

Eaton RG, Malerich MM: Volar plate arthroplasty of the proximal interphalangeal joint: a review of ten years' experience. J Hand Surg 5:260, 1980.

Swanson AB: Silastic HP 100 Swanson finger joint implant for metacarpophalangeal and proximal interphalangeal joint arthroplasty and Dow Corning Wright Swanson finger joint Grommet II for metacarpophalangeal implant arthroplasty. Grand Rapids, Dow Corning Wright, 1988.

Swanson AB: Flexible implant arthroplasty for arthritic finger joints. J Bone Joint Surg 54A:435, 1972.

Swanson AB, Leonard JB, deGroot Swanson G: Implant resection arthroplasty of the finger joints. Hand Clin 2:107, 1986.

Swanson AB, Maupin BK, Gajjar NV, Swanson GD: Flexible implant arthroplasty in the proximal interphalangeal joint of the hand. J Hand Surg 10A:796, 1985.

Thumb Carpometacarpal Joint Arthroplasty

Burton RI, Pellegrini VD: Surgical management of basal joint arthritis of the thumb. II. Ligament reconstruction with tendon interposition arthroplasty. J Hand Surg 11A:324, 1986.

Cannon NM: Diagnosis and Treatment Manual for Physicians and Therapists, 3rd ed. Indianapolis, The Hand Rehabilitation Center of Indiana, PC, 1991.

Creighton JJ, Steichen JB, Strickland JW: Long-term evaluation of Silastic trapezial arthroplasty in patients with osteoarthritis. J Hand Surg 16A:510, 1991.

Dell PC, Brushart TM, Smith RJ: Treatment of trapeziometacarpal arthritis: results of resection arthroplasty. J Hand Surg 3:243, 1978.

Eaton RG, Littler JW: Ligament reconstruction for the painful thumb carpometacarpal joint. J Bone Joint Surg 55A:1655, 1973.

Kleinman WB, Eckenrode JF: Tendon suspension sling arthroplasty for thumb trapeziometacarpal arthritis. J Hand Surg 16A:983, 1991.

Hofammann DY, Ferlic DC, Clayton ML: Arthroplasty of the basal joint of the thumb using a silicone prosthesis. J Bone Joint Surg 69A:993, 1987.

Pellegrini VD, Burton RI: Surgical management of basal joint arthritis of the thumb. I. Long-term results of silicone implant arthroplasty. J Hand Surg 11A:309, 1986.

Wrist and Distal Radioulnar Joint Disorders

Radius Fractures

Alffram PA, Bauer GCH: Epidemiology of fractures of the forearm: a biomechanical investigation of bone strength. J Bone Joint Surg 44A:158, 1962.

Anderson DD, Bell AL, Gaffney MB, Imbriglia JE: Contact stress distributions in malreduced intraarticular distal radius fractures. J Orthop Trauma 10:331, 1996.

Fernandez DL: Acute and chronic derangement of the distal radio-ulnar joint after fractures of the distal radius. EFORT J 1:41, 1999.

Fernandez DL: Fractures of the distal radius: operative treatment. Instr Course Lect 42:73, 1993.

Fernandez DL: Smith Frakturen. Z Unfallmed Berufskrankheiten 3:110, 1980.

Fernandez DL, Geissler WB: Treatment of displaced articular fractures of the radius. J Hand Surg 16A:375, 1991.

Fernandez DL, Jupiter JB: Fractures of the distal radius. A practical approach to management. New York, Springer-Verlag, 1995.

Friberg S, Lundstrom B: Radiographic measurements of the radiocarpal joint in normal adults. Acta Radiol Diagn 17:249, 1976.

Gartland JJ, Werley CW: Evaluation of healed Colles' fractures. J Bone Joint Surg 33A:895, 1951.

Gelberman RH, Szabo RM, Mortensen WW: Carpal tunnel pressures and wrist position in patients with Colles' fractures. J Trauma 24:747, 1984.

Kaempffe FA, Wheeler DR, Peimer CA, et al: Severe fractures of the distal radius: effect of amount and duration of external fixator distraction on outcome. J Hand Surg 18A:33, 1993.

Kozin SH: Early soft-tissue complications after fractures of the distal part of the radius. J Bone Joint Surg 75A:144, 1993.

Melone CP: Open treatment for displaced articular fractures of the distal radius. Clin Orthop 202:103, 1988.

Melone CP: Articular fractures of the distal radius. Orthop Clin North Am 15:217, 1984.

Newport ML: Colles fracture: managing a common upper extremity injury. J Musculoskel Med 17(1):292, 2000.

Pattee GA, Thompson GH: Anterior and posterior marginal fracture-dislocation of the distal radius. Clin Orthop 231:183, 1988.

Short WH, Palmer AK, Werner FW, Murphy DJ: A biomechanical study of distal radius fractures. J Hand Surg 12A:529, 1987.

Simpson NS, Jupiter JB: Delayed onset of forearm compartment syndrome: a complication of distal radius fracture in young adults. J Orthop Trauma 9:411, 1995.

Talesnick J, Watson HK: Midcarpal instability caused by malunited fractures of the distal radius. J Hand Surg 9A:350, 1984.

Trumble T, Glisson RR, Seaber AV, Urbaniak JR: Forearm force transmission after surgical treatment of distal radioulnar joint disorders. J Hand Surg 12A:196, 1987.

Viegas SF, Tencer AF, Cantrell J, et al: Load transfer characteristics of the wrist. Part II. Perilunate instability. J Hand Surg 12A:978, 1987.

Triangular Fibrocartilage Complex Tears

Adams BD: Partial excision of the triangular fibrocartilage complex articular disc: biomechanical study. J Hand Surg 18A:919, 1993.

Bednar M, Arnoczky S, Weiland A: The microvasculature of the triangular fibrocartilage complex: its clinical significance. J Hand Surg 16A:1101, 1991.

Bowers WH, Zelouf DS: Treatment of chronic disorders of the distal radioulnar joint. In Lichtman DM, Alexander AH (eds): The Wrist and Its Disorders, 2nd ed. Philadelphia, WB Saunders, 1997, pp 475–477.

Byrk FS, Savoie FH III, Field LD: The role of arthroscopy in the diagnosis and management of cartilaginous lesions of the wrist. Hand Clin 15(3):423, 1999.

Chidgey LK, Dell PC, Bittar ES, Spanier SS: Histologic anatomy of the triangular fibrocartilage complex. J Hand Surg 16A:1084, 1991.

Cooney WP, Linscheid RL, Dobyns JH: Triangular fibrocartilage tears. J Hand Surg 19A:143, 1994.

Corso SJ, Savoie FH, Geissler WB, et al: Arthroscopic repair of peripheral avulsions of the triangular fibrocartilage complex of the wrist: a multicenter study. Arthroscopy 13:78, 1997.

Feldon P, Terrono AL, Belsky MR: Wafer distal ulna resection for triangular fibrocartilage tears and/or ulna impaction syndrome. J Hand Surg 17A:731, 1992.

Fellinger M, Peicha G, Seibert FJ, Grechenig W: Radial avulsion of the triangular fibrocartilage complex in acute wrist trauma: a new technique for arthroscopic repair. Arthroscopy 13:370, 1997.

Jantea CL, Baltzer A, Ruther W: Arthroscopic repair of radial-sided lesions of the fibrocartilage complex. Hand Clin 11:31, 1995.

Johnstone DJ, Thorogood S, Smith WH, Scott TD: A comparison of magnetic resonance imaging and arthroscopy in the investigation of chronic wrist pain. J Hand Surg 22B(6):714, 1997.

Kleinman WB, Graham TJ: Distal ulnar injury and dysfunction. In Peimer CA (ed): Surgery of the Hand and Upper Extremity, vol 1. New York, McGraw-Hill, 1996, pp 667–709.

Lester B, Halbrecht J, Levy IM, Gaudinez R: "Press test" for office diagnosis of triangular fibrocartilage complex tears of the wrist. Ann Plast Surg 35:41, 1995.

Levinsohn EM, Rosen ID, Palmer AK: Wrist arthrography: Value of the three-compartment injection method. Radiology 179:231, 1991.

Lichtman DM: The Wrist and Its Disorders. Philadelphia, WB Saunders, 1988.

Loftus JB, Palmer AK: Disorders of the distal radioulnar joint and triangular fibrocartilage complex: an overview. In Lichtman DM, Alexander AH (eds): The Wrist and Its Disorders, 2nd ed. Philadelphia, WB Saunders, 1997, pp 385–414.

Mikic ZDJ: Age changes in the triangular fibrocartilage in the wrist joint. J Anat 126:367, 1978.

Palmer AK: Triangular fibrocartilage complex lesions: A classification. J Hand Surg 14A:594, 1989.

Palmer AK, Glisson RR, Werner FW. Ulnar variance determination. J Hand Surg 7A:376, 1982.

Palmer AK, Werner FW: Biomechanics of the distal radial ulnar joint. Clin Orthop 187:26, 1984.

Palmer AK, Werner FW: The triangular fibrocartilage complex of the wrist: anatomy and function. J Hand Surg 6A:153, 1981.

Palmer AK, Werner FW, Glisson RR, Murphy DJ: Partial excision of the triangular fibrocartilage complex. J Hand Surg 13A:403, 1988.

Palmer AK: Triangular fibrocartilage complex lesions: a classification. J Hand Surg 14A:594, 1989.

Pederzini L, Luchetti R, Soragni O, et al: Evaluation of the triangular fibrocartilage complex tears by arthroscopy, arthrography and magnetic resonance imaging. Arthroscopy 8:191, 1992.

Peterson RK, Savoie FH, Field LD: Arthroscopic treatment of sports injuries to the triangular fibrocartilage. Sports Med Artho Rev 6:262, 1998.

Potter HG, Asnis-Ernberg L, Weiland AJ, et al: The utility of high-resolution magnetic resonance imaging in the evaluation of the triangular fibrocartilage complex of the wrist. J Bone Joint Surg 79A:1675, 1997.

Reagan DS, Linscheid RL, Dobyns JH: Lunotriquetral sprains. J Hand Surg 9A:502, 1984.

Roth JH, Haddad RG: Radiocarpal arthroscopy and arthrography in the diagnosis of ulnar wrist pain. Arthroscopy 2:234, 1986.

Sagerman SD, Short W: Arthroscopic repair of radial-sided triangular fibrocartilage complex tears. Arthroscopy 12:339, 1996.

Savoie FH: The role of arthroscopy in the diagnosis and management of cartilaginous lesions of the wrist. Hand Clin 11:1, 1995.

Savoie FH, Grondel RJ: Arthroscopy for carpal instability. Orthop Clin North Am 26:731, 1995.

Savoie FH, Whipple TL: The role of arthroscopy in athletic injuries of the wrist. Clin Sports Med 15:219, 1996.

Thuri-Pathi RG, Ferlic DC, Clayton ML, McLure DC: Arterial anatomy of the triangular fibrocartilage of the wrist and its surgical significance. J Hand Surg 11A:258, 1986.

Trumble TE, Gilbert M, Bedder N: Arthroscopic repair of the triangular fibrocartilage complex. Arthroscopy 12:588, 1996.

Viegas SF, Patterson RM, Hokanson JA, et al: Wrist anatomy: incidence, distribution and correlation of anatomic variations, tears and arthrosis. J Hand Surg 18A:463, 1993.

de Quervain's Disease

Edwards EG: deQuervain's stenosing tendo-vaginitis at the radial styloid process. South Surg 16:1081, 1950.

Jackson WT, et al: Anatomical variations in the first extensor compartment of the wrist. J Bone Joint Surg 68A:923, 1986.

Minamikawa Y, Peimer CA, Cox WL, Sherwin FS: deQuervain's syndrome: surgical and anatomical studies of the fibroosseous canal. Orthopaedics 14:545, 1991.

Strickland JW, Idler RS, Creighton JC: Hand clinic deQuervain's stenosing tenovitis. Indiana Med 83(5):340, 1990.

Totten PA: Therapist's management of deQuervain's disease. In Hunter JM (ed): Rehabilitation of the Hand, Surgery and Therapy. St. Louis, Mosby, 1990.

Intersection Syndrome

Grundberg AB, Reagan DS: Pathologic anatomy of the forearm: intersection syndrome. J Hand Surg 10A:299, 1985.

Wrist Ligament Injury

Blatt G: Capsulodesis in reconstructive hand surgery. Hand Clin 3:81, 1987.

Lavernia CJ, Cohen MS, Taleisnik J: Treatment of scapholunate dissociation by ligamentous repair and capsulodesis. J Hand Surg 17A:354, 1992.

Watson HK, Ballet FL: The SLAC wrist: scapholunate advanced collapse pattern of degenerative arthritis. J Hand Surg 9A:358, 1984.

Evaluation

We typically take an anatomically oriented approach to identifying and treating elbow injuries. With few exceptions, pain in a particular area of the elbow is caused by the surrounding or underlying physical structures (Fig. 2–1). Injuries should also be classified into **acute** (such as a radial head fracture or posterior elbow dislocation) or **progressive overuse** with repetitive microtrauma. The athlete should be able to localize his or her primary symptoms into one of five areas.

Differential Diagnosis of Elbow Pain According to Symptom Location (Figs. 2–2 to 2–5)

Location	Possible Disorders
Anterior	Anterior capsular strain
	Distal biceps tendon rupture/tendinitis
	Dislocation of the elbow
	Pronator syndrome (throwers)
Medial	Medial epicondylitis
	Ulnar collateral ligament injury (MCL)
	Ulnar neuritis or ulnar nerve subluxation
	Flexor pronator muscle strain
	Fracture
	Little League elbow in skeletally immature throwers
	Valgus extension overload overuse symptoms

continued

Differential Diagnosis of Elbow Pain According to Symptom Location (Figs. 2–2 to 2–5) *(Continued)*

Posteromedial	Olecranon tip stress fracture
	Posterior impingement in throwers
	Trochlear chondromalacia
Posterior	Olecranon bursitis
	Olecranon process stress fracture
	Triceps tendinitis
Lateral	Capitellum fracture
	Cervical radiculopathy—referred pain
	Lateral epicondylitis
	Lateral collateral injury
	Osteochondral degenerative changes
	Osteochondritis dessicans (Panner's disease)
	Posterior interosseous nerve syndrome
	Radial head fracture
	Radial tunnel syndrome
	Synovitis

MCL, medial collateral ligament.
Modified from Conway JE: Clinical evaluation of elbow injuries in the athlete. J Musculoskel Med 10(3):20–28, 1988.

Thrower's History

In a throwing athlete, the examiner should seek out details, including:

- Acute versus progressive injury.
- Intensity of symptoms.
- Duration of symptoms.

- Throwing schedule:
  - Frequency of throwing.
  - Intensity.
  - Duration.
  - Types and proportion of pitches delivered.
  - Delivery style (sidearm versus overhead—the former more injurious to the elbow).
  - Types and proportions of throws delivered (e.g., curves are more deleterious than fastballs).
  - Rest periods employed.
  - Warm-up and cool-down regimens employed.
  - Phase the pain manifests in (e.g., early cocking, acceleration, follow-through).
  - Restriction of motion.
  - Locking or checkrein-type symptoms.

Common Complaints in Throwing Athletes

Medial elbow pain from ulnar collateral ligament (UCL) valgus overload (UCL injury) may present with an acute "pop" or progressive medial elbow discomfort after heavy throwing. These athletes complain of losing significant speed of their throw. Ulnar nerve signs (including numbness and paresthesias radiating into the ulnar two fingers) occur with UCL injury in up to 40% of athletes. Instability of the ligament allows traction injury to the ulnar nerve.

Posterior elbow pain often is present with **valgus extension overload syndrome.**

Lateral   Medial

Humerus

Lateral supracondyle ridge

Coronoid fossa

Lateral epicondyle

Medial epicondyle

Radial fossa

Capitellum

Trochlear groove

Trochlea

Radial head

Radial neck

Coronoid process

Radial tuberosity

Ulnar tuberosity

Radius

Ulna

Figure 2–1. Osseous structures of the humeroradial and humeroulnar joints.

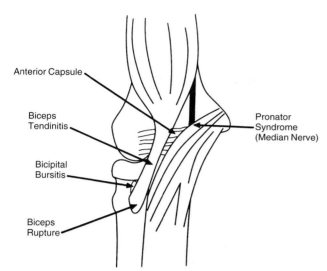

Figure 2–2. Anterior elbow pain. (From Mellion MB, Walsh WM, Shelton GL: The Team Physician's Handbook, 3rd ed. Philadelphia, Hanley and Belfus, 2000, pp. 419–420.)

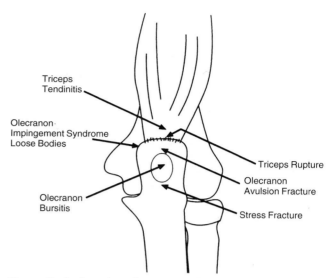

Figure 2–4. Posterior elbow pain. (From Mellion MB, Walsh WM, Shelton GL: The Team Physician's Handbook, 3rd ed. Philadelphia, Hanley and Belfus, 2002, pp. 419–420.)

Lateral elbow pain in throwers is produced by **compression** and subsequent lesions of the radial head or capitellum or resultant loose bodies.

Physical Examination

Physiologic/pathologic changes often noted in throwers include:

- Flexion contracture of elbow (loss of extension).
- Cubitus valgus.
- Flexor-pronator muscular hypertrophy.
- Anterior capsular contracture.
- Olecranon hypertrophy.
- Posterior or anterior compartment loose bodies.

Medial Joint Examination

- Point tenderness at the medial epicondyle or musculoskeletal junction indicates flexor-pronator strain (rarely a defect is noted, indicating a tear).
- Tenderness on palpation of the anterior band of the UCL **differentiates pathology of the flexor-pronator group from UCL laxity or tear.**
- Pain or asymmetrical laxity on valgus stress testing of the UCL should be noted. Valgus stress testing is done by flexing the elbow 20 to 30 degrees to unlock the olecranon, with a comparison of the affected with the asymptomatic elbow. This can be performed in the supine, prone, or seated position.

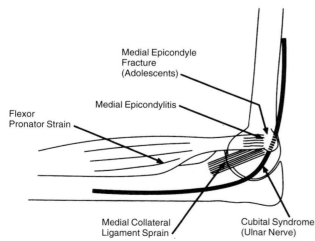

Figure 2–3. Medial elbow pain. (From Mellion MB, Walsh WM, Shelton GL: The Team Physician's Handbook, 3rd ed. Philadelphia, Hanley and Belfus, 2002, pp. 419–420.)

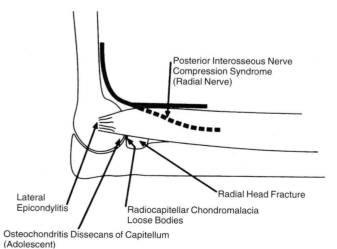

Figure 2–5. Lateral elbow pain. (From Mellion MB, Walsh WM, Shelton GL: The Team Physician's Handbook, 3rd ed. Philadelphia, Hanley and Belfus, 2002, pp. 419–420.)

- The **valgus extension snap maneuver** is performed by placing a firm valgus stress on the elbow, then snapping the elbow into extension. Reproduction of pain during this test is indicative of **valgus extension overload syndrome of the elbow.**
- The posteromedial ulnohumeral joint is palpated for tenderness or osteophytes found in valgus extension overload syndrome.
- Inflammation of the ulnar nerve can be identified by Tinel examination.
- An attempt is made to sublux the ulnar nerve in its cubital tunnel.
- The fifth finger and ulnar half of the ring finger are checked for paresthesias or sensory loss.

Lateral Joint Examination

- The radiocapitellar joint is palpated to check for osteophytes.
- Joint effusion may be palpable at the posterolateral aspect of the joint.

- The stability of the lateral ligament complex is tested with varus stressing.
- The lateral epicondyle is palpated for possible lateral epicondylitis or "tennis elbow," typically from a late or mechanically poor backhand.

Posterior Joint Examination

- The olecranon is palpated for spurs, fractures, or loose bodies.
- The triceps insertion is palpated for tendinitis or a partial tear.

Anterior Joint Examination

- Anterior capsulitis produces poorly localized tenderness that can be identified by palpation.
- The biceps tendon and brachialis are palpated for tendinitis or a partial tear.
- The "checkrein phenomenon" may produce symptoms and coronoid hypertrophy anteriorly.

Findings in Common Conditions of the Elbow and Forearm

Valgus Extension Overload Syndrome

Tenderness around the tip of the olecranon (posterior elbow)

Pain with forced passive elbow extension

Increased valgus laxity (variable)

Cubital Tunnel Syndrome

Tenderness over the course of the ulnar nerve

Abnormal Tinel sign over the ulnar nerve as it passes through the cubital tunnel (at the elbow medially)

Ulnar nerve compression test abnormal

Elbow flexion test abnormal (variable)

Abnormal sensation (two-point discrimination or light touch), little finger (fifth finger); ulnar aspect of ring finger (fourth finger); ulnar aspect of hand (variable)

Weakness and atrophy of the ulnar-innervated intrinsic muscles of the hand (variable)

Weakness of flexor digitorum profundus to the little finger (variable)

Signs of concomitant ulnar nerve instability, elbow instability, or elbow deformity (occasionally)

Lateral Epicondylitis (Extensor Origin Tendinitis)

Tenderness at the lateral epicondyle and at the origin of the involved tendons

Pain produced by resisted wrist extension (see Lateral Epicondylitis section)

Pain with passive flexion of the fingers and the wrist with the elbow fully extended (variable)

Radial Tunnel Syndrome

Tenderness in the extensor muscle mass of the forearm at the arcade of Frohse (distal to lateral epicondyle)

Long finger extension test reproduces familiar pain

Weakness of finger and thumb extensors and extensor carpi ulnaris (unusual); see text

Pronator Teres Syndrome

Tenderness in the proximal forearm over pronator teres

Abnormal sensation (two-point discrimination or light touch) in the thumb, index finger, long finger, and radial side of ring finger (variable)

Prolonged resisted pronation reproduces symptoms

Weakness of median innervated muscle (variable)

Rare, but **often incorrectly diagnosed as carpal tunnel**

Resisted elbow flexion and forearm supination reproduces symptoms (compression at the lacertus fibrosus)

Resisted long finger proximal interphalangeal joint flexion reproduces symptoms (compression by the flexor digitorum superficialis)

Weakness of median innervated muscles (variable)

Anterior Interosseous Nerve Syndrome

Weakness of flexor pollicis longus and flexor digitorum profundus to index finger (O sign)

Weakness of pronator quadratus (variable)

Medial Epicondylitis (Flexor-Pronator Tendinitis)

Tenderness over the common flexor origin

Resisted wrist flexion test reproduces pain

Resisted forearm pronation reproduces pain

Differentiate this from UCL tear and/or cubital tunnel syndrome (ulnar nerve)

Distal Biceps Tendon Rupture

Swelling

Ecchymosis

Palpable gap in the biceps tendon

Weak or absent supination and elbow flexion

Findings in Common Conditions of the Elbow and Forearm *(Continued)*

Ulnar Collateral Ligament (UCL) Strain or Tear

Medial elbow joint pain in a thrower

Complete tears open on valgus stress testing with the elbow flexed at 25 degrees (compared to the uninvolved side)

Incomplete tears are tender on palpation of the UCL, but don't open on valgus stressing

Differentiate this from a flexor-pronator strain or medial epicondylitis (see text)

Nursemaid's Elbow (Pulled Elbow Syndrome)

Mean age is 2 to 3 years old

History of longitudinal traction on an extended elbow

A partial slippage of the annular ligament over the head of the radius and into the radiocapitellar joint

History is critical to making diagnosis

Child typically holds the arm at the side with the hand pronated (palm down)

Closed reduction is highly successful (86 to 98%). First supinate (palm up) the forearm. Then hyperflex the elbow.

Keep the examiner's thumb over the radial head laterally to feel the snap of the ligament reduction

Little League Elbow

Term encompasses a spectrum of pathologies about the elbow joint in young developing (pediatric) throwers

Four distinct vulnerable areas to throwing stress: (1) medial elbow tension overload; (2) lateral articular surface compression overload; (3) posterior medial shear forces; and (4) extension overload of the lateral restraints

May present as Panner's disease (necrosis of the capitellum), OCD, medial epicondylar fracture, medial apophysitis, medial ligament rupture, posterior osteophyte formation at the tip of the olecranon

This subset of pediatric throwing athletes should be evaluated by a pediatric orthopaedic surgeon

Osteoarthritis

Restricted flexion or extension

Effusion (variable)

Modified from Reider B: The Orthopaedic Physical Examination. Philadelphia, WB Saunders, 1999.

Rehabilitation Rationale for Throwers

Repetitive throwing results in muscular and bony hypertrophic changes about the elbow. Slocum was one of the first to classify throwing injuries of the elbow into medial tension and valgus compression overload injuries. ***Valgus stress plus forced extension is the major pathologic mechanism of the thrower's elbow.*** Tension (Fig. 2–6) is produced on the medial aspect of the elbow during throwing. *Compression* is produced on the lateral aspect of the elbow.

Classification of Injuries of the Elbow in Throwing Athletes

Medial Stress

Flexor muscle strain or tear

Avulsion of the medial epicondyle

Attenuation or tear of the MCL

Ulnar nerve traction

Lateral Compression

Hypertrophy of the radial head and capitellum

Avascular necrosis of the capitellum

Osteochondral fractures of the radial head or capitellum

Forced Extension

Olecranon osteophyte formation on tip of the olecranon process

Loose body formation

Scarring and fibrous tissue deposition in the olecranon fossa

MCL, medial collateral ligament.

General Rehabilitation Principles

Rehabilitation of the elbow complex in a throwing athlete requires a carefully directed program to ensure full restoration of motion and function. Frequently after surgery, motion is lost as a result of the elbow's high degree of joint congruency, capsular anatomy, and soft tissue changes. To obtain full function without complications, a sequential, progressive treatment program must be developed. This program requires that specific criteria be met at each stage before advancement to the next one. The final goal is to return the athlete to the sport as quickly and as safely as possible.

Several key principles should be considered during the rehabilitation of a throwing athlete with an elbow disorder. **(1) The effects of immobilization must be minimized. (2) Healing tissue must never be overstressed. (3) The patient must fulfill specific criteria before progressing from one phase to the next during the rehabilitation process. (4) The rehabilitation program must be based on current clinical and scientific research. (5) The rehabilitation program should be adaptable to each patient and the patient's specific goals.** Finally, these basic treatment principles should be followed throughout the rehabilitation process.

Elbow rehabilitation in throwing athletes generally follows a **four-phase progression.** It is important that certain criteria be met at each level before advancement to the next stage. This allows athletes to progress at their own pace based on tissue-healing constraints.

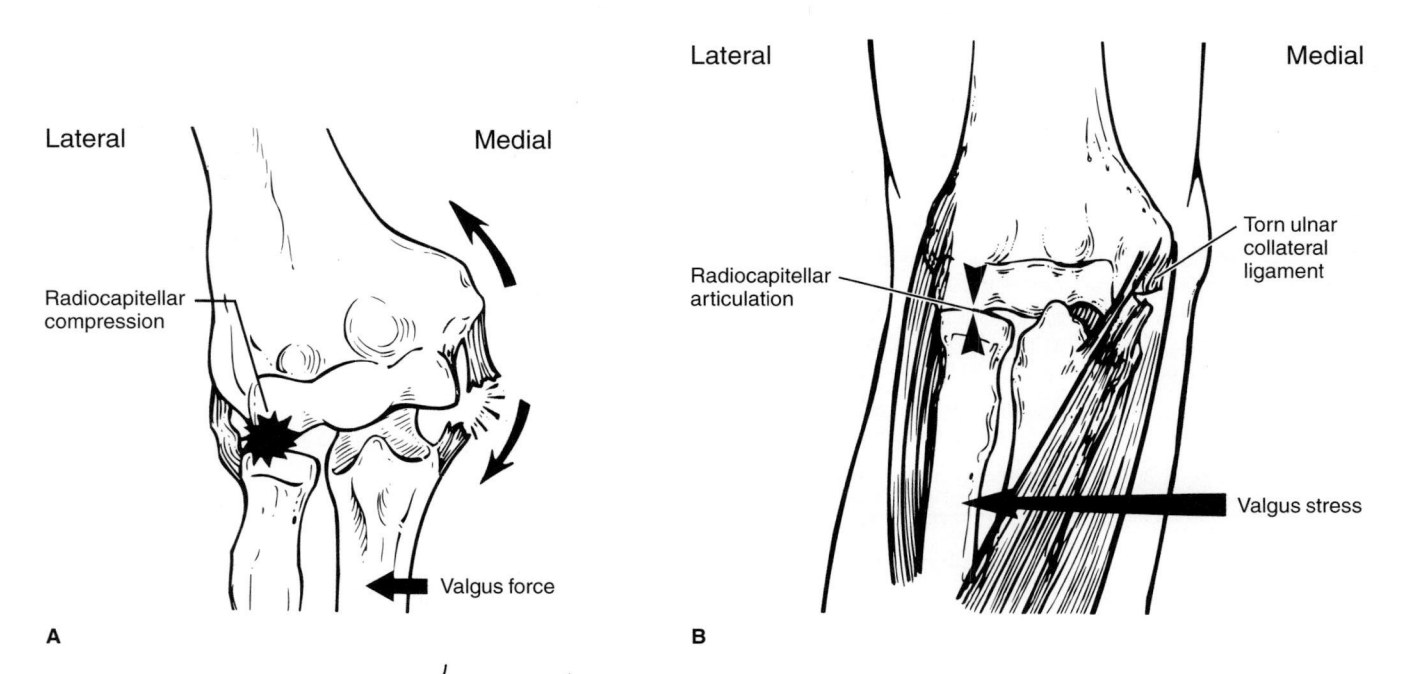

Lateral   Medial

Radiocapitellar
compression

Valgus force

A

Lateral   Medial

Radiocapitellar
articulation

Torn ulnar
collateral
ligament

Valgus stress

B

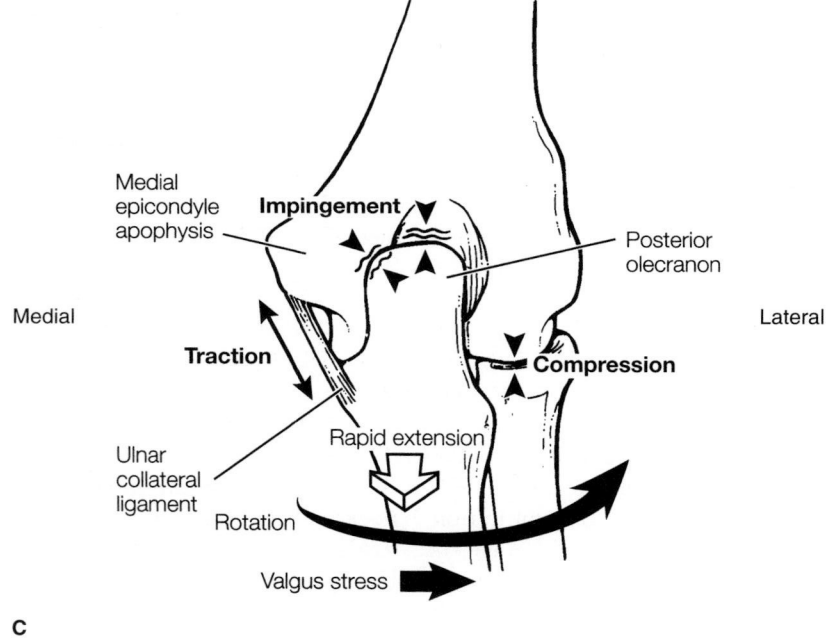

Medial
epicondyle
apophysis

Impingement

Posterior
olecranon

Medial

Traction

Compression

Ulnar
collateral
ligament

Rapid extension

Rotation

Valgus stress

C

Lateral

Figure 2–6. *A,* Valgus forces at the elbow injure the ulnar collateral ligament (UCL) and
compress the radiocapitellar joint. *B,* Patients
who have medial elbow instability with throwing are subject to lateral compression forces (ar-
rowheads) on the radiocapitellar articulation and
medial valgus stress (arrow). This can lead to a
torn UCL. *C,* Valgus extension overload syndrome. Rapid elbow extension with valgus stress
and rotation causes medial traction, lateral compression, and intra-articular posterior impingement. Such stress can injure the ulnar collateral
ligament, medial epicondyle apophysis, lateral
compartment, and posterior olecranon. (*A,* From
Nirsahl RP, Kraushaar BS: Assessment and treatment guidelines for elbow injuries. Physician
Sports Med 24[5]:230, 1996; *B,* from Harding
WG: Use and misuse of the tennis elbow strap.
Physician Sports Med 20[8]:430, 1992; *C,* from
Fox GM, Jebson PT, Orwin JF: Over-use injuries
of the elbow. Physician Sports Med
23[8]:58–73.)

Phase 1: Regaining Motion

The first phase involves *regaining motion* lost during immobilization after surgery. Pain, inflammation, and muscle atrophy also are treated. Common regimens for inflammation and pain involve modalities such as cryotherapy, high-voltage galvanic stimulation (HVGS), ultrasound, and whirlpool. Joint mobilization techniques can also be used to help minimize pain and promote motion.

To minimize muscular atrophy, submaximal isometric exercises for elbow flexors and extensors, as well as for the forearm pronators and supinators, are started early. Strengthening of the shoulder should also begin relatively early to prevent functional weakness. **Care should be taken early in the rehabilitation program to restrict shoulder external rotation movements that may place valgus stress on the medial structures of the elbow.**

Elbow flexion contracture is common after an elbow injury or surgery when range of motion (ROM) is not treated appropriately. **Fifty percent of baseball pitchers have been found to have flexion contractures of the elbow,** and 30% have cubitus valgus deformities. Prevention of these contractures is the key. Early ROM is vital to nourish the articular cartilage and promote proper collagen fiber alignment. A gradual increase in and early restoration of full passive elbow extension are essential to prevent flexion contraction. Several popular techniques to improve limited ROM are joint mobilization, contract-relax stretching, and low-load, long-duration stretching for the restoration of full elbow extension.

Joint mobilizations can be performed to the humeroulnar, humeroradial, and radioulnar joints. Limited elbow extension tends to respond to posterior glides of the ulna on the humerus. The grade of the mobilization depends on the phase of rehabilitation in effect.

Another technique to restore full elbow extension is *low-load, long-duration stretching* (Fig. 2–7). A good passive overpressure stretch can be achieved by having the patient hold a 2- to 4-pound weight or use an elastic band with the upper extremity resting on a fulcrum just proximal to the elbow joint to allow for greater extension. This stretch should be performed for 10 to 12 minutes to incorporate a long-duration, low-intensity stretch. Stretching of this magnitude has been found to elicit a plastic collagen tissue response, resulting in permanent soft tissue elongation. It is important to note that if the intensity of this stretch is too great, pain and/or a protective muscle response may result, which could inhibit collagen fiber elongation.

Phase 2: Regaining Strength and Endurance

The **intermediate phase** consists of improving the patient's overall *strength, endurance, and elbow mobility.* To progress to this phase, the patient must demonstrate full elbow ROM (0–135 degrees), minimal or no pain or tenderness, and a "good" (4/5) muscle grade for the elbow flexor and extensor groups. During this phase, isotonic strengthening exercises are emphasized for the entire arm and shoulder complex.

Phase 3: Return to Functional Participation

The third phase is the **advanced strengthening phase.** The primary goal in this phase is to prepare the athlete for *the return to functional participation* and initiation of throwing activities. A total arm strengthening program is used to improve the power, endurance, and neuromuscular control of the entire limb. Advancement to phase 3 requires demonstration of full, pain-free ROM, no pain or tenderness, and 70% strength compared with the contralateral side.

Plyometric exercises are most beneficial in this phase; these drills closely simulate functional activities, such as throwing and swinging, and are performed at higher speeds. They also teach the athlete to transfer energy and stabilize the involved area. Plyometrics use a stretch-shortening cycle of muscle, thus using eccentric/concentric muscle extension. For instance, greater emphasis is placed on the biceps musculature in this phase of rehabilitation because it plays a vital role eccentrically during the deceleration and follow-through phases of the throwing motion by preventing hyperextension. One specific plyometric activity involves exercise tubing. Starting with the elbow flexed and the shoulder in 60 degrees of flexion, the patient releases the isometric hold, initiating an eccentric phase. As full extension is approached, the athlete quickly flexes the elbow again, going into a concentric phase. The eccentric activity produces a muscular stretch, thus activating the muscle spindles and producing a greater concentric contraction.

The primary targets for strengthening in this phase are the biceps, triceps, and wrist flexor/pronator muscles. The biceps, the wrist flexors, and pronators greatly reduce valgus stresses on the elbow during the throwing motion. Other key muscle groups stressed in this phase are the triceps and rotator cuff. The triceps are used in the acceleration phase of the throwing motion, whereas attention to the rotator cuff helps to establish the goal of total arm strengthening.

Figure 2–7. Low-load, long-duration stretching of the elbow for restoration of full elbow extension.

To improve shoulder strength, the throwing athlete is introduced to a set of exercises known as the **"Thrower's Ten"** program, later in this chapter.

Rehabilitation of an injured elbow is different from any other rehabilitation program for throwing athletes. Initially, elbow extension ROM must be obtained to prevent elbow flexion contracture. Next, valgus stress needs to be minimized through the conditioning of elbow and wrist flexors, as well as the pronator muscle group. Finally, the shoulder, especially the rotator cuff musculature, must be included in the rehabili-

tation process. The rotator cuff is vital to the throwing pattern and, if not strengthened, can lead to future shoulder problems.

Phase 4: Return to Activity

The final stage of the rehabilitation program for the throwing athlete is *return to activity*. This stage uses a progressive interval throwing program to gradually increase the demands on the upper extremity by controlling throwing distance, frequency, and duration.

Rehabilitation Protocol
Posterior Rehabilitation after Elbow Arthroscopy (Posterior Compartment or Valgus Extension Overload Surgery)

Phase I: Immediate Motion Phase
Goals
- Improve or regain full ROM.
- Decrease pain or inflammation.
- Retard muscular atrophy.

Days 1–4
- ROM to tolerance (extension-flexion and supination-pronation). Often full elbow extension is not possible because of pain.
- Gentle overpressure into extension Fig.(2–8).

Figure 2–8. Gentle elbow overpressure into extension.

- Wrist flexion-extension stretches.
- Gripping exercises with putty.
- Isometrics, wrist extension-flexion.
- Isometrics, elbow extension-flexion.
- Compression dressing, ice four to five times daily.

Days 5–10
- ROM exercises to tolerance (at least 20–90 degrees).
- Overpressure into extension.
- Joint mobilization to reestablish ROM.
- Wrist flexion-extension stretches.
- Continue isometrics.

- Continue use of ice and compression to control swelling.

Days 11–14
- ROM exercises to tolerance (at least 10–100 degrees).
- Overpressure into extension (three to four daily).
- Continue joint mobilization techniques.
- Initiate light dumbbell program (progressive resistance exercise for biceps, triceps, wrist flexors, extensors, supinators, and pronators).
- Continue use of ice postexercise.

Phase II: Intermediate Phase
Goals
- Improve strength, power, and endurance.
- Increase ROM.
- Initiate functional activities.

Weeks 2–4
- Full ROM exercises (four to five times daily).
- Overpressure into elbow extension.
- Continue progressive resistance exercise program for elbow and wrist musculature.
- Initiate shoulder program (external rotation and rotator cuff).
- Continue joint mobilization.
- Continue ice after exercise.

Weeks 5–7
- Continue all exercises listed above.
- Initiate light upper body program.
- Continue use of ice after activity.

Phase III: Advanced Strengthening Program
Goals
- Improve strength, power, and endurance.
- Gradual return to functional activities.

Criteria to Enter Phase III
- Full, nonpainful ROM.
- Strength 75% or more of contralateral side.
- No pain or tolerance.

Rehabilitation Protocol
**Posterior Rehabilitation after Elbow Arthroscopy
(Posterior Compartment or Valgus Extension Overload Surgery)** *(Continued)*

Weeks 8–12
- Continue progressive resistance exercise program for elbow and wrist.
- Continue shoulder program.

- Continue stretching for elbow and shoulder.
- Initiate interval throwing program and gradually return to sports activities.

From Wilk KE, Arrigo CA, Andrews JR, Azar FM: Rehabilitation following elbow surgery in the throwing athlete. Operative Tech Sports Med 4:114–132, 1996.

Medial Collateral Ligament (Ulnar Collateral Ligament) Injuries

David W. Altchek, MD, and Michael Levinson, PT

Important Rehabilitation Points

- The medial collateral ligament (MCL or UCL) of the elbow has been clearly documented as a frequent site of serious injury in overhead throwers.
- Pitching generates a large valgus force at the elbow. These forces peak at the medial elbow during the late cocking and early acceleration phases of throwing as the elbow moves from flexion and extension, at speeds that have been estimated to reach 3000 degrees/sec.
- Dillman and coworkers estimated that the typical fastball thrown by an elite pitcher produces a load that approaches the actual tensile strength of the MCL.

Anatomy and Biomechanics

The **MCL** has two bundles of primary importance, **anterior and posterior** (Fig. 2–9). These bundles tighten in reciprocal fashion as the elbow is flexed and extended. The anterior bundle tightens in extension and loosens in flexion. The posterior bundle tightens in flexion and loosens in extension.

Most MCL tears cause pain during the acceleration phase of throwing.

Treatment

- **The anterior bundle of the MCL is the primary focus of MCL reconstruction.**
- The most common graft is the ipsilateral palmaris longus; other options are the gracilis or semitendinosis, or plantaris tendon.

Figure 2–9. UCL complex of the elbow, consisting of three bundles: anterior, posterior, and transverse oblique. (From Wilk KE, Arrigo CA, Andrews JR: Rehabilitation of the elbow in the throwing athlete. J Orthop Sports Phys Ther 17:305, 1993.)

- Altchek recently described a "docking procedure" for MCL reconstruction. The reconstruction is done through a muscle-splitting approach that preserves the flexor-pronator origin. This generally avoids ulnar nerve transposition and minimizes the number of bony tunnels required.

Rehabilitation after MCL reconstruction emphasizes early, controlled ROM to avoid excessive stretching. The patient is encouraged to wear the postoperative brace at all times to avoid any chance of valgus stress being placed on the graft. Passive stretching by the therapist should also be avoided.

Rehabilitation Protocol
Conservative Treatment of Medial (Ulnar) Collateral Sprains
Wilk, Arrigo, and Andrews

Phase 1: Immediate Motion Phase

Goals
- Increase ROM.
- Promote healing of UCL.
- Retard muscular atrophy.
- Decrease pain and inflammation.

Range of Motion
- Brace (optional) nonpainful ROM (20–90 degrees).
- Active-assisted ROM, passive ROM elbow and wrist (nonpainful range).

Exercises
- Isometrics—wrist and elbow musculature.
- Shoulder strengthening (**no external rotation strengthening**).

Ice and Compression

Phase 2: Intermediate Phase

Goals
- Increase ROM.
- Improve strength and endurance.
- Decrease pain and inflammation.
- Promote stability.

Range of Motion
- Gradually increase motion 0–135 degrees (increase 10 degrees/wk).

Exercises
- Initiate isotonic exercises
  - Wrist curls.
  - Wrist extension.
  - Pronation-supination.
  - Biceps-triceps.

- Dumbbells: external rotation, deltoid, supraspinatus, rhomboids, internal rotation.

Ice and Compression

Phase 3: Advanced Phase

Criteria for Progression to Phase 2
- Full ROM.
- No pain or tenderness.
- No increase in laxity.
- Strength $^4/_5$ of elbow flexors-extensors.

Goals
- Improve strength, power, and endurance.
- Improve neuromuscular control.

Exercises
- Initiate exercise tubing, should program
  - "Thrower's Ten" Program.
  - Biceps-triceps program.
  - Supination-pronation.
  - Wrist extension-flexion.

Phase 4: Return to Activity Phase

Criteria for Progression to Return to Throwing
- Full, nonpainful ROM.
- No increase in laxity.
- Isokinetic test fulfills criteria.
- Satisfactory clinical examination.

Exercises
- Initiate interval throwing.
- Continue "Thrower's Ten" program.
- Continue plyometrics.

Rehabilitation Protocol
After Chronic Ulnar Collateral Ligament Injury: Reconstruction Using Autogenous Graft

Phase 1: Immediate Postoperative Phase (1–3 Weeks)

Goals
- Protect healing tissue.
- Decrease pain/inflammation.
- Retard muscular atrophy.

Week 1

Brace
- Posterior splint at 90 degrees elbow flexion.
- Elbow compression dressing (2–3 days).

Range of Motion
- Wrist active ROM extension-flexion.

Exercises
- Gripping exercises.
- Wrist ROM.
- Shoulder isometrics (**no shoulder external rotation**).
- Biceps isometrics.

Rehabilitation Protocol
After Chronic Ulnar Collateral Ligament Injury:
Reconstruction Using Autogenous Graft *(Continued)*

Cryotherapy

Week 2

Brace
- Application of functional brace set at 30–100 degrees.

Exercises
- Initiate wrist isometrics.
- Initiate elbow flexion-extension isometrics.
- Continue all exercises listed above.

Week 3

Brace
- Advance brace 15–110 degrees (gradually increase ROM—5 degrees extension and 10 degrees flexion/wk).

Exercises
- Continue all exercises listed above.

Phase 2: Intermediate Phase (Weeks 4–8)

Goals
- Gradual increase in ROM.
- Promote healing of repaired tissue.
- Regain and improve muscular strength.

Week 4

Brace
- Functional brace set 10–120 degrees.

Exercises
- Begin light resistance exercises for arm (1 pound)
  - Wrist curls, extensions, pronation, supination.
  - Elbow extension-flexion.
- Progress shoulder programs emphasize rotator cuff strengthening (**avoid external rotation of shoulder until week 6**).

Week 6

Brace
- Functional brace set (0–130 degrees); active ROM (0–145 degrees without brace).

Exercises
- Progress elbow strengthening exercises.

- Initiate shoulder external rotation strengthening.
- Progress shoulder program.

Phase 3: Advanced Strengthening Phase (Weeks 9–13)

Goals
- Increase strength, power, endurance.
- Maintain full elbow ROM.
- Gradually initiate sporting activities.

Week 9

Exercises
- Initiate eccentric elbow flexion-extension.
- Continue isotonic program; forearm and wrist.
- Continue shoulder program—"Thrower's Ten" Program.
- Manual resistance diagonal patterns.
- Initiate plyometric exercise program.

Week 11

Exercises
- Continue all exercises listed above.
- Begin light sport activities (e.g., golf, swimming).

Phase 4: Return to Activity Phase (Weeks 14–26)

Goals
- Continue to increase strength, power, and endurance of upper extremity musculature.
- Gradual return to sport activities.

Week 14

Exercises
- Initiate interval throwing program (phase 1).
- Continue strengthening program.
- Emphasis on elbow and wrist strengthening and flexibility exercises.

Weeks 22–26

Exercises
- Gradual return to competitive throwing.

Ulnar Nerve Injury at the Elbow (Cubital Tunnel) (Fig. 2–10)

Repetitive valgus stresses to the elbow during throwing often produce medial traction on the ulnar nerve. Ulnar nerve injury results from repetitive traction combined with elbow ligament laxity, recurrent subluxation or dislocation of the nerve outside of the ulnar groove, compression of the nerve, or direct trauma.

Deficiency or laxity of the anterior bundle of the UCL of the elbow commonly causes stress on the ulnar nerve, and in throwers, these are often found concomi- **tantly.** Throwers often have a hypertrophied forearm flexor mass (attaching to the medial epicondyle) that compresses the nerve during muscle contraction.

Initial treatment of ulnar nerve symptoms in throwers is relative rest, cryotherapy, nonsteroidal anti-inflammatory drugs (NSAIDs), and modification of biomechanical throwing errors. Surgical transposition of the nerve may eventually be required (use of fasciodermal sling) for recalcitrant symptoms.

The physician must examine for concomitant elbow pathology (unstable UCL) in throwers with ulnar nerve symptoms. If found, these other pathologies must be addressed.

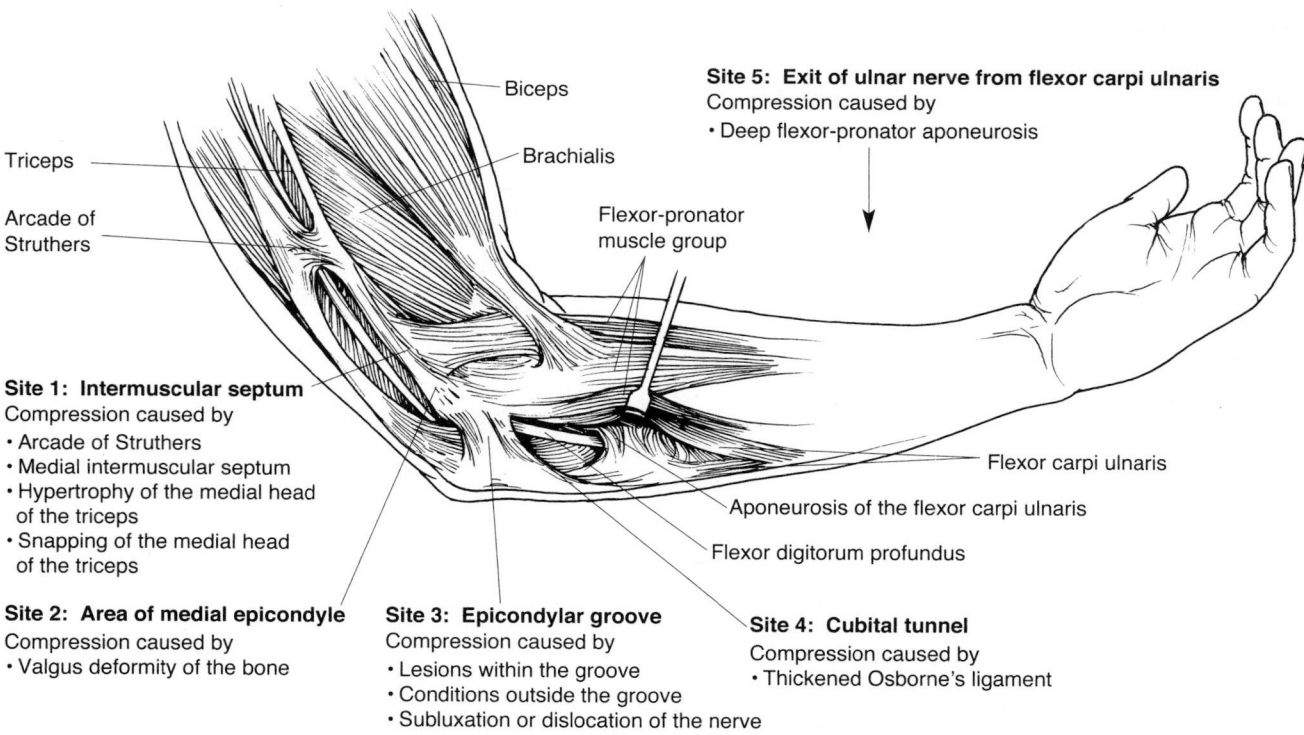

Site 5: Exit of ulnar nerve from flexor carpi ulnaris
Compression caused by
• Deep flexor-pronator aponeurosis

Biceps

Triceps

Brachialis

Arcade of
Struthers

Flexor-pronator
muscle group

Site 1: Intermuscular septum
Compression caused by
• Arcade of Struthers
• Medial intermuscular septum
• Hypertrophy of the medial head
of the triceps
• Snapping of the medial head
of the triceps

Flexor carpi ulnaris

Aponeurosis of the flexor carpi ulnaris

Flexor digitorum profundus

Site 2: Area of medial epicondyle
Compression caused by
• Valgus deformity of the bone

Site 3: Epicondylar groove
Compression caused by
• Lesions within the groove
• Conditions outside the groove
• Subluxation or dislocation of the nerve

Site 4: Cubital tunnel
Compression caused by
• Thickened Osborne's ligament

Figure 2–10. The five sites for potential ulnar nerve compression and the causes of compression at each site. (Adapted from Amadio PC: Anatomical basis for a technique of ulnar nerve transposition. Surg Radiol Anat 8:155–201, 1986.)

Rehabilitation Protocol
After Ulnar Nerve Transposition

Phase 1: Immediate Postoperative Phase (Week 1–2)

Goals
• Allow soft tissue healing of relocated nerve.
• Decrease pain and inflammation.
• Retard muscular atrophy.

Week 1
• Posterior splint at 90 degrees elbow flexion with wrist free for motion (sling for comfort).
• Compression dressing.
• Exercises: gripping exercises, wrist ROM, shoulder isometrics.

Week 2
• Remove posterior splint for exercise and bathing.
• Progress elbow ROM (passive ROM 15–120 degrees).
• Initiate elbow and wrist isometrics.
• Continue shoulder isometrics.

Phase 2: Intermediate Phase (Weeks 3–7)
Goals
• Restore full pain-free ROM.
• Improve strength, power, endurance of upper extremity musculature.

• Gradually increase functional demands.

Week 3
• Discontinue posterior splint.
• Progress elbow ROM, emphasize full extension.
• Initiate flexibility exercises for
  • Wrist extension-flexion.
  • Forearm supination-pronation.
  • Elbow extension-flexion.
• Initiate strengthening exercises for
  • Wrist extension-flexion.
  • Forearm supination-pronation.
  • Elbow extension-flexion.
  • Shoulder program.

Week 6
• Continue all exercises listed above.
• Initiate light sport activities.

Phase 3: Advanced Strengthening Phase (Weeks 8–11)

Goals
• Increase strength, power, and endurance.
• Gradually initiate sporting activities.

Rehabilitation Protocol
After Ulnar Nerve Transposition *(Continued)*

Week 8
- Initiate eccentric exercise program.
- Initiate plyometric exercise drills.
- Continue shoulder and elbow strengthening and flexibility exercises.
- Initiate interval throwing program.

Phase 4: Return to Activity Phase (Weeks 12–16)

Goals
Gradual return to sporting activities.

Week 12
- Return to competitive throwing.
- Continue "Thrower's Ten" program.

From Wilk KE, Arrigo CA, Andrews JR, Azar FM: Rehabilitation following elbow surgery in the throwing athlete. Operative Tech Sports Med 4:114–132, 1996.

Treating Flexion Contracture (Loss of Extension) in Throwing Athletes

- Gelinas and colleagues reported that 50% of professional baseball pitchers they tested had a flexion contracture (loss of extension) of the elbow.
- Typically a loss of up to 10 degrees of extension is unnoticed by the athlete and is not required for "functional" elbow ROM.
- Joint mobilization and **low-load, long-duration stretching** (see Fig. 2–7) are advocated for restoration of extension.
- High-intensity, short-duration stretching is **contraindicated** for limited elbow ROM (may produce myositis ossificans).

- Initial treatment includes moist heat and ultrasound, dynamic splinting at night during sleep (low-load, long-duration stretch), joint mobilizations, and ROM exercises at end ranges, done several times a day.
- If nonoperative measures fail in the rare patient with *loss of functional motion*, arthroscopic arthrolysis may be required.
- Accelerated rehabilitation after this surgery is required, but overly aggressive rehabilitation must be avoided to avoid inflammation (and thus reflex splinting and stiffening) of the elbow.

Rehabilitation Protocol
After Arthroscopic Arthrolysis of the Elbow

Phase 1: Immediate Motion Phase

Goals
- Improvement of ROM.
- Reestablishing full passive extension.
- Retard muscular atrophy.
- Decrease pain/inflammation.

Days 1–3
- ROM to tolerance (elbow extension-flexion) (two sets of 10/hour).
- Overpressure into extension (at least 10 degrees).
- Joint mobilization.
- Gripping exercise with putty.
- Isometrics for wrist and elbow.
- Compression and ice hourly.

Days 4–9
- ROM extension-flexion (at least 5–120 degrees).
- Overpressure into extension—5-pound weight, elbow in full extension (four to five times daily).

- Joint mobilization.
- Continue isometrics and gripping exercises.
- Continue use of ice.

Days 10–14
- Full passive ROM.
- ROM exercises (two sets of 10/hour).
- Stretch into extension.
- Continue isometrics.

Phase 2: Motion Maintenance Phase

Goals
- Maintain full ROM.
- Gradually improve strength.
- Decrease pain/inflammation.

Weeks 2–4
- ROM exercises (four to five times daily).
- Overpressure into extension—stretch for 2 minutes (three to four times daily).

continued

Rehabilitation Protocol
After Arthroscopic Arthrolysis of the Elbow *(Continued)*

- Initiate progressive resistance exercise (PRE) program (light dumbbells)
  - Elbow extension-flexion.
  - Wrist extension-flexion.
- Continue use of ice postexercise.

Weeks 4–6
- Continue all exercises listed above.
- Initiate interval sport program.

From Wilk KE, Arrigo CA, Andrews JR, Azar FM: Rehabilitation following elbow surgery in the throwing athlete. Operative Tech Sports Med 4:114–132, 1996.

A Basic Elbow Exercise Program (Performed Three Times a Day)

Kevin Wilk, PT

1. **Deep Friction Massage**
   Deep transverse friction across the area of the elbow that is sore; 5 minutes, several times daily (not shown).
2. **Grip**
   Grip apparatus, putty, small rubber ball, and the like. Use as continuously as possible all day long (not shown).
3. **Stretch Flexors** (Fig. 2–11)
   Straighten elbow completely. With palm facing up, grasp the middle of the hand and thumb. Pull the wrist down as far as possible. Hold for 10 counts. Release and repeat 5 to 10 times before and after each exercise session.
4. **Stretch Extensors**
   Straighten elbow completely. With the palm facing down, grasp the back of the hand and pull the wrist down as far as possible. Hold for a 10 count. Release and repeat 5 to 10 times, before and after each exercise session.

Progressive Resistance Elbow Exercises

Begin each PRE with one set of 10 repetitions without weight, progressing to five sets of 10 repetitions as tolerable. When you are able to easily perform five sets of 10 repetitions, you may begin adding weight. Begin each PRE with one set of 10 repetitions with 1 pound, progressing to five sets of 10 as tolerable. When you are able to easily perform five sets of 10 repetitions with 1 pound, you may begin to progress your weight in the same manner.

In a preventative elbow maintenance program (excluding specific rotator cuff exercises), it is permissible to advance weight as tolerable with strengthening exercises, taking care to emphasize proper lifting technique.

5. **Wrist Curls** (Fig. 2–12)
   The forearm should be supported on a table with the hand off the edge; the palm should face upward. Using a weight or hammer, lower that hand as far as possible and then curl it up as high as possible. Hold for a two count.

Figure 2–11. Flexor stretching. (From Wilk KE: Elbow Exercises. Health South Handout, 1993.)

Figure 2–14. Neutral wrist curls. (From Wilk KE: Elbow exercises. HealthSouth Handout, 1993.)

Figure 2–12. Wrist Curls. (From Andrews JR, Wilk KE: The Athlete's Shoulder New York, Churchill Livingstone, 1994, p. 707.)

6. **Reverse Wrist Curls** (Fig. 2–13)
   The forearm should be supported on a table with the hand off the edge; the palm should face downward. Using a weight or hammer, lower the hand as far as possible and then curl the wrist up as high as possible. Hold for a two count.

7. **Neutral Wrist Curls** (Fig. 2–14)
   The forearm should be supported on a table with the wrist in neutral position and the hand off the edge. Using a weight or hammer held in a normal hammering position, lower the wrist into ulnar deviation as far as possible. Then bring into radial deviation as far as possible. Hold for a two count. Relax.

8. **Pronation** (Fig. 2–15)
   The forearm should be supported on a table with the wrist in neutral position. Using a weight or hammer held in a normal hammering position, roll the wrist and bring the hammer into pronation as far as possible. Hold for a two count. Raise back to the starting position.

9. **Supination** (Fig. 2–16)
   The forearm should be supported on the table with the wrist in neutral position. Using a weight or

hammer held in a normal hammering position, roll the wrist bringing the hammer into full supination. Hold for a two count. Raise back to the starting position.

10. **Broomstick Curl-up** (Fig. 2–17A)
    Use a 1- to 2-foot broom handle with a 4- to 5-foot cord attached in the middle with a 1- to 5-pound weight tied in the center.
    - Extensors (see Fig. 2–17B)
      Grip the stick on either side of the rope with the palms down. Curl the cord up by turning the stick toward you (the cord is on the side of the stick, away from you). Once the weight is pulled to the top, lower the weight by unwinding the stick, rotating it away from you. Repeat three to five times.
    - Flexors
      Same as above exercise (extensors), but have the palms facing upward.

11. **Bicep Curl** (Fig. 2–18)
    Support the arm on the opposite hand. Bend the elbow to full flexion, then straighten the arm completely.

12. **French Curl** (Fig. 2–19)
    Raise the arm overhead. Take the opposite hand and give support at the elbow. Straighten the elbow over the head, hold for a two count.

Figure 2–13. Reverse wrist curls. (From Wilk KE: Elbow exercises. HealthSouth Handout, 1993.)

Figure 2–15. Pronation exercises. (From Andrews JR, Wilk KE: The Athlete's Shoulder. New York, Churchill Livingstone, 1994, p. 387.)

Figure 2–16. Supination exercises. (From Wilk KE: Elbow exercises. HealthSouth Handout, 1993.)

Figure 2–17. Broomstick curl-up. (From Wilk KE: Elbow exercises. HealthSouth Handout, 1993.)

A.

B.

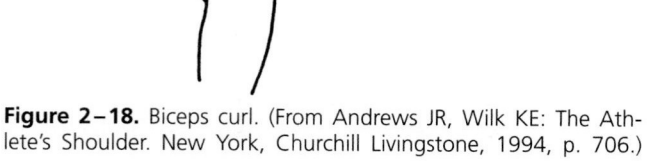

Figure 2–18. Biceps curl. (From Andrews JR, Wilk KE: The Athlete's Shoulder. New York, Churchill Livingstone, 1994, p. 706.)

Figure 2–19. French curl. (From Wilk KE: Elbow exercises. HealthSouth Handout, 1993.)

Eccentric Elbow Pronation (Fig. 2–20)

Holding a hammer in the hand (tied to a rubber band), start with the hand supinated, pronate against the rubber band. Then slowly allow the rubber band to overpower the wrist into supination.

Eccentric Elbow Supination (Fig. 2–21)

Holding a hammer in pronation (tied to a rubber band), supinate against the rubber band resistance. Then slowly allow the rubber band to overpower the wrist into pronation. ■

Figure 2–20. Eccentric elbow pronation exercise. (From Andrews JR, Wilk KE: The Athlete's Shoulder. New York, Churchill Livingstone, 1994, p. 708.)

Figure 2–21. Eccentric elbow supination exercise. (From Andrews JR, Wilk KE: The Athlete's Shoulder. New York, Churchill Livingstone, 1994, p. 708.)

Treatment and Rehabilitation of Elbow Dislocations

Kevin Wilk, PT, James R. Andrews, MD

Rehabilitation Considerations

- Elbow dislocations constitute 10 to 25% of all injuries to the elbow.
- Ninety percent of elbow dislocations produce **posterior** or posterolateral displacement of the forearm relative to the distal humerus.
- Fractures associated with elbow dislocations most frequently involve the radial head and the coronoid process of the elbow.
- The distal radioulnar joint (wrist) and the interosseous membrane of the forearm should be examined for tenderness and stability to rule out a possible Essex-Lopresti injury.
- When intra-articular fractures of the radial head, olecranon, or coronoid process occur with elbow dislocation, this is termed a **complex dislocation.**
- Associated neurologic injury is very uncommon, with the ulnar nerve the most commonly injured (stretch neurapraxia).

- A minor (but permanent) **loss of terminal elbow extension (5–15 degrees) is the most common sequela after posterior elbow dislocation.**
- Pronation and supination are characteristically unaffected after this injury.
- Elbow flexion returns first, with maximal improvement usually taking 6 to 12 weeks. Elbow extension returns more slowly and may continue to improve for 3 to 5 months.

Prolonged rigid immobilization has been associated with the least satisfactory arc of elbow motion and should be avoided.

- Heterotopic ossification (calcification) is common after elbow dislocation (up to 75% of patients) but rarely limits motion (fewer than 5% of patients). The most common sites for periarticular calcification are the anterior elbow region and the collateral ligaments.
- Mechanical testing confirms a 15% average loss of elbow strength after elbow dislocation.
- Approximately 60% of patients do not believe the injured elbow is as "good" as the uninvolved elbow at the end of treatment.

Classification

The traditional classification of elbow dislocations divides injuries into **anterior** (2%) and **posterior** dislocations. *Posterior* dislocations are further subdivided according to the final resting position of the olecranon in relation to the distal humerus: **posterior, posterolateral (most common), posteromedial (least common), and pure lateral.**

Morrey makes a clinical distinction between complete dislocation and **perched** dislocation (Fig. 2–22). Because perched dislocations have less ligament tearing, they have a more rapid recovery and more rapid rehabilitation. For a complete elbow dislocation, the anterior capsule must be disrupted. The brachialis must also be torn or significantly stretched.

Many elbow dislocations are accompanied by some type of UCL involvement. More specifically, the anterior oblique band of the UCL is affected. Tullos and colleagues found that the anterior oblique band of the UCL was torn in 34 of 37 patients who had previously experienced a posterior elbow dislocation. Repair of this ligament is sometimes indicated in athletes if the injury occurs in the dominant arm. This optimizes the chance for full return to the athlete's previous level of competition.

Evaluation, Work-up, and Reduction

- Swelling and deformity are noted on initial inspection.
- Concomitant upper extremity injuries should be ruled out by palpation of the shoulder and wrist.

Figure 2–22. Simplified classification of elbow dislocation has prognostic implications. *A*, Perched (subluxed). *B*, Complete (dislocated). (*A* and *B*, From Morrey BF: Biomechanics of the elbow and forearm. Orthop Sports Med 17:840, 1994.)

- Complete neurovascular examinations should be done before and after reduction.
- For posterior dislocations:

    The player is removed from the field with the arm supported.

    A neurovascular examination is done, and the patient is placed prone with the arm flexed at 90 degrees over the edge of the table (Fig. 2–23).

    Any medial or lateral translation of the proximal ulna is gently corrected.

    The physician grasps the wrist and applies traction and slight supination of the forearm to distract

    and unlock the coronoid process from the olecranon fossa.

    An assistant places countertraction on the arm. Pressure is applied to the olecranon while the arm is pronated (i.e., palm down) to complete the reduction.

    An obvious "clunk" indicates reduction.

    Neurovascular examination is repeated and elbow instability is evaluated by placing the elbow through a gentle ROM, watching for instability as the elbow is extended. Instability noted at a certain degree of extension (e.g., 20 degrees)

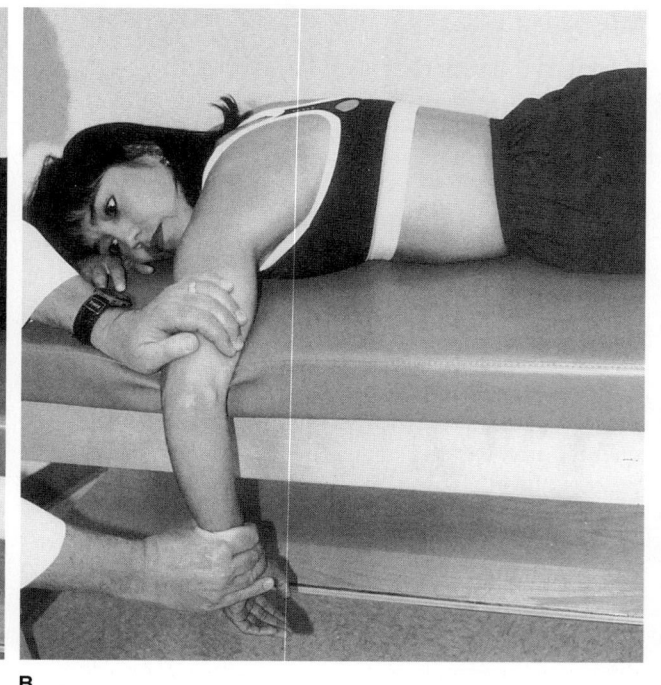

Figure 2–23. *A*, Reduction of a simple posterior elbow dislocation can be done with the patient lying prone and the injured elbow flexed about 90 degrees over the edge of the table. *B*, After correcting any medial or lateral translation of the proximal ulna, the clinician applies downward traction to the forearm and gentle pressure to the olecranon.

should be documented and conveyed to the therapist.

The arm is placed in a sling (at 90 degrees) and iced and elevated.

If an immediate on-the-field reduction cannot be performed, muscle relaxation in the emergency room is of great importance.

Radiographs (anteroposterior [AP] and lateral) of the elbow, forearm, and wrist are obtained to ensure that no associated fractures are present.

Surgical Indications

- For acute elbow dislocations when flexion of the elbow beyond 50 to 60 degrees is required to maintain reduction.
- When the dislocation is associated with an unstable fracture about the joint.

Recurrent Instability after Elbow Dislocation

- Recurrent elbow instability is extremely rare, occurring in fewer than 1 to 2% of patients.
- The MCL has been identified as the primary stabilizer of the elbow joint. Exam and repair of the MCL complex and flexor-pronator musculotendinous origin is recommended.

- The lateral elbow ligaments play a role in stability, keeping the elbow from subluxing posteriorly and rotating away (**posterolateral rotatory instability**).

Important Rehabilitation Points

- **Early *active* mobilization (within the first 2–3 weeks) is needed to avoid post-traumatic stiffness (*not passive mobilization*).**
- Dynamic elbow splints or patient-adjusted progressive static splints should be used if motion is not steadily improving at 4 to 6 weeks after injury.
- **Valgus stressing should be avoided during rehabilitation because it can lead to instability or repeat dislocation.**
- Excessive early passive ROM should be avoided because it increases swelling and inflammation.
- Beginning at week 1, a hinged ROM elbow brace preset from 30 to 90 degrees is worn.
- Each week, motion in the brace is increased by 5 degrees of extension and 10 degrees of flexion.
- **Forced terminal extension should be avoided.** Full elbow extension is less critical for the non-throwing patient and is preferable to recurrent instability.

Rehabilitation Protocol
After Elbow Dislocation
Wilk and Andrews

Phase 1 (Days 1–4)

- Immobilization of elbow at 90 degrees of flexion in a well-padded posterior splint for 3–4 days.
- Begin light gripping exercises (putty or tennis ball).
- **Avoid any passive ROM**
  (patient to perform active ROM when the posterior splint is removed and replaced with a hinged elbow brace or sling).
- **Avoid valgus stresses to the elbow.**
- Use cryotherapy and HVGS.

Phase 2 (Days 4–14)

- Replace the posterior splint with a hinged elbow brace initially set at 15–90 degrees.
- Wrist and finger active ROM in all planes.
- Active elbow ROM (*avoid* valgus stress).
  - Flexion-extension-supination-pronation.
- Multiangle flexion isometrics.
- Multiangle extension isometrics (avoid valgus stress).
- Wrist curls/reverse wrist curls.
- Light biceps curls.

- Shoulder exercises (*avoid external rotation of shoulder, because this places valgus stress at the elbow). The elbow is stabilized during shoulder exercises.

Phase 3 (Weeks 2–6)

- Hinged brace settings 0 degrees to full flexion.
- PRE progression of elbow and wrist exercises.
- Okay to initiate some gentle low-load, long-duration stretching (see Fig. 2–7) around 5–6 weeks for the patient's loss of extension.
- Gradual progression of weight with curls, elbow extension, and so on.
- Sports-specific exercises and drills initiated.
- External rotation and internal rotation exercises of the shoulder may be incorporated at 6–8 weeks.
- Around 8 weeks in the **asymptomatic** patient, start interval throwing program.
- No return to play until strength is 85 to 90% of the uninvolved limb.

Lateral and Medial Epicondylitis

Champ L. Baker Jr., MD, and Mark Baker, PT

Lateral Epicondylitis (Tennis Elbow)

Background

Lateral epicondylitis (tennis elbow) is defined as a pathologic condition of the wrist extensor muscles at their origin on the lateral humeral epicondyle. The tendinous origin of the extensor carpi radialis brevis (ECRB) is the area of most pathologic change. Changes can also be found in the musculotendinous structures of the extensor carpi radialis longus, extensor carpi ulnaris, and extensor digitorum communis (Fig. 2–24A). Overuse or repetitive trauma in this area causes fibrosis and microtears in involved tissues. Nirschl referred to the microtears and the vascular ingrowth of the involved tissues as **angiofibroblastic hyperplasia.** He also suggested the degenerative process should be termed tendinosis rather than tendinitis.

Most patients with lateral epicondylitis are between the ages of 30 and 55 years, and many have poorly conditioned muscles. Ninety-five percent of tennis elbow occurs in *non*–tennis players. Ten to 50% of regular tennis players experience tennis elbow symptoms of varying degree some time in their tennis lives. The most common cause of tennis elbow in tennis players is a "late," mechanically poor backhand (Fig. 2–25) that places excess force across the extensor wad, that is, the elbow "leads" the arm. Other contributing factors include incorrect grip size, string tension, poor racquet "dampening," and underlying weak muscles of the shoulder, elbow, and arm. Tennis grips that are too small often exacerbate or cause tennis elbow.

Often a history of repetitive flexion-extension or pronation-supination activity and overuse is obtained (e.g., twisting a screw driver, lifting heavy luggage with the palm down). Tightly gripping a heavy briefcase is a very common cause. Raking leaves, baseball, golfing, gardening, and bowling can also cause lateral epicondylitis.

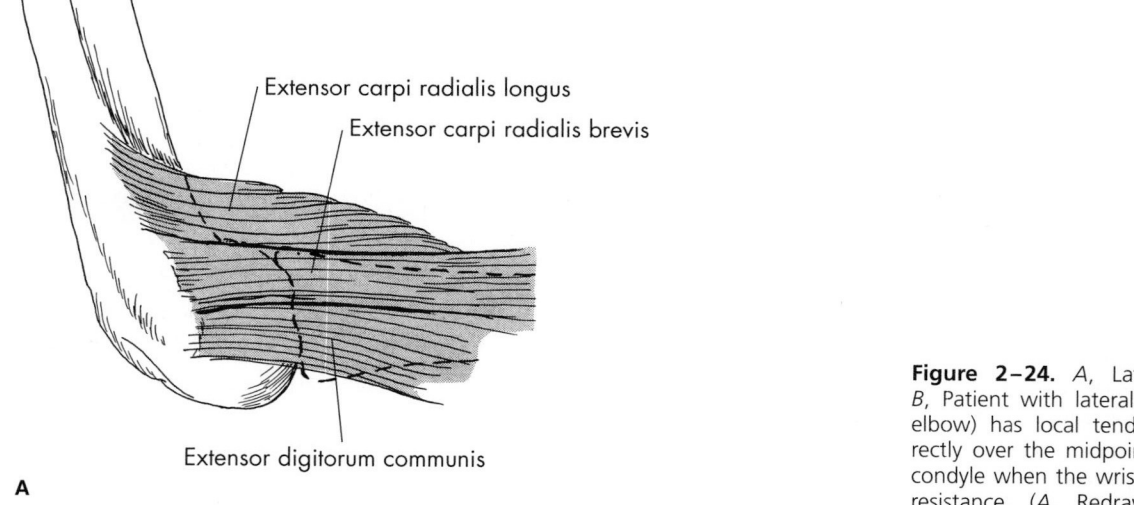

Extensor carpi radialis longus

Extensor carpi radialis brevis

Extensor digitorum communis

A

B

Figure 2–24. *A,* Lateral extensor wad. *B,* Patient with lateral epicondylitis (tennis elbow) has local tenderness and pain directly over the midpoint of the lateral epicondyle when the wrist is extended against resistance. (*A,* Redrawn from Tullos H, Schwab G, Bennett JB, Woods GW: Factors influencing elbow instability. Instr Course Lect 30:185–99, 1981; *B,* from Shaffer B, O'Mara J: Common elbow problems, part 2: management specifics. J Musculoskel Med 14[4]:30, 1997.)

A   **B**

Figure 2–25. *A,* "Late" backhand or "leading with the elbow" causes excessive repetitive force across the extensor wad of the elbow. This results in lateral epicondylitis (tennis elbow). *B,* In the correct position, the arm strikes the ball early, in front of the body, and the arm is raised and extended in follow-through. (From Harding WG: Use and misuse of the tennis elbow strap. Physician Sports Med 20[8]:40, 1992.)

Physical Examination

- Point tenderness typically occurs over the ECRB origin at the lateral epicondyle (see Fig. 2–24B).
- The tenderness may be more generalized over the common extensor wad insertion at the lateral epicondyle (just distal and anterior to the lateral epicondyle).
- The pain is often exacerbated by wrist extension against resistance with the forearm pronated (palm down).
- Elbow extension may be mildly limited.
- *Mill's test* may be positive. With this test, pain occurs over the lateral epicondyle when the wrist and fingers are completely flexed (Fig. 2–26).
- With *Maudsley's test,* the patient may feel pain on resisted extension of the middle finger at the MCP joint when the elbow is fully extended (Fig. 2–27).
- Evaluation should note possible sensory paresthesias in the superficial radial nerve distribution to rule out a *radial tunnel syndrome.* **Radial tunnel syndrome** (Fig. 2–28) is the most common cause of refractory lateral pain and coexists with lateral epicondylitis in 10% of patients.
- The *cervical nerve roots* should be examined to rule out cervical radiculopathy.
- Other conditions that should be considered include bursitis of the bursa below the conjoined tendon, chronic irritation of the radiohumeral joint or capsule, radiocapitellar chondromalacia or arthritis, radial neck fracture, Panner's disease, Little League elbow, and osteochondritis dissecans of the elbow.

Figure 2–26. Mill test. Pain occurs over the lateral epicondyle when the wrist and fingers are completely flexed.

Differential Diagnosis of Lateral Elbow Pain

	Type, Site of Pain	Provocative Test	Neurologic Findings
Lateral epicondylitis	Well localized point tenderness over lateral epicondyle, pain increases with use	Resisted wrist extension; resisted forearm pronation; chair-lift test	None
Intra-articular pathology	Generalized elbow pain	Axial compression test	None
Cervical radiculopathy	Diffuse lateral arm pain; neck pain and/or stiffness	Limited neck ROM; Spurling test positive	Abnormal reflex, sensory, or motor examination results; abnormal EMG/NCS
Radial tunnel syndrome	Vague, diffuse forearm ache; pain more distal than in lateral epicondylitis; pain present at rest	Resisted long-finger extension; resisted forearm supination; positive differential lidocaine injection	Paresthesias in the first dorsal web space of hand (5–10%); abnormal EMG/NCS (10%)

EMG, electromyography; NCS, nerve conduction study.
From Warhold LG, Osterman AL, Shirven T: Lateral epicondylitis: how to test it and prevent recurrence. J Musculoskel Med June 10(10):243, 1993.

Nonoperative Treatment

Activity Modification

- In nonathletes, **elimination of the activities that are painful** is key to improvement (e.g., repetitive valve opening).
- Treatments such as ice and NSAIDs may lessen the inflammation, but continued repetition of the aggravating motion will prolong any recovery.
- Often, repetitive pronation-supination motions and lifting heavy weights at work can be modified or eliminated. Activity modifications such as avoidance of grasping in pronation (Fig. 2–29) and substituting controlled supination lifting instead may relieve symptoms (Fig. 2–30).

- Lifting should be done with the palms *up* (supination) whenever possible, and *both* upper extremities should be used in a manner that reduces forcible elbow extension, supination, and wrist extension.

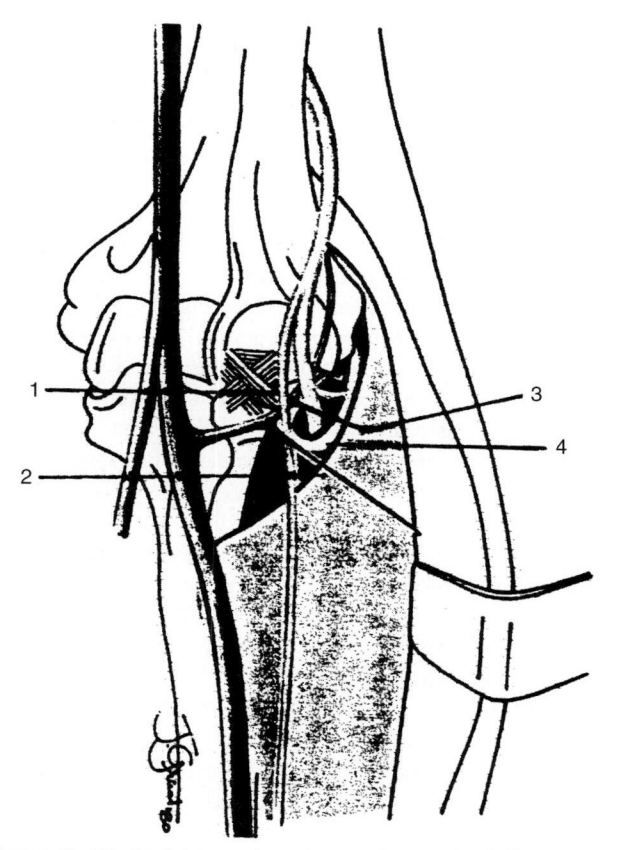

Figure 2–28. Radial tunnel syndrome. Four potentially compressive anatomic elements: (1) Fibrous bands overlying the radial head and capsule. (2) Fibrous origin of the extensor carpi radialis brevis (ECRB). (3) Radial recurrent arterial fan. (4) Arcade of Frohse. (From Moss S, Switzer H: Radial tunnel syndrome: a spectrum of clinical presentations. J Hand Surg 8:415, 1983.)

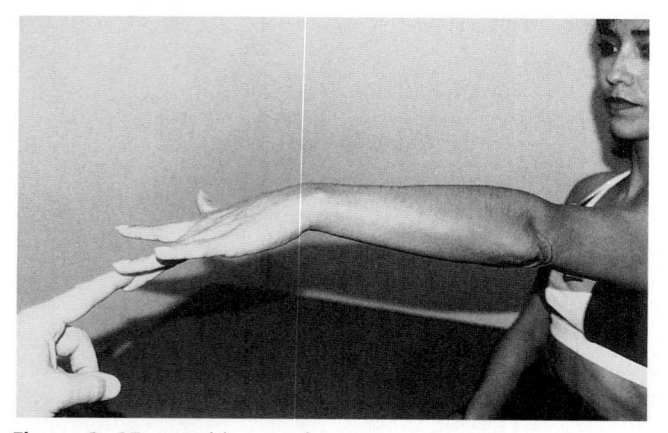

Figure 2–27. Maudsley test for lateral epicondylitis. Pain on resisted extension of the middle finger at the metacarpophalangeal (MCP) I joint when the elbow is fully extended.

Figure 2–29. Modify activity by avoiding grasping heavy objects in pronation (i.e., incorrectly).

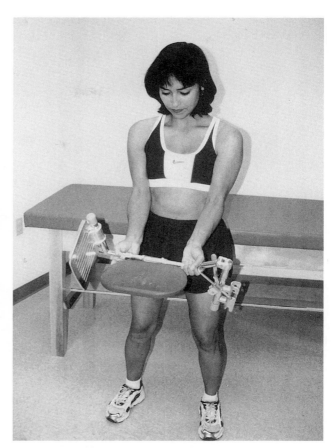

Figure 2–30. Lifting in supination (palm up) with both upper extremities. This is the correct way to avoid pain in patients with lateral epicondylitis of the extensor wad.

Correction of Mechanics

- If a late or poor backhand causes pain, **correction of the mechanics of the stroke** is warranted.
- Avoidance of ball impact that lacks a forward body weight transference is stressed.
- If typing with unsupported arms exacerbates the pain, placing the elbows on stacked towels for support will help.

Nonsteroidal Anti-inflammatory Drugs

- If not contraindicated, we use Cox-2 inhibitors (rofe-coxib [Vioxx], celecoxib [Celebrex]) for their improved safety profile.

Icing

- Ten to 15 minutes of ice, four to six times a day.

Stretching

- ROM of exercises emphasizing end-range and passive stretching (elbow in full extension and wrist in flexion with slight ulnar deviation) (Figs. 2–31 and 2–32).

Counterforce Bracing

- Bracing is used only during actual play or aggravating activity.

- The tension is adjusted to comfort while the muscles are relaxed so that maximal contraction of the finger and wrist extensors is inhibited by the band (Fig. 2–33).
- The band is placed two fingerbreadths distal to the painful area of the lateral epicondyle.
- Some authors recommend 6 to 8 weeks' use of a **wrist splint** positioned in 45 degrees of dorsiflexion.
- Tennis players may reduce racquet string tension, change the size of the grip (usually to a larger grip), and change to a better dampening racquet. For grip size, Nirschl recommended measuring the length from the proximal palmar crease to the tip of the ring finger with a ruler (Fig. 2–34). If the distance is 4.5 inches, the grip should be a $4\frac{1}{2}$.

Cortisone Injection

- We have had excellent results with injection of cortisone for tennis elbow.
- We recommend injecting no more often than every 3 months, and no more than three injections a year to avoid possible tendon rupture.

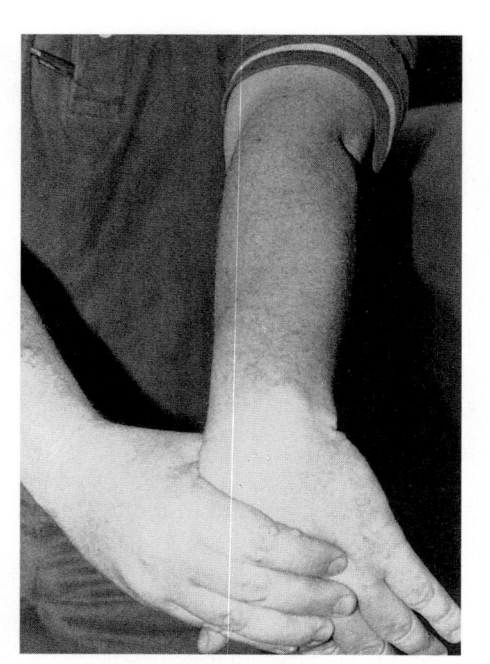

Figure 2–31. Wrist extensor stretch for lateral epicondylitis. With the elbow in extension and the wrist in flexion and slight ulnar deviation, the patient performs five or six stretches, holding for 30 seconds. Repeat two or three times a day.

Figure 2–32. Wrist flexor wad stretching for medial epicondylitis. With the elbow in extension and the wrist in extension and slight radial deviation, the patient performs five or six stretches, holding for 30 seconds. Repeat two or three times a day.

Technique

- Use 2 ml of lidocaine in a 25-gauge 1-inch needle centered at the point of maximal tenderness at the ECRB origin, not entering the tendon.
- The needle is left in place, and then the syringe is changed and 0.5 ml of betamethasone (Celestone) is injected. This is preferred rather than skin infiltration with cortisone to avoid skin and subcutaneous tissue atrophy from the steroid.

Range of Motion Exercises (see Figs. 2–31 and 2–32)

- Exercises emphasize end-range and passive stretching (elbow in full extension and wrist in flexion with slight ulnar deviation).
- Soft tissue mobilization is done with and perpendicular to the tissue involved.
- Phonophoresis or iontophoresis may be helpful.

Tennis elbow strap

Lateral epicondyle

Extensor carpi radialis brevis

Figure 2–33. Lateral counterforce brace for elbow (lateral epicondylitis). Place the brace two fingerbreadths distal to the lateral epicondyle (snug). This attempts to work as a counterforce brace that places some stress at the brace itself rather than causing proximal insertional pain at the lateral epicondyle.

Figure 2–34. Nirschl technique for proper handle size measured from the proximal palmar crease to the tip of the ring finger. Place the measuring rule between the ring and the long fingers for proper ruler placement on the palmar crease. The measurement obtained is the proper handle size—that is, if this distance is 4½ inches, the proper handle size is 4½ inches. (By permission of the Mayo Foundation for Medical Education and Research.)

Strengthening Exercises

- A **gentle strengthening program** should be used for grip strength, wrist extensors, wrist flexors, biceps, triceps, and rotator cuff strengthening.

- *However, the acute inflammatory phase must have resolved first, with 2 weeks of no pain before initiation of graduated strengthening exercises.*
- Development of symptoms (i.e., pain) modifies the exercise progression, with a lower level of intensity and more icing if pain recurs.
- The exercise program includes:
  - Active motion and submaximal isometrics.
  - Isotonic eccentric hand exercises with graduated weights not to exceed 5 pounds.
- Wrist curls

    Sit with the hand over the knee. With palm up (supination), bend the wrist 10 times holding a 1- to 2-pound weight. Increase to two sets of 10 daily; then increase the weight by 1 pound up to 5–6 pounds. Repeat this with the palm down (pronation), but progress to only 4 pounds.
- Forearm strengthening

    Hold the arm out in front of the body, palm down. The patient clenches the fingers, bends the wrist up (extension), and holds it tight for 10 seconds. Next, with the other hand, the patient attempts to push the hand down. Hold for 10 seconds, 5 repetitions, slowly increasing to 20 repetitions two to three times a day.

    Weight on the end of a rope (Fig. 2–35) can be used to strengthen wrist flexors and extensors. The patient rolls up a string with a weight tied on the end. The weight can be progressively increased. Flexors are worked with the palms up; extensors with the palm down.

Figure 2–35. Wrist flexors and extensors. The patient rolls up a string with a weight tied on the end. The weight may be progressively increased. Flexors are worked with the palms up, the extensors with the palms down. (From Galloway M, De Maio M, Mangine R: Rehabilitative techniques in the treatment of medial and lateral epicondylitis. Orthopedics 15[9]:1089, 1992.)

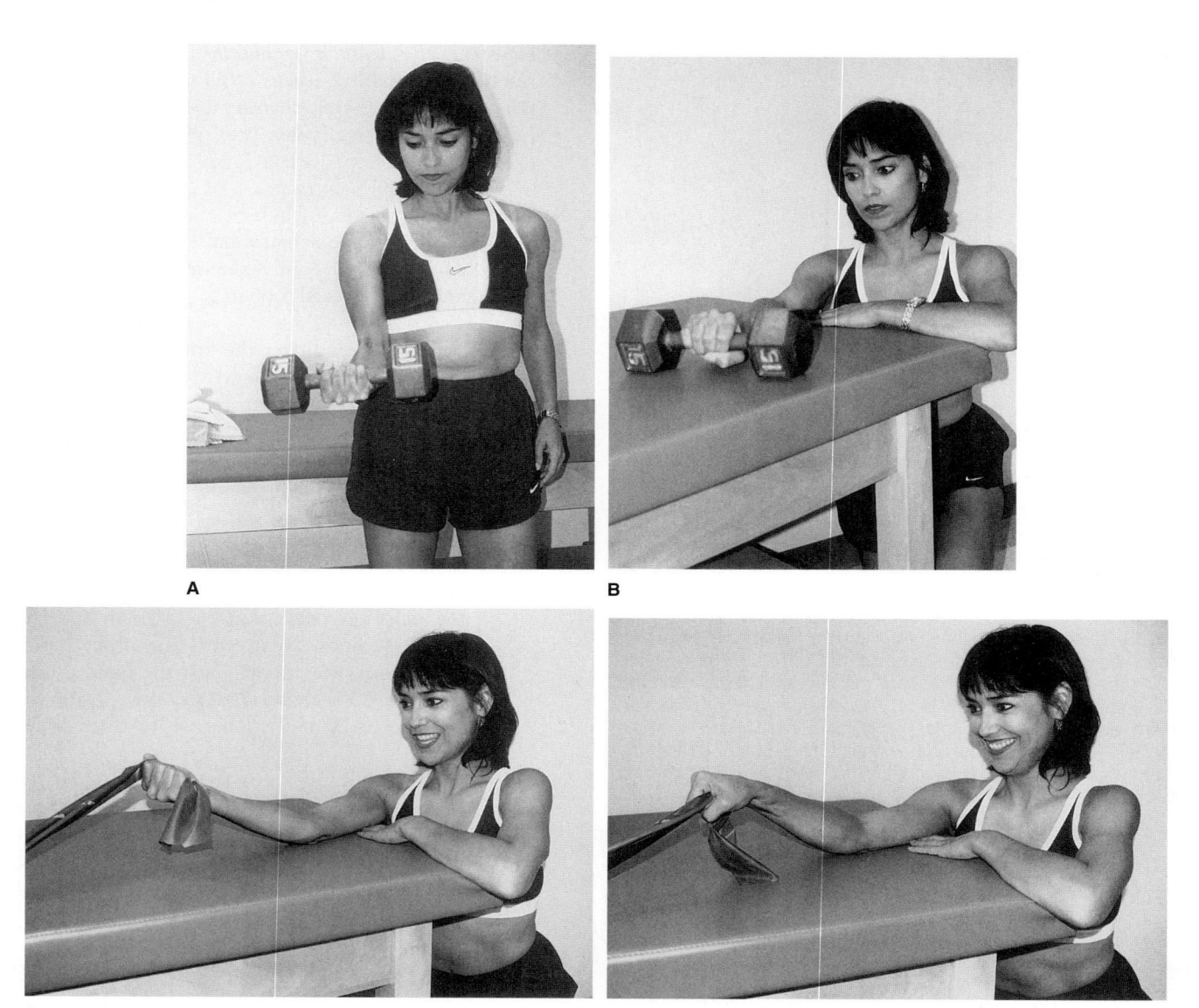

Figure 2–36. *A*, Wrist flexion-resistive training. *B*, Wrist extension-resistive training. *C*, Elbow flexion-Theraband training. *D*, Elbow extension-Theraband training.

Elbow flexion and extension exercises (Figs. 2–36 and 2–37).

Squeeze a racquetball repetitively for forearm and hand strength.

• Progress strength, flexibility, and endurance in a *graduated* fashion with slow-velocity exercises involving application of gradually increasing resistance. A "no-pain–no-gain" philosophy is incorrect here.

Galloway, DeMaio, and Mangine also divide their approach to patients with epicondylitis (medial or lat-

eral) into three stages: The *initial phase* is directed toward reducing inflammation, preparing the patient for phase 2. The *second phase* emphasizes return of strength and endurance. Specific inciting factors are identified and modified. *Phase 3* involves functional rehabilitation designed to return the patient to the desired activity level. This protocol is also based on the severity of the initial symptoms and objective findings at initiation of treatment.

Rehabilitation Protocol
Evaluation-based Rehabilitation of Medial and Lateral Epicondylitis
Galloway, DeMaio, and Mangine

Rationale: Patients begin a rehabilitation protocol based on their symptoms and objective physical findings. The *initial phase* of each protocol is directed toward restoring ROM at the wrist and elbow. *Phase 2* involves strength training and a structured return to activity. First, obtain relief of acute pain and then increase forearm extensor power, flexibility, and endurance.

	Protocol 1 (Severe Symptoms)	Protocol 2 (Mild/Moderate Symptoms)	Protocol 3 (Symptoms Resolved)
When	• Pain at rest. • Point tenderness. • Pain with minimally re-sisted wrist extension. • Swelling. • Grip strength difference (GSD) > 50%. • > 5 degrees motion loss at wrist or elbow.	• Pain with activity only. • Minimal point tenderness. • Minimal pain with resisted wrist flexion-extension. • GSD > 50%. • No motion loss.	• No pain with daily activity. • No referred pain. • Full ROM. • GSD < 10%.
Evaluation	• Duration of symptoms. • Referred pain. • Grip strength measure-ment. • Elbow palpation. • Motion measurement. • History of injury or incit-ing activity. • Differential diagnosis.	• Duration of symptoms. • Referred pain. • Grip strength measure-ment. • Elbow palpation. • Motion measurement. • History of injury or incit-ing activity. • Differential diagnosis.	• Review initial injury or inciting activity. • Identify requirements for returning to desired activ-ity. • Identify remaining func-tional deficits.

Treatment	**Phase 1 (Reduce Inflammation)**
	• Rest.
	• Passive ROM.
	• Cold therapy.
	• Medications.
	
	Phase 2 (Rehabilitation)
	• Limit activity.
	• Cold therapy.
	• Stretching (static).
	• Strengthening (isometric).
	• Ultrasound.
	• HVGS.
	• Proceed to protocol 2 when tolerating above.
	• Surgical indications.
		Phase 1 (Reduce Inflammation)
		• Rest.
		• Passive ROM.
		• Cold therapy.
		• Medications.
		
		Phase 2 (Rehabilitation)
		• Limit activity.
		• Flexibility.
		• Strengthening.
		• Transverse friction massage.
		• Cold therapy.
		• HVGS.
		• Ultrasound.
		• Proceed to protocol 3.
			• Preactivity flexibility.
			• Strengthening
			  • Isokinetics.
			  • Isotonic.
			• Modalities
			  • Whirlpool.
			  • Ice after activity.
			• Technique modification.
			• Equipment modification.
			• Counterforce bracing.
			• Friction massage.
			• Gradual return to activity.

Goals	• Resolution of pain at rest. • Tolerate stretching/strengthening with mini-mal discomfort. • Improve ROM. • Maintain cardiovascular conditioning.	• No pain with daily activity. • No pain with stretch-ing/(PREs). • Full ROM. • Prepare for functional rehabilitation. • Maintain cardiovascular conditioning.	• Pain-free return to activity. • Prevent recurrence—maintenance program of stretching.

Rehabilitation Protocol
After Lateral Epicondylitis Surgery
Baker and Baker

Days 1–7

- Position the extremity in a sling for comfort.
- Control edema and inflammation: apply ice for 20 minutes two or three times a day.
- Gentle hand, wrist, and elbow ROM exercises. Exercises should be done in a pain-free range.
- Active shoulder ROM (glenohumeral joint), lower trapezius setting.

Weeks 2–4

- Remove sling.
- Advance ROM passive motion. Passive motion should be continued and combined with active-assisted motion within the patient's pain tolerance.
- Gentle strengthening exercises with active motion and submaximal isometrics.
- Edema and inflammation control: continue ice application 20 minutes two or three times a day.
- Shoulder strengthening: manual D1 and D2 proprioceptive neuromuscular facilitation to the glenohumeral

joint with the patient supine. Scapular strengthening with manual resistance and continued lower trapezius setting.

Weeks 5–7

- Advance strengthening as tolerated to include weights or rubber tubing.
- ROM with contined emphasis on end-range and passive overpressure.
- Edema and inflammation control with ice application for 20 minutes after activity.
- Modified activities in preparation for beginning functional training.
- Gentle massage along and against fiber orientation.
- Counterforce bracing.

Weeks 8–12

- Continue counterforce bracing if needed.
- Begin task-specific functional training.
- Return to sport or activities.

Surgical Treatment

Surgical treatment of tennis elbow is not considered unless the patient has recalcitrant symptoms for more than 1 year despite the nonoperative treatment previously discussed. Various operations have been described for tennis elbow pain. Many authors have recommended excision of torn, scarred ECRB origin, removal of granulation tissue, and subchondral bone drilling for neovascularization stimulation. The elbow capsule is not violated unless intra-articular pathology exists. We prefer to treat these patients arthroscopically whenever possible. Arthroscopic release of the ECRB tendon and decortication of the lateral epicondyle are analagous to the open procedure. Arthroscopic treatment of lateral epicondylitis offers several potential advantages over open procedures, and its success rate is comparable. The lesion is addressed directly, and the common extensor origin is preserved. Arthroscopy also allows for an intra-articular examination for other disorders. It also permits a shorter postoperative rehabilitation period and an earlier return to work or sports.

Postoperatively, we encourage our patients to begin active ROM within the first 24 to 48 hours. The patient is usually seen for follow-up within the first 72 hours. At this time, she or he is encouraged to begin extension and flexion exercises. After the swelling subsides, usually 2 to 3 weeks after surgery, the patient can rapidly regain full ROM and begin strengthening exercises. Return to throwing sports is allowed when the patient has regained full strength.

Medial Epicondylitis (Golfer's Elbow)

Medial epicondylitis (golfer's elbow) is far less frequent than lateral epicondylitis, but it also requires a detailed examination because of the proximity to other medial structures that may mimic medial epicondylitis. Exclusion of other etiologies of medial elbow pain is important for appropriate treatment.

Medial epicondylitis (often called golfer's elbow) is defined as a pathologic condition that involves the pronator teres and flexor carpi radialis origins at the medial epicondyle. However, abnormal changes in the flexor carpi ulnaris and palmaris longus origins at the elbow may also be present.

Repetitive trauma resulting in microtears is a causative factor. Throwing athletes who have repetitive valgus stress on the elbow and repetitive flexor forearm musculature pull develop an overuse syndrome that affects the medial common flexor origin. Medial epicondylitis is an example of medial tension overload of the elbow. Tennis, racquetball, squash, and throwing often produce this condition. The serve and forearm strokes are the most likely to bring on pain.

A   B

Figure 2–37. Elbow Theraband strengthening exercises.

Examination

Medial epicondylitis is diagnosed clinically by pain and tenderness to palpation localized to the medial epicondyle with wrist flexion and pronation against resistance (Fig. 2–38). Medial pain is often elicited after making a tight fist, and grip strength is usually decreased.

It is *extremely important* to differentiate medial epicondylitis from UCL rupture and instability. In the latter, valgus stress testing reveals UCL pain and opening (instability) of the elbow joint (Fig. 2–39). Concomitant ulnar neuropathy at the elbow may be present with either of these conditions.

Differential Diagnosis

UCL Rupture in Throwers

• Valgus stress testing of the elbow identifies injury to the UCL.

Figure 2–38. Medial epicondylitis may be diagnosed clinically by pain localized to the medial epicondyle during wrist flexion and pronation against resistance. Pain is often elicited after making a tight fist, and grip strength is usually diminished on the affected side. (From Morrey BF: The Elbow and Its Disorders. Philadelphia, WB Saunders, 1985.)

Figure 2–39. *A,* Medial joint pain elicited by placing a valgus stretch to the elbow identifies injury to the UCL. *B,* To test for valgus instability, the patient's elbow is supinated and flexed 20 to 25 degrees to release the olecranon. The examiner stabilizes the humerus by grasping above the condyles with one hand. The other hand applies valgus stress to the elbow with an abduction force to the distal ulna. (*A,* From Morrey BF: The Elbow and Its Disorders. Philadelphia, WB Saunders, 1985; *B,* from Nirschl RP, Kraushaar BS: Assessment and treatment guidelines for elbow injuries. Physician Sports Med 24[5]:230, 1996.)

- A valgus stress is applied to the arm with the elbow slightly flexed and the forearm supinated (see Fig. 2–39B). Opening of the joint is indicative of UCL rupture and instability.

Ulnar Neuropathy

- Tinel sign is positive at the elbow over the ulnar nerve in the cubital tunnel (elbow) with chronic neuropathy.
- Concomitant compression neuropathy symptoms are often present, with numbness and tingling into the ulnar two (fourth and fifth) fingers.
- Ulnar neuropathy in throwers is seldom isolated and is often found concomitantly with the UCL injury or medial epicondylitis because of traction on the nerve in the unstable elbow.
- Other causes of medial elbow pain to be considered are osteochondritis dissecans of the elbow and osteoarthritis.

Nonoperative Treatment

- Nonoperative treatment of medial epicondylitis is similar to that of lateral epicondylitis and begins with modifying or stopping activities that produce tension overload, the underlying etiology of medial epicondyli-

tis, and correction of training errors (overuse) and throwing mechanics causing the tension overload.
- NSAIDs and icing are used for control of edema and inflammation.
- Braces exist that provide counterforce bracing to the medial flexor wad, but we have had little success with these.
- Stretching and ROM exercises are the same as those described for lateral epicondylitis.
- After the acute pain and inflammation subside, strengthening exercises of the elbow, forearm, wrist, and rotator cuff are begun, concentrating on strengthening of the wrist flexors (see Lateral epicondylitis Protocol).
- For persistent symptoms, cortisone injection (0.5 ml of betamethasone) into the area of maximal tenderness may be useful, but should be given no more frequently than every 3 months and no more than three injections per year (see section on injection technique for lateral epicondylitis). The needle must stay anterior to the medial epicondyle to avoid the ulnar nerve (posterior to the injection site). *If the patient has radiating pain down into the forearm or fingers (accidental nerve injection), do not inject.*
- Surgical intervention may be indicated for symptoms that persist longer than 1 year.

Rehabilitation Protocol
Lateral or Medial Epicondylitis
Wilk and Andrews

Phase 1—Acute Phase

- Goals
  - Decrease inflammation/pain.
  - Promote tissue healing.
  - Retard muscle atrophy.
- Cryotherapy.
- Whirlpool.
- Stretching to increase flexibility
  - Wrist extension-flexion.
  - Elbow extension-flexion.
  - Forearm supination-pronation.
- HVGS.
- Phonophoresis.
- Friction massage.
- Iontophoresis (with an anti-inflammatory such as dexamethasone).
- Avoid painful movements (such as gripping).

Phase 2—Subacute Phase

- Goals
  - Improve flexibility.
  - Increase muscular strength and endurance.
  - Increase functional activities and return to function.
  - Emphasize concentric-eccentric strengthening.
  - Concentrate on involved muscle group(s).
  - Wrist extension-flexion.
  - Forearm pronation-supination.
- Elbow flexion-extension.
- Initiate shoulder strengthening (if deficiencies are noted).
- Continue flexibility exercises.
- Use counterforce brace.
- Continue use of cryotherapy after exercise or function.
- Initiate gradual return to stressful activities.
- Gradually reinitiate previously painful movements.

Phase 3—Chronic Phase

- Goals
  - Improve muscular strength and endurance.
  - Maintain/enhance flexibility.
  - Gradually return to sport high-level activities.
- Continue strengthening exercises (emphasize eccentric-concentric).
- Continue to emphasize deficiencies in shoulder and elbow strength.
- Continue flexibility exercises.
- Gradually diminish use of counterforce brace.
- Use cryotherapy as needed.
- Initiate gradual return to sport activity.
- Equipment modifications (grip size, string tension, playing surface).
- Emphasize maintenance program.

A patient is advanced to high-level functional activities when elbow ROM is normal and pain free and strength is within 10% of the uninvolved extremity. It is imperative to monitor these criteria closely to avoid the tendency of lateral and medial epicondylitis to become chronic.

Summary of Elbow Rehabilitation Principles for Epicondylitis

The guidelines for rehabilitation are centered on tissue healing constraints and the constraints of pain and activity. The strengthening phase of rehabilitation begins with active motion and submaximal isometrics. When these activities are tolerated for 1.5 weeks without complications, the patient is progressed with PREs.

We recommend a low load for lower repetitions two times a day initially, progressing to moderate intensity for higher repetitions three times a day. ROM is very important during the entire rehabilitation process; however, increased emphasis should be placed on ROM during the first 4 weeks to prevent fibrosis of the healing tissues. The therapist must also take into consideration the factor of irritation, which, if ignored, will lead to further fibrosis owing to inflammation.

The differences in the rehabilitation protocols for medial and lateral epicondylitis are, of course, due to the anatomy. However, this protocol can guide the clinician in developing a specific program to meet the patient's needs. One thing remains constant: we must limit harmful forces that can cause further degeneration of the involved tissue during the nonoperative or postoperative rehabilitation period. A factor that should always be considered in the patient undergoing postoperative rehabilitation is the realization that the patient's condition was unresponsive to conservative treatment. Therefore, timelines and progression should always be presentation specific. If these guidelines are followed with core general principles, patients should return to modification-free activities. ■

Isolated Fracture of the Radial Head

Mason's classification of radial head fractures is the most widely accepted and useful for determining treatment

TYPE I

TYPE II

TYPE III

TYPE IV

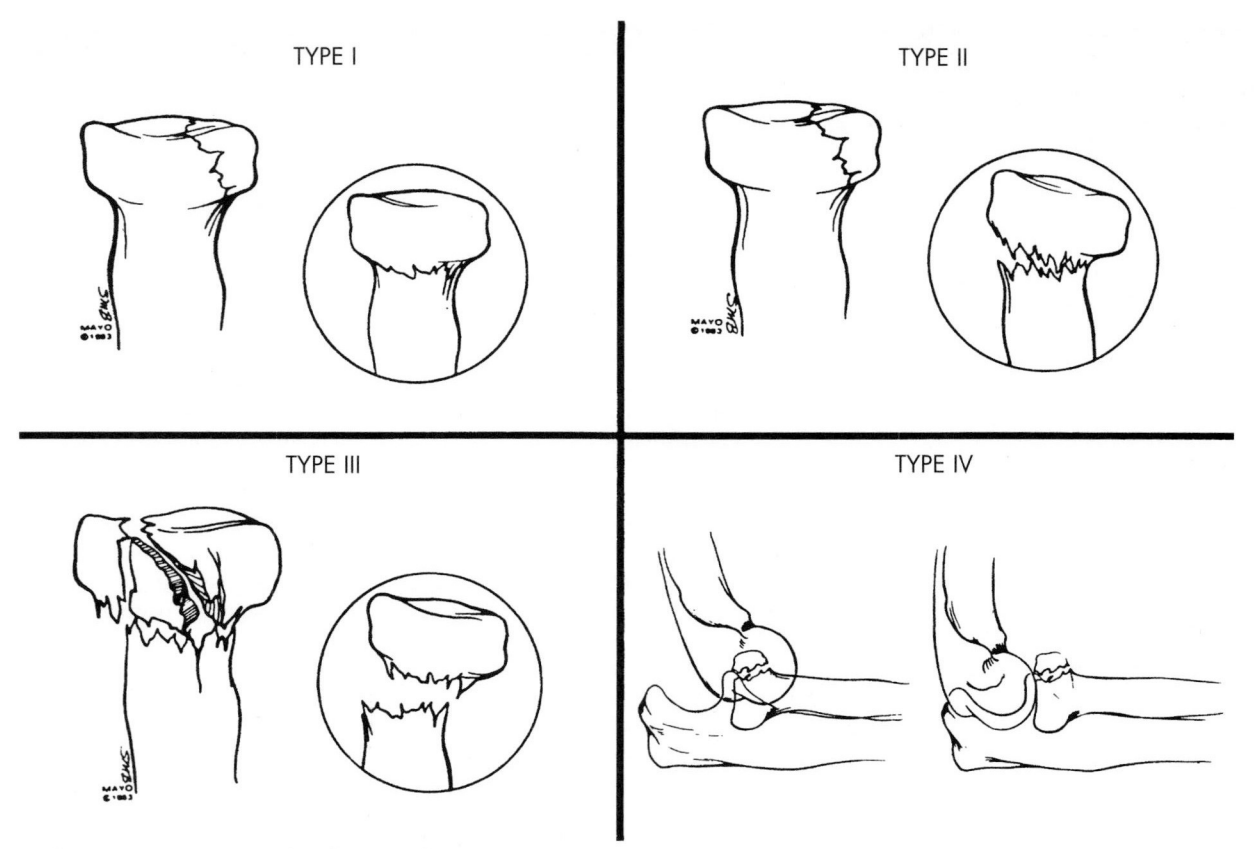

Figure 2–40. Mason's classification of radial head fractures. (From Broberg MA, Morrey BF: Results of treatment of fracture dislocations of the elbow. Clin Orthop 216:109, 1987.)

(Fig. 2–40; Table 2–1). Rehabilitation is also based on this classification.

Table 2–1

Mason Classification of Radial Head Fractures

Type	Description	Treatment
I	Nondisplaced fracture Often missed on radiograph Positive posterior fat pad sign	Minimal immobilization and early motion
II	Marginal radial head fracture with displacement, depression, or angulation	ORIF, early motion
III	Comminuted fracture of the entire radial head	Open reduction and internal fixation, early motion if possible
IV	Concomitant dislocation of the elbow or other associated injuries	Radial head resection Check distal wrist joint (Essex-Lopresti injury) Guarded prognosis for return to sports

ORIF, open reduction and internal fixation.

Rehabilitation Principles

- *Nondisplaced type I* fractures require little or no immobilization.
- Active and passive ROM can begin immediately after injury to promote full ROM.
- Conditioning in the form of elbow flexion and extension, supination and pronation isometrics, and wrist and shoulder isotonics can be implemented immediately (usually within the first week) after injury.
- Stress (e.g., heavy lifting) to the radial head is minimized.
- Three to 6 weeks of active elbow flexion and extension can be used, along with wrist isotonics.
- *Types II and III* fractures usually require ORIF. Frequently, immobilization is required for a brief time, followed by active and passive ROM exercises.
- *Type IV* comminuted fractures frequently require stabilization of the elbow joint and excision of fragments and usually cause some functional limitation.

Full ROM rarely returns in type IV injuries and chronic elbow pain often persists.

Rehabilitation Protocol
After Radial Head Fracture
(Type I Fracture of Type II or III Fracture Stabilized with ORIF)

Phase 1—Immediate Motion Phase

- Goals
  - Decrease pain and inflammation.
  - Regain full wrist and elbow ROM.
  - Retard muscular atrophy.

Week 1
- Begin elbow active ROM and active-assisted ROM; minimal accepted ROM (15–105 degrees) by 2 weeks.
- Begin putty/gripping exercises.
- Begin isometric strengthening exercises (elbow and wrist).
- Begin isotonic strengthening exercises for wrist.

Phase 2—Intermediate Phase

- Goals
  - Maintain full elbow ROM.
  - Progress elbow strengthening exercises.
  - Gradually increase functional demands.

Week 3
- Initiate shoulder strengthening exercises; concentrate on rotator cuff.
- Continue ROM exercises for elbow (full flexion-extension).

- Initiate light-resistance elbow flexion-extension (1 pound).
- Initiate active-assisted ROM and passive ROM supination-pronation to tolerance.

Week 6
- Continue active-assisted ROM and passive ROM supination-pronation to full range.
- Progress shoulder program.
- Progress elbow strengthening exercises.

Phase 3—Advanced Strengthening Phase

- Goals
  - Maintain full elbow ROM.
  - Increase strength, power, endurance.
  - Gradually initiate sporting activities.

Week 7
- Continue active-assisted ROM and passive ROM to full supination-pronation.
- Initiate eccentric elbow flexion-extension.
- Initiate plyometric exercise program.
- Continue isotonic program for forearm, wrist, and shoulder.
- Continue until 12 weeks.

Elbow Arthroplasty

Indications for elbow arthroplasty include:

- Pain, instability, and bilateral ankylosis, such as in patients with advanced stage 3 or 4 rheumatoid arthrosis that is unresponsive to medical management.
- Failed interpositional or anatomic arthroplasty.
- Failed prosthetic arthroplasty.
- Arthrodesis in poor functional position.
- After en bloc resection for tumor.
- Degenerative arthrosis after failed débridement and loose body excision.
- Rheumatoid arthrosis in which synovectomy and radial head excision have failed.

Contraindications to elbow arthroplasty include:

- Active infection.
- Absent flexors or flail elbow from motor paralysis.
- Noncompliant patient with respect to activity limitations.
- Inadequate posterior skin quality.
- Inadequate bone stock or ligamentous instability with resurfacing inplants.
- Neurotrophic joint.

Elbow prostheses are classified as **semiconstrained** (loose-hinge or sloppy-hinge), **nonconstrained** (minimally constrained), or **fully constrained.** Fully constrained prostheses are no longer used because of their unacceptable failure rate.

Rehabilitation Protocol
After Total Elbow Replacement

3 Days
- Remove bulky dressing and replace with light compressive dressing.

- Begin active ROM exercises for the elbow and forearm six times a day for 10 to 15 minutes. *Active ROM exercises should be performed with the elbow close to the body to*
  continued

Rehabilitation Protocol
After Total Elbow Replacement (*Continued*)

avoid excessive stretch of the reconstructed elbow collateral ligaments.
- Fit an elbow extension splint to be worn between exercise sessions and at night.

Week 2
- Passive ROM exercises may be initiated to the elbow.
- Functional electrical stimulation (FES) may be initiated to stimulate biceps or triceps or both.

Week 6
- Discontinue elbow extension splint during the day if elbow stability is adequate.

- ROM exercises may now be performed with the elbow away from body.

Week 8
- Discontinue elbow extension splint at night.
- Initiate gradual, gentle strengthening exercises for the hand and forearm. Light resistance may be begun to the elbow.
- Perform therapy within the patient's comfort level.

From Cannon NM: Diagnosis and Treatment Manual for Physicians and Therapists, 3rd ed. Indianapolis, The Hand Rehabilitation Center of Indiana, PC, 1991.

Olecranon Bursitis

Olecranon bursitis, inflammation (or infection) of the subcutaneous bursa overlying the posterior olecranon process, may be acute (traumatic) or chronic, aseptic or septic. Because the bursa is not developed until after the age of 7 years, this condition is rare in children. The mechanism of injury may be a direct blow (fall on playing surface) or chronic repeated trauma with gradual fluid accumulation. Infection can result from hematogenous seeding (*Staphylococcus aureus*) or direct inoculation (cut or injection).

Physical examination usually reveals posterior elbow swelling and tenderness with a palpable, often large, bursa. In septic bursitis, the area often is warm and erythematous. Although there is no intra-articular involvement, extreme flexion may be limited.

Treatment of aseptic bursitis includes a compression dressing, icing, and a soft elbow pad to avoid constant irritation. We employ a Hayes universal elbow pad manufactured by Hely and Weber (1-800-221-5465). These measures should allow gradual resorption of the fluid. If motion of the elbow is severely affected, the bursa is aspirated and the aspirate is sent for Gram stain and culture studies. Septic bursitis requires incision and drainage, open wound management, and antibiotic therapy based on culture results. Gentle active ROM can be initiated, but excessive ROM should be avoided until the wound is stable.

Post-Traumatic Elbow Stiffness

Michael L. Lee, MD, and Melvin P. Rosenwasser, MD

Evaluation and Management

Stiffness of the elbow can result from congenital deformities, paralytic deformities, degenerative arthrosis, burns, or infections, but by far the most common is post-traumatic.

The "normal" arc of motion of the elbow, as defined by the American Academy of Orthopaedic Surgeons, is 0 degrees extension to 146 degrees flexion, and 71 degrees pronation to 84 degrees supination. Morrey and coworkers (1981) have determined that the ROM required for activities of daily living, the "functional ROM," is extension-flexion 30 degrees and 130 degrees and pronation-supination 50 to 50 degrees. Terminal flexion is more important to activities of daily living than is terminal extension.

Classification

Post-traumatic elbow stiffness has been divided by Morrey (1993) into extrinsic (extra-articular), intrinsic (intra-articular), and mixed causes.

Extrinsic (Extra-articular) Causes of Elbow Stiffness

Skin, subcutaneous tissue
Capsule (posterior or anterior)
Collateral ligament contracture
Myostatic contracture (posterior or anterior)
Heterotopic ossification (HO)

Intrinsic (Intra-articular) Causes of Elbow Stiffness

Articular deformity
Articular adhesions
Impinging osteophytes
  Olecranon
  Coronoid
Impinging fibrosis
  Olecranon fossa
  Coronoid fossa
Loose bodies
Mixed

Extrinsic causes include everything about the elbow except the articular surface itself, from the skin down to the capsule and collateral ligaments. Skin contractures or subcutaneous scarring from incisions or burns can limit elbow motion. Direct elbow capsular injury, injury to the brachialis, or injury to the triceps causes hematoma resulting in scarring in a contracted position with limitation of motion. Collateral ligament injury with subsequent healing in the contracted position can alter the normal axis of motion, further inhibiting the arc of motion.

In addition, acute pain induces both a voluntary and an involuntary guarding of the elbow against motion—thus promoting contracture of the elbow capsule and brachialis muscle—and is thought to be the mechanism behind elbow stiffness in minor trauma to the elbow with minimal soft tissue injury. Entrapment neuropathies, most commonly of the ulnar nerve, but also reported in the radial and median nerve, can cause pain resulting in guarding against motion.

Intrinsic causes can result from articular incongruity, loss of articular cartilage, hypertrophic callus on the articular surface, intra-articular adhesions, fibrosis within the normal fossa (coronoid or olecranon), or hypertrophic impinging osteophytes.

Evaluation of the Stiff Elbow

History

The two most important answers to be gleaned from the history are

1. The perceived deficits in motion.
2. Whether or not the elbow is painful.

Deficits in pronation-supination imply radiocapitellar pathology, and deficits in flexion-extension imply ulnohumeral pathology. Unless there is severe HO ossification or complete ankylosis, either pronation-supination or flexion-extension will predominate in the patient's complaints. Deficits in extension less than 30 degrees or deficits of less than 100 degrees total arc of motion are within the functional ROM, and surgical correction is unlikely to be of benefit.

Normally, post-traumatic elbow stiffness is not painful. Pain implies arthrosis, impingement, entrapment neuropathy, or less frequently, instability.

Physical Examination

Physical examination begins with inspection of skin, noting scars and areas of fibrosis in the preoperative planning of surgical approach. The nature of skin loss, fibrosis, or adherence and its contribution to stiffness should be evaluated for the need of a flap. The ROM—passive, active, and active-assisted—should be carefully documented. The endpoint of restricted motion should be noted, with a *soft endpoint* implying soft tissue constraint and a *hard endpoint* implying bony impingement. Unfortunately, this distinction is usually not obvious. The strength and control of major muscle groups about the elbow should be assessed to determine whether the patient would be able to cooperate with the vigorous physical therapy program that will be necessary, whether treated operatively or nonoperatively. Neurovascular examination should focus on the ulnar and median nerves, which may show clinical or subclinical signs and symptoms of entrapment in scar or bony callus.

Radiographic Evaluation

Radiographic evaluation serves three purposes:

1. To evaluate the degree of degenerative changes.
2. To rule out impinging hardware.
3. To rule out heterotopic ossification.

In most patients, AP elbow, lateral elbow, and radiocapitellar oblique views will suffice. For severe deformity or for bridging HO, an axial CT scan or lateral tomograms may be necessary to evaluate the joint. MRI does not provide more information than CT, but may be useful in assessing MCL and lateral collateral ligament integrity. It should be noted that focal articular cartilage loss can be difficult to appreciate with any preoperative imaging modality and may become apparent only at surgery.

Treatment

Nonoperative Treatment

The management of elbow stiffness begins with prevention via early motion and treatments related to achieving early motion, including stable internal fixation of fractures. Conditions creating inflammation in or around the elbow should be corrected. Anti-inflammatory medications are helpful in decreasing swelling. Heat prior to exercise, icing afterward, and physical therapy modalities like iontophoresis, ultrasound, massage, and electrostimulation can help to increase motion. Muscle weakness or imbalance should be corrected with strengthening exercises.

After elbow trauma, whether treated surgically or not, it is crucial to recognize when the patient's elbow motion is not progressing and to initiate more aggressive treatment.

Acute Treatment

The first-line treatment for elbow stiffness is gradual, patient-controlled, physical therapy–directed stretching exercises. If motion still does not progress, splinting becomes the next step.

Dynamic hinged elbow splints with spring or rubberband tension are useful to assist with deficits of elbow flexion. Dynamic splints are often poorly tolerated by patients because they impart continuous stretch that may cause cocontraction and spasm of antagonistic muscles, leaving the patient with no reprieve other than removing the splint.

Adjustable static (turnbuckle) splints are better tolerated for resistant flexion or extension deficits. If deficits are present in both directions, an adjustable turnbuckle orthosis can be used in alternating directions.

Finally, static splints that exceed the maximum passive extension or flexion capacity by 20 degrees can be made for nighttime use.

FES has met with limited success and cannot be recommended at this time. Continuous passive motion machines also have a limited role in established contractures.

Chronic Treatment

Once the elbow becomes nonpainful, yet a motion deficit exists despite splinting (generally after 6 months), further conservative treatment is unlikely to be of benefit.

Closed manipulation under anesthesia, previously thought to be of benefit, is believed to worsen elbow stiffness by inducing new inflammation and tearing the soft tissue capsule and brachialis muscle, thus causing more hematoma and additional fibrosis. Forceful leveraging can also cause articular cartilage that has been encased in adhesions to delaminate.

Operative Treatment

If conservative measures fail and the patient has reasonable expectations as to the expected results and can cooperate with the arduous postoperative rehabilitation, operative management can be considered.

The degree of degenerative changes within the elbow joint determines the surgical intervention of posttraumatic elbow stiffness. For patients with **no or minimal degenerative changes,** soft tissue releases with or without distraction are indicated. Patients with **moderate degenerative changes** can be treated with limited bony arthroplasties: débridement arthroplasty or Outerbridge-Kashiwagi ulnohumeral arthroplasty. Younger patients with severe degenerative changes can be treated with distraction fascial arthroplasty. For older patients (>60 years), low-demand elbows, or those who have failed soft tissue or limited bony procedures, total elbow arthroplasty may be the only option.

For patients with minimal or no degenerative changes, soft tissue releases combined with removal of bony impingement can be helpful.

Surgical Indications

A patient who perceives significant functional deficits from the stiffness and is both cooperative and motivated enough to participate in the extensive physical therapy program is a candidate for operative release. In most cases, surgery offers improvement with flexion contractures greater than 30 degrees and maximum flexion is less than 100 degrees. There are no absolute patient age limits for operative release, although young children may be unable to participate in physical therapy and the elderly may have confounding medical problems.

Timing

When the early phase of soft tissue healing has resolved, which can be as early as 3 months following injury, patients can be considered for a soft tissue release.

Approaches

In selecting the approach to the elbow, the existing scars and the condition of the skin about the elbow must be considered along with the direction of motion restriction.

If both flexion and extension are limited, then access to both the front and the back of the ulnohumeral joint can be achieved through either a lateral (Kocher) approach or a medial approach. It is helpful to approach the elbow on the side with significant bony impingement. The medial approach is favored if the ulnar nerve requires exploration or release. Both approaches may also be concurrently used.

If there is adequate flexion and only extension is limited (flexion contracture), then an anterior approach will allow access to release the anterior capsule, brachialis muscle, and rarely, biceps tendon. With this approach, the olecranon fossa is not visualized, and one must be certain that there are no posterior impediments.

If flexion is limited and extension is good (extension contracture), often the result of postsurgical casting in extension or impinging olecranon fixation, then a direct posterior approach can be used allowing access to the triceps muscle, posterior capsule, and olecranon fossa.

If the pronation-supination motion is limited, then the extended lateral (Kocher) approach allows good visualization of the radiocapitellar joint in addition to both the anterior and the posterior ulnohumeral joints.

Release

After arthrotomy of the elbow joint, the release must be tailored to the offending structures. If the brachialis muscle is tight, it should be released or recessed off the humerus. If the triceps or the biceps is tight, then a tendolysis or more proximal mobilization of the muscle should be carried out, with tenotomy or Z-lengthening being reserved for more severe cases. If the anterior or posterior capsule is contracted, a capsulotomy or capsulectomy should be performed. Bridging or impinging heterotopic ossification should be excised. Within the joint, impinging marginal osteophytes or hypertrophic callus should be removed. The coronoid and olecranon fossa must be débrided of the fibrofatty tissue, which can serve as a block to motion. If either collateral ligament is contracted, it may be released and Z-lengthened. Morrey (1993) believes that if the collateral ligaments are released, then a distraction device should be applied to stabilize the elbow during soft tissue healing.

If the radial head is blocking pronation-supination or flexion, the radial head should be excised at the head-neck junction, with care taken to preserve the annular ligament.

For medial approaches, the ulnar nerve must be identified and protected. The stiffer the elbow joint, the more necessary it becomes to transpose the ulnar nerve to allow for nerve gliding and prevent traction injury. It is usually transposed subcutaneously, but if the subcutaneous tissue bed is scarred, then submuscular transposition is more appropriate. The wound is closed in layers over suction drains to lessen the hematoma.

Stiff Elbow with Moderate Articular Degenerative Changes

For stiff elbows with moderate degenerative changes, limited bony arthroplasties are necessary in addition to soft tissue releases to help restore motion: débridement arthroplasty or an Outerbridge-Kashiwagi ulnohumeral arthroplasty may be operative options. For symptomatic (painful) arthrosis, radial head excision, olecranon ostectomy, osteophyte excision, olecranon-coronoid fossa débridement, and capsular release through a lateral incision may increase motion and diminish pain. One must be careful not to sacrifice the collateral ligaments, which will result in instability.

Débridement Arthroplasty

Débridement arthroplasty has been described as a treatment for advanced primary osteoarthrosis of the elbow, but it may be considered for post-traumatic stiffness with osteoarthrosis.

The elbow is approached through a posterolateral skin incision as allowed by existing scars. The distal humerus is approached between the triceps and the brachioradialis. The radial collateral ligament is Z-lengthened. The joint is opened with flexion and varus. The olecranon and olecranon fossa are débrided of osteophytes. The coronoid and radial head and their corresponding fossa are likewise débrided. They did not recommend resection of the radial head. The radial collateral ligament is repaired, and the wound closed over drains. Continuous passive motion is used immediately after surgery.

Outerbridge-Kashiwagi Ulnohumeral Arthroplasty

Kashiwagi employs a technique of débridement arthroplasty that allows exploration and débridement of the anterior and posterior compartments with less extensive soft tissue dissection.

The elbow is approached through a small posterior midline incision. The triceps muscle is split, and the posterior capsule is opened. The tip of the olecranon is excised. The olecranon fossa is first fenestrated with a dental burr, then opened up to 1 cm in diameter, allowing removal of anterior compartment loose bodies and débridement of the coronoid and radial head. Morrey (1992) modified this procedure, recommending elevation of the triceps (rather than splitting the triceps) and use of a trephine to open the olecranon fossa.

Advanced Articular Degenerative Changes

The operative options for younger patients with elbow stiffness and severe degenerative changes, which unfortunately make up the largest group of patients with post-traumatic elbow stiffness, are quite limited because of the high demands placed on the elbow. Fascial arthroplasty and total elbow arthroplasty are the two operative options. Because there is no single good position for the elbow, arthrodesis is not an option. Resection arthroplasty usually results in intolerable instability or weakness or both.

For older patients, total elbow arthroplasty becomes a more attractive option. Total elbow arthroplasty can also be the salvage procedure for patients who have undergone previous unsuccessful soft tissue or limited bony débridement arthroplasties.

Distraction Fascial Arthroplasty

According to Morrey (1992), **there are three indications for interpositional arthroplasty:**

1. Loss of more than half of the articular surface.
2. Significant adhesions that avulse more than half of the articular surface.
3. Malunion causes significant incongruity of the articular surface.

An extensile-type posterior approach to the elbow is made through existing scars. Any restrictive capsule, ligaments, and muscles are released to obtain elbow motion. The radial head and any impinging bone are then excised, which may afford additional motion. The humeral condyles and olecranon joint surfaces are then recontoured ("anatomic arthroplasty") to provide a smooth surface for rotation. A cutis graft or fascia lata graft (currently most common) may be used as the interpositional material. The graft is stretched over the distal humerus and proximal ulna and securely sutured in place, often through bone tunnels.

To protect and give some degree of stability to the elbow, an external distraction device allowing motion is applied. The distraction device is carefully centered about the projected center of elbow rotation in the distal humerus. The landmarks for the center are the anteroinferior aspect of the medial epicondyle and the center of the capitellum. The distraction device is then attached to the humerus and ulna, and the joint is distracted approximately 3 to 5 mm. Any deficient collateral ligaments should be reconstructed.

Total Elbow Arthroplasty

In general, total elbow arthroplasty in post-traumatic arthrosis has not been able to give the same satisfactory results as those performed for rheumatoid arthritis. Total elbow arthroplasty probably should be reserved for patients older than 60 years with low-demand elbows. Nonconstrained implants are not recommended because post-traumatic elbows often lack the ligamentous stability necessary for their success. Semiconstrained total elbow arthroplasty has shown moderate success but may not be durable.

The elbow is approached posteriorly or posteromedially as allowed by existing scars. The ulnar nerve is identified medially and mobilized to allow for anterior transposition. The Bryan-Morrey exposure begins with medial elevation of the triceps muscle and tendon in continuity with a periosteal sleeve off the ulna to allow for elbow subluxation. The anterior and posterior capsules are excised or released. The distal humerus and proximal ulna are prepared with bone cuts specific to the implant, with care taken to preserve the medial and lateral humeral columns. The implant is cemented, adequate hemostasis is achieved, and the wound is closed over drains. Motion begins when the wound is sealed.

Heterotopic Ossification

A thorough discussion of HO about the elbow is beyond the scope of this review. Direct trauma in the forms of intramuscluar bleeding and displaced fracture fragments is the most common cause of HO about the elbow. Other risk factors include neural axis trauma (thought to be due to some humoral mediator or systemic cascade), thermal injury "usually related to the degree, but not necessarily the site of burn," and forceful passive manipulation of stiff joints.

There appears to be a direct correlation between the frequency of HO and the magnitude of the injury. The incidence in the elbow ranges from 1.6 to 56% and generally increases with fracture severity and fracture-dislocations.

Clinically, patients present with swelling, hyperemia, and diminished motion between 1 and 4 months following injury. The differential diagnosis includes infection, thrombophlebitis, and reflex sympathetic dystrophy. In patients with spinal cord injuries, HO is found distal to the level of the lesion and thus occurs most commonly in the lower extremities. When the upper extremity is involved, it is usually on the side of spasticity, most commonly in the flexor muscles or posterolateral elbow. HO is diffuse and does not necessarily follow anatomic structures or planes.

HO can be detected radiographically within the first 4 to 6 weeks. It is important to differentiate periarticular calcifications, indicative of MCL or LCL injury, from true HO. The technetium bone scan turns positive before the plain films. Sensitivity increases with the triple-phase bone scan. CT scan may help define the internal architecture of the HO to assess its maturity, and can be helpful in determining the anatomic location of the HO.

Upper extremity HO has been classified by Hastings and Graham into three types:

> Class I — radiographic HO without functional limitation
>
> Class II — subtotal limitation
>
> > Class IIA — limitation in flexion-extension plane
> >
> > Class IIB — limitation in pronation-supination axis
> >
> > Class IIC — limitation in both planes of motion
>
> Class III — complete bony ankylosis

Treatment

HO can be inhibited pharmacologically. Diphosphonates inhibit the crystallization of hydroxyapatite, thus diminishing the mineralization of the osteoid. NSAIDs, particularly indomethacin, are thought to decrease HO by interrupting the synthesis of prostaglandin E_2 and also by inhibiting differentiation of precursor cells into active osteoblasts, and should be initiated in the early postoperative or postinjury period. External beam radiation is advocated for use about the hip to prevent HO and after excision of HO (700–800 rads in a single dose) within 48 to 72 hours after resection to prevent recurrence.

Obviously, not all patients require surgical intervention. There is evidence that HO may resorb, especially in children and in those with neurologic recovery. For increasing limitation of motion and functional impairment unresponsive to physical therapy, surgery can be considered. The timing of surgery is critical. The HO should be metabolically quiescent at the time of surgery, based on physical appearance of the limb (decreased swelling and erythema) and mature appearance on radiographs. Progressive soft tissue contracture if surgery is delayed must be balanced against the increased risk of recurrence if excised too early.

Summary

In summary, post-traumatic elbow stiffness can be classified into that resulting from intrinsic causes, extrinsic causes, or a combination of the two. Prevention with modalities aimed at early motion is crucial to the management of stiffness. Treatment of post-traumatic elbow stiffness begins with supervised physical therapy often combined with splinting. Patients with less than functional motion, 30 to 130 degrees of extension-flexion or 50 to 50 degrees of pronation-supination, and who are willing to cooperate with the aggressive, prolonged physical therapy are candidates for operative management.

For patients with no or mild degenerative changes, soft tissue releases are appropriate. The direction of motion limitation will dictate the operative approach and the capsuloligamentous structures to be released. Continuous passive motion postoperatively seems to be of benefit. Results show consistent improvement in the motion arc.

For patients with moderate degenerative changes, limited bony arthroplasty (débridement arthroplasty or Outerbridge-Kashiwagi ulnohumeral arthroplasty) have high satisfaction rates and reliable improvement in the motion arc.

For patients with advanced degenerative changes, distraction fascial arthroplasty can be done in younger patients or a total elbow arthroplasty in an older patient, although the results are acceptable but not excellent. Fascial arthroplasty outcomes are often unpredictable, and total elbow arthroplasty results have a high rate of loosening (up to 20%), complications (up to 25%), and revisions (up to 18%), but they seem to be improving with refinement of prosthesis design and implantation techniques. ■

Bibliography

Dillman CJ, Fleisig GS, Andrews JR, Escamilla RF: Kinetics of baseball pitching with implications about injury mechanisms. Am J Sports Med 23(2):233, 1995.

Forster MC, Clark DI, Lunn PG: Elbow osteoarthritis: prognostic indicators in ulnohumeral debridement—the Outerbridge-Kashiwagi procedure. J Shoulder Elbow Surg 10(6):557, 2001.

Galloway M, De Maio M, Mangine R: Rehabilitation techniques in the treatment of medial and lateral epicondylitis. Orthopedics 15(9):1089, 1992.

Gelinas JJ, Faber KJ, Patterson SD, King GJ: The effectiveness of turnbuckle splinting for elbow contractures. J Bone Joint Surg [Br] 82(1):74, 2000.

Hastings H 2nd, Graham TJ: The classification and treatment of heterotopic ossification about the elbow and forearm. Hand Clinics 10(3):417, Review 1994.

Hyman J, Breazeale NM, Altcheck DW: Valgus instability of the elbow in athletes. Clin Sports Med 20(1):25, Review 2001.

Mason ML: Some observations on fractures of the head of the radius with a review of one hundred cases. Br J Surg 42:123, 1954.

Morrey BF, Askew LJ, An KN, Chao EY: A biomechanical study of normal functional elbow motion. J Bone Joint Surg [Am] 63:872–877, 1981.

Morrey BF: Biomechanics of the elbow and forearm. Orthop Sports Med 17:840, 1994.

Morrey BF: Post-traumatic stiffness: distraction arthroplasty. In Morrey BF (ed): The Elbow and Its Disorders, 2nd ed. Philadelphia, WB Saunders, 1993, pp. 476–491.

Morrey BF: Primary degenerative arthritis of the elbow: treatment by ulnohumeral arthroplasty. J Bone Joint Surg [Br] 74:409–413, 1992.

Nirschl, RP, Chumbley EM, O'Connor FG: Evaluation of overuse elbow injuries. Am Fam Physician 61(3):691, 2000.

Peters T, Baker CL: Lateral epicondylitis. Review Clin Sports Med 20(3):549, Review 2001.

Slocum DB: Classification of elbow injuries from baseball pitching. Tex Med 64(3):48, 1968.

Tullos HS, Bennett J, Shepard D: Adult elbow dislocations: mechanisms of instability. Instr Course Lect 35:69, 1986.

Wilk, KE: Stretch-shortening drills for the upper extremities: theory and clinical application. J Orthop Sports Phys Ther 17(5):225, 1993.

Brian S. Cohen, MD, Anthony A. Romeo, MD,
and Bernard R. Bach Jr., MD

Background

Normal function of the "shoulder complex" requires the coordinated movements of the sternoclavicular (SC), acromioclavicular (AC), and glenohumeral (GH) joints, as well as the scapulothoracic articulation and the motion interface between the rotator cuff and the overlying coracoacromial arch. Successful elevation of the arm requires a minimum of 30 to 40 degrees of clavicular elevation and at least 45 to 60 degrees of scapula rotation. Motion across these articulations is accomplished by the interaction of approximately 30 muscles. Pathologic changes in any portion of the complex may disrupt the normal biomechanics of the shoulder.

The **primary goal** of the shoulder complex is to position the hand in space for activities of daily living. Secondarily, during overhead athletic activities such as throwing and serving, the shoulder functions as the "funnel" through which the forces from the larger, stronger muscles of the legs and trunk are passed to the muscles of the arm, forearm, and hand, which have finer motor skills. The ability to execute these actions successfully comes from the inherent mobility and functional stability of the GH joint.

"Unrestricted" motion occurs at the GH joint as a result of its osseous configuration (Fig. 3–1). A large humeral head articulating with a small glenoid socket allows extremes of motion at the expense of the stability that is seen in other joints (Table 3–1). Similarly, the scapula is very mobile on the thoracic wall. This enables it to follow the humerus, positioning the glenoid appro-

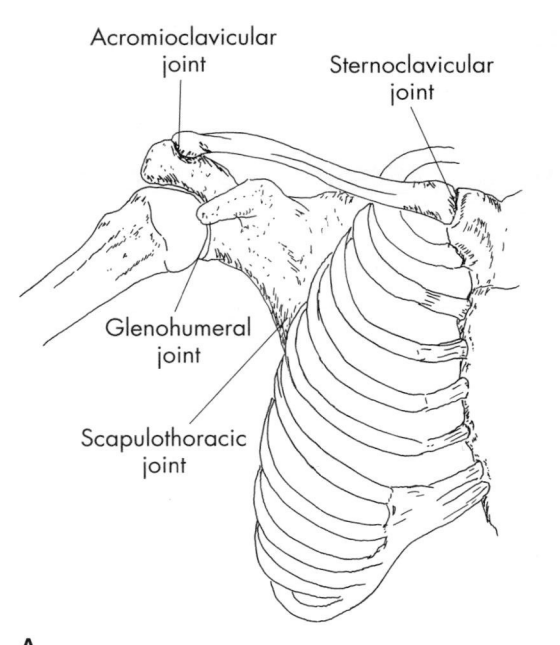

Acromioclavicular joint

Sternoclavicular joint

Glenohumeral joint

Scapulothoracic joint

A

Figure 3–1. *A,* Shoulder joint osteology. *B,* Shoulder musculature. The shallow glenohumeral (GH) joint (*i, anterior view*) derives some stability from the surrounding tendons and musculature, most significantly the rotator cuff (*ii, posterior view*), which consists of the supraspinatus, infraspinatus, teres minor, and subscapularis tendons. The acromioclavicular (AC) articulation (*iii, anterior view*) is surrounded by the AC and coracoclavicular (CC) ligaments. *C,* The AC ligament gives anterior-posterior and medial-lateral stability to the AC joint, and the CC ligaments provide vertical stability. The sternoclavicular joint has little bony stability but strong ligaments—primarily the costoclavicular, sternoclavicular, and interclavicular—that contribute to joint stability. (*B,* From Sartoris DJ: Diagnosing shoulder pain: what's the best imaging approach? Physician Sports Med 20[9]:150, 1992; *C,* from Hutchinson MR, Ahuja GS: Diagnosing and treating clavicle fractures. Physician Sports Med 24[3]:26–35, 1996.)

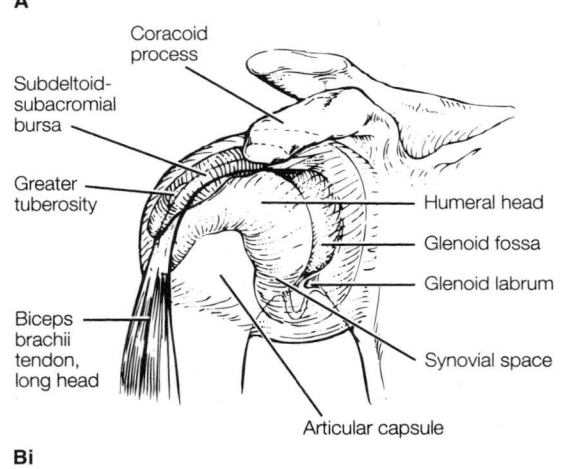

Coracoid process

Subdeltoid-subacromial bursa

Greater tuberosity

Biceps brachii tendon, long head

Humeral head

Glenoid fossa

Glenoid labrum

Synovial space

Articular capsule

Bi

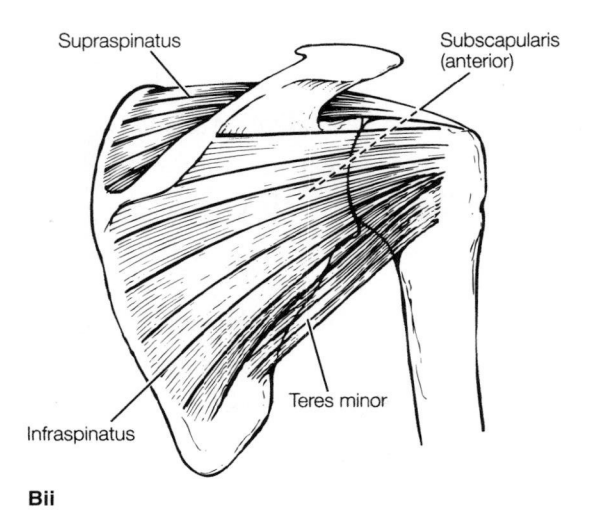

Supraspinatus

Subscapularis (anterior)

Teres minor

Infraspinatus

Bii

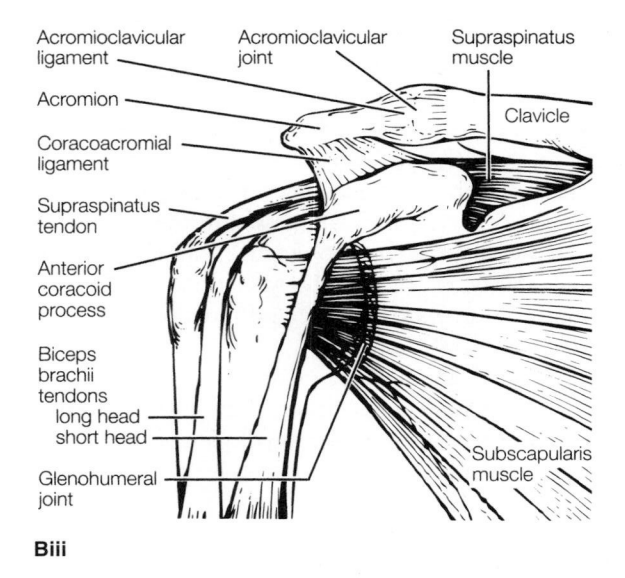

Acromioclavicular ligament

Acromion

Coracoacromial ligament

Supraspinatus tendon

Anterior coracoid process

Biceps brachii tendons
    long head
    short head

Glenohumeral joint

Acromioclavicular joint

Supraspinatus muscle

Clavicle

Subscapularis muscle

Biii

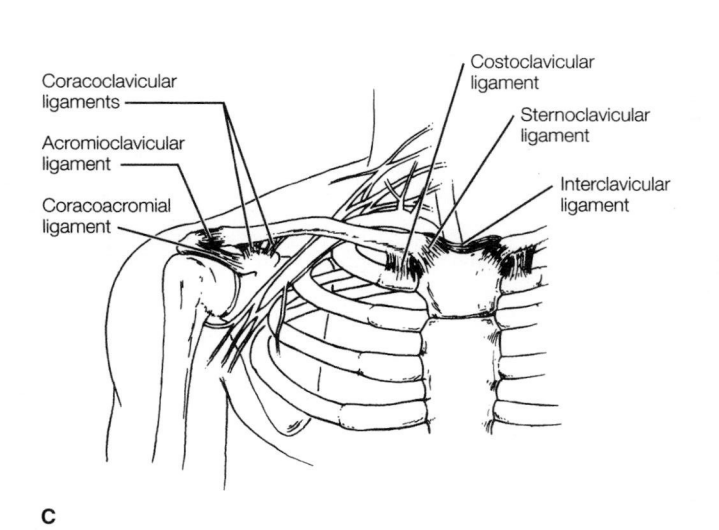

Coracoclavicular ligaments

Acromioclavicular ligament

Coracoacromial ligament

Costoclavicular ligament

Sternoclavicular ligament

Interclavicular ligament

C

Table 3-1

Normal Joint Motions and Bony Positions around the Shoulder Joint

Scapula
Rotation through arc of 65 degrees with shoulder abduction
Translation on thorax up to 15 cm

Glenohumeral Joint

Abduction	140 degrees
Internal/external rotation	90/90
Translation	
Anterior-posterior	5–10 mm
Inferior-superior	4–5 mm
Total rotations	
Baseball	185 degrees
Tennis	165 degrees

priately while avoiding humeral impingement on the acromion. Osseous stability of the GH joint is enhanced by the fibrocartilaginous labrum, which functions to enlarge and deepen the socket while increasing the conformity of the articulating surfaces. However, the majority of the stability at the shoulder is determined by the soft tissue structures that cross it. The ligaments and capsule form the static stabilizers and function to limit translation

and rotation of the humeral head on the glenoid. The **superior GH ligament** has been shown to be an important inferior stabilizer. The **middle GH ligament** imparts stability against anterior translation with the arm in external rotation, and abduction less than 90 degrees. The **inferior GH ligament** is the most important anterior stabilizer with the shoulder in 90 degrees of abduction and external rotation, which represents the most unstable position of the shoulder (Fig. 3–2).

The muscles make up the dynamic stabilizers of the GH joint and impart stability in a variety of ways. During muscle contraction, they provide increased capsuloligamentous stiffness, which increases joint stability. They act as dynamic ligaments when their passive elements are put on stretch (Hill, 1951). Most importantly, they make up the components of force couples that control the position of the humerus and scapula, helping to appropriately direct the forces crossing the GH joint (Poppen and Walker, 1978) (Table 3–2).

Proper scapula motion and stability are critical for normal shoulder function. The scapula forms a stable base from which all shoulder motion occurs, and correct positioning is necessary for efficient and powerful GH joint movement. Abnormal scapula alignment and movement, or **scapulothoracic dyskinesis,** can result in clinical findings consistent with instability and/or impingement syndrome. Strengthening of the scapular stabilizers is an important component of the rehabilitation protocol after all

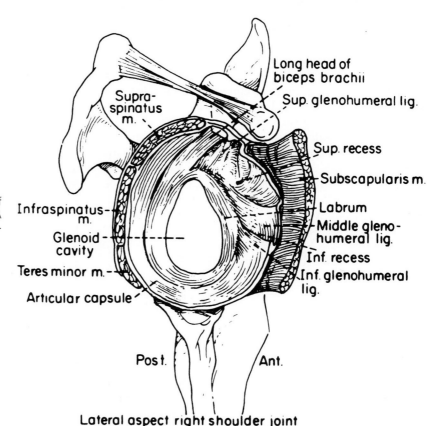

Figure 3–2. GH ligaments and the rotator cuff stabilizers of the GH joint. (From Rockwood CA Jr, Matsen FA III: The Shoulder, 2nd ed. Philadelphia, WB Saunders, 1988, p. 255.)

Table 3-2

Forces and Loads on the Shoulder in Normal Athletic Activity

Rotational Velocities

Baseball	7000 degrees/sec
Tennis serve	1500 degrees/sec
Tennis forehand	245 degrees/sec
Tennis backhand	870 degrees/sec

Angular Velocities

Baseball	1150 degrees/sec

Acceleration Forces

Internal rotation	60 Nm
Horizontal adduction	70 Nm
Anterior shear	400 Nm

Deceleration Forces

Horizontal abduction	80 Nm
Posterior shear	500 Nm
Compression	70 Nm

shoulder injuries and is essential for a complete functional recovery of the shoulder complex.

In most patients, rehabilitation after a shoulder injury should initially focus on pain control and regaining the coordinated motion throughout all components of the shoulder complex. Once motion is regained, attention is shifted to strengthening and re-educating the muscles around the shoulder to perform their normal tasks. To reproduce the precision with which the shoulder complex functions, the muscles need to be re-educated through "learned motor patterns." These patterns position the shoulder complex in "predetermined" ways and activate the muscles in precise synchronization to maximize recovery of function. Associated conditioning of the lower extremities and trunk muscles is extremely important because over 50% of the kinetic energy during throwing and serving is generated from the legs and trunk muscles. Therefore, rehabilitation of all components of the kinetic chain is required before the successful return of competitive or strenuous overhead athletic activities.

General Principles of Shoulder Rehabilitation

Many pathologic conditions can affect the shoulder complex. As in other parts of the musculoskeletal system, the problem can be the result of an acute traumatic injury with disruption of one or more portions of the system or the result of repetitive microtrauma that slowly alters the normal mechanics of the entire complex. *Motion, strength,* and *stability* are the three components of shoulder function that can be disrupted by an acute or chronic injury. All three can be treated effectively with therapeutic rehabilitation.

Obvious findings of gross instability, massive muscle tears, or severe losses of motion are easily diagnosed, but not necessarily easily treated. Subtle findings, such as increased humeral translation due to a loss of GH joint internal rotation, superior humeral head migration as a result of rotator cuff weakness, or abnormal scapular positioning secondary to weakness of the trapezius or serratus anterior muscles, are more difficult to diagnose and just as difficult to treat. For successful rehabilitation, recognition and treatment of the pathology are as important as understanding its impact on normal shoulder function. The goal of rehabilitation, regardless of the pathology, is always a functional recovery.

The most important factor that determines the success or failure of a particular shoulder rehabilitation protocol is establishing the correct diagnosis.

It is not unusual in the present healthcare delivery environment for a primary care physician to be treating difficult musculoskeletal injuries and referring patients for therapy. If the rehabilitation program does not match the correct diagnosis, the treating therapist should request a more thorough evaluation of the patient. For example, a patient diagnosed with a "shoulder contusion" may be referred for physiotherapy. After 1 to 2 weeks without any progress, the patient should be carefully reevaluated. With reevaluation, including appropriate radiographs (e.g., an axillary lateral radiograph) the cause of the failed rehabilitation may be as ominous as a locked posterior dislocation of the humeral head, a diagnosis that is missed 80% of the time by the initial treating physician.

In general, shoulder rehabilitation after an injury or surgery should begin with early active motion to help restore normal shoulder mechanics. The benefits of early joint mobilization have been well documented in other areas of the body. For example, accelerated rehabilitation programs for the knee after anterior cruciate ligament reconstruction have resulted in earlier restoration of motion, strength, and function without compromising stability. Strict immobilization has been shown to be responsible for the development of "functional" instability in the shoulder secondary to rotator cuff inhibition, muscular atrophy, and poor neuromuscular control. A lack of active motion within the shoulder complex compromises the normal kinematic relationship between the GH and the scapulothoracic joints and can lead to rotator cuff abnormalities or impingement syndrome. Concerns about early active motion in patients with shoulder pathology are the fear of aggravating an already painful condition and the risk of compromising a surgical repair. The timing of motion and strengthening exercises needs to be well documented by the treating physician and clearly outlined for the patient and physical therapist.

One therapeutic modality, which is making advances in shoulder rehabilitation because it puts less stress on the tissues, is aquatic physical therapy (see Chapter 7, Special Topics). The benefit of aquatic rehabilitation is related to the buoyancy effect that the water provides for the upper extremity, decreasing the weight of the arm to as little as one eighth its original weight at 90 degrees of abduction or forward flexion. The apparent decrease in weight of the arm or the shoulder puts less stress on the repaired or inflamed tissues during active exercises. This allows early restoration of active movement in a protected environment instituting the early return of normal motor patterns.

Intake Evaluation

Before therapy of the shoulder begins, a general intake evaluation is performed. The intake survey begins with a thorough evaluation of all the components of the shoulder complex, as well as all parts of the "kinematic" chain. The examination starts with a general assessment of the patient's active motion. Movement of both scapulae along the thoracic wall should be monitored from behind the patient. Scapula motion should be both smooth and symmetrical. Evidence of scapular winging or asymmetri-

cal movements should alert the examiner to a potential nerve injury, or more often, weakness of the muscles that stabilize the scapula. As discussed earlier, abnormal scapula motion can cause symptoms consistent with anterior instability or impingement. Analysis of the AC joint for areas of tenderness, as well as degrees of motion, is also important because this small joint can be the source of extremely painful pathology. The evaluation of the shoulder complex is completed with a thorough examination of the GH joint for range of motion (ROM), stability, and muscle strength. Once the shoulder complex has been thoroughly evaluated, other areas that function during overhead activities need to be evaluated. Examination of the patient's hips and knees is performed, with close attention to hip flexion and rotation. ROM and strength of the lumbar spine should be well documented. It is not uncommon to see a loss of motion in the hips, knees, or lower back contributing to abnormal shoulder mechanics in a throwing athlete. Evidence of kyphosis or scoliosis of the thoracic spine should be recorded, because both of these conditions have been associated with altering spine motion during throwing, as well as disrupting normal scapular rhythm.

Differential Diagnosis of Shoulder Pain

Rotator cuff or biceps tendon
  Strain
  Tendinitis
  Tear
GH instability
  Anterior
  Posterior
  Multidirectional
GH instability with secondary impingement
Primary impingement of the cuff or biceps tendon
Calcific tendinitis
AC joint pathology
  Arthritis
  Separation
  Weight-lifter's osteolysis
GH arthritis
  Rheumatoid arthritis
  Septic arthritis
  Inflammatory arthritis
  Neuropathic (Charcot) arthritis
  Crystaline arthritis (gout, pseudogout)
  Hemophilic arthritis
  Osteochondromatosis
Thoracic outlet syndrome
Cervical spine/root/brachial plexus injury with referred pain
Suprascapular nerve neuropathy
Shoulder dislocation
  Acute
  Chronic (missed)
SC injury
Adhesive capsulitis (frozen shoulder)

SLAP lesion
Fracture
  Humerus
  Clavicle
  Scapula
Scapular winging
Little League shoulder
Reflex sympathetic dystrophy
Tumor
  Metastatic
  Primary
  Multiple myeloma
  Soft tissue neoplasm
Bone disorders
  Osteonecrosis (AVN)
  Paget's disease
  Osteomalacia
  Hyperparathyroid disease
Infection
Intrathoracic disorders (referred pain)
  Pancoast's tumor
  Diaphragmatic irritation, esophagitis
  Myocardial infarction
Psychogenic disorders
Polymyalgia rheumatica
Neuralgic amyotrophy (Parsonage-Turner syndrome)
Abdominal disorders (referred pain)
  Gastric ulcer
  Gall bladder
  Subphrenic abscess

AVN, avascular necrosis; SLAP, superior labrum from anterior to posterior.

The Importance of History-Taking in Evaluating Shoulder Pain

It is important to determine whether the shoulder pain results from acute, traumatic events or from chronic, repetitive overuse. For example, an AC joint separation can be ruled out in a pitcher who has AC joint pain that has developed over 2 months with no history of trauma or direct blow to the shoulder. The anatomic location of the pain should be pinpointed (e.g., rotator cuff insertion, posterior shoulder) rather than settling for "the whole shoulder hurts."

The patient should be questioned about neck pain or neurologic symptoms indicative of **referred** shoulder pain (e.g., C5–6 lesion or suprascapular nerve). The patient's chief complaint is important and often a good differentiator: weakness, stiffness, pain, catching, popping, subluxation, "dead-arm" impingement, loss of motion, crepitance, radiation into hand.

In our institution we try to determine which category of shoulder pain the patient falls into. For **referred neck pain** to the shoulder, are the complaints more radicular in nature with an unimpressive shoulder exam? Is the cause of pain a **frozen shoulder** from not using the arm, with a block that equally restricts active and passive motion? And was there an underlying cause (e.g., rotator cuff tear) that made the patient initially stop using the shoulder?

Is the etiology an **unstable shoulder** after a previous dislocation or in a very ligamentously loose individual (torn loose or born loose)? Is the cause of pain a **rotator cuff tear** with pain and weakness on overhead activities, or does the pain originate from the spectrum of rotator cuff tendinitis, partial thickness tearing, bursitis, impingement, etc.? Did the patient have trauma to the shoulder with a fracture or AC joint tenderness and radiographic evidence of osteolysis of the AC joint? A thorough history and physical exam must be employed to avoid sending the patient to the therapist with a prescription of "shoulder pain—evaluate and treat."

Important History in Throwing Athletes with Shoulder Pain

General information
  Age
  Dominant handedness
  Years throwing
  Level of competition
Medical information
  Chronic or acute medical problems
  Review of systems
  Pre-existing or recurrent shoulder problems
  Other musculoskeletal problems (acute or distant)
Shoulder complaints
  Symptoms
    Pain
    Weakness, fatigue
    Instability
    Stiffness
    Functional catching
  Injury pattern
    Sudden or acute onset

Shoulder complaints (*Cont'd*)
    Gradual or chronic onset
    Traumatic fall or blow
    Recurrent
  Symptom characteristics
    Location
    Character and severity
    Provocation
    Duration
    Paraesthesias
    Phase of throwing
    Related activities, disability
  Related symptoms
    Cervical
    Peripheral nerve
    Brachial plexus
    Entrapment

From Andrews JR, Zarins B, Wilk KE: Injuries in Baseball. Philadelphia, Lippincott-Raven, 1998.

Examination of the Shoulder

Physical Examination of the Throwing Shoulder

Sitting Position

Inspection
Palpation
  SC, clavicle, AC joint
  Acromion, coracoid
  Bicipital groove
  Scapula
  Musculature

ROM
  Crepitus
  GH motion
  Scapulothoracic motion
Rotator cuff, scapular muscle testing
  Isolated muscle testing
  Supraspinatus testing
Scapular winging

Physical Examination of the Throwing Shoulder (*Continued*)

Stability testing
  Anterior-posterior Lachman
  Anterior-posterior apprehension
Ligamentous laxity (thumb to wrist, "double-jointed"
fingers)
  Inferior sulcus sign
Impingement signs
Biceps testing

Supine Position

Motion
Anterior instability tests
  Anterior shoulder drawer
  Apprehension
  Relocation test

Posterior instability tests
  Posterior shoulder drawer
  Apprehension
Labral testing
  Clunk test

Prone Position

Palpation of posterior structures
Motion re-evaluation
Stability—anterior apprehension

Neurologic and Cervical Examination

Rule out referred or neurologic origin of shoulder pain

Radiographic Examination

From Andrews JR, Zarins B, Wilk KE: Injuries in Baseball. Philadelphia, Lippincott-Raven, 1998.

Inspection of the shoulder:

- The presence of atrophy, hypertrophy, scapular wing-ing, asymmetry of shoulders, swelling, deformity, ery-thema, or the patient supporting the shoulder with the other arm.
- Isolated **atrophy** of
  - Supraspinatus and infraspinatus fossa (possible ro-tator cuff disease, entrapment or injury to the suprascapular nerve, disuse).
  - Deltoid or teres minor muscle atrophy (possible axillary nerve injury).
  - Winging of the scapula (long thoracic nerve injury).
- "Popeye" bulge of the biceps (evidence of proximal tear of the long head of the biceps) worsened with flexion of the elbows (Fig. 3–3).
- Deformity of the AC joint (grade 2 or 3 AC joint separation).
- Deformity of shoulder (probable dislocation and/or fracture).

Figure 3–3. Rupture of the long head of the biceps tendon, of-ten referred to as a "Popeye" deformity. (From Reider B: The Orthopaedic Physical Examination. Philadelphia, WB Saunders, 1999.)

Palpation of the shoulder begins with palpation of the sternoclavicular (SC) joint and proximal clavicle.

- Prominence, asymmetry, or tenderness to palpation indicates SC dislocation (traumatic), subluxation (traumatic), or arthritis (insidious).
- The **clavicle** is palpated for possible claviclar fracture.
- The **AC** joint is palpated for pain or prominence.
  - A prominence indicates a traumatic grade 2 or 3 AC joint separation.
  - Tenderness, with no prominence (*no* trauma) is in-dicative of weight-lifter's osteolysis or arthritis of the AC joint.
- If palpation of the **bicipital groove** identifies tender-ness, biceps tendinitis is suggested.
  - Biceps tendinitis often results from the biceps hav-ing to "overwork" in its secondary role as a humeral head depressor because of concomitant rotator cuff pathology (biceps tendinitis seldom ex-ists alone, with the exception of a weight-lifter performing too many biceps curls).
  - An absence of the biceps in the groove indicates a rupture of the long head of the biceps.
- Palpation of the **anterior GH joint** and **coracoid** may identify anterior shoulder tenderness, which is a common and a *very nonspecific finding*.
- Tenderness to palpation in the **greater tuberosity** and insertion site of the **rotator cuff insertion** (just distal to the anterolateral border of the acromion) in-dicates
  - Rotator cuff tendinitis or tear.
  - Primary or secondary impingement.
  - Subacromial bursitis.
- Palpation of the **scapulothoracic muscles** and medial border of the **scapula** checks for
  - Winging of the scapula, indicative of injury to the long thoracic nerve or weakness of the scapulotho-racic muscles (possible scapular dyskinesis).

- Crepitance, which is found with snapping scapula syndrome or tender scapulothoracic bursitis.

Range of Motion Testing of the Glenohumeral and Scapulothoracic Joints

The **throwing athlete's** shoulder often demonstrates a functional adaptation of **increased external rotation** of the throwing arm (Fig. 3–4) and decreased internal

Figure 3–4. Functional adaptation (increased external rotation) in a thrower. (From McCluskey GM: Classification and diagnosis of glenohumeral instability in athletes. Sports Med Arthroscopy Rev 8[2]:158–169, 2000.)

Figure 3–6. ROM testing: forward flexion.

rotation. Testing of the symmetry of active and passive ROM of the shoulder should include

- Internal and external rotation (Fig. 3–5).
- Abduction.
- Forward flexion (Fig. 3–6).
- Extension (Fig. 3–7).

Evaluation of scapulothoracic motion should note subtle scapular winging or lag.

Adhesive capsulitis (frozen shoulder) causes **both restricted active (patient lifts arm) and passive (examiner lifts arm)** shoulder motion, compared with an acute rotator cuff tear, which results in restricted active motion but near-normal passive motion.

A   **B**

Figure 3–5. Range of motion (ROM) testing: internal (*A*) and external (*B*) rotation.

Figure 3–7. ROM testing: extension.

Figure 3–9. Roos test for thoracic outlet syndrome.

Neurologic Testing

Reflexes, motor strength, sensation, and neck ROM are evaluated. Specific tests are used to rule out thoracic outlet syndrome (TOS) and encroachment on a cervical nerve root.

- **Adson test** (Fig. 3–8) is used to rule out TOS.
  - The arm of the standing (or seated) patient is abducted 30 degrees at the shoulder and maximally extended.
  - The radial pulse is palpated and the examiner grasps the patient's wrist.

Figure 3–8. Adson test for thoracic outlet syndrome.

- The patient then turns the head toward the symptomatic shoulder and is asked to take a deep breath and hold it.
- The quality of the radial pulse is evaluated in comparison to the pulse taken while the arm is resting at the patient's side.
- Diminution or disappearance of the pulse suggests a TOS.
- Some clinicians have patients turn their heads **away** from the side tested in a modified test.
- **Wright maneuver** is a similar test in which the shoulder is abducted to 90 degrees and fully externally rotated.
- **Roos test** (Fig. 3–9) is also used to rule out TOS.
  - The patient abducts the shoulder 90 degrees while flexing the elbow to 90 degrees.
  - The hand is opened and closed 15 times.
  - Numbness, cramping, weakness, or inability to complete the repetitions is suggestive of TOS.
- **Spurling test** (Fig. 3–10) detects encroachment on a cervical nerve root (cervicular radiculopathy).
  - The neck is extended and rotated toward the involved side before axial compression.
  - The maneuver is designed to exacerbate encroachment on a cervical nerve root by decreasing the dimensions of the neural foramen.
  - Radicular pain (positive result) radiates into the upper extremity in a specific dermatomal distribution (typically radiates below the elbow).
- Suprascapular nerve compression is difficult to diagnose. Posterior pain and posterior scapular atrophy (infraspinatous fossa) often are present.

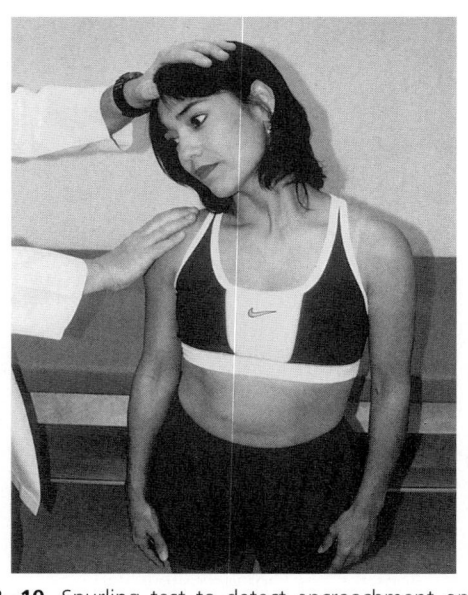

Figure 3–10. Spurling test to detect encroachment on a cervical nerve root.

Figure 3–12. Yergason test for biceps pathology.

- Suprascapular notch tenderness is variable. Electromyography (EMG) studies should confirm diagnosis.

Biceps Testing

- With **Speed test,** the examiner resists forward elevation of the athlete's arm with approximately 60 degrees of forward flexion and 45 degrees of abduction with the elbow fully extended and supinated (Fig. 3–11). The test is positive for proximal biceps tendon involvement if the patient complains of pain.
- For **Yergason test** (Fig. 3–12), the examiner resists the athlete's attempted supination (palm up) from a starting position of elbow flexion of 90 degrees and pronation (palm down). The test is positive when the patient experiences pain about the bicipital groove.
- The **biceps load test** tests for a superior labrum from anterior to posterior (SLAP) lesions of the attachment of the long head of the biceps at the superior glenoid area (see p. 235).
  - With the patient supine on the table, the examiner gently grasps the patient's wrist and elbow.
  - The patient's arm is abducted 90 degrees with the forearm supinated.
  - An anterior apprehension test is performed on the relaxed patient.
  - When the patient becomes apprehensive during external rotation of the shoulder, the external rotation is stopped.

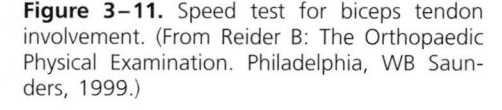

Figure 3–11. Speed test for biceps tendon involvement. (From Reider B: The Orthopaedic Physical Examination. Philadelphia, WB Saunders, 1999.)

- The patient is then asked to flex the elbow while the examiner resists the flexion with one hand.
- The examiner asks how the apprehension has changed, if at all. If the apprehension has lessened or the patient feels more comfortable, the test is considered negative for a SLAP lesion.
- If apprehension is unchanged or has become more painful, the test is considered positive for a SLAP lesion.
- The examiner must sit adjacent to the shoulder at the same height as the patient and should face the patient at a right angle.
- This test has a sensitivity of 90.9%, a specificity of 96.9%, a positive predictive value of 83%, and a negative predictive value of 98% according to Kim and colleagues (2001).
- The **SLAP test** is done with the patient's arm abducted 90 degrees and the hand supinated.
  - The examiner places one hand on the patient's shoulder with the thumb in the 6 o'clock position in the axilla.
  - The examiner's opposite hand exerts a downward force on the patient's hand, thus creating a fulcrum to shift the humeral head superiorly.
  - Crepitation or pain constitutes a positive test.

Ligamentous Laxity Testing

- **Ligamentous laxity is indicated by the sulcus sign** (Fig. 3–13).
  - The patient sits comfortably on the examination table with his or her arms hanging free down by the side.

- The examiner stands in front of the patient and applies a traction force along the longitudinal axis of the humerus by pulling it in an inferior direction.
- Both arms are pulled simultaneously or individually.
- The distance between the acromion and the humeral head is recorded in centimeters.
- **A sulcus of 2 cm or more under the acromion** or an asymmetrical sulcus is positive for inferior subluxation or laxity.
- The second portion of this test is to have the seated, relaxed patient place the arm in 90 degrees of abduction and resting on the examiner's shoulder. The examiner then applies a caudally directed force to the proximal humerus. Excessive inferior translation with a sulcus defect at the acromion and a feeling of subluxation are considered a positive test.
- An additional maneuver is to place the patient's arm in maximum external rotation while the longitudinal force is reapplied. The sulcus sign is measured again and compared with the sulcus that is observed when the arm is in the neutral, relaxed position. With external rotation, the anterior capsule and rotator interval are tightened, which should reduce the amount of inferior translation of the head and produce a smaller measurable sulcus sign.

Patients with generalized ligamentous laxity usually demonstrate a positive sulcus sign, elbow hyperextension, finger hyperextension ("double-jointed"), and a positive thumb-to-forearm test (ability to place the abducted thumb on the ipsilateral forearm). This laxity may at times contribute to multidirectional instability (born loose).

Figure 3–13. Sulcus sign (see text). *A,* The inferior instability test. Best conducted with the patient standing, this test establishes the sulcus sign, a measure of the inferior translation of the humeral head. *B,* Positive sulcus sign of the shoulder. Note the inferior subluxation. (*A,* From Backer M, Warren RF: Recognizing and treating shoulder instability in female athletes. Women's Health Orthop Ed 3[3]:37–40, 2000.)

A   B

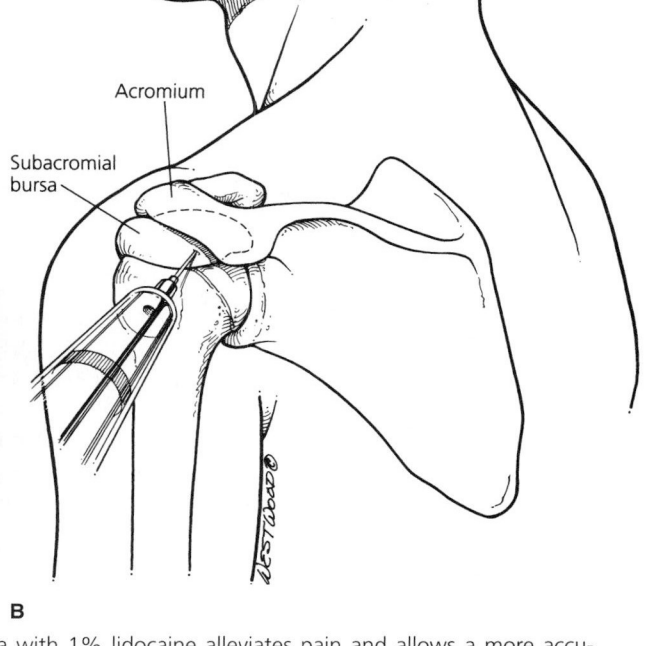

A

B

Figure 3–14. *A* and *B,* Injection of the subacromial bursa with 1% lidocaine alleviates pain and allows a more accurate testing of the strength of the rotator cuff. (*B,* From Idler RS: Rotator cuff disease: diagnosing a common cause of shoulder pain. J Musculoskel Med 6[2]:63–69, 1998.)

Rotator Cuff Testing

Differentiation between rotator cuff tendinitis, bursitis, or a torn rotator cuff (weakness on motor testing) often is aided by a **lidocaine test** (Fig. 3–14). Injection of lidocaine into the subacromial bursa often improves the patient's pain and allows better assessment of *true* motor strength (now not limited by pain).

The **infraspinatus** is tested for weakness by resisted external rotation (Fig. 3–15). With the elbows at the side (taking the deltoid out of the examination), the arms are compared for asymmetry of strength.

Internal rotation against resistance tests the **subscapularis** portion of the rotator cuff. The **"lift-off" test** is also used to test the subscapularis. The patient's hand is placed behind the back and lifted away from the body against resistance (Fig. 3–16).

The **supraspinatus** portion of the rotator cuff **is the most commonly torn portion of the cuff.** With the arm

Figure 3–15. External rotation testing of the rotator cuff (infraspinatus portion).

Figure 3–16. "Lift-off" test to evaluate the subscapularis portion of the rotator cuff.

Figure 3–17. Supraspinatus isolation test is done by resisting the athlete's abduction from the starting position of 90 degrees abduction and about 30 degrees of forward flexion. The examiner applies a downward force toward the floor and the athlete resists.

slightly abducted, forward flexed, and internally rotated, the patient attempts to maintain the arm's position while the examiner pushes downward on the patient's hand (Fig. 3–17). This is called the **supraspinatous isolation test.**

The **"drop-arm" test** (Fig. 3–18) may **suggest a full-thickness rotator cuff tear.**

- The patient is asked to lower the arm from full elevation to 90 degrees of abduction (with the arm extended straight out to the side).
- Patients with large, full-thickness rotator cuff tears often cannot perform this exercise and are unable to smoothly lower the arm to their side. Instead it "drops," even with repeated attempts.

Impingement Tests

Secondary impingement often results in a "relative narrowing" of the subacromial space producing inflammation and tenderness at the rotator cuff, which gets "banged on" by the overlying acromial arch in overhead throwing. The painful, weakened rotator cuff is not as able to perform its humeral head depressor role, thus allowing less subacromial "clearance" during throwing or overhead activities and secondary impingement and a vicious circle is begun.

In **Neer test,** the examiner performs forward elevation of the internally rotated humerus. Pain on this test indicates rotator cuff impingement and/or inflammation (often positive with rotator cuff tendinitis, tears, and primary and secondary subacromial impingement) (Fig. 3–19).

Hawkins test is done with across-the-chest adduction of the internally rotated, forward-flexed arm (Fig. 3–20); pain indicates coracoacromial arch impingement on the rotator cuff. The differential diagnosis is the same as with Neer test (rotator cuff tendinitis, tear, subacromial impingement).

Assessment of underlying shoulder stability is very important in rotator cuff evaluation because rotator cuff signs and symptoms (e.g., tender rotator cuff insertion, RTC tendinitis, etc.) are often a secondary manifestation of an underlying problem in shoulder instability.

The **internal rotation resistance strength test** is used to differentiate internal impingement from external impingement (Fig. 3–21).

- The examiner stands behind the standing patient.
- The patient's arm is abducted 90 degrees and externally rotated 80 degrees.

Figure 3–18. "Drop-arm" test. A positive test indicates a full-thickness rotator cuff tear.

Figure 3–19. Neer impingement test (see text).

Figure 3–20. Hawkins impingement test (see text).

- An isometric manual muscle test is performed for external rotation and is compared with a similar test performed for internal rotation strength.
- Good strength in external rotation and weakness in internal rotation is considered a positive test.
- A positive internal rotation resistance strength test with a positive impingement sign is indicative of **internal impingement (SLAP lesion)**. A negative internal rotation resistance strength test with a positive impingement sign is indicative of external impingement. This test has a sensitivity of 88%, a specificity of 96%, a positive predictive value of 88%, a negative predictive value of 96%, and an accuracy of 94% according to Zaslar (1999).

Figure 3–21. Internal rotation resistance strength test.

Anterior Instability Testing

The **anterior drawer test** (Lachman test of the shoulder) is used to determine whether the patient has anterior instability (i.e., anterior GH joint laxity). The humeral head is passively translated anteriorly on the glenoid with the shoulder as shown in Figure 3–22.

The **anterior apprehension test (crank test)** (Fig. 3–23) is used to assess recurrent anterior instability.

- The patient lies supine on the table with the shoulder at the edge of the table.
- With the arm at 90 degrees of abduction, the elbow is grasped by the examiner with one hand and slowly externally rotated.
- The other hand is placed with fingertips posterior to the humeral head and a gentle anterior force is applied to the humeral head.
- The test is considered positive for anterior instability if the patient expresses apprehension by verbal communication, facial expression, or reflex contracture of the shoulder muscles.
- The test also can be done at 45 and 135 degrees of abduction. At 45 degrees of abduction, the test stresses the subscapularis and middle GH ligament complex. At more than 90 degrees of abduction, the test stresses the inferior GH ligament complex.

The **anterior release test** (Fig. 3–24) evaluates possible anterior instability.

- The patient lies supine on a table with the affected arm over the edge of table.
- The patient abducts the arm 90 degrees while the examiner applies a posteriorly directed force on the humeral head.
- The posterior force is maintained while the arm is brought into extreme external rotation.
- The humeral head is then released suddenly.
- The test is considered positive when the patient experiences sudden pain or a distinct increase in pain or when symptoms that occurred during athletic or work activities are reproduced.
- This test has a sensitivity of 91.9%, a specificity of 88.9%, a positive predictive value of 87.1%, a negative predictive value of 93%, and an accuracy of 90.2% according to Gross and Distefano (1997).

The **shoulder relocation test** (Fig. 3–25) evaluates the patient for internal impingement, recurrent anterior subluxation, and recurrent anterior inferior instability.

- The test is done with the patient supine on the table and usually after an anterior apprehension test.
- *This test can be used to differentiate between anterior instability and impingement.*
- The supine patient's arm is placed in abduction, external rotation, and hyperextension (the apprehension

Figure 3–22. Anterior shoulder drawer test. *A,* The examiner stands at the athlete's axilla with the athlete's arm in 80 to 90 degrees of abduction, and 10 to 20 degrees of external rotation. The athlete's hand is placed between the examiner's outside arm and flank, thereby freeing both examining hands. The examiner should adduct her or his arm against the side to hold the patient's hand in place. *B,* Next, the examiner places her or his hand that is closest to the athlete on the shoulder to be examined with the thumb anteriorly on the coracoid and the finger posteriorly on the scapular spine. This position will allow the examiner to stabilize the scapula and feel the motion of the shoulder translation. With her or his outside hand (the one holding the athlete's hand in the axilla), the examiner grasps the athlete's upper arm just distal to the deltoid insertion. *C,* The examiner applies an anteriorly directed force similar to that used in performing an anterior drawer test in the knee. She or he should maintain a counterforce on the scapula and coracoid with the other hand. This technique allows the examiner to feel the degree of anterior translation of the humeral head and compare it with the opposite shoulder. (*A–C,* From Andrews J, Zarins R, Wilk KE: Injuries in Baseball. Philadelphia, Lippincott-Raven, 1998.)

position), and a posteriorly directed force is applied to the proximal humerus.

- Diminished pain or apprehension with the posteriorly directed force is considered a positive relocation test.
- **If *apprehension is eliminated,*** the test is more specific for anterior instability.
- **If *pain is eliminated,*** the test is more specific for internal impingement.
- Patients with external impingement generally do not have pain in this position. If they do, the relocation test is negative and does not relieve pain.

The **load-and-shift test** (Fig. 3–26) defines passive anterior and posterior translation of the humeral head on the glenoid in patients with hyperlaxity or instability of the shoulder The test can be done with the patient sitting or supine.

Figure 3–23. Anterior apprehension ("crank") test to evaluate recurrent anterior instability. (From Backer M, Warren RF: Recognizing and treating shoulder instability in female athletes. Women's Health Orthop Ed 3[3]:37–40, 2000.)

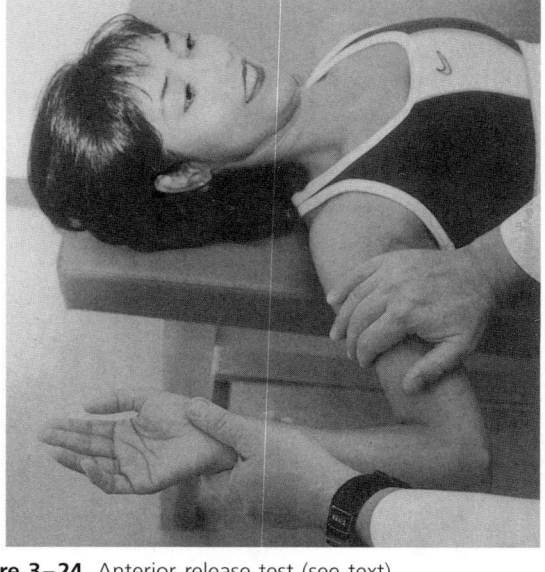

Figure 3–24. Anterior release test (see text).

- Sitting position
  - The examiner stands behind the patient and places one hand over the acromion and scapula to stabilize the shoulder while the other hand cups the proximal humerus with the thumb on the posterior joint line and the index finger on the anterior aspect of the shoulder.
  - The humeral head is loaded by pushing it into the glenoid fossa and is moved relative to the glenoid in the anterior posterior direction (shifting).
  - The degree of translation is recorded along with pain, crepitation, and apprehension.
- Supine position
  - With the patient supine and the shoulder over the edge of the table, the arm is abducted

Figure 3–25. Relocation test for anterior instability (see text).

45 degrees in the scapular plane with neutral rotation.
- While one hand cups the proximal humerus and one hand cups the elbow, an axial load is applied to the humerus with the hand grasping the elbow to compress the humeral head into the glenoid fossa (loading).
- The other hand then shifts the proximal humerus in the anteroposterior direction relative to the glenoid fossa.
- The degree of translation, crepitation, pain, or apprehension is noted.

Posterior Instability and Labral Testing

Posterior instability is evaluated with the **posterior apprehension test** (Fig. 3–27) and the **posterior shoulder drawer test** (Fig. 3–28).

The "clunk" test (Fig. 3–29) is used to assess for labral tears.

- The examiner places one hand on the humeral head with the fingers posterior while the other hand grasps the athlete's humeral condyles at the elbow, providing a back-and-forth motion between internal and external rotation.
- The athlete's shoulder is brought into overhead abduction past 120 degrees, and the examiner's hand on the humeral head provides an anteriorly directed levering force while rotating the humerus with the other hand.
- The examiner is attempting to capture any labral tear with the humeral head and make it snap or pop with the humeral head circumduction motion.
- The test is positive if a "clunk" or reproducible intra-articular pop is appreciated.

The **labral crank test** (Fig. 3–30) to assess for superior labral tear can be done with the patient standing or supine.

- The patient's arm is elevated to 160 degrees in the scapular plane.
- An axial load is applied along the humerus while the arm is rotated maximally in internal rotation and in external rotation.
- The test is considered positive if pain is elicited during this maneuver (usually in external rotation), with or without a click, or if there is reproduction of symptoms (catching or pain) that is similar to the pain felt by the patient during athletic or work activities.
- This test has a sensitivity of 91% and a specificity of 93% according to Liu and coworkers (1996).

O'Brien test (Fig. 3–31) (active compression test), used to evaluate superior labral tears, SLAP lesions, AC joint pathology, and intra-articular biceps pathology, is done with the patient standing.

Figure 3–26. Load-and-shift test. *A*, Standard position. *B*, Anterior translation. *C*, Posterior translation. *D*, Alternative technique. *E*, Anterior translation. *F*, Posterior translation. These tests define passive shoulder translation (increased instability or hyperlaxity). (*A–F*, From Reider B: The Orthopaedic Physical Examination. Philadelphia, WB Saunders, 1999.)

- The patient forward flexes the arm 90 degrees with the elbow in complete extension and then adducts the arm 10 degrees to 15 degrees medial to the sagittal plane of the body.
- The arm is placed in maximal internal rotation so that the thumb is down.
- The examiner stands behind the patient and applies a downward force to the arm while the patient resists this downward motion.
- The second portion of the test is done with the arm in the same position but the patient fully supinates

the forearm with the palm facing the ceiling. The same maneuver is repeated.
- The test is considered positive if pain is elicited during the first step and reduced or eliminated with the second step of this maneuver.
- A click or pop is sometimes heard.
- The test is also considered positive for AC joint pathology when the pain is localized to the top of the shoulder.
- This test is more commonly positive with the palm toward the ceiling.

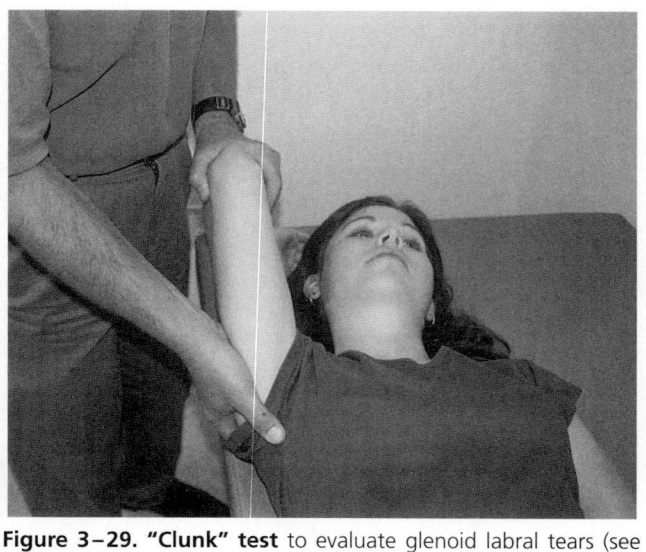

Figure 3–27. Posterior apprehension test. The athlete's shoulder is flexed to at least 90 degrees and internally rotated while the examiner applies a posteriorly directed force on the humerus while increasing the degree of adduction. He or she should use greater forward flexion to 120 degrees to evaluate for posterior and inferior apprehension.

Acromioclavicular Joint Testing

Passive cross-chest adduction (Fig. 3–32) may reproduce AC joint pain if AC joint injury, arthritis, or weight-lifter's osteolysis is present.

    O'Brien test was originally conceived as a test for the AC joint, but may indicate tears of the glenoid labrum as well (see p. 140).

Figure 3–29. "Clunk" test to evaluate glenoid labral tears (see page 140).

General Shoulder Rehabilitation Goals

Motion

Once the intake evaluation is completed, the therapist should be more comfortable anticipating the patient's response to the therapeutic regimen. The key to recovery is motion. The main deterrent to motion is pain, which also is responsible for a high degree of muscle inhibition. Pain can result from injury or surgery. Pain relief can be achieved

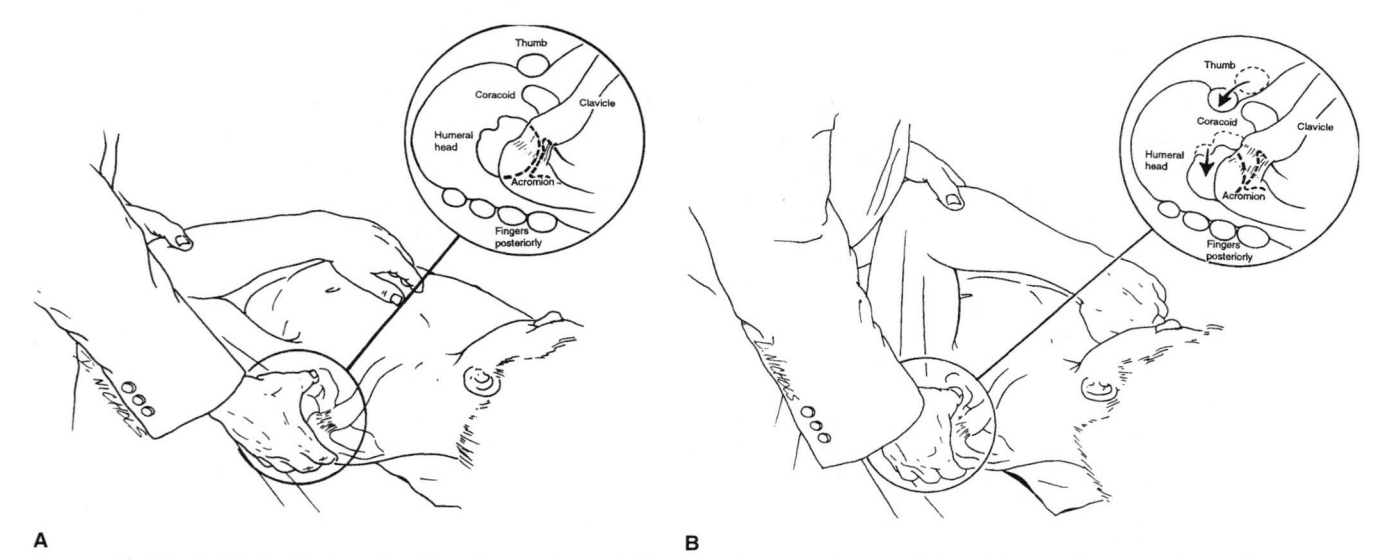

A

B

Figure 3–28. Posterior shoulder drawer test. *A,* The examiner uses her or his hand that is closest to the athlete to grasp the elbow and position the shoulder in about 90 to 120 degrees of abduction and 30 degrees of forward flexion. The examiner's other hand is placed on the athlete's shoulder with the fingers posteriorly on the scapular spine and the thumb on the coracoid (*inset*). *B,* The examiner's thumb on the coracoid is then brought down over the anterior humeral head and a posteriorly directed force is applied (*inset*) as the shoulder is brought into greater flexion and internal rotation. The amount of posterior translation can be appreciated by the motion of the examiner's thumb and by the feeling of the humeral head moving toward the fingers placed posteriorly on the shoulder (*A* and *B,* From Andrews JR, Zarins B, Wilk KE: Injuries in Baseball. Philadelphia, Lippincott-Raven, 1998. Artist: D. Nichols.)

Figure 3–30. "Crank" test. The examiner abducts the arm to 90 degrees, translating the humeral head anteriorly by posterior force, and palpates and feels for crepitus, or grinding, on the anterior rim of the glenoid. (From Andrews JR, Wilk KE: The Athlete's Shoulder. New York, Churchill Livingstone, 1994.)

by a variety of modalities including rest, avoidance of painful motions, cryotherapy, ultrasound, galvanic stimulation, and medications (Fig. 3–33). Once the discomfort is controlled, motion exercises can be started. **Early motion should focus on pain-free ranges below 90 degrees of abduction or 90 degrees of forward flexion.** For most patients, **the early goal is to achieve 90 degrees of elevation and 45 degrees of external rotation with the arm comfortably at the side.** These positions of the shoulder are consistent with most skilled-length and force-dependent motor patterns. For surgical patients, it is the responsibility of the surgeon to obtain at least 90 degrees of stable elevation in the operating room in order for the therapist to be able to gain this motion soon after surgery. Exercises that are used to regain motion around the shoulder include active-assisted pulley or wand maneuvers and passive joint mobilization and stretching. (Figs. 3–34 and 3–35).

We initially begin ROM exercises with the patient supine, the arm comfortably at the side with a small cushion or towel under the elbow, and the elbow bent. This reduces the forces crossing the shoulder joint by decreasing the effect of gravity and **shortening the lever arm** of the upper extremity. As the patient begins to recover pain-free motion, the exercises are done in the seated and standing positions.

Figure 3–31. O'Brien test (active compression test) is used to evaluate superior labral tears, superior labrum from anterior to posterior (SLAP) lesions, AC joint pathology, and intra-articular biceps pathology. *A,* The patient forward flexes the arm to 90 degrees with the elbow extended and adducted 15 degrees medial to the midline of the body and with the thumb pointed down. The examiner applies a downward force to the arm that the patient resists. *B,* Next, the test is performed with the arm in the same position, but the patient fully supinates the arm with the palm facing the ceiling. The same maneuver is repeated. The test is positive for a superior labral injury if pain is elicited in the first step and reduced or eliminated in the second step of this maneuver. (*A* and *B,* From Cannon WD, DeHaven KE: Evaluation and diagnosis of shoulder problems in the throwing athletes. Sports Med Arthroscopy Rev 8[2]:168, 2000.)

Figure 3–32. Passive cross-chest adduction to test for **AC joint pathology.**

Muscle Strengthening

The timing at which muscle strengthening enters the rehabilitation regimen is related to the diagnosis and treatment. For instance, patients who have had a rotator cuff repair generally should avoid active motion and muscle strengthening of the rotator cuff muscles for 6 weeks after surgery, allowing the repaired tendon time to heal securely to the bone of the greater tuberosity of the humerus.

Strengthening of the muscles around the shoulder can be accomplished through different exercises. Initially, basic **closed-chain exercises** are the safest strengthening exercises (Fig. 3–36). The advantage of closed-chain exercises is a cocontraction of both the agonist and the antagonist muscle groups. These exercises closely replicate normal physiologic motor patterns and function to stabilize the shoulder and limit the amount of shear forces crossing the joint. A closed-chain exercise is one in which the distal segment is stabilized against a fixed object. In the shoulder, this can include a wall, a door, or a table. The goal is to generate resistance through motion of the shoulder and scapula. One example of this is the "clock" exercise in which the hand is stabilized against a wall or table, depending on the amount of abduction allowed, and the hand is rotated to different positions of the clock face. This motion effectively stimulates rotator cuff activity. Initially, the maneuvers are done with the shoulder in less than 90 degrees of abduction or flexion. As the tissues heal and motion is recovered, strengthening progresses to greater amounts of abduction and forward flexion.

Strengthening of the scapular stabilizers is very important early on in the rehabilitation program. Scapular strengthening begins with closed-chain exercises (Fig. 3–37) and advances to open-chain exercises (Fig. 3–38).

Recovery can be enhanced by utilizing **proprioceptive neuromuscular facilitation (PNF) exercises.** The therapist can apply specific sensory inputs to facilitate a specific activity or movement pattern. One example of this is the **D2 flexion-extension pattern for the upper extremity.** During this maneuver, the therapist applies

A   B   C

Figure 3–33. Modalities for pain relief. *A,* Ultrasound. *B,* Galvanic stimulation. *C,* Cryotherapy.

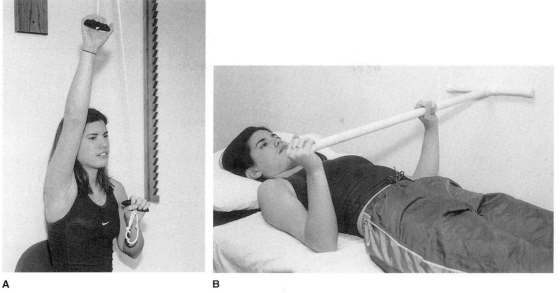

Figure 3–34. Exercises to regain motion. Active-assisted ROM exercises using a pulley system (*A*) and a dowel stick (*B*).

Figure 3–35. Passive joint mobilization. *A*, Forward flexion. *B*, External rotation with the arm at the side. *C*, External rotation with the arm in 90 degrees of abduction. *D*, Cross-body adduction.

A   **B**

Figure 3–36. Closed-chain shoulder exercises. *A,* Isometric strengthening of the rotator cuff in abduction (pushing out against the wall). *B,* Isometric strengthening of the rotator cuff in external rotation.

rhythmic stabilization at different positions of arm elevation, such as 30 degrees, 60 degrees, 90 degrees, and 120 degrees. This results in improved stability of the GH joint through isometric strengthening of the dynamic stabilizers.

As recovery continues and more motion is regained, more aggressive strengthening can be instituted. Closed-

chain exercises can be advanced to open-chain exercises, in which the hand is no longer stabilized against a fixed object. This results in increased shear forces crossing the shoulder joint. Internal and external rotation exercises are one form of open-chain activity and should be done with the shoulder positioned in the scapular plane (Fig. 3–39). **The scapular plane position** is re-created with the arm situated between 30 degrees and 60 degrees anterior to the coronal plane of the thorax, or approximately at the halfway point between directly out to the side (coronal plane) and directly in front (sagittal plane) of the patient. This orientation has been shown to put minimal stress on the joint capsule and orient the shoulder in the position of functional movement. Rotational exercise should begin with the arm comfortably at the patient's side, and advanced to 90 degrees based on the patient's healing stage and level of discomfort. The variation in position positively stresses the dynamic stabilizers by altering the stability of the GH joint from maximum stability with the arm at the side to minimum stability with the arm at 90 degrees of abduction.

The most functional of the open-chain exercises are the **plyometric exercises.** Plyometric activities are defined by a stretching and a shortening cycle of the muscle. This is a component of all athletic activity. Initially, the muscle is eccentrically stretched and then slowly loaded. The higher level of stress that these exercises place on the tissue requires that they be incorporated into the rehabilitation program only after healing is com-

A

Figure 3–37. Closed-chain strengthening exercises of the scapula stabilizers. *A,* Scapular protraction. *B* and *C,* Scapular retraction.

B

C

Figure 3–38. Open-chain strengthening exercises of the scapula stabilizers without (*A–D*) and with (*E–H*) light-weight dumbbells.

pleted and full motion is attained. Plyometric exercises are successful in helping the muscle to recover strength and power. Theraband tubing, a medicine ball, or free weights are all acceptable plyometric devices (Fig. 3–40).

These exercises require close observation by the therapist to help the patient avoid injury.

It is important that while rehabilitation of the shoulder is being done, the remainder of the musculoskeletal

A

B

C

Figure 3–39. Open-chain isotonic strengthening of the rotator cuff (internal rotation) using Theraband tubing (*A*), lightweight dumbbells (*B*), and external rotation strengthening (*C*).

system is not neglected. **Overall conditioning** including stretching, strengthening, and endurance training of the other components of the kinematic chain should be performed simultaneously with shoulder rehabilitation.

Patient motivation is a critical component of the rehabilitation program. Without self-motivation, any treatment plan is destined to fail. For complete recovery, most rehabilitation protocols will require the patient to perform some of the exercises on his or her own at home. This requires not only an understanding of the maneuvers but also the discipline for the patient to execute them on a regular basis. **Patient self-motivation** is even more crucial in the present medical environment with increased attention directed at cost control. Many insurance carriers limit coverage for physical therapy. As a result, a comprehensive home exercise program should also be out-

lined for the patient early in the rehabilitation process. This allows patients to augment their rehabilitation exercises at home and gives them a feeling of responsibility for their own recovery.

Impingement Syndrome

The term "impingement syndrome" was popularized by Neer in 1972 as a clinical entity in which the rotator cuff was pathologically compressed against the anterior structures of the coracoacromial arch, the anterior third of the acromion, the coracoacromial ligament, and the AC joint (Fig. 3–41).

Irritation of the rotator cuff muscle compromises its function as a depressor of the humeral head during overhead activities

A   **B**

Figure 3–40. Plyometric shoulder strengthening exercises using Theraband tubing *(A)* and an exercise ball *(B)*.

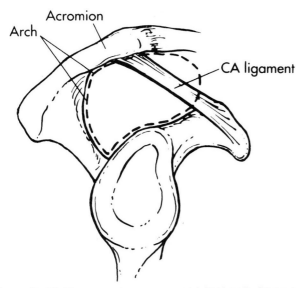

Figure 3–41. The normal coracoacromial (CA) arch. (From Jobe FW [ed]: Operative Techniques in Upper Extremity Sports Injuries. St. Louis, Mosby, 1996.)

(i.e., less clearance of the humeral head under the arch), which further intensifies the impingement process (Fig. 3–42).

A reactive progression of this syndrome is defined by a narrowing of the subacromial outlet by spur formation in the coracoacromial ligament and on the undersurface of the anterior third of the acromion (Fig. 3–43). All of these factors result in an increase in pressure on the rotator cuff, which can lead to chronic wearing and subsequent tearing of the rotator cuff tendons. Neer also defined three stages of impingement relating patient age, physical findings, and clinical course.

Progressive Stages of Shoulder Impingement

Stage 1: Edema and Inflammation

Typical age	Younger than 25 yr, but may occur at any age.
Clinical course	Reversible lesion.
Physical signs	• Tenderness to palpation over the greater tuberosity of the humerus.
	• Tenderness along anterior ridge or acromion.
	• Painful arc of abduction between 60 and 120 degrees, increased with resistance at 90 degrees.
	• Positive impingement sign.
	• Shoulder ROM may be restricted with significant subacromial inflammation.

Stage 2: Fibrosis and Tendinitis

Typical age	25–40 yr.
Clinical course	Not reversible by modification of activity.
Physical signs	Stage 1 signs plus the following:
	• Greater degree of soft tissue crepitus may be felt because of scarring in the subacromial space.
	• Catching sensation with lowering of arm at approximately 100 degrees.
	• Limitation of active and passive ROM.

Stage 3: Bone Spurs and Tendon Ruptures

Typical age	Greater than 40 yr.
Clinical course	Not reversible.

continued

Progressive Stages of Shoulder Impingement
(Continued)

Physical signs	Stages 1 and 2 signs plus the following: • Limitation of ROM, more pronounced with active motion. • Atrophy of infraspinatus. • Weakness of shoulder abduction and external rotation. • Biceps tendon involvement. • AC joint tenderness.

Patients with subacromial impingement often complain of shoulder pain, weakness, and possible paresthesias in the upper arm. It is very important to rule out other causes of these symptoms, such as cervical spine pathology. When subacromial impingement is suspected, **it is necessary to differentiate primary from secondary impingement.** Correct identification of the etiology of the problem is essential for successful treatment.

Primary Impingement

Primary subacromial impingement is the result of an abnormal mechanical relationship between the rotator cuff and the coracoacromial arch. It also includes other "primary" factors that can lead to narrowing of the subacromial outlet (Table 3–3). Patients with primary impinge-

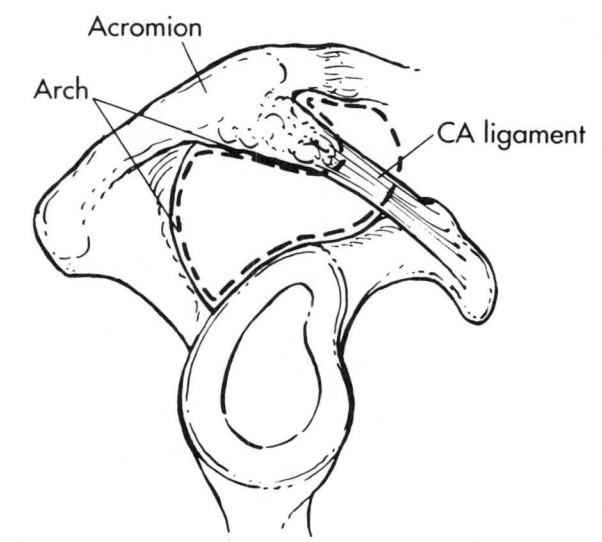

Figure 3–43. Pathologic narrowing of the CA arch. (From Jobe FW [ed]: Operative Techniques in Upper Extremity Sports Injuries. St. Louis, Mosby, 1996.)

ment are usually older than 40 years, complain of anterior shoulder and upper lateral arm pain, with an inability to sleep on the affected side. They have complaints of "shoulder weakness," and difficulty performing overhead activities. On physical examination, patients may exhibit a loss of motion or weakness of rotator cuff strength secondary to pain. They will usually have a positive Hawkins sign (see Fig. 3–20) and a positive impingement

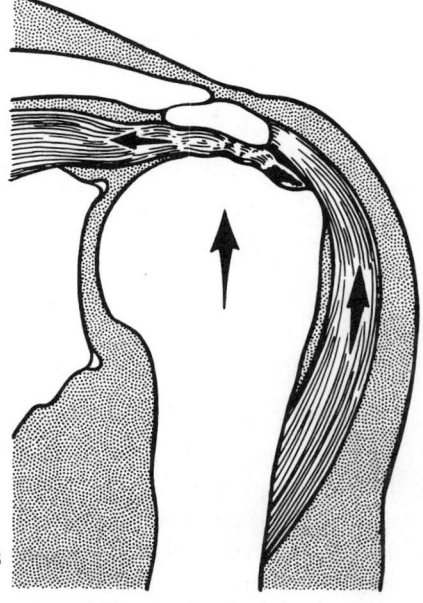

Figure 3–42. The supraspinatus tendon (rotator cuff) helps to stabilize the head of the humerus against the upward pull of the deltoid. *A,* Subacromial impingement is prevented by the normal cuff rotator function. *B,* Deep surface tearing of the supraspinatus tendon weakens the ability of the cuff to hold the humeral head down (i.e., depress the humeral head to allow clearance under the acromion) resulting in impingement of the tendon at the acromion with overhead activities. (*A* and *B,* Redrawn from Matsen FA III, Arntz CT: Subacromial impingement. In Rockwood CA Jr, Matsen FA III [eds]: The Shoulder. Philadelphia, WB Saunders, 1990, p. 624.)

Table 3-3

Structural Factors That May Increase Subacromial Joint Impingement

Structure	Abnormal Characteristics
Acromioclavicular joint	Congenital anomaly Degenerative spur formation
Acromion	Unfused acromion Degenerative spurs on undersurface Malunion/nonunion of fracture
Coracoid	Congenital anomaly Abnormal shape after surgery or trauma
Rotator cuff	Thickening of tendon from calcific deposits Tendon thickening after surgery or trauma Upper surface irregularities from partial or complete tears
Humerus	Increased prominence of greater tuberosity from congenital anomalies or malunions

Modified from Matsen FA III, Arntz CT: Subacromial Impingement. In Rockwood CA Jr, Matsen FA III (eds): The Shoulder. Philadelphia, WB Saunders, 1990.

Figure 3-44. Approach for an AC joint injection.

sign as described by Neer (see Fig. 3–19). The **impingement test** is performed by injecting 10 ml of 1% lidocaine (Xylocaine) into the subacromial space (see Fig. 3–14). Patients with primary impingement may have associated AC joint arthritis, which may contribute to their symptoms and compression of their rotator cuff. These patients may report additional discomfort in the AC joint area with internal rotation maneuvers, such as scratching their back, or experience pain superiorly with abduction of their shoulder. Findings on physical examination that confirm the diagnosis of AC joint arthritis include "point" tenderness at the AC joint with palpation, worsening of the pain at the AC joint with cross-body adduction (see Fig. 3–32), and resolution of the pain with an injection of lidocaine into the AC joint (Fig. 3–44). Radiologic evaluation including an axillary and supraspinatus outlet view may support the diagnosis of primary or "outlet" impingement by demonstrating an os acromiale or a type III acromion (large, hooked acromial spur), respectively (Fig. 3–45).

Secondary Impingement

Secondary impingement is a clinical phenomenon that results in a "relative narrowing" of the subacromial space. This often results from GH or scapulothoracic joint instability. In patients who have underlying GH instability, the symptoms are those of rotator cuff dysfunction (which occur from an overuse injury of the cuff from the increased work the muscles are performing to stabilize the shoulder). The loss of the stabilizing function of the rotator cuff muscles also leads to an abnormal superior translation of the humeral head (decreased depression

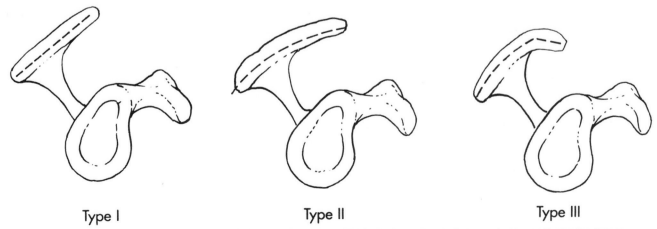

Type I   Type II   Type III

Figure 3-45. Different acromion morphologies. (From Jobe FW [ed]: Operative Techniques in Upper Extremity Sports Injuries. St. Louis, Mosby, 1996.)

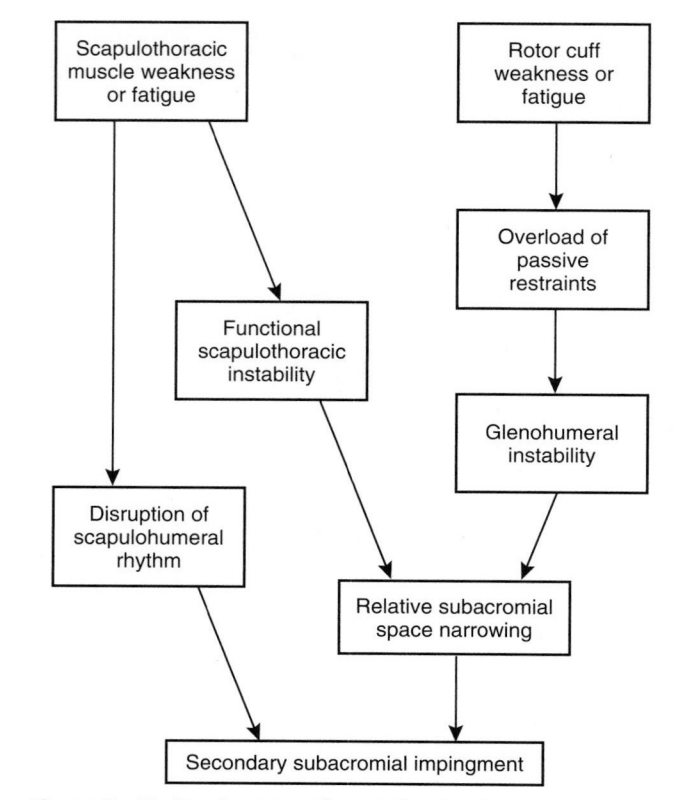

Figure 3–46. Development of secondary impingement.

of the humeral head during throwing and less "clear-ance") and mechanical impingement of the rotator cuff on the coracoacromial arch (see Fig. 3–42). In patients who have scapular instability, impingement results from **improper positioning of the scapula with relation to the humerus.** The instability leads to insufficient retraction of the scapula, which allows for earlier abutment of the coracoacromial arch on the underlying rotator cuff (Fig. 3–46).

Patients with secondary impingement are usually younger and often participate in overhead sporting activities such as baseball, swimming, volleyball, or tennis. They complain of pain and weakness with overhead motions and may even describe a feeling of the arm going "dead." On physical examination, the examiner should look for possible associated pathology, including GH joint instability with a positive apprehension (see Fig. 3–23) and relocation (see Fig. 3–25) test or abnormal scapular function such as scapular winging or asymmetrical scapular motion. **Patients with tightening of the posterior capsule have a loss of internal rotation. Posterior capsular tightness leads to an obligate translation of the humeral head and rotator cuff in an anterior and superior direction, which contributes to the impingement problem.**

In patients with secondary impingement, treatment of the underlying problem should result in resolution of

the "secondary impingement" symptoms. **Often, the recognition of the underlying GH joint instability or scapular instability is missed, and the "secondary impingement" is incorrectly treated as a "primary" (large spur) impingement. A subacromial decompression here worsens the symptoms because the shoulder is rendered even more "unstable."**

Treatment

The key to the successful treatment of subacromial impingement is defining the underlying cause of the impingement symptoms, whether they are primary or secondary to the pathologic relationship between the coracoacromial arch and the rotator cuff. This factor becomes more critical when conservative management fails and surgical intervention is indicated, because the operative procedures for these two clinical entities may be entirely different. **For primary impingement, surgical treatment involves widening the subacromial outlet by performing a subacromial decompression (acromioplasty). The surgical treatment for secondary impingement is directed toward the *etiology* of the symptoms.** For example, if the symptoms of impingement are secondary to anterior GH joint instability, **the surgical treatment is an anterior stabilization, not an acromioplasty.** Performing an acromioplasty in this setting may provide short-term benefit, but as the activities related to the onset of the problem resume, the instability symptoms will persist.

Nonoperative Treatment

Nonoperative treatment is very successful and involves a combination of treatment modalities including anti-inflammatory medications and a well-organized rehabilitation program. In general, the comprehensive rehabilitative protocols for both primary and secondary impingement syndrome are similar and follow the postoperative rehabilitation plan for patients who have had a subacromial decompression with a normal rotator cuff. The initial goals of the rehabilitative process are to obtain pain relief and regain motion. Along with oral medications, judicious use of subacromial injections with a corticosteroid may help to control the discomfort in the acute stages of the inflammatory process. Other modalities such as cryotherapy and ultrasound are also effective in controlling pain. Improving comfort will allow more successful advances in motion and strengthening. Because the rotator cuff tendon is intact, ROM exercises can be both passive and active. Initially, these are done with the arm below 90 degrees of abduction to avoid impingement of the rotator cuff. As symptoms improve, the ROM is increased.

Initially, strengthening exercises begin with the arm at the side. The program begins with closed-chain exercises (see Fig. 3–36), with open-chain exercises initiated after advancing the closed-chain exercises without aggravating shoulder discomfort (see Fig. 3–39). **These exercises help restore the ability of the rotator cuff to dynamically depress and stabilize the humeral head, resulting in a gradual relative increase in the subacromial space.** In patients with secondary impingement, strengthening is started with the arm comfortably at the patient's side to avoid positions that provoke symptoms of instability, such as abduction combined with external rotation. As the dynamic stabilizers respond to the strengthening program, exercises can be added in higher planes of abduction. In general, **strengthening of the deltoid muscle is not emphasized early in the rehabilitation program to avoid a disproportionate increase in the upward force on the humerus.**

Scapula stabilizing exercises are important for patients with primary or secondary impingement (see Figs. 3–37 and 3–38). The scapula forms the base from which the rotator cuff muscles originate. Reciprocal motion is required between the GH and scapulothoracic joint articulations for proper cuff function and correct positioning of the coracoacromial arch.

Abnormal scapular movement or dyskinesia can be treated with a scapular taping program as part of the exercise regimen (Fig. 3–47). Scapular taping can improve the biomechanics of the scapulohumeral and scapulothoracic joints, helping to relieve patient's symptoms.

Historically, nonoperative treatment was considered unsuccessful if no improvement occurred after a year of proper conservative management. **Today, nonoperative treatment should be considered unsuccessful if the patient shows no improvement after 3 months of a comprehensive and coordinated medical and rehabilitative program.** Furthermore, **after 6 months of appropriate conservative treatment, most patients have achieved maximal improvement from the nonoperative treatment program.** Failed conservative management or a plateau in recovery at an undesirable level of function is an indication for surgical intervention.

Operative Treatment

The success of operative treatment is determined by the choice of an appropriate operative procedure and the technical skill of the surgeon. **For primary impingement, the current procedure of choice** is arthroscopic subacromial decompression, although comparable long-term results can be obtained with a traditional open acromioplasty. Rehabilitation after the surgery focuses on pain control, improved ROM, and muscle strengthening.

When GH joint instability is the reason for secondary impingement, surgical treatment is a stabilization procedure. In our practice, we see numerous patients whose impingement was secondary (due to underlying GH joint instability) but were incorrectly treated with subacromial decompression. This only worsens the underlying instability.

The most commonly performed procedure is an open stabilization, with either a repair of a torn or avulsed labrum or a capsular shift (capsulorrhaphy), depending on the etiology. With technologic advances in arthroscopic instrumentation, fixation devices, and electrothermal technology, many surgeons are now performing arthroscopic stabilization procedures. The potential advantages of arthroscopic procedures include decreased operative time, less operative morbidity, less loss of motion, and a quicker recovery. Currently, the **literature reflects a higher failure rate after arthroscopic stabilization than after open stabilization.** Arthroscopic procedures require advanced arthroscopic skills, complete recognition of the pathoanatomy, challenging fixation techniques, and appropriate diagnosis-related rehabilitation programs. The rehabilitation principles after an arthroscopic stabilization procedure that includes a labral repair or suture capsulorrhaphy are similar to those after an open stabilization. The biology of healing tissue is the same whether the procedure is done open or arthroscopically, unless the tissue has been treated with thermal energy. **Electrothermal arthroscopic capsulorrhaphy, or "shrinking" the shoulder capsule, requires a protective period of approximately 3 weeks after the treatment.** If the rehabilitation program is advanced too early, before the healing response has been adequately initiated, there is a high risk that the capsule will be "stretched" and the procedure will not correct the capsular laxity. The rehabilitation protocol after an open or arthroscopic Bankart repair for anterior shoulder instability is fundamentally the same, except for the 3-week delay for patients who have been treated with an electrothermal capsulorrhaphy.

Figure 3–47. Example of scapular taping.

Rehabilitation Protocol
Conservative (Nonoperative) Treatment of Shoulder Impingement
Wilk and Andrews

Impingement is a chronic inflammatory process produced as the rotator cuff muscles (supraspinatus, infraspinatus, teres major, and subscapularis) and the subdeltoid bursa are "pinched" against the coracoacromial ligament and the anterior acromion when the arm is raised above 80 degrees. The supraspinatus-infraspinatus portion of the rotator cuff is the most common area of impingement. This syndrome is commonly seen in throwing sports, in racquet sports, and in swimmers; but can be present in anyone who uses the arm repetitively in a position over 90 degrees of elevation.

Phase 1: Maximal Protection—Acute Phase

Goals
- Relieve pain and swelling.
- Decrease inflammation.
- Retard muscle atrophy.
- Maintain/increase flexibility.

Active Rest
- Eliminate any activity that causes an increase in symptoms (e.g., throwing).

Range of Motion
- Pendulum exercises.
- Active-assisted ROM—limited symptom-free available range
  - Rope and pulley
    - Flexion.
  - L-bar
    - Flexion.
    - Neutral external rotation.

Joint Mobilizations
- Grades 1 and 2.
- Inferior and posterior glides in scapular plane.

Modalities
- Cryotherapy.
- Transcutaneous electrical stimulation (TENS), high-voltage galvanic stimulation (HVGS).

Strengthening Exercises
- Isometrics—submaximal (see p. 146)
  - External rotation.
  - Internal rotation.
  - Biceps.
  - Deltoid (anterior, middle, posterior).

Patient Education and Activity Modification
- Regarding activity, pathology, and avoidance of overhead activity, reaching, and lifting activity.

Phase 2: Motion Phase—Subacute Phase

Criteria for Progression to Phase 2
- Decreased pain and/or symptoms.
- Increased ROM.

- Painful arc in abduction only.
- Improved muscular function.

Goals
- Reestablish nonpainful ROM.
- Normalize athrokinematics of shoulder complex.
- Retard muscular atrophy without exacerbation of pain.

Range of Motion
- Rope and pulley
  - Flexion.
  - Abduction (symptom-free motion only).
- L-bar
  - Flexion.
  - Abduction (symptom-free motion).
  - External rotation in 45 degrees of abduction, progress to 90 degrees of abduction.
  - Internal rotation in 45 degrees of abduction, progress to 90 degrees of abduction.
- Initiate anterior and posterior capsular stretching (Fig. 3–48).

Joint Mobilizations
- Grades 2, 3, and 4.
- Inferior, anterior, and posterior glides.
- Combined glides as required.

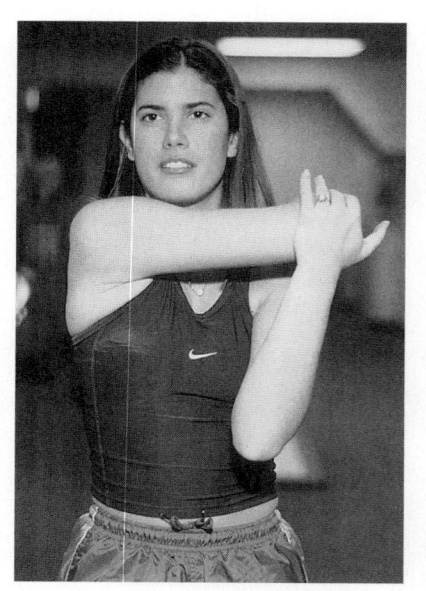

Figure 3–48. Stretching of the posterior capsule.

Rehabilitation Protocol
Conservative (Nonoperative) Treatment of Shoulder Impingement *(Continued)*
Wilk and Andrews

Modalities
- Cryotherapy.
- Ultrasound/phonophoresis.

Strengthening Exercises
- Continue isometrics exercises.
- Initiate scapulothoracic strengthening exercises (see scapulothoracic section).
- Initiate neuromuscular control exercises.

Phase 3: Intermediate Strengthening Phase

Criteria for Progression to Phase 3
- Decrease in pain and symptoms.
- Normal active-assisted ROM.
- Improved muscular strength.

Goals
- Normalize ROM.
- Symptom-free normal activities.
- Improve muscular performance.

Range of Motion
- Aggressive L-bar active-assisted ROM in all planes.
- Continue self-capsular stretching (anterior-posterior).

Strengthening Exercises
- Initiate isotonic dumbbell program
  - Side-lying neutral
    - Internal rotation (p. 148).
    - External rotation (p. 148).
  - Prone
    - Extension.
    - Horizontal abduction.
  - Standing
    - Flexion to 90 degrees.
    - Supraspinatus.
- Initiate serratus exercises
  - Wall push-ups.
- Initiate tubing progression in slight abduction for internal and external rotation strengthening.
- Initiate arm ergometer for endurance.

Phase 4: Dynamic Advanced Strengthening Phase

Criteria for Progression to Phase 4
- Full, nonpainful ROM.
- No pain or tenderness.
- 70% of contralateral strength.

Goals
- Increase strength and endurance.
- Increase power.
- Increase neuromuscular control.

Isokinetic Testing
- Internal and external rotation modified neutral.
- Abduction-adduction.

Initiate "Thrower's Ten" Exercise Program (see Thrower's Ten section)
Isokinetics
- Velocity spectrum 180 degrees/sec to 300 degrees/sec.
- Progress from modified neutral to 90/90 position as tolerated.

Initiate Plyometric Exercises (late in this phase) (see p. 149)

Phase 5: Return to Activity Phase

Criteria for Progression to Phase 5
- Full, nonpainful ROM.
- No pain or tenderness.
- Isokinetic test that fulfills criteria.
- Satisfactory clinical examination.

Goal
- Unrestricted symptom-free activity.

Isokinetic Test
- 90/90 internal and external rotation, 180 degrees/sec, 300 degrees/sec.
- Abduction-adduction, 180 degrees/sec, 300 degrees/sec.

Initiate Interval Throwing Program
- Throwing.
- Tennis.
- Golf.

Maintenance Exercise Program

Flexibility Exercises
- L-bar
  - Flexion.
  - External rotation.
  - Self-capsular stretches.

Isotonic Exercises
- Supraspinatus.
- Prone extension.
- Prone horizontal abduction.

Theratubing Exercises
- Internal and external rotation.
- Neutral or 90/90 position.
- D2 proprioceptive neuromuscular facilitation (PNF) pattern.

Serratus Push-ups
Interval Throwing Phase II for Pitchers

Rehabilitation Protocol
After Arthroscopic Subacromial Decompression—Intact Rotator Cuff (Distal Clavicle Resection)
Bach, Cohen, and Romeo

Phase 1: Weeks 0–4

Restrictions
- ROM
  - 140 degrees of forward flexion.
  - 40 degrees of external rotation.
  - 60 degrees of abduction.
- ROM exercises begin with the arm comfortably at the patient's side, progress to 45 degrees of abduction and eventually 90 degrees. Abduction is advanced slowly depending on patient comfort level.
- No abduction or rotation until 6 wk after surgery—this combination re-creates the impingement maneuver.
- No resisted motions until 4 wk postoperative.
- (No cross-body adduction until 8 wk postoperatively if distal clavicle resection.)

Immobilization
- Early motion is important.
- Sling immobilization for comfort only during the first 2 wk.
- Sling should be discontinued by 2 wk after surgery.
- Patients can use sling at night for comfort.

Pain Control
- Reduction of pain and discomfort is essential for recovery
  - Medications
    - Narcotics—10 day–2 wk following surgery.
    - Nonsteroidal anti-inflammatory drugs (NSAIDs)–for patients with persistent discomfort following surgery.
  - Therapeutic modalities
    - Ice, ultrasound, HVGS.
    - Moist heat before therapy, ice at end of session.

Motion: Shoulder
- Goals
  - 140 degrees of forward flexion.
  - 40 degrees of external rotation.
  - 60 degrees of abduction.
- Exercises
  - Begin with Codman pendulum exercises to promote early motion.
  - Passive ROM exercises (see Fig. 3–35).
  - Capsular stretching for anterior, posterior, and inferior capsule, using the opposite arm (see Fig. 3–48).
  - Active-assisted ROM exercises (see Fig. 3–34)
    - Shoulder flexion.
    - Shoulder extension.
    - Internal and external rotation.
  - Progress to active ROM exercises as comfort improves.

Motion: Elbow
- Passive—progress to active
  - 0–130 degrees.
  - Pronation and supination as tolerated.

Muscle Strengthening
- Grip strengthening with racquetball, putty, Nerf ball.

Phase 2: Weeks 4–8

Criteria for Progression to Phase 2
- Minimal pain and tenderness.
- Nearly complete motion.
- Good "shoulder strength" $^4/_5$ motor.

Restrictions
- Progress ROM goals to
  - 160 degrees of forward flexion.
  - 45 degrees of internal rotation (vertebral level L1).

Immobilization
- None.

Pain Control
- NSAIDs—for patients with persistent discomfort.
- Therapeutic modalities
  - Ice, ultrasound, HVGS.
  - Moist heat before therapy, ice at end of session.
- Subacromial injection: lidocaine/steroid—for patients with acute inflammatory symptoms that do not respond to NSAIDs.

Motion
- Goals
  - 160 degrees of forward flexion.
  - 60 degrees of external rotation.
  - 80 degrees of abduction.
  - 45 degrees of internal rotation (vertebral level L1).
- Exercises
  - Increasing active ROM in all directions.
  - Focus on prolonged, gentle passive stretching at end ranges to increase shoulder flexibility.
  - Utilize joint mobilization for capsular restrictions, especially the posterior capsule (see Fig. 3–48).

Muscle Strengthening
- Rotator cuff strengthening (only three times per week to avoid rotator cuff tendinitis)
  - Begin with closed-chain isometric strengthening (see Fig. 3–36)
    - Internal rotation.
    - External rotation.
    - Abduction.
  - Progress to open-chain strengthening with Therabands (see Fig. 3–38)
    - Exercises performed with the elbow flexed to 90 degrees.
    - Starting position is with the shoulder in the neutral position of forward flexion, abduction, and external rotation (arm comfortably at the patient's side).
    - Exercises are performed through an arc of 45 degrees in each of the five planes of motion.

Rehabilitation Protocol
After Arthroscopic Subacromial Decompression—Intact Rotator Cuff (Distal Clavicle Resection) *(Continued)*
Bach, Cohen, and Romeo

- Six color-coded Theraband bands are available; each provides increasing resistance from 1 to 6 pounds, at increments of one pound.
- Progression to the next band occurs usually in 2- to 3-wk intervals. Patients are instructed not to progress to the next band if there is any discomfort at the present level.
- Theraband exercises permit both **concentric and eccentric strengthening** of the shoulder muscles and are a form of isotonic exercises (characterized by variable speed and fixed resistance)
  - Internal rotation.
  - External rotation.
  - Abduction.
  - Forward flexion.
  - Extension.
- Progress to light isotonic dumbbell exercises (see Fig. 3–39B)
  - Internal rotation.
  - External rotation.
  - Abduction.
  - Forward flexion.
  - Extension.
- Scapular stabilizer strengthening
  - Closed-chain strengthening exercises (see Fig. 3–37)
    - Scapular retraction (rhomboideus, middle trapezius).
    - Scapular protraction (serratus anterior).
    - Scapular depression (latissimus dorsi, trapezius, serratus anterior).
  - Progress to open-chain scapular stabilizer strengthening (see Fig. 3–38).

Note: Do not perform more than 15 repetitions for each set, or more than three sets of repetitions. If this regimen is easy for the patient, then increase the resistance, not the repetitions. Upper body strengthening with excessive repetitions is counterproductive.

Phase 3: Weeks 8–12
Criteria for Progression to Phase 3
- Full painless ROM.
- Minimal or no pain.
- Strength at least 50% of contralateral shoulder.
- "Stable" shoulder on clinical examination—no impingement signs.

Goals
- Improve shoulder strength, power, and endurance.
- Improve neuromuscular control and shoulder proprioception.
- Prepare for gradual return to functional activities.

Motion
- Achieve motion equal to contralateral side.
- Utilize both active and passive ROM exercises to maintain motion.

Muscle Strengthening
- Advance strengthening of rotator cuff and scapular stabilizers as tolerated.
- Eight to 15 repetitions for each exercise, for three sets.
- Continue strengthening only three times per week to avoid rotator cuff tendinitis from overtraining.

Functional Strengthening
- Plyometric exercises (see Fig. 3–40).

For Patients with Concomitant Distal Clavicle Resections
- Now begin cross-body adduction exercises
  - First passive, advance to active motion when AC joint pain is minimal.

Phase 4: Weeks 12–16
Criteria for Progression to Phase 4
- Full, painless ROM.
- No pain or tenderness.
- Shoulder strength that fulfills established criteria.
- Satisfactory clinical examination.

Goals
- Progressive return to unrestricted activities.
- Advancement of shoulder strength and motion with a home exercise program that is taught throughout rehabilitation.

Progressive, Systematic Interval Program for Returning to Sports
- Throwing athletes (see p. 190).
- Tennis players (see p. 192).
- Golfers (see p. 195).
- Institute "Thrower's Ten" program (p. 165) for overhead athlete.

Maximum improvement is expected by 4–6 mo following an acromioplasty, and 6–12 mo following an acromioplasty combined with a distal clavicle resection.

Warning Signals
- Loss of motion—especially internal rotation.
- Lack of strength progression—especially abduction.
- Continued pain—especially at night.

Treatment of above "Problems"
- These patients may need to move back to earlier routines.
- May require increased utilization of pain control modalities as outlined above.
- If no improvement, patients may require repeat surgical as outlined
  - It is important to determine that the appropriate surgical procedure was done initially.
  - Issues of possible secondary gain must be evaluated.

Rehabilitation Protocol
After Arthroscopic Subacromial Decompression and/or Partial Rotator Cuff Débridement
Wilk

This rehabilitation program's goal is to return the patient/athlete to activity/sport as quickly and safely as possible. The program is based on muscle physiology, biomechanics, anatomy, and healing response.

Phase 1: Motion Phase

Goals
- Reestablish nonpainful ROM.
- Retard muscular atrophy.
- Decrease pain/inflammation.

Range of Motion
- Pendulums exercise.
- Rope and pulley.
- L-Bar exercises
    - Flexion-extension.
    - Abduction-adduction.
    - Internal and external rotation (begin at 0 degrees abduction, progress to 45 degrees abduction, then 90 degrees abduction).
- Self-stretches (capsular stretches).

Strengthening Exercises
- Isometrics.
- May initiate tubing for internal and external rotation at 0 degrees abduction late phase.

Decrease Pain and Inflammation
- Ice, NSAIDs, modalities.

Phase 2: Intermediate Phase

Criteria for Progression to Phase 2
- Full ROM.
- Minimal pain and tenderness.
- "Good" manual muscle testing (MMT): internal and external rotation and flexion.

Goals
- Regain and improve muscular strength.
- Normalize arthrokinematics.
- Improve neuromuscular control of shoulder complex.

Exercises
- Initiate isotonic program with dumbbells.
- Shoulder musculature.
- Scapulothoracic musculature.
- Initiate neuromuscular control exercises.
- Initiate trunk exercises.
- Initiate upper extremity endurance exercises.

Normalize Athrokinematics of Shoulder Complex
- Joint mobilization.
- Control L-bar ROM.

Decrease Pain and Inflammation
- Continue use of modalities, ice, as needed.

Phase 3: Dynamic (Advanced) Strengthening Phase

Criteria for Progression to Phase 3
- Full nonpainful ROM.
- No pain or tenderness on examination.
- Strength 70% of contralateral side.

Goals
- Improve strength, power, and endurance.
- Improve neuromuscular control.
- Prepare athlete to begin to throw, and similar activities.

Emphasis of Phase 3
- High-speed, high-energy strengthening exercises.
- Eccentric exercises.
- Diagonal patterns.

Exercises
- Continue dumbbell strengthening (supraspinatus, deltoid).
- Initiate tubing exercises in the 90/90 position for internal and external rotation (slow/fast sets).
- Tubing exercises for scapulothoracic musculature.
- Tubing exercises for biceps.
- Initiate plyometrics for rotator cuff.
- Initiate diagonal patterns (PNF).
- Initiate isokinetics.
- Continue endurance exercises: neuromuscular control exercises.

Phase 4: Return to Activity Phase

Criteria for Progression to Phase 4
- Full ROM.
- No pain or tenderness.
- Isokinetic test that fulfills criteria to throw.
- Satisfactory clinical examination.

Goal
- Progressively increase activities to prepare patient for full functional return.

Exercises
- Initiate interval throwing program (see p. 190).
- Continue all exercises as in phase 3
    - Throw and train on same day.
    - Lower extremity and ROM on opposite days.
- Progress interval program.

Follow-up Visits
- Isokinetic tests.
- Clinical examination.

Rotator Cuff Tendinitis in the Overhead Athlete

Overhead athletic activities can be classified as those movements that require repetitive motions with the arm in at least 90 degrees of forward flexion or abduction or a combination of the two. Athletes who participate in activities such as swimming, tennis, or throwing sports experience this type of repetitive trauma to the shoulder and, as a result, are prone to shoulder disorders. The frequency of injury is related to the athlete's age and level of competition. These patients present a significant diagnostic and treatment challenge to the physician. They usually demonstrate a degree of *hyperlaxity of the GH joint* resulting from *an increased anterior laxity of their shoulder capsule*, which is required to perform these overhead motions, as well as a *compensatory tightening of the posterior capsule*. **Symptom-free function in the setting of substantial GH joint "laxity" or looseness is accomplished by the proper development of the dynamic stabilizers crossing the GH joint.**

During overhead sports, the rotator cuff is continually being challenged to keep the humeral head centered in the glenoid and prevent pathologic displacement owing to the extreme forces acting on the shoulder (see Table 3–2). As a result of this highly stressed environ-

ment, the joint capsule and rotator cuff can develop a secondary inflammatory response. Prolonged rotator cuff tendinitis can result in decreased muscular efficiency with loss of dynamic stability, with a final pathway of functional instability and progressive tissue failure. **Posterior capsular tightness, which manifests as a loss of internal rotation, is often present in overhead throwers and may lead to anterior-superior humeral head translation, further contributing to irritation of the rotator cuff.**

The biomechanics of throwing has been closely analyzed. As a result, it serves as an appropriate model to examine the motions and arm positions of overhead athletic activities. The **throwing motion** and its related biomechanics is divided into **six stages:** wind-up, early-cocking, late-cocking, acceleration, deceleration, and follow-through (Fig. 3–49).

- **Wind-up:** Serves as the preparatory phase. Includes body rotation and ends when the ball leaves the nondominant hand.
- **Early-cocking:** As the ball is released from the glove hand, the shoulder abducts and externally rotates. The body starts moving forward, generating momentum. Early-cocking terminates as the forward foot contacts the ground.
- **Late-cocking:** As the body rapidly moves forward, the dominant shoulder achieves maximal abduction

Figure 3–49. Six phases of throwing. (From Jobe FW [ed]: Operative Techniques in Upper Extremity Sports Injuries. St. Louis, Mosby, 1996.)

and external rotation. Significant torques and forces are placed on the shoulder restraints at this extreme range of motion.

- **Acceleration:** Begins with further forward body motion, internal rotation of the humerus leading to internal rotation of the throwing arm. Acceleration ends with ball release.
- **Deceleration:** Begins after ball release and constitutes 30% of the time required to dissipate the excess kinetic energy of the throwing motion.
- **Follow-through:** Completes the remaining 70% of the time required to dissipate the excess kinetic energy. All major muscle groups must eccentrically contract to accomplish this result. Follow-through ends when all motion is complete.

Athletes who experience **pain in the late-cocking phase** usually localize the symptoms to the **anterior aspect of their shoulder.** The position of the arm during the late-cocking phase is maximal abduction and external rotation, which challenges the anterior stability of the GH joint. Pain during this stage can be the result of anterior instability or from the rotator cuff owing to secondary impingement related to the anterior instability. **Discomfort during the late-cocking and early ac-** **celeration stages can be experienced posteriorly,** and may be secondary to the irritation of the posterior capsule and rotator cuff as it tries to balance out the increased anterior laxity. Another potential cause is **trauma to the posterior-superior glenoid labrum** and associated articular surface of the rotator cuff related to the hyperabduction and rotation that occurs during overhead sports. This condition has been labeled **"internal impingement"** and may be another consequence of subtle increases in anterior GH joint laxity. Furthermore, a considerable amount of energy is absorbed during the follow-through stage of throwing. The posterior shoulder structures and the eccentrically contracting muscles experience an enormous amount of repetitive stress during this phase and as a result are at risk for injury.

These patients are a diagnostic challenge to the physician. A considerable amount of information can be obtained from the history (see the Importance of History-Taking section). It is important to identify the specific throwing phase associated with the onset of symptoms.

- Localization of pain is important, as well as documenting any recent change in the athlete's training

CLASSIFICATION SYSTEM

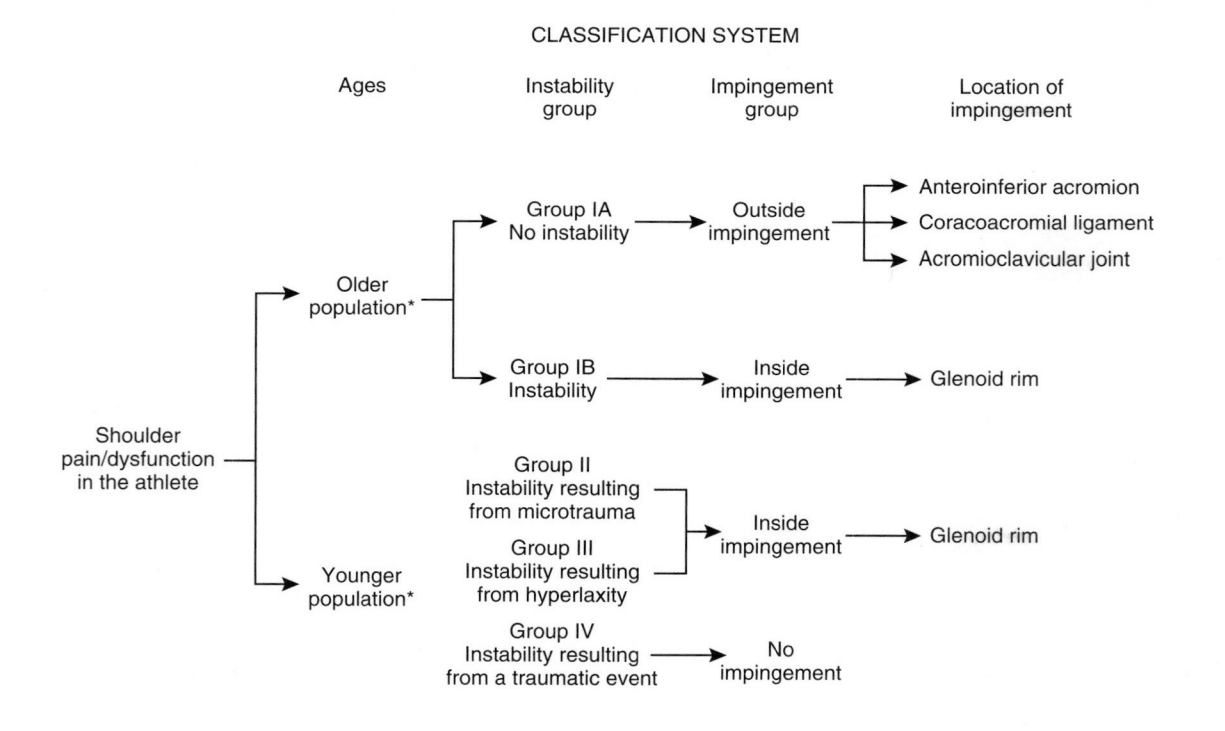

* There is some overlap between the two age groups.

Figure 3–50. Classification of shoulder pain and dysfunction in the overhead athlete. (From Jobe FW [ed]: Operative Techniques in Upper Extremity Sports Injuries. St. Louis, Mosby, 1996.)

routine. This includes both the general conditioning program and the throwing regimen.

- **On physical examination, one needs to examine for shoulder instability, posterior capsular tightness, primary impingement, and rotator cuff tendinitis.**
- Findings on physical examination that are indicative of a rotator cuff tendinitis include tenderness and possibly weakness with resisted external rotation or abduction in the scapular plane.
- Pain with resistance is known as "tendon signs" and at a minimum represents inflammation of the cuff tendons. Resolution of the symptoms and recovery of strength after injection of lidocaine in the subacromial space strongly suggest cuff tendinitis rather than a cuff tear.

Rotator cuff tendinitis can lead to a secondary type impingement and also make a primary impingement syndrome more symptomatic. Rehabilitation focuses on resolution of the inflammation, recovery of motion, and careful strengthening of the rotator cuff muscles and the scapular stabilizers.

Figure 3–50 depicts a classification system for shoulder pain and dysfunction in the overhead athlete. Rehabilitation programs for pitchers, position players, tennis players, and golfers are included in the Interval Throwing section. **These programs should be implemented for all patients returning to their sport after a period of inactivity.** For sports-specific rehabilitation programs to be successful, the entire body must be re-educated in a stepwise fashion to perform the various activities related to the sport. This encourages a smooth transition for the athlete back to sport. These protocols are appropriate for all patients recovering from a shoulder injury, regardless of their treatment. Diagnosis and treatment will dictate when patients can begin sport-specific exercises and at what level they enter into the rehabilitation program.

Table 3–4		
Isokinetic Criteria for Return to Throwing*		
Bilateral compression	ER	98–105%
Bilateral compression	IR	105–115%
Bilateral compression	ABD	98–103%
Bilateral compression	ADD	110–125%
Unilateral ratio	ER/IR	66–70%
Unilateral ratio	ABD/ADD	78–85%
Peak torque:body weight ratio	ER	18–22%
Peak torque:body weight ratio	IR	28–32%
Peak torque:body weight ratio	ABD	24–30%
Peak torque:body weight ratio	ADD	32–38%

*All data represent 180% test speed.
ABD, abduction; ADD, adduction; ER, external rotation; IR, internal rotation.
Modified from Wilk KE, Andrews JK, Arrigo CA: The abductor and adductor strength characteristics of professional baseball pitchers. Am J Sports Med 23(3):307, 1995.

The important factor requires the treatment team to begin these exercises after the patient has recovered the appropriate motion and strength in the shoulder following the more traditional physical therapy programs as outlined in this chapter. The team has to advance the patient appropriately. If discomfort develops as the result of "too much" being done, the athlete should take a few days rest. Additional treatment may be required to decrease inflammation, and a return to the previous exercise level may be needed until symptoms have resolved. The details outlined in these protocols are to help the athlete and the trainer move along a progressive course to achieve a full recovery and return to competition. Objective data that can be acquired before resumption of throwing is outlined in Table 3–4.

Common Causes of Injuries to the Pitching Arm*

Even with excellent conditioning, good gradual warm-up, adequate rest, and proper throwing mechanics, the upper extremity of a thrower experiences great stresses.

The causes of pitching arm injuries may be divided into four categories: **conditioning problems, fatigue, overuse** (or **overload**), and **mechanical faults.**

Conditioning Problems

The lack of being properly conditioned

- Lack of total body fitness.
- Lack of arm strengthening via a structured progressive preseason throwing program.

The lack of the development of good arm strength and stamina over a long period of time (months to years)

- Need for an off-season throwing program.
- Need of a supervised and structured preseason and in-season throwing program.

continued

Common Causes of Injuries to the Pitching Arm* *(Continued)*

Improper strengthening and/or weight training program causing

- A restricted ROM in the shoulder and/or trunk.
- An imbalance of antagonistic muscle strength.
- The shortening or bulking-up of muscle fibers involved in the throwing mechanism.

Overstretching the shoulder joint causing too much laxity.
Lack of proper warm-up and stretching program before pitching.
Experimenting with new pitches at full velocity, full distance, or throwing too hard for too long early in the season.
Pitching in games before being properly conditioned and prepared for competitive situations.

Fatigue, Overuse, and/or Overload Factors

Throwing too many pitches during one outing.
Throwing when tired, fatigued, or with tight muscle fibers.
Not getting adequate rest and recovery time between pitching turns.
Lack of an active in-season maintenance program of running, stretching, light strengthening work, and a controlled throwing program.
Playing or practicing at other positions between pitching turns, resulting in overuse.
Strength work that is too fatiguing or strenuous between pitching turns causing a general body or specific muscle fatigue.

Mechanical faults

Usually negatively affect control and velocity and cause added stress on the throwing arm.

*For an outstanding review of pitching faults and their correction, we recommend Injuries in Baseball by Wilk, Andrews, and Zarins.
From Wilk KE, Andrews JR, Zarins B: Injuries in Baseball. Philadelphia, Lippincott-Raven, 1998.

Prevention of Arm Injuries in Throwers

Coaches and trainers can help prevent arm injuries in throwers by

- Making sure pitchers are properly conditioned (total body) before throwing full velocity or pitching competitively.
- Making sure pitchers have and use a proper stretching and warm-up and cool-down program before throwing a baseball.
- Developing a year-round throwing program to maintain arm strength and stamina, flexibility, and normal ROM. We recommend a 2- to 3-wk rest period at the end of a long season, followed by a limited and modified off-season throwing program.
- Teaching and supervising a proper weight and resistance program. Coaches or medical personnel should be responsible for this program. Many pitchers restrict their flexibility and ROM by improper use of weights. Other pitchers have actually weakened themselves by overstretching the shoulder joint, causing too much laxity.
- Having the pitcher throw at reduced velocity and shorter distances when learning new mechanical techniques or new pitches.
- Making certain a pitcher pitches with proper throwing mechanics. Although each pitcher throws somewhat within his or her own style, through the critical phase of throwing (from hand-break through the deceleration phase), most successful, injury-free pitchers use very similar, time-proven techniques.
- Limiting the amount of throwing the pitcher does during drills and practices if he or she plays another defensive position. The defensive positions that would cause the least amount of stress on the arm are first base or the outfield.
- Making certain the pitcher dresses properly for warmth during cold temperatures, or for prevention of early heat exhaustion during very hot weather. Also, be aware of proper intake of fluids to prevent early dehydration and muscle fatigue.
- Finally, even though lightweight, full ROM conditioning and strength work are recommended, the best method to build throwing arm strength and stamina is to throw a baseball, and throw it biomechanically correctly.

From Wilk KE, Andrews JR, Zarins B: Injuries in Baseball. Philadelphia, Lippincott-Raven, 1998.

Our **throwers rehab regimen** includes:

- Self-stretching techniques for pathologic changes in "tightness" of the capsule (see Fig. 3–51).
- Off-season adherence to rotator cuff, scapulothoracic, and shoulder girdle strengthening with the **"Thrower's Ten"** program (Fig. 3–52).

- Excellent conditioning of the "entire" athlete.
- Warm-up and cool-down period with practice and games.
- Avoidance of "overuse"—throwing while fatigued.
- Use of the throwing program described in Wilk and coworkers (1998).

A, **Inferior capsular stretch.** Hold the involved arm overhead with the elbow bent and the arm straight ahead. Using the uninvolved arm, stretch the arm farther overhead. When a stretching sensation is felt, hold for 5 sec and repeat.

A

B, **Posterior capsular stretch.** With the uninvolved arm, grasp the elbow of the involved arm. Pull the involved arm across the chest to stretch the back of the involved shoulder. Hold at the end point for 5 sec and repeat. This is very important in throwers because of a tight posterior capsule.

B

C, **Anterior capsular stretch.** Standing in a doorway, the patient holds on to the doorframe with the elbow straight and the shoulder abducted to 90 degrees and externally rotated. Walk through the doorway until a stretch is felt at the front of the shoulder. Hold for 5 sec and repeat. Avoid this stretch in patients with generalized ligamentous laxity or multidirectional instability.

C

Figure 3–51. Self-stretching of the shoulder. (*A–F,* From Wilk KE, Andrews JR: The Athlete's Shoulder. New York, Churchill Livingstone, 1994.)

D, **Pectoralis minor stretch.** Lie on the back, pushing the shoulders toward the ceiling with a partner giving resistance. Relax and have the partner stretch the shoulder down. Hold the stretch for 5 sec.

D

E, **Pectoralis major corner stretch.** Stand facing a corner. Position one arm on each side of the corner with the arms approximately 90 degrees away from the side and the forearms resting on the wall. Lean forward into the corner until a stretch is felt on the front of the shoulders. Hold____sec. Repeat____times.

E

F, **Biceps stretch.** Sit with the elbow extended and resting on the leg. With the uninvolved arm pushing on the forearm, straighten the elbow and hold the stretch for 5 sec.

F

A, **Diagonal pattern D2 extension.** Grip the tubing handle overhead and out to the side with the hand of the involved arm. Pull the tubing down and across the body to the opposite side of the leg. During the motion, lead with the thumb. Perform ＿＿ sets of ＿＿ repetitions ＿＿ times daily.

Diagonal pattern D2 flexion. Grip the tubing handle in the hand of the involved arm, beginning with the arm 45 degrees out from the side and the palm facing backward. After turning the palm forward, flex the elbow and bring the arm up and over the uninvolved shoulder. Turn the palm down and reverse to take the arm to the starting position. The exercise should be performed in a controlled manner. Perform ＿＿ sets of ＿＿ repetitions ＿＿ times daily.

B, **Dumbbell exercises for deltoid and supraspinatus deltoid strengthening.** Stand with the arm at the side with the elbow straight and the palm against the side. Raise the arm to the side, palm down, until the arm reaches 90 degrees. Perform ＿＿ sets of ＿＿ repetitions ＿＿ times daily.

Supraspinatus strengthening. Stand with the elbow straight and the thumb up. Raise the arm to shoulder level at a 30-degree angle in front of the body. Do not go above shoulder height. Hold for 2 sec and lower slowly. Perform ＿＿ sets of ＿＿ repetitions ＿＿ times daily.

Figure 3–52. *A–J,* **"Thrower's Ten" program.** The "Thrower's Ten" program is designed to exercise the major muscles necessary for throwing. The program's goal is to be an organized and concise exercise program. In addition, all exercises included are specific to the thrower and are designed to improve strength, power, and endurance of the shoulder complex musculature. (From Andrews JR, Wilk KE: The Athlete's Shoulder. New York, Churchill Livingstone, 1994.)

C, **Prone shoulder abduction for rhomboids: diagonal pattern D2 flexion.** With the involved hand, grip the tubing handle across the body and against the thigh of the opposite leg. Starting with the palm down, rotate the palm up to begin. Flex the elbow and bring the arm up and over the involved shoulder with the palm facing inward. Turn the palm down and reverse to take the arm to the starting position. The exercise should be performed in a controlled manner. Perform _____ sets of _____ repetitions _____ times daily.

C

D, **Prone shoulder extension for latissimus dorsi.** Lie on the table, face down, with the involved arm hanging straight to the floor and the palm facing down. Raise the arm straight back as far as possible. Hold for 2 sec and lower slowly. Perform _____ sets of _____ repetitions _____ times daily.

D

E, **Internal rotation at 90 degrees abduction.** Stand with the shoulder abducted to 90 degrees and externally rotated 90 degrees and the elbow bent to 90 degrees. Keep the shoulder abducted and rotate the shoulder forward, keeping the elbow at 90 degrees. Return the tubing and the hand to the start position slowly and controlled.
Left, Slow-speed sets: perform _____ sets of _____ repetitions _____ times daily.
Right, Fast-speed sets: perform _____ sets of _____ repetitions _____ times daily.

External rotation at 90 degrees abduction. Stand with the shoulder abducted to 90 degrees and the elbow flexed to 90 degrees. Grip the tubing handle while the other hand is fixed straight ahead. Keep the shoulder abducted and rotate the shoulder back, keeping the elbow at 90 degrees. Return the tubing and the hand to the start position slowly and controlled.
Left, Slow-speed sets: perform _____ sets of _____ repetitions _____ times daily.
Right, Fast-speed sets: perform _____ sets of _____ repetitions _____ times daily.

E

F, **Biceps strengthening with tubing.** Stand with one end of the tubing securely in the involved hand and the opposite end under the foot of the involved side, controlling tension. Assist with the opposite hand, flexing the arm through full ROM. Return to the starting position with a slow 5-count. Repeat three to five sets of 10 repetitions.

F

G, **Dumbbell exercises for triceps and wrist extensors-flexors. Triceps curls:** Raise the involved arm overhead. Provide support at the elbow from the uninvolved hand. Straighten the arm overhead. Hold for 2 sec and lower slowly. Perform _____ sets of _____ repetitions _____ times daily.
Wrist flexion. Support the forearm on a table with the hand off the edge, the palm facing upward. Hold a weight or hammer in the involved hand and lower it as far as possible; then curl it up as high as possible. Hold for a 2-count. Perform _____ sets of _____ repetitions _____ times daily.
Wrist extension. Support the forearm on a table with the hand off the edge, the palm facing downward. Hold a weight or hammer in the involved hand and lower it as far as possible, then curl it up as high as possible. Hold for a 2-count. Perform _____ sets of _____ repetitions _____ times daily.
Forearm pronation. Support the forearm on a table with the wrist in neutral position. Hold a weight or hammer in a normal hammering position and roll the wrist and bring the hammer into pronation as far as possible. Hold for a 2-count. Raise to the starting position. Perform _____ sets of _____ repetitions _____ times daily.
Forearm supination. Support the forearm on a table with the wrist in neutral position. Hold a weight or hammer in a normal hammering position and roll the wrist, bringing the hammer into full supination. Hold for a 2-count. Raise back to the starting position. Perform _____ sets of _____ repetitions _____ times daily.

G

H, **Serratus anterior strengthening.** Start with a push-up into the wall. Gradually progress to the tabletop and eventually to the floor as tolerable. Perform _____ sets of _____ repetitions _____ times daily.

H

I, **Press-ups.** Sit on a chair or a table and place both hands firmly on the sides of the chair or table, the palm down and the fingers pointed outward. The hands should be placed as far apart as the width of the shoulders. Slowly push downward through the hands to elevate the body. Hold the elevated position for 2 sec. Repeat. Perform _____ sets of _____ repetitions _____ times daily.

I

J, **Rowing.** Lie on the stomach with the involved arm hanging over the side of a table, the dumbbell in the hand and the elbow straight. Slowly raise the arm, bending the elbow, and bring the dumbbell as high as possible. Hold at the top for 2 sec, then lower slowly. Repeat. Perform _____ sets of _____ repetitions _____ times daily.

J

• Use of the Fundamental Shoulder Exercises program developed by Health-South Sports Medicine and Rehabilitation of Birmingham, Alabama (Fig. 3–53).

Rotator Cuff Tears

Rotator cuff tears and subacromial impingement are among the most common causes of shoulder pain and disability. The frequency of rotator cuff tears increases with age, with full-thickness tears uncommon in patients younger than 40 years. The **rotator cuff "complex"** refers to the tendons of **four muscles: subscapularis, supraspinatus, infraspinatus, and teres minor.** These four muscles originate on the scapula, cross the GH joint, then transition into tendons that insert onto the tuberosities of the proximal humerus. **The rotator cuff has three well-recognized functions: rotation of the humeral head, stabilization of the humeral head in the glenoid socket by compressing the round head into the shallow socket, and the ability to provide "muscular balance," stabilizing the GH joint when other larger muscles crossing the shoulder contract.** Injury to the rotator cuff may occur in progressive stages (see box p. 149). Rotator cuff tears can be classified as either *acute* or *chronic*, based on their timing, and as *partial* (articular or bursal side) or *complete*, based on the depth of the tear. Complete tears can be classified based on the size of the tear in square centimeters as described by Post (1983): **small** (0–1 cm^2), **medium** (1–3 cm^2), **large** (3–5 cm^2), or

A, **Rope and pulley, flexion.** The overhead rope and pulley should be positioned in a doorway. Sit in a chair with your back against the door, directly underneath the pulley. With the elbow straight and the thumb facing upward, raise the involved arm out to the front of the body as high as possible. Assist as needed by pulling down with the uninvolved arm. Hold overhead ____ sec and repeat ____ times.

A

B

B, **L-bar flexion.** Lie on the back and grip the L-bar between the index finger and the thumb, with the elbows straight. Raise both arms overhead as far as possible, keeping the thumbs up. Hold for ____ sec and repeat ____ times.

C, **L-bar external rotation, scapular plane.** Lie on the back with the involved arm 45 degrees from the body and the elbow at 90 degrees. Grip the L-bar in the hand of the involved arm and keep the elbow stabilized. Using the uninvolved arm, push the involved arm into external rotation. Hold for ____ sec, return to the starting position. Repeat ____ times.

C

D, **L-bar internal rotation, scapular plane.** Lie on the back with the involved arm 45 degrees from the body and the elbow at 90 degrees. Grip the L-bar in the hand of the involved arm and keep the elbow in the flexed position. Using the uninvolved arm, push the involved arm into internal rotation. Hold for ____ sec, return to the starting position. Repeat ____ times.

D

E, **Tubing, external rotation.** Stand with the involved elbow fixed at the side, the elbow at 90 degrees, and the involved arm across the front of the body. Grip the tubing handle; the other end of the tubing should be fixed. Pull out with the arm, keeping the elbow at the side. Return the tubing slowly and controlled. Perform ____ sets of ____ repetitions.

E

Figure 3–53. The **fundamental shoulder exercise program.** *(A–J, From Wilk KJ: Handout on Shoulder Exercises. Birmingham, Ala, HealthSouth Sports Medicine and Rehabilitation, 1993.)*

F, **Tubing, internal rotation.** Stand with the involved elbow fixed at the side, the elbow at 90 degrees, and the shoulder rotated out. Grip the tubing handle; the other end of the tubing should be fixed. Pull the arm across the body, keeping the elbow at the side. Return the tubing slowly and controlled. Perform _____ sets of _____ repetitions.

F

G, **Lateral raises to 90 degrees.** Stand with the involved arm at the side, the elbow straight, and the palm against the side. Raise the arm, rotating the palm up as the arm reaches 90 degrees. Do not go above shoulder height. Hold for _____ sec and lower slowly. Perform _____ sets of repetitions.

G

H, **"Empty can."** Stand with the involved elbow straight and the thumb down. Raise the arm to shoulder height at a 30-degree angle in front of the body. Do not go above shoulder height. Hold _____ sec and lower slowly. Perform _____ sets of _____ repetitions.

H

I, **Prone horizontal abduction.** Lie on the table, face down, with the involved arm hanging straight to the floor and the palm facing down. Raise the arm out to the side, parallel to the floor. Hold _____ sec and lower slowly. Perform _____ sets of _____ repetitions.

I

J, **Biceps curls.** Stand with the involved arm against the side and the palm facing inward. Bend the elbow upward, turning the palm up as you progress. Return to the starting position, lowering slowly. Perform _____ sets of _____ repetitions.

J

massive (>5 cm^2). All these factors, as well as the patient's demographic and medical background, play a role in determining the treatment plan.

Surgical repair of a torn rotator cuff is done in an effort to decrease pain, increase function, and improve ROM. Postoperative care must strike a precarious balance between restrictions that allow for tissue healing, activities that return ROM, and gradual restoration of muscle function and strength. It is not uncommon to have residual postoperative stiffness and pain despite an excellent operative repair if the postop rehabilitation is not correct.

Wilk and Andrews described multiple factors that significantly affect the postoperative rehabilitation program after repair of rotator cuff tears.

Factors Affecting Rehabilitation after Repair of Rotator Cuff Tears

Type of Repair

Open
Mini-open
Arthroscopic

Size of Tear

Absolute size
Number of tendons involved

Patient's Tissue Quality

Good, fair, poor

Factors Affecting Rehabilitation after Repair of Rotator Cuff Tears *(Continued)*

Location of Tear

Superior tear
Superoposterior
Superoanterior

Surgical Approach

Onset of Tissue Failure

Acute or gradual onset
Timing of repair

Patient Variables

Age
Dominant or nondominant arm
Preinjury level
Desired level of function (work and sports)
Work situation
Patient compliance with therapy regimen

Rehabilitation Situation

Supervised or unsupervised

Physician's Philosophic Approach

From Wilk KE, Crockett HC, Andrews JR: Rehabilitation after rotator cuff surgery. Tech Shoulder Elbow Surg 1(2):128–144, 2000.

Type of Repair

Patients who have had deltoid muscle detachment or release from the acromion or clavicle (e.g., **traditional open rotator cuff repair**) may not perform active muscle contractions of the deltoid for 6 to 8 weeks. This is avoided to prevent avulsion of the deltoid.

Arthroscopic repair of the cuff actually has a slightly *slower* rate of rehabilitation progression owing to the weaker fixation of the repair compared with that of the open procedure. A **mini-open** procedure, involving a vertical split with the orientation of the deltoid fibers, allows mild, earlier deltoid muscular contractions. Regardless of the surgical approach performed, the underlying biology of healing tendons must be respected for all patients.

Size of the Tear

Functional outcome and expectation after rotator cuff surgery are directly related to the size of the tear repaired. Wilk and Andrews (2002) base the rate of rehab on the size and extent of the tear (see Rehabilitation Protocol, p. 184).

Tissue Quality

The quality of the tendon, muscular tissue, and bone helps determine speed of rehabilitation. Thin,

fatty, or weak tissue is progressed slower than excellent tissue.

Location of the Tear

Tears that involve posterior cuff structures require a slower progression in external rotation strengthening. Rehabilitation after subscapularis repair (anterior structure) should limit resisted internal rotation for 4 to 6 weeks. Restriction of the amount of passive external rotation motion should also be restricted until early tissue healing has occurred. Most tears occur and are confined to the supraspinatus tendon, the critical site of wear, often corresponding to the site of subacromial impingement.

Onset of the Rotator Cuff Tear and the Timing of the Repair

Acute tears with *early* repair may have a slightly greater propensity to develop stiffness, and we are a little more aggressive in the ROM program. Cofield (2001) noted that patients who underwent an early repair progressed more rapidly with rehabilitation than those with a late repair.

Patient Variables

Several authors have reported a less successful outcome in older patients than young. This may be due to older patients' typically having larger and more complex tears, probably affecting outcome.

Several studies have noted no difference in outcome based on arm dominance. Hawkins and associates (1991) noted that worker's compensation patients required twice as long to return to work compared with their non–worker's compensation cohorts.

Finally, researchers have noted a correlation between preoperative shoulder function and outcome after surgical repair. Generally, patients who have an active lifestyle before surgery return to the same postop.

Rehabilitation Situation and Surgeon's Philosophic Approach

We recommend treatment with a skilled shoulder therapist rather than a home therapy program. Lastly, some physicians prefer more aggressive progression, whereas others remain very conservative in their approach.

Rehabilitation after rotator cuff surgery emphasizes immediate motion, early dynamic GH joint stability, and gradual restoration of rotator cuff strength. Throughout rehabilitation, overstressing of the healing tissue is to be avoided, striking a balance between regaining shoulder mobility and promoting soft tissue healing.

Basic Rehabilitation Goals after Rotator Cuff Repair

Goal 1	Maintain integrity of the repaired rotator cuff. *Never overstress healing tissue.*
Goal 2	Reestablish full passive ROM as quickly and safely as possible.
Goal 3	Reestablish dynamic humeral head control. *Do not work through a shoulder shrug!*
Goal 4	Improve external rotation muscular strength. *Reestablish muscular balance.*
Goal 5	Initiate resisted shoulder abduction and flexion when muscular balance is restored.
Goal 6	Caution against overaggressive activities (tissue-healing constraints).
Goal 7	Restore patient's functional use of shoulder, but do so gradually.
Goal 8	Activate rotator cuff muscles through inhibition of pain.

From Wilk KE, Crockett HC, Andrews JR: Rehabilitation after rotator cuff surgery, Tech Shoulder Elbow Surg 1(2):128–144, 2000.

Figure 3–54. Radiologic evaluation of the shoulder: lateral view in the plane of the scapula. (From Rockwood CA Jr, Matsen FA III: The Shoulder, 2nd ed. Philadelphia, WB Saunders, 1988.)

Acute Tears

Patients with acute tears of the rotator cuff usually present to their physician after a traumatic injury. They have complaints of pain and sudden weakness, which may be manifested by an inability to elevate the arm. On physical examination, they have a weakness in shoulder motion of forward elevation, external rotation, or internal rotation depending on which cuff muscles are involved. Passive motion is usually intact depending on the timing of presentation. If the injury is chronic and the patient has been avoiding using the shoulder because of pain, there may be concomitant adhesive capsulitis (limitation of passive shoulder motion) and weakness of active ROM (underlying rotator cuff tear).

Radiographs

A standard radiologic evaluation or "trauma shoulder series" should be obtained, including an **anteroposterior (AP) view** in the plane of the scapula ("true AP" of GH joint) (Fig. 3–54), a **lateral view** in the plane of the scapula (Fig. 3–55), and **an axillary lateral view** (Fig. 3–56). These radiographs help to eliminate other potential pathologic entities such as a fracture or dislocation. MRI can provide direct imaging of the rotator cuff, helping to confirm the clinical diagnosis.

It is important to remember that **the likelihood of an associated rotator cuff tear with a shoulder dislocation increases with age.** In patients older than 40 years of age, an associated rotator cuff tear is present with shoulder dislocation in more than 30%; in patients older than 60 years, it is present in more than 80%. Therefore,

serial examinations of the shoulder are necessary after a dislocation to evaluate the integrity of the rotator cuff. If significant symptoms of pain and weakness persist after 3 weeks, an imaging study of the rotator cuff is required. A

Figure 3–55. Radiologic evaluation of the shoulder: lateral view in the plane of the scapula. (From Rockwood CA Jr, Matsen FA III: The Shoulder, 2nd ed. Philadelphia, WB Saunders, 1988.)

Figure 3–56. Radiologic evaluation of the shoulder: axillary lateral view. This view is important to avoid missing acute or chronic shoulder dislocation. (From Rockwood CA Jr, Matsen FA III: The Shoulder, 2nd ed. Philadelphia, WB Saunders, 1988.)

torn rotator cuff after a dislocation is a surgical problem, so once the diagnosis is made, surgical repair is indicated.

Treatment

The recommended treatment for active patients with acute tears of the rotator cuff is surgical repair. Advantages of early operative repair include mobility of the rotator cuff, which allows technically easier repairs, good quality of the tendon, which allows a more stable repair, and in the patients with cuff tears associated with a dislocation, the repair will improve GH joint stability.

Chronic Tears

Chronic rotator cuff tears may be an asymptomatic pathologic condition that has an association with the normal aging process. A variety of factors, including poor vascularity, a "hostile" environment between the coracoacromial arch and the proximal humerus, decreased use, or gradual deterioration in the tendon, contribute to the senescence of the rotator cuff, especially the supraspinatus. Lehman and colleagues (1995) found rotator cuff tears in 30% of cadavers older than 60 years and in only 6% of those younger than 60 years. In a study by Romeo and coworkers (1999), **the average age of their patients treated for a rotator cuff tear was 58 years.** Many patients with a chronic rotator cuff tears are over the age of 50 years, have no history of shoulder trauma,

and have vague complaints of intermittent shoulder pain that has become progressively more symptomatic. These patients may also have a history that is indicative of a primary impingement etiology.

Examination

- On physical examination, some evidence of muscular atrophy may be seen in the supraspinatus fossa.
- Depending on the size of the tear, there may also be atrophy in the infraspinatus fossa.
- Passive motion is usually maintained, but may be associated with subacromial crepitance.
- Smooth active motion is diminished, and symptoms are reproduced when the arm is lowered from an overhead position.
- Muscle weakness is related to the size of the tear and the muscles involved.
- A subacromial injection of lidocaine may help to differentiate weakness that is caused by associated painful inflammation from that caused by a cuff tendon tear.
- Provocative maneuvers including the Neer impingement sign (see Fig. 3–19) and the Hawkins sign (see Fig. 3–20) may be positive but are nonspecific because they may be positive with other conditions such as rotator cuff tendinitis, bursitis, or partial-thickness rotator cuff tears.
- It is important that other potential etiologies be investigated. Patients with cervical radiculopathy at the C5–6 level can have an insidious onset of shoulder pain, rotator cuff weakness, and muscular atrophy in the supraspinatus and infraspinatus fossa.

Imaging

Imaging studies may be helpful in confirming the diagnosis of a chronic rotator cuff tear and may help to determine the potential success of operative treatment.

- A "trauma shoulder series" (p. 172) may show some proximal (superior) humeral migration, which is indicative of chronic rotator cuff insufficiency.
- Plain radiographs can also show degenerative conditions or bone collapse consistent with a cuff tear arthropathy in which both the cuff deficiency and the arthritis contribute to the patient's symptoms.
- An MRI examination of the shoulder may help to demonstrate a rotator cuff tear, its size, and degree of retraction. The MRI can also help assess the rotator cuff musculature. Evidence of fatty or fibrous infiltration of the rotator cuff muscles is consistent with a long-standing cuff tear and is a poor prognostic indicator for a successful return of cuff function.
- Ultrasound and double-contrast shoulder arthrography are additional studies that are occasionally used to diagnose rotator cuff tears, but are less helpful for determining the age of the tear.

Treatment

Treatment of most patients with a chronic tear of the rotator cuff follows a conservative rehabilitation program. Operative intervention in this patient population is indicated for patients who are unresponsive to conservative management or demonstrate an acute tearing of a chronic injury. The primary goal of surgical management of rotator cuff tears is to obtain pain relief. Additional goals, which are easier to achieve with acute rotator cuff tears than chronic rotator cuff tears, include improved ROM, improved strength, and return of function.

Rehabilitation Protocol
For Patients with Chronic Rotator Cuff Tears—Treated Conservatively (Nonoperatively)
Bach, Cohen, and Romeo

Phase 1: Weeks 0–4

Restrictions
- Avoid provocative maneuvers or exercises that cause discomfort
  - Includes both offending ROM exercises and strengthening exercises.
- Patients may have an underlying subacromial bursitis, therefore ROM exercises, and muscle strengthening exercises should begin with the arm in less than 90 degrees of abduction.
- **Avoid** abduction-rotation—re-creates impingement maneuver.
- **Avoid** "empty-can" exercises.

Immobilization
- Brief sling immobilization for comfort only.

Pain Control
- Reduction of pain and discomfort is essential for recovery.
- Medications
  - NSAIDs—for the older population with additional comorbidities, consider newer cyclooxygenase-2 (COX-2) inhibitors.
  - Subacromial injection of corticosteroid and local anesthetic; judicious use for patients with acute inflammatory symptoms of a concomitant bursitis; limit of three injections.
- Therapeutic modalities
  - Ice, ultrasound, HVGS.
  - Moist heat before therapy, ice at end of session.

Shoulder Motion

Goals
- Internal and external rotation equal to contralateral side, with the arm positioned in less than 90 degrees of abduction.

Exercises
- Begin with Codman pendulum exercises to gain early motion.
- Passive ROM exercises (see Fig. 3–35)
  - Shoulder flexion.
  - Shoulder extension.
  - Internal and external rotation.

- Capsular stretching for anterior, posterior, and inferior capsule by using the opposite arm (see Fig. 3–48).
- **Avoid** assisted motion exercises (see Fig. 3–34)
  - Shoulder flexion.
  - Shoulder extension.
  - Internal and external rotation.
- Progress to active ROM exercises
  - "Wall-walking" (Fig. 3–57).

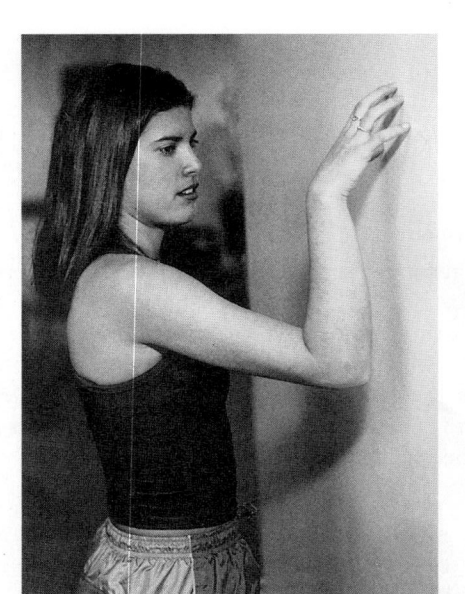

Figure 3–57. Demonstration of active ROM of the shoulder, "Wall walking."

Elbow Motion
- Passive to active motion, progress as tolerated
  - 0–130 degrees.
  - Pronation to supination as tolerated.

Muscle Strengthening
- Grip strengthening (putty, Nerf ball, racquetball).
- Use of the arm for activities of daily living **below shoulder level.**

Rehabilitation Protocol
For Patients with Chronic Rotator Cuff Tears—Treated Conservatively (Nonoperatively) *(Continued)*
Bach, Cohen, and Romeo

Phase 2: Weeks 4–8

Criteria for Progression to Phase 2
- Minimal pain and tenderness.
- Improvement of passive ROM.
- Return of functional ROM.

Goals
- Improve shoulder complex strength, power, and endurance.

Restrictions
- Avoid provocative maneuvers or exercises that cause discomfort for the patient.
- Includes both ROM exercises and strengthening exercises.

Immobilization
- None.

Pain Control
- Reduction of pain and discomfort is essential for recovery.
- Medications
  - NSAIDs—for older population with additional co-morbidities, consider newer COX-2 inhibitor formulas.
  - Subacromial injection of corticosteroid and local anesthetic; judicious use for patients with acute inflammatory symptoms of a concomitant bursitis; limit of three injections.
- Therapeutic modalities
  - Ice, ultrasound, HVGS.
  - Moist heat before therapy, ice at end of session.

Motion
Goal
- Equal to contralateral shoulder in all planes of motion.

Exercises
- Passive ROM.
- Capsular stretching.
- Active-assisted motion exercises.
- Active ROM exercises.

Muscle Strengthening
- Three times per week, 8 to 12 repetitions, for three sets.
- Strengthening of the remaining muscles of the rotator cuff.
- Begin with closed-chain isometric strengthening (see Fig. 3–36)
  - Internal rotation.
  - External rotation.
  - Abduction.
- Progress to open-chain strengthening with Therabands (see Fig. 3–39)
  - Exercises performed with the elbow flexed to 90 degrees.
  - Starting position is with the shoulder in the neutral position of 0 degrees of forward flexion, abduction, and external rotation.

- Exercises are done through an arc of 45 degrees in each of the five clinical planes of motion.
- Six color-coded bands are available, each provides increasing resistance from 1 to 6 pounds, at increments of 1 pound.
- Progression to the next band occurs usually in 2- to 3-wk intervals. Patients are instructed not to progress to the next band if there is any discomfort at the present level.
- Theraband exercises permit concentric and eccentric strengthening of the shoulder muscles and are a form of isotonic exercises (characterized by variable speed and fixed resistance)
  - Internal rotation.
  - External rotation.
  - Abduction.
  - Forward flexion.
  - Extension.
- Progress to light isotonic dumbbell exercises (see Fig. 3–39B)
  - Internal rotation.
  - External rotation.
  - Abduction.
  - Forward flexion.
  - Extension.
- Strengthening of deltoid (Fig. 3–58).
- Strengthening of scapular stabilizers
  - Closed-chain strengthening exercises (see Fig. 3–37)
    - Scapular retraction (rhomboideus, middle trapezius).
    - Scapular protraction (serratus anterior).
    - Scapular depression (latissimus dorsi, trapezius, serratus anterior).
    - Shoulder shrugs (upper trapezius).
  - Progress to open-chain scapular stabilizer strengthening (see Fig. 3–38).

Phase 3: Weeks 8–12

Criteria for Progression to Phase 3
- Full painless ROM.
- No pain or tenderness with strengthening exercises.

Goals
- Improve neuromuscular control and shoulder proprioception.
- Prepare for gradual return to functional activities.
- Establish a home exercise maintenance program that is performed at least three times per week for both stretching and strengthening.

Functional Strengthening
- Plyometric exercises (see Fig. 3–40).

continued

Rehabilitation Protocol
For Patients with Chronic Rotator Cuff Tears—Treated Conservatively (Nonoperatively) (Continued)
Bach, Cohen, and Romeo

A   **B**

Figure 3–58. Strengthening of the anterior deltoid. *A,* Closed-chain isometric. *B,* Open-chain isotonic.

Progressive, Systematic Interval Program for Returning to Sports
- Throwing athletes—see p. 190.
- Tennis players—see p. 193.
- Golfers—see p. 195.

Maximal improvement is expected by 4–6 mo.

Warning Signals
- Loss of motion—especially internal rotation.
- Lack of strength progression—especially abduction, forward elevation.
- Continued pain—especially at night.

Treatment of Warning Signals
- These patients may need to move back to earlier routines.
- May require increased utilization of pain control modalities as outlined above.
- May require surgical intervention.

Rehabilitation Protocol
After Surgical Repair of the Rotator Cuff
Bach, Cohen, and Romeo

Phase 1: Weeks 0–6

Restrictions
- No active ROM exercises.
- Active ROM exercises initiation based on size of tear
  - Small tears (0–1 cm)—no active ROM before 4 wk.
  - Medium tears (1–3 cm)—no active ROM before 6 wk.

- Large tears (3–5 cm)—no active ROM before 8 wk.
- Massive tears (>5 cm ROM)—no active ROM before 12 wk.
- Delay active-assisted ROM exercises for similar time periods based on size of tear.

Rehabilitation Protocol
After Surgical Repair of the Rotator Cuff (Continued)
Bach, Cohen, and Romeo

- Passive ROM only
  - 140 degrees of forward flexion.
  - 40 degrees of external rotation.
  - 60–80 degrees of abduction without rotation.
- No strengthening/resisted motions of the shoulder until 12 wk after surgery
  - For tears with high healing potential (small tears, acute, patients younger than 50 years, nonsmoker), isometric strengthening progressing to Theraband exercises may begin at 8 wk. Strengthening exercises before 12 wk should be performed with the arm at less than 45 degrees of abduction.

Immobilization
- Type of immobilization depends on amount of abduction required to repair rotator cuff tendons with little or no tension.
- Use of sling—if tension of repair is minimal or none with arm at the side
  - Small tears—1–3 wk.
  - Medium tears—3–6 wk.
  - Large and massive tears—6–8 wk.
- Abduction orthosis—if tension of repair is minimal or none with the arm in 20–40 degrees of abduction
  - Small tears—6 wk.
  - Medium tears—6 wk.
  - Large and massive tears—8 wk.

Pain Control
- Patients treated with arthroscopic rotator cuff repair experience less postoperative pain than patients treated with mini-open or open repairs (but more tenuous repair).
- Medications
  - Narcotic—for 7–10 day following surgery.
  - NSAIDs—for patients with persistent discomfort following surgery. In the older population with additional comorbidities, consider newer COX-2 inhibitor formulas.
- Therapeutic modalities
  - Ice, ultrasound, HVGS.
  - Moist heat before therapy, ice at end of session.

Shoulder Motion
- Passive only
  - 140 degrees of forward flexion.
  - 40 degrees of external rotation.
  - 60–80 degrees of abduction.
- For patients immobilized in abduction pillow, avoid adduction (i.e., bringing arm toward midline).
- Exercises should begin "above" the level of abduction in the abduction pillow
  - Begin Codman pendulum exercises to promote early motion.
  - Passive ROM exercises only (see Fig. 3–35).

Elbow Motion
- Passive—progress to active motion
  - 0–130 degrees.
  - Pronation and supination as tolerated.

Muscle Strengthening
- Grip strengthening only in this phase.

Phase 2: Weeks 6–12
Criteria for Progression to Phase 2
- At least 6 wk of recovery has elapsed.
- Painless passive ROM to
  - 140 degrees of forward flexion.
  - 40 degrees of external rotation.
  - 60–80 degrees of abduction.

Restrictions
- **No strengthening/resisted motions of the shoulder until 12 wk after surgery.**
- During phase 2, no active ROM exercises for patients with massive tears.

Immobilization
- Discontinuation of sling or abduction orthosis.
- Use for comfort only.

Pain Control
- NSAIDs for patients with persistent discomfort following surgery.
- Therapeutic modalities
  - Ice, ultrasound, HVGS.
  - Moist heat before therapy, ice at end of session.

Shoulder Motion
Goals
- 140 degrees of forward flexion—progress to 160 degrees.
- 40 degrees of external rotation—progress to 60 degrees.
- 60–80 degrees of abduction—progress to 90 degrees.

Exercises
- Continue with passive ROM exercises to achieve above goals (see Fig. 3–35).
- Begin active-assisted ROM exercises for the above goals (see Fig. 3–34).
- Progress to active ROM exercises as tolerated after full motion achieved with active-assisted exercises.
- Light passive stretching at end ROMs.

Muscle Strengthening
- Begin rotator cuff and scapular stabilizer strengthening for small tears with excellent healing potential—as outlined below in phase 3.
- Continue with grip strengthening.

continued

Rehabilitation Protocol
After Surgical Repair of the Rotator Cuff (Continued)
Bach, Cohen, and Romeo

Phase 3: Months 4–6
Criteria for Progression to Phase 3
- Painless active ROM.
- No shoulder pain or tenderness.
- Satisfactory clinical examination.

Goals
- Improve shoulder strength, power, and endurance.
- Improve neuromuscular control and shoulder proprioception.
- Prepare for gradual return to functional activities.
- Establish a home exercise maintenance program that is performed at least three times per week for strengthening.
- Stretching exercises should be performed daily.

Motion
- Achieve motion equal to contralateral side.
- Use passive, active-assisted **and active** ROM exercises.
- Passive capsular stretching at end ROMs, especially cross-body (horizontal) adduction and internal rotation to stretch the posterior capsule.

Muscle Strengthening
- Strengthening of the rotator cuff
  - Begin with closed-chain isometric strengthening (see Fig. 3–36)
    - Internal rotation.
    - External rotation.
    - Abduction.
    - Forward flexion.
    - Extension.
  - Progress to open-chain strengthening with Therabands (see Fig. 3–39)
    - Exercises performed with the elbow flexed to 90 degrees.
    - Starting position is with the shoulder in the neutral position of 0 degrees of forward flexion, abduction, and external rotation. The arm should be comfortable at the patient's side.
    - Exercises are performed through an arc of 45 degrees in each of the five planes of motion.
    - Six color-coded bands are available; each provides increasing resistance from 1 to 6 pounds, at increments of 1 pound.
    - Progression to the next band occurs usually in 2- to 3-wk intervals. Patients are instructed not to progress to the next band if there is any discomfort at the present level.
    - Theraband exercises permit concentric and eccentric strengthening of the shoulder muscles and are a form of isotonic exercises (characterized by variable speed and fixed resistance)
      - Internal rotation.
      - External rotation.

- Abduction.
- Forward flexion.
- Extension.
- Progress to light isotonic dumbbell exercises (see Fig. 3–39B)
  - Internal rotation.
  - External rotation.
  - Abduction.
  - Forward flexion.
  - Extension.
- Strengthening of deltoid—especially anterior deltoid (see Fig. 3–58).
- Strengthening of scapular stabilizers
  - Closed-chain strengthening exercises (Fig. 3–59; see also Fig. 3–37)
    - Scapular retraction (rhomboideus, middle trapezius).
    - Scapular protraction (serratus anterior).
    - Scapular depression (latissimus dorsi, trapezius, serratus anterior).
    - Shoulder shrugs (trapezius, levator scapulae).
  - Progress to open-chain scapular stabilizer strengthening (see Fig. 3–38).

Goals
- Three times per week.
- Begin with 10 repetitions for one set, advance to 8 to 12 repetitions for three sets.
- Functional strengthening: (begins after 70% of strength recovered)
  - Plyometric exercises (see Fig. 3–40).
- Progressive, systematic interval program for returning to sports
  - Throwing athletes—see p. 190
  - Tennis players—see p. 193
  - Golfers—see p. 195

Maximal Improvement
- Small tears—4–6 mo.
- Medium tears—6–8 mo.
- Large and massive tears—8–12 mo.

Patients will continue to show improvement in strength and function for at least 12 mo.

Warning Signals
- Loss of motion—especially internal rotation.
- Lack of strength progression—especially abduction.
- Continued pain—especially at night.

Treatment
- These patients may need to move back to earlier routines.
- May require increased utilization of pain control modalities as outlined above.
- May require repeat surgical intervention.

Rehabilitation Protocol
After Surgical Repair of the Rotator Cuff *(Continued)*
Bach, Cohen, and Romeo

 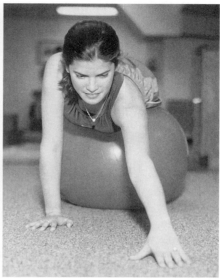

A   B

Figure 3–59. Additional closed-chain scapular stabilizer strengthening. *A,* Start. *B,* Finish (the right arm is the focus of rehabilitation).

- Indications for repeat surgical intervention
  - Inability to establish more than 90 degrees forward elevation by 3 mo.
  - Steady progress interrupted by a traumatic event and/or painful pop during the healing phase with a lasting loss of previously gained active motion.

- Radiographic evidence of loosened intra-articular implants (e.g., corkscrews) after an injury in the postoperative rehabilitation period. The patient has a loss of active motion and/or crepitance of the joint as well.

Rotator Cuff Tears in Overhead Athletes

Overhead athletes are at an increased risk for rotator cuff injuries because of the repetitive, high-velocity, mechanical stresses placed on their shoulders. **Those athletes who have an underlying degree of instability may experience compression of the cuff as well as the posterior-superior glenoid labrum along the upper third of the posterior glenoid.** This condition, known as *internal impingement,* **is a contributing factor to the development of articular-sided partial-thickness tears and full-thickness tears in overhead athletes.**

Successful treatment of this patient population depends on the recognition of the underlying instability.

The diagnosis requires a comprehensive history focusing on the timing and quality of the pain and a complete physical examination performing provocative maneuvers that test for instability.

- Radiologic evaluation with an arthrogram-enhanced MRI may identify partial-thickness tears.

- In this population, patients with partial-thickness tears **rarely require operative repair** because of resolution of symptoms after proper shoulder rehabilitation (see p. 174) and/or an operative stabilization procedure.
- **Overhead athletes diagnosed with a full-thickness rotator cuff tear in the setting of anterior instability should be treated aggressively with surgical repair of the rotator cuff and a stabilization procedure.** This recommendation is at odds with historical recommendations for older patients to treat the rotator cuff tear, then evaluate the need for additional treatment of the instability.
- Maximal athletic performance requires an intact rotator cuff and a stable shoulder.
- **Aggressive débridement of partial-thickness tears is discouraged because of the risk of thinning of the tendons and propagation to a full-thickness tear.**

Rehabilitation for patients with partial tears treated nonoperatively is similar to the program on p. 174. Patients treated with operative stabilization procedures follow the postoperative routine on p. 203, and patients who have an associated cuff repair follow the rehabilitation on p. 183. Once the overhead athlete has completely healed the repair, recovered full ROM and a significant amount of strength, he or she can advance to the sport-specific rehabilitation program (see Interval Throwing section).

Rehabilitation after Arthroscopically Assisted Mini-open Repair of the Rotator Cuff

We use three different rehabilitation programs based on the size of the tear and the condition of the repaired tissues (Table 3–5). The three programs differ mainly in their rates of progression:

- The **type 1 program** is used for small tears in younger patients with good to excellent tissues. This program is much more progressive than type 2 or 3.
- The **type 2 program** is used for medium to large tears in active individuals with good tissues.
- The **type 3 program** is used for patients with large to massive tears with a tenuous repair and fair to poor tissue quality.

Important General Points for Rehabilitation after Rotator Cuff Repair*

- Reestablishing early passive ROM is considered paramount.
- On postoperative day 1, the patient's arm is *passively* moved through a ROM (flexion in the scapular plane and internal and external rotation in the scapular plane at 45 degrees of abduction).
- Allow active-assisted external and internal rotation with L-bar (Breg Corp., Vista, Calif) in the scapular plane (Fig. 3–60). The patient moves the arm to tolerance but no farther and gently progresses ROM over subsequent days.

*From Wilk KE, Meister K, Andrews JR: Current concepts in the rehabilitation of the overhead throwing athlete. Am J Sports Med 30(1): 136, Review 2002.

- Active-assisted arm elevation with the L-bar in the scapular plane is allowed at 7 to 10 days. The therapist must provide assistance or support as the patient lowers the arm from 80 to 30 degrees of elevation or the patient will have pain secondary to his or her inability to control the arm while lowering it.
- As motion progresses, exercises are done with the arm abducted to 75 degrees during external and internal rotation active-assisted ROM stretching.
- The patient is then progressed to 90 degrees of abduction for these ROM exercises.
- Finally, the arm is placed at the side (0 degrees of abduction) during external and internal rotation.

Goals for obtaining **full passive motion of the shoulder** after rotator cuff repair
    Type 1—3–4 wk
    Type 2—4–6 wk
    Type 3—6–8 wk

- **The restoration of *active* motion is much slower because of healing constraints, pain inhibition, and weakness of the rotator cuff.**
- Motions such as excessive shoulder extension, adduction behind the back, and horizontal adduction are **prohibited** for at least 6 to 8 weeks.
- Cryotherapy is used four to eight times a day for the first 7 to 10 days to suppress inflammation, decrease muscle spasm, and enhance analgesia.
- Active **submaximal, pain-free multiangle isometrics** are used for the internal and external rotators, abductors, flexors, and elbow flexor muscle groups.
- **Rhythmic stabilization exercises** (in the supine position) are begun at 10 to 14 days postoperative (type 2 protocol) to restore the dynamic stabilization of the GH joint through cocontractions of the surrounding musculature. These exercises are designed to prevent and treat the **"shrug" sign** (Fig. 3–61).
- These exercises are done in the **"balanced position,"** defined as 100 to 110 degrees of elevation and 10 degrees of horizontal abduction (Fig. 3–62).
- In this position, the therapist provides an **extremely low** (3–4 pounds of force) isometric force to resist

Table 3-5		

Criteria for Rehabilitation after Mini-open Repair of the Rotator Cuff

Size of Tear	Guidelines	Rehabilitation Program
Small (≤1 cm)	Sling 7–10 days Restore full ROM within 4–6 wk	Type 1
Medium to large (2–4 cm)	Sling 2–3 wk Restore ROM within 8–10 wk	Type 2
Large to massive (≥5 cm)	Abduction pillow 1–2 wk Sling 2–3 wk Restore full ROM within 10–14 wk	Type 3

A, Lie on the back with the involved arm against the body and the elbow at 90 degrees. Grip the T-bar handle in the hand of the involved arm, and with the uninvolved arm, push the involved shoulder into external rotation. Hold for 5 sec. Return to the starting position and repeat.

B, Lie on the back with the involved arm 45 degrees from the body and the elbow at 90 degrees. Grip the T-bar in the hand of the involved arm and keep the elbow in the flexed position. Using the opposite arm, push the involved arm into external rotation. Hold for 5 sec. Return to the starting position and repeat.

Figure 3–60. Active-assisted ROM exercises, external rotation. (*A* and *B,* From Andrews JR, Wilk KE: The Athlete's Shoulder. New York, Churchill Livingstone, 1994.)

flexion and extension and horizontal abduction and adduction.

- The **"balanced position"** (100–110 degrees of elevation) is used so that the deltoid muscle generates a more horizontal (and thus compressive) force (Fig. 3–63). This exercise at 100 to 125 degrees activates the rotator cuff with assistance from the deltoid to **avoid superior migration** of the humeral head.
- The **shrug sign** occurs with a **strong deltoid muscle overpowering the weakened rotator cuff, causing the humeral head to superiorly migrate** (see Fig. 3–42). This is related to a lack of humeral head control. At initiation of arm elevation to 25 to 30 degrees, the entire shoulder elevates or "shrugs." Dynamic stabilization drills should alleviate this.
- As GH joint control is regained and reestablished, the drills can be done at lower flexion angles (30, 60, 90 degrees). The progression is (1) supine (scapula support) to (2) side-lying (Fig. 3–64), and then (3) seated.
- Rhythmic stabilization drills (low 3- to 4-pound force) are done for the internal and external rotators in the plane of the scapula (start at 7 to 10 days) (Fig. 3–65).

Figure 3–61. "Shrug" sign. Note superior displacement of the humerus and compensatory scapular muscle activity.

- At 3 weeks, isotonic tubing is used for external and internal rotator muscles with the arm at the side (see Fig. 3–39). As strength improves, side-lying external rotator strengthening is begun. External rotation strength is emphasized.
- **Emphasis is on external rotation strength** because this strength is critical in reestablishing functional use of the arm.

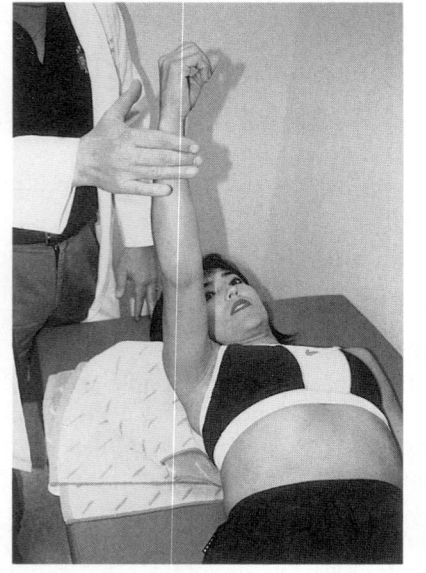

Figure 3–62. Rhythmic stabilization exercise drills. The patient's arm is placed in the balanced position and reciprocal static isometric contractions are done to resist shoulder flexion and horizontal abduction and adduction.

Deltoid alone

Figure 3–63. Deltoid muscle resultant vectors. With the arm at the side, the line of the deltoid muscle insertion into the humerus is 27 degrees. Thus, the resultant vector is superior migration of the humeral head. **At 90 to 100 degrees of arm elevation, the deltoid muscle generates a compressive force into the glenoid.** (From Andrews JR, Zarins B, Wilk KE: Injuries in Baseball. Philadelphia, Lippincott-Raven, 1997.)

- The patient is not allowed to progressively exercise through a shrug sign (deleterious to the repair). Emphasis should be on reestablishing dynamic stabilization.
- **Once external rotation strength is achieved, active abduction and flexion are allowed.**
- At 8 weeks, light isotonic strengthening and flexibility exercises are begun, with low weight and high repetition for muscle endurance and strength.

Figure 3–64. Rhythmic stabilization drills to reestablish dynamic glenohumeral joint stability.

Figure 3–65. Rhythmic stabilization drills to resist external and internal rotation of the glenohumeral joint.

- At 3 months, the patient can progress to the fundamental shoulder exercise program (see p. 169).
- Tennis players
  - Ground strokes are allowed at 5 to 6 months.
  - Serving is allowed when pain-free (10 to 12 months).
  - Interval training tables are on p. 193.
- Golfers
  - Golf swing is begun at 16 weeks.
  - Gradual return to play is allowed at 6 to 7 months.
  - Interval training figures are on p. 195.

- Internal training programs for overhead athletes should be employed after periods of prolonged inactivity or after the surgically repaired athlete has healed and is cleared to play. These programs encourage a gradual resumption of activity rather than immediate full velocity throwing that may produce injury (see Interval Throwing section).
- Patients with **arthroscopic repairs** are generally progressed **2 to 3 weeks slower** than those with arthroscopically-assisted mini-open procedures because the fixation is not as strong.

Rehabilitation Protocol
After Rotator Cuff Surgery Type 1 Rotator Cuff Repair (Arthroscopy Assisted Mini-open Repair for Small to Medium Tears [<1 cm]
Wilk, Crockett, and Andrews

Candidates for Type 1 Protocol

- **Young patient.**
- **Excellent tissue quality.**
- **Small tear (<1 cm).**

Phase 1: Immediate Postsurgical Phase (Days 1–10)

Goals

- Maintain integrity of repair.
- Gradually increase passive ROM.
- Diminish pain and inflammation.
- Prevent muscular inhibition.

Days 1–6

- Sling.
- Pendulum exercises.
- Active-assisted ROM exercise (L-bar)
  - External and internal rotation in scapular plane.
- Passive ROM
  - Flexion to tolerance.
  - External and internal rotation in scapular plane.

continued

Rehabilitation Protocol
After Rotator Cuff Surgery Type 1 Rotator Cuff Repair (Arthroscopy Assisted Mini-open Repair for Small to Medium Tears [<1 cm] *(Continued)*
Wilk, Crockett, and Andrews

- Elbow/hand gripping and ROM exercises.
- Submaximal pain-free isometrics
  - Flexion.
  - Abduction.
  - External rotation.
  - Internal rotation.
  - Elbow flexors.
- Cryotherapy for pain and inflammation (ice 15–20 min every hour).
- Sleeping (in sling).

Days 7–10
- Discontinue sling at days 7–10.
- Pendulum exercises (e.g., flexion, circles).
- Progress passive ROM to tolerance
  - Flexion to at least 115 degrees.
  - External rotation in scapular plane to 45–55 degrees.
  - Internal rotation in scapular plane to 45–55 degrees.
- Active-assisted ROM exercises (L-bar)
  - External and internal rotation in scapular plane.
  - Flexion to tolerance (therapist provides assistance by supporting arm).
- Continue elbow/hand ROM and gripping exercises.
- Continue isometrics
  - Flexion with bent elbow.
  - Extension with bent elbow.
  - Abduction with bent elbow.
  - External and internal rotation with arm in scapular plane.
  - Elbow flexion.
  - May initiate external and internal rotation tubing at 0 degrees abduction, if patient exhibits necessary active ROM.
- Continue use of ice for pain control (use ice at least six to seven times daily).
- Sleeping (continue sleeping in sling until physician instructs [usually day 7]).

Precautions
- No lifting of objects.
- No excessive shoulder motion behind back.
- No excessive stretching or sudden movements.
- No supporting of body weight by hands.
- Keep incision clean and dry.

Phase 2: Protection Phase (Day 11–Week 5)
Goals
- Allow healing of soft tissue.
- Do not overstress healing tissue.
- Gradually restore passive ROM (weeks 2–3).
- Reestablish dynamic shoulder stability.
- Decrease pain and inflammation.

Days 11–14
- Passive ROM to tolerance
  - Flexion 0–145/160 degrees.
  - External rotation at 90 degrees abduction: at least 75–80 degrees.
  - Internal rotation at 90 degrees abduction: at least 55–60 degrees.
- Active-assisted ROM to tolerance
  - Flexion.
  - External and internal rotation in scapular plane.
  - External and internal rotation at 90 degrees abduction.
- Dynamic stabilization drills (i.e., rhythmic stabilization drills [see Fig. 3–65])
  - External and internal rotation in scapular plane.
  - Flexion-extension at 100 degrees flexion.
- Continue isotonic external and internal rotation with tubing.
- Initiate prone rowing, elbow flexion.
- Initiate active exercise (flexion-abduction).
- Continue use of cryotherapy.

Weeks 3–4
- Patient should exhibit full passive ROM, nearing full active ROM.
- Continue all exercises listed above.
- Initiate scapular muscular strengthening program.
- Initiate side-lying external rotation strengthening (light dumbbell).
- Initiate isotonic elbow flexion.
- Continue use of ice as needed.
- May use pool for light ROM exercises.

Week 5
- Patient should exhibit full active ROM.
- Continue active-assisted ROM and stretching exercises.
- Progress isotonic strengthening exercise program
  - ER tubing
    - Side-lying internal rotation.
    - Prone rowing.
    - Prone horizontal abduction.
    - Shoulder flexion (scapular plane).
    - Shoulder abduction.
    - Biceps curls.

Precautions
- No lifting of heavy objects.
- No supporting of body weight by hands and arms.
- No sudden jerking motions.

Phase 3: Intermediate Phase (Weeks 6–11)
Goals
- Gradual restoration of shoulder strength and power.
- Gradual return to functional activities

Rehabilitation Protocol
After Rotator Cuff Surgery Type 1 Rotator Cuff Repair (Arthroscopy-Assisted Mini-open Repair for Small to Medium Tears [<1 cm] *(Continued)*
Wilk, Crockett, and Andrews

- Continue stretching and passive ROM (as needed to maintain full ROM).
- Continue dynamic stabilization drills.
- Progress isotonic strengthening program
  - External and internal rotation tubing.
  - External rotation side-lying.
  - Lateral raises.
  - Full can in scapular plane.
  - Prone rowing.
  - Prone horizontal abduction.
  - Prone extension.
  - Elbow flexion.
  - Elbow extension.
- If physician permits, the patient may initiate *light* functional activities.

Weeks 8–10
- Continue all exercises listed above.
- Progress to fundamental shoulder exercises.
- Initiate interval golf program (slow rate of progression).

Phase 4: Advanced Strengthening Phase (Weeks 12–19)
Goals
- Maintain full nonpainful active ROM.
- Enhance functional use of upper extremity.
- Improve muscular strength and power.
- Gradual return to functional activities.

Week 12
- Continue ROM exercises and stretching to maintain full ROM.
- Self-capsular stretches.
- Progress shoulder strengthening exercises to fundamental shoulder exercises.
- Initiate swimming or tennis program (if appropriate).

Week 15
- Continue all exercises listed above.
- Progress golf program to playing golf (if appropriate).

Phase 5: Return to Activity Phase (Weeks 20–26)
Goals
- Gradual return to strenuous work activities.
- Gradual return to recreational sport activities.

Week 20
- Continue fundamental shoulder exercise program (at least four times/wk) (see p. 169).
- Continue stretching, if motion is tight.
- Continue progression to sport participation.

Rehabilitation Protocol
After Rotator Cuff Surgery Type 2 Rotator Cuff Repair (Arthroscopy-Assisted Mini-open Repair for Medium to Large Tears [>1 cm, <5 cm]
Wilk, Crockett, and Andrews

Candidates for Type 2 Rehabilitation
- **Medium to large tear.**
- **Active patient.**
- **Good tissue quality.**

Phase 1: Immediate Postsurgical Phase (Days 1–10)
Goals
- Maintain integrity of the repair.
- Gradually increase passive ROM.
- Diminish pain and inflammation.
- Prevent muscular inhibition.

Days 1–6
- Sling or abduction brace (physician's decision).
- Pendulum stretches.
- Active-assisted ROM exercises (L-bar)
  - External and internal rotation in scapular plane.
- Passive ROM
  - Flexion to tolerance.
  - External and internal rotation in scapular plane.
- Elbow/hand gripping and ROM exercises.
- Submaximal pain-free isometrics
  - Flexion.
  - Abduction.
  - External rotation.
  - Internal rotation.
  - Elbow flexors.
- Cryotherapy for pain and inflammation (ice 15–20 min every hour).
- Sleeping in sling or brace.

continued

Rehabilitation Protocol
After Rotator Cuff Surgery Type 2 Rotator Cuff Repair (Arthroscopy-Assisted Mini-open Repair for Medium to Large Tears [>1 cm, <5 cm] *(Continued)*
Wilk, Crockett, and Andrews

Days 7–10
- Discontinue brace at days 10–14.
- Pendulum exercises (e.g., flexion, circles).
- Progress passive ROM to tolerance
  - Flexion to at least 105 degrees.
  - External rotation in scapular plane to 35–45 degrees.
  - Internal rotation in scapular plane to 35–45 degrees.
- Active-assisted ROM exercises (L-bar)
  - External and internal rotation in scapular plane.
  - Flexion to tolerance (therapist provides assistance by supporting arm).
- Continue elbow/hand ROM and gripping exercises.
- Continue isometrics
  - Flexion with bent elbow.
  - Extension with bent elbow.
  - Abduction with bent elbow.
  - External and internal rotation with arm in scapular plane.
  - Elbow flexion.
- Continue use of ice for pain control (at least six to seven times daily).
- Sleeping (in brace until physician instructs).

Precautions
- No lifting of objects.
- No excessive shoulder extension.
- No excessive stretching or sudden movements.
- No supporting of body weight by hands.
- Keep incision clean and dry.

Phase 2: Protection Phase (Day 11–Week 6)
Goals
- Allow healing of soft tissue.
- Do not overstress healing tissue.
- Gradually restore full passive ROM (weeks 4–5).
- Reestablish dynamic shoulder stability.
- Decrease pain and inflammation.

Days 11–14
- Discontinue use of sling or brace.
- Passive ROM to tolerance
  - Flexion 0–125/145 degrees.
  - External rotation at 90 degrees abduction: at least 45 degrees.
  - Internal rotation at 90 degrees abduction: at least 45 degrees.
- Active-assisted ROM to tolerance
  - Flexion.
  - External and internal rotation in scapular plane.
  - External and internal rotation at 90 degrees abduction.
- Dynamic stabilization drills (i.e., rhythmic stabilization drills [see Fig. 3–65])
  - External and internal rotation in scapular plane.
  - Flexion-extension at 100 degrees flexion.

- Continue all isometric contractions.
- Continue use of cryotherapy as needed.
- Continue all precautions.

Weeks 3–4
- Patient should exhibit full passive ROM.
- Continue all exercises listed above.
- Initiate gentle external and internal rotation strengthening using exercise tubing at 0 degrees of abduction.
- Initiate manual resistance external rotation supine in scapular plane.
- Initiate prone rowing to neutral arm position.
- Initiate isotonic elbow flexion.
- Continue use of ice as needed.
- May use heat before ROM exercises.
- May use pool for light ROM exercises.

Weeks 5–6
- May use heat prior to exercises.
- Continue active-assisted ROM and stretching exercises.
- Initiate active ROM exercises
  - Shoulder flexion scapular plane.
  - Shoulder abduction.
- Progress isotonic strengthening exercise program
  - External rotation tubing.
  - Side-lying internal rotation.
  - Prone rowing.
  - Prone horizontal abduction.
  - Biceps curls.

Precautions
- No heavy lifting of objects.
- No excessive behind-the-back movements.
- No supporting of body weight by hands and arms.
- No sudden jerking motions.

Phase 3: Intermediate Phase (Weeks 7–14)
Goals
- Full active ROM (weeks 8–10).
- Full passive ROM.
- Dynamic shoulder stability.
- Gradual restoration of shoulder strength and power.
- Gradual return of functional activities.

Week 7
- Continue stretching and passive ROM (as needed to maintain full ROM).
- Continue dynamic stabilization drills.
- Progress strengthening program
  - External and internal rotation tubing.
  - External rotation side-lying.
  - Lateral raises.*
  - Full can in scapular plane.*
  - Prone rowing.
  - Prone horizontal abduction.

Rehabilitation Protocol
After Rotator Cuff Surgery Type 2 Rotator Cuff Repair (Arthroscopy-Assisted Mini-open Repair for Medium to Large Tears [>1 cm, <5 cm] *(Continued)*
Wilk, Crockett, and Andrews

- Prone extension.
- Elbow flexion.
- Elbow extension.

Week 8
- Continue all exercises listed above.
- If physician permits, may initiate *light* functional activities.

Week 14
- Continue all exercises listed above.
- Progress to fundamental shoulder exercises (see p. 169).

Phase 4: Advanced Strengthening Phase (Weeks 15–22)

Goals
- Maintain full nonpainful ROM.
- Enhance functional use of upper extremity.
- Improve muscular strength and power.
- Gradual return to functional activities.

Week 15
- Continue ROM and stretching to maintain full ROM.
- Self-capsular stretches.

- Progress shoulder strengthening exercises to fundamental shoulder exercises.
- Initiate interval golf program (if appropriate).

Week 20
- Continue all exercises listed above.
- Progress golf program to playing golf (if appropriate).
- Initiate interval tennis program (if appropriate).
- May initiate swimming.

Phase 5: Return to Activity Phase (Weeks 23–30)

Goals
- Gradual return to strenuous work activities.
- Gradual return to recreational sport activities.

Week 23
- Continue fundamental shoulder exercises program (at least four times/wk).
- Continue stretching, if motion is tight.
- Continue progression to sport participation.

*Patient must be able to elevate arm without shoulder or scapular hiking before initiating isotonics; if unable, continue GH joint exercises.

Rehabilitation Protocol
After Rotator Cuff Surgery Type 3 Rotator Cuff Repair (Arthroscopy-Assisted Mini-open Repair for Large to Massive Tears [>5 cm]
Wilk, Crockett, and Andrews

Candidates for Type 3 Rehabilitation
- **Large to massive tear.**
- **Poor tissue quality.**
- **Tenuous repair.**

Phase 1: Immediate Postsurgical Phase (Days 1–10)

Goals
- Maintain integrity of the repair.
- Gradually increase passive ROM.
- Diminish pain and inflammation.
- Prevent muscular inhibition.

Days 1–6
- Sling or slight abduction brace (physician's decision).
- Pendulum exercises.
- Active-assisted ROM exercise (L-bar)
  - External and internal rotation in scapular phase.

- Passive ROM
  - Flexion to tolerance.
  - External and internal rotation in scapular plane (gentle ROM).
- Elbow/hand gripping and ROM exercises.
- Submaximal gentle isometrics
  - Flexion.
  - Abduction.
  - External rotation.
  - Internal rotation.
  - Elbow flexors.
- Cryotherapy for pain and inflammation (ice 15–20 min every hour).
- Sleeping (in sling or brace).

Days 7–10
- Continue use of brace or sling.
- Pendulum exercises (e.g., flexion, circles).

continued

Rehabilitation Protocol
After Rotator Cuff Surgery Type 3 Rotator Cuff Repair (Arthroscopy-Assisted Mini-open Repair for Large to Massive Tears [>5 cm] *(Continued)*
Wilk, Crockett, and Andrews

- Progress passive ROM and gripping exercises
  - Flexion to at least 90 degrees.
  - External rotation in scapular plane to 35 degrees.
  - Internal rotation in scapular plane to 35 degrees.
- Continue elbow/hand ROM and gripping exercises.
- Continue submaximal isometrics
  - Flexion with bent elbow.
  - Extension with bent elbow.
  - Abduction with bent elbow.
  - External and internal rotation with arm in scapular plane.
  - Elbow flexion.
- Continue use of ice for pain control (at least six to seven times daily).
- Sleeping (in brace until physician instructs).

Precautions
- Maintain arm in brace, remove only for exercise.
- No lifting of objects.
- No excessive shoulder extension.
- No excessive or aggressive stretching or sudden movements.
- No supporting of body weight by hands.
- Keep incision clean and dry.

Phase 2: Protection Phase (Day 11–Week 6)
Goals
- Allow healing of soft tissue.
- Do not overstress healing tissue.
- Gradually restore full passive ROM (weeks 4–5).
- Reestablish dynamic shoulder stability.
- Decrease pain and inflammation.

Days 11–14
- Continue use of brace.
- Passive ROM to tolerance
  - Flexion 0–approximately 125 degrees.
  - External rotation at 90 degrees abduction: at least 45 degrees.
  - Internal rotation at 90 degrees abduction: at least 45 degrees.
- Active-assisted ROM to tolerance
  - External and internal rotation in scapular plane.
  - Flexion-extension at 100 degrees flexion.
- Continue all isometric contractions.
- Continue use of cryotherapy as needed.
- Continue all precautions.

Weeks 3–4
- Initiate active-assisted ROM flexion in supine (therapist supports arm during motion).
- Continue all exercises listed above.
- Initiate external and internal rotation strengthening using exercise tubing at 0 degrees of abduction.

- Progress passive ROM till approximately full ROM at weeks 4–5.
- Initiate prone rowing to neutral arm position.
- Initiate isotonic elbow flexion.
- Continue use of ice as needed.
- May use heat prior to ROM exercises.
- May use pool for light ROM exercises.
- Continue use of brace during sleeping until end of week 4.
- Discontinue use of brace at end of week 4.

Weeks 5–6
- May use heat prior to exercises.
- Continue active-assisted ROM and stretching exercises.
- Initiate active ROM exercises
  - Shoulder flexion scapular plane.
  - Shoulder abduction.
- Progress isotonic strengthening exercise program
  - External rotation tubing.
  - Side-lying internal rotation.
  - Prone rowing.
  - Prone horizontal abduction.
  - Biceps curls.

Precautions
- No lifting.
- No excessive behind-the-back movements.
- No supporting of body weight by hands and arms.
- No sudden jerking motions.

Phase 3: Intermediate Phase (Weeks 7–14)
Goals
- Full active ROM (weeks 10–12).
- Maintain full passive ROM.
- Dynamic shoulder stability.
- Gradual restoration of shoulder strength and power.
- Gradual return to functional activities.

Week 7
- Continue stretching and passive ROM (as needed to maintain full ROM).
- Continue dynamic stabilization drills.
- Progress strengthening program
  - External and internal rotation tubing.
  - External rotation side-lying.
  - Lateral raises* (active ROM only).
  - Full can in scapular plane* (active ROM only).
  - Prone rowing.
  - Prone horizontal abduction.
  - Elbow flexion.
  - Elbow extension.

Week 10
- Continue all exercises listed above.
- If physician permits, may initiate *light* functional activities.

Rehabilitation Protocol
After Rotator Cuff Surgery Type 3 Rotator Cuff Repair (Arthroscopy-Assisted Mini-open Repair for Large to Massive Tears [>5 cm] *(Continued)*
Wilk, Crockett, and Andrews

Week 14
- Continue all exercises listed above.
- Progress to fundamental shoulder exercises.

Phase 4: Advanced Strengthening Phase (Weeks 15–22)

Goals
- Maintain full nonpainful ROM.
- Enhance functional uses of upper extremity.
- Improve muscular strength and power.
- Gradual return to functional activities.

Week 15
- Continue ROM and stretching to maintain full ROM.
- Self-capsular stretches.
- Progress shoulder strengthening exercises to fundamental shoulder exercises.

Week 20
- Continue all exercises listed above.
- Continue to perform ROM stretching, if motion is not complete.

Phase 5: Return to Activity Phase (Weeks 23–30)

Goals
- Gradual return to strenuous work activities.
- Gradual return to recreational sport activities.

Week 23
- Continue fundamental shoulder exercise program (at least four times/wk).
- Continue stretching, if motion is tight.

Week 26
- May initiate interval sport program (e.g., golf).

*Patient must be able to elevate arm without shoulder or scapular hiking before initiating isotonics; if unable, continue GH joint exercises.

Rehabilitation Protocol
Interval Throwing Program for Pitchers
Wilk

Step 1

Toss the ball (no wind-up) against a wall on alternate days. Start with 25–30 throws, build up to 70 throws, and gradually increase the throwing distance.

Number of Throws	Distance (ft)
20	20 (warm-up phase)
25–40	30–40
10	20 (cool-down phase)

Step 2

Toss the ball (playing catch with easy wind-up) on alternate days.

Number of Throws	Distance (ft)
10	20 (warm-up)
10	30–40
30–40	50
10	20–30 (cool-down)

Step 3

Continue increasing the throwing distance while still tossing the ball with an easy wind-up.

Number of Throws	Distance (ft)
10	20 (warm-up)
10	30–40
30–40	50–60
10	30 (cool-down)

Step 4

Increase throwing distance to a maximum of 60 feet. Continue tossing the ball with an occasional throw at no more than half speed.

Number of Throws	Distance (ft)
10	30 (warm-up)
10	40–45
30–40	60–70
10	30 (cool-down)

Step 5

During this step, gradually increase the distance to 150 feet maximum.

continued

Rehabilitation Protocol
Interval Throwing Program for Pitchers (Continued)
Wilk

Phase 5–1

Number of Throws	Distance (ft)
10	40 (warm-up)
10	50–60
15–20	70–80
10	50–60
10	40 (cool-down)

Phase 5–2

Number of Throws	Distance (ft)
10	40 (warm-up)
10	50–60
20–30	80–90
20	50–60
10	40 (cool-down)

Phase 5–3

Number of Throws	Distance (ft)
10	40 (warm-up)
10	60
15–20	100–110
20	60
10	40 (cool-down)

Phase 5–4

Number of Throws	Distance (ft)
10	40 (warm-up)
10	60
15–20	120–150
20	60
10	40 (cool-down)

Step 6
Progress to throwing off the mound at one-half to three-fourths speed. Try to use proper body mechanics, especially when throwing off the mound.
- Stay on top of the ball.
- Keep the elbow up.
- Throw over the top.
- Follow through with the arm and trunk.
- Use the legs to push.

Phase 6–1

Number of Throws	Distance (ft)
10	60 (warm-up)
10	120–150 (lobbing)
30	45 (off the mound)
10	60 (off the mound)
10	40 (cool-down)

Phase 6–2

Number of Throws	Distance (ft)
10	50 (warm-up)
10	120–150 (lobbing)
20	45 (off the mound)
20	60 (off the mound)
10	40 (cool-down)

Phase 6–3

Number of Throws	Distance (ft)
10	50 (warm-up)
10	60
10	120–150 (lobbing)
10	45 (off the mound)
30	60 (off the mound)
10	40 (cool-down)

Phase 6–4

Number of Throws	Distance (ft)
10	50 (warm-up)
10	120–150 (lobbing)
10	45 (off the mound)
40–50	60 (off the mound)
10	40 (cool-down)

At this time, if the pitcher has successfully completed phase 6–4 without pain or discomfort and is throwing approximately three-fourths speed, the pitching coach and trainer may allow the pitcher to proceed to step 7: "up/down bullpens." Up/down bullpens is used to simulate a game. The pitcher rests between a series of pitches to reproduce the rest period between innings.

Step 7
Up/down bullpens (one-half to three-fourths speed)

Day 1

Number of Throws	Distance (ft)
10 warm-up throws	120–150 (lobbing)
10 warm-up throws	60 (off the mound)
40 pitches	60 (off the mound)
Rest 10 min	
20 pitches	60 (off the mound)

Day 2
Off

Day 3

Number of Throws	Distance (ft)
10 warm-up throws	120–150 (lobbing)
10 warm-up throws	60 (off the mound)
30 pitches	60 (off the mound)

Rehabilitation Protocol
Interval Throwing Program for Pitchers (Continued)
Wilk

Rest 10 min

10 warm-up throws	60 (off the mound)
20 pitches	60 (off the mound)

Rest 10 min

10 warm-up throws	60 (off the mound)
20 pitches	60 (off the mound)

Day 4
Off

Day 5

Number of Throws	Distance (ft)
10 warm-up throws	120–150 (lobbing)
10 warm-up throws	60 (off the mound)
30 pitches	60 (off the mound)

Rest 8 min

20 pitches	60 (off the mound)

Rest 8 min

20 pitches	60 (off the mound)

Rest 8 min

20 pitches	60 (off the mound)

At this point, the pitcher is ready to begin a normal routine, from throwing batting practice to pitching in the bullpen. This program can and should be adjusted as needed by the trainer or physical therapist. Each step may take more or less than listed, and the program should be monitored by the trainer, physical therapist, and physician. The pitcher should remember that it is necessary to work hard but not overdo it.

Rehabilitation Protocol
Interval Throwing Program for Catchers, Infielders, and Outfielders
Wilk

Note: Perform each step three times. All throws should have an arc or "hump." The maximum distance thrown by infielders and catchers is 120 feet. The maximum distance thrown by outfielders is 200 feet.

Step 1

Toss the ball with no wind-up. Stand with your feet shoulder-width apart and face the player to whom you are throwing. Concentrate on rotating and staying on top of the ball.

Number of Throws	Distance (ft)
5	20 (warm-up)
10	30
5	20 (cool-down)

Step 2

Stand sideways to the person to whom you are throwing. Feet are shoulder-width apart. Close up and pivot onto your back foot as you throw.

Number of Throws	Distance (ft)
5	30 (warm-up)
5	40
10	50
5	30 (cool-down)

Step 3

Repeat the position in step 2. Step toward the target with your front leg and follow through with your back leg.

Number of Throws	Distance (ft)
5	50 (warm-up)
5	60
10	70
5	50 (cool-down)

Step 4

Assume the pitcher's stance. Litt and stride with your lead leg. Follow through with your back leg.

Number of Throws	Distance (ft)
5	60 (warm-up)
5	70
10	80
5	60 (cool-down)

Step 5

Outfielders: Lead with your glove-side foot forward. Take one step, crow-hop and throw the ball.

continued

Rehabilitation Protocol
Interval Throwing Program for Catchers, Infielders, and Outfielders
(Continued)
Wilk

Infielders: Lead with your glove-side foot forward. Take a shuffle step and throw the ball. Throw the last five throws in a straight line.

Number of Throws	Distance (ft)
5	70 (warm-up)
5	90
10	100
5	80 (cool-down)

Step 6

Use the throwing technique used in step 5. Assume your playing position. Infielders and catchers do not throw farther than 120 feet. Outfielders do not throw farther than 150 feet (midoutfield).

Number of Throws	Infielders' and Catchers' Distance (ft)	Outfielders' Distance (ft)
5	80 (warm-up)	80 (warm-up)
5	80–90	90–100
5	90–100	110–125
5	110–120	130–150
5	80 (cool-down)	80 (cool-down)

Step 7

Infielders, catchers, and outfielders all may assume their playing positions.

Number of Throws	Infielders' and Catchers' Distance (ft)	Outfielders' Distance (ft)
5	80 (warm-up)	80–90 (warm-up)
5	80–90	110–130
5	90–100	150–175
5	110–120	180–200
5	80 (cool-down)	90 (cool-down)

Step 8

Repeat step 7. Use a fungo bat to hit to the infielders and outfielders while in their normal playing positions.

Rehabilitation Protocol
Interval Program for Tennis Players
Wilk

This tennis protocol is designed to be performed every other day. Each session should begin with the warm-up exercises as outlined below. Continue with your strengthening, flexibility, and conditioning exercises on the days you are not following the tennis protocol.

Warm-up

Lower Extremity
- Jog four laps around the tennis court.
- Stretches
  - Gastrocnemius.
  - Achilles tendon.
  - Hamstring.
  - Quadriceps.

Upper Extremity
- Shoulder stretches
  - Posterior cuff.
  - Inferior capsule.
  - Rhomboids.
  - Forearm/wrist stretches.
  - Wrist flexors.
  - Wrist extensors.

Trunk
- Side bends.
- Extension.
- Rotation.

Forehand Ground Strokes

Hit toward the fence on the opposite side of the court. Do not worry about getting the ball in the court.

During all of the strokes listed above, remember these key steps:

- Bend your knees.
- Turn your body.
- Step toward the ball.
- Hit the ball when it is out in front of you.

Avoid hitting with an open stance because this places undue stress on your shoulder. This is especially more stressful during the forehand stroke if you have had anterior instability or impingement problems. This is also true during the backhand if you have had problems of posterior instability.

Rehabilitation Protocol
Interval Program for Tennis Players *(Continued)*
Wilk

On the very first day of these sport-specific drills, start with bouncing the ball and hitting it. Try to bounce the ball yourself and hit it at waist level. This will allow for consistency in the following:

- How the ball comes to you.
- Approximating your timing between hits.
- Hitting toward a target to ensure follow-through and full extension.
- Employing the proper mechanics, thereby placing less stress on the anterior shoulder.

Week 1

Day 1
- 25 forehand strokes.
- 25 backhand strokes.

Day 2
If there are no problems after the first-day workout, increase the number of forehand and backhand strokes

- 50 forehand strokes.
- 50 backhand strokes.

Day 3
- 50 forehand strokes (waist level).
- 50 backhand strokes (waist level).
- 25 high forehand strokes.
- 25 high backhand strokes.

Week 2

Progress to having the ball tossed to you in a timely manner, giving you enough time to recover from your deliberate follow-through (i.e., wait until the ball bounces on the other side of the court before tossing another ball). Always aim the ball at a target or at a spot on the court.

If you are working on basic ground strokes, have someone bounce the ball to you consistently at waist height.

If you are working on high forehands, have the ball bounced to you at shoulder height or higher.

Day 1
- 25 high forehand strokes.
- 50 waist-high forehand strokes.
- 50 waist-high backhand strokes.
- 25 high backhand strokes.

Day 2
- 25 high forehand strokes.
- 50 waist-high forehand strokes.
- 50 waist-high backhand strokes.
- 25 high backhand strokes.

Day 3
Alternate hitting the ball cross-court and down-the-line, using the waist-high and high forehand and backhand strokes
- 25 high forehand strokes.
- 50 waist-high forehand strokes.

- 50 waist-high backhand strokes.
- 25 high backhand strokes.

Week 3
Continue the three-times-per-week schedule. Add regular and high forehand and backhand volleys. At this point, you may begin having someone hit tennis balls to you from a basket of balls. This will allow you to get the feel of the ball as it comes off another tennis racket. Your partner should wait until the ball that you hit has bounced on the other side of the court before hitting another ball to you. This will give you time to emphasize your follow-through and not hurry to return for the next shot. As always, emphasis is placed on proper body mechanics.

Day 1
- 25 high forehand strokes.
- 50 waist-high forehand strokes.
- 50 waist-high backhand strokes.
- 25 high backhand strokes.
- 25 low backhand and forehand volleys.
- 25 high backhand and forehand volleys.

Day 2
Same as day 1, week 3.

Day 3
Same as day 2, week 3 with emphasis on direction (i.e., down-the-line and cross-court). Remember, good body mechanics is still a must:
- Keep knees bent.
- Hit the ball on the rise.
- Hit the ball in front of you.
- Turn your body.
- Do not hit the ball with an open stance.
- Stay on the balls of your feet.

Week 4

Day 1
Continue having your partner hit tennis balls to you from out of a basket. Alternate hitting forehand and backhand strokes with lateral movement along the baseline. Again, emphasis is on good mechanics as described previously.

Alternate hitting the ball down-the-line and cross-court. This drill should be done with a full basket of tennis balls (100–150 tennis balls).

Follow this drill with high and low volleys using half a basket of tennis balls (50–75 balls). This drill is also performed with lateral movement and returning to the middle of the court after the ball is hit.

Your partner should continue allowing enough time for you to return to the middle of the court before hitting the next ball. This is to avoid your rushing the stroke and using faulty mechanics.

Day 2
Same drill as day 1, week 4.

continued

Rehabilitation Protocol
Interval Program for Tennis Players (Continued)
Wilk

Day 3
Same drills as day 2, week 4.

Week 5

Day 1
Find a partner able to hit consistent ground strokes (able to hit the ball to the same area consistently, e.g., to your forehand with the ball bouncing about waist high).

Begin hitting ground strokes with this partner alternating hitting the ball to your backhand and to your forehand. Rally for about 15 min, then add volleys with your partner hitting to you from the baseline. Alternate between backhand and forehand volleys and high and low volleys. Continue volleying another 15 min. You will have rallied for a total of 30 to 40 min.

At the end of the session, practice a few serves while standing along the baseline. First, warm up by shadowing for 1 to 3 min. Hold the tennis racquet loosely and swing across your body in a figure 8. Do not swing the racquet hard. When you are ready to practice your serves using a ball, be sure to keep your toss out in front of you, get your racquet up and behind you, bend your knees, and hit up on the ball. Forget about how much power you are generating, and forget about hitting the ball between the service lines. Try hitting the ball as if you are hitting it toward the back fence.

Hit approximately 10 serves from each side of the court. Remember, this is the first time you are serving, so do not try to hit at 100% of your effort.

Day 2
Same as day 1, week 5, but now increase the number of times you practice your serve. After working on your ground strokes and volleys, return to the baseline and work on your second serve. Hit up on the ball, bend your knees, follow through, and keep the toss in front of you. This time hit 20 balls from each side of the court (i.e., 20 into the deuce court and 20 into the ad court).

Day 3
Same as day 2, week 5, with ground strokes, volleys, and serves. Do not add to the serves. Concentrate on the following:

- Bending your knees.
- Preparing the racket.
- Using footwork.
- Hitting the ball out in front of you.
- Keeping your eyes on the ball.
- Following through.
- Getting in position for the next shot.
- Keeping the toss in front of you during the serve.

The workout should be the same as day 2, but if you emphasize the proper mechanics listed previously, you should feel as though you had a harder workout than in day 2.

Week 6

Day 1
After the usual warm-up program, start with specific ground-stroke drills, with you hitting the ball down-the-line and your partner on the other side hitting the ball cross-court. This will force you to move quickly on the court. Emphasize good mechanics as mentioned previously.

Perform this drill for 10 to 15 min before reversing the direction of your strokes. Now have your partner hit down-the-line while you hit cross-court.

Proceed to the next drill with your partner hitting the ball to you. Return balls using a forehand, then a backhand, then a put-away volley. Repeat this sequence for 10 to 15 min. End this session by serving 50 balls to the ad court and 50 balls to the deuce court.

Day 2
Same as day 1, week 6, plus returning serves from each side of the court (deuce and ad court). End with practicing serves, 50 to each court.

Day 3
Perform the following sequence: warm-up; cross-court and down-the-line drills; backhand, forehand, and volley drills; return of serves; and practice serves.

Week 7

Day 1
Perform the warm-up program. Perform drills as before and practice return of serves. Before practicing serving, work on hitting 10–15 overhead shots. Continue emphasizing good mechanics. Add the approach shot to your drills.

Day 2
Same as day 1, week 7, except double the number of overhead shots (25–30 overheads).

Day 3
Perform warm-up exercises and cross-court drills. Add the overhead shot to the backhand, forehand, and volley drill, making it the backhand, forehand, volley and overhead drill.

If you are a serious tennis player, you will want to work on other strokes or other parts of your game. Feel free to gradually add them to your practice and workout sessions. Just as in other strokes, the proper mechanics should be applied to drop volley, slice, heavy topspin, drop shots, and lobs, offensive and defensive.

Week 8

Day 1
Warm-up and play a simulated one-set match. Be sure to take rest periods after every third game. Remember, you will have to concentrate harder on using good mechanics.

Day 2
Perform another simulated game but with a two-set match.

Rehabilitation Protocol
Interval Program for Tennis Players *(Continued)*
Wilk

Day 3
Perform another simulated game, this time a best-of-three-set match.

If all goes well, you may make plans to return to your regular workout and game schedule. You may also practice or play on consecutive days if your condition allows it.

Rehabilitation Protocol
Interval Program for Golfers
Wilk

This sport-specific protocol is designed to be performed every other day. Each session should begin with the warm-up exercises outlined here. Continue the strengthening, flexibility, and conditioning exercises on the days you are not playing or practicing golf. Advance one stage every 2–4 wk, depending on the severity of the shoulder problem, as each stage becomes pain free in execution.

Warm-up

Lower extremities: Jog or walk briskly around the practice green area three or four times; stretch the hamstrings, quadriceps, and Achilles tendon.

Upper extremities: Stretch the shoulder (posterior cuff, anterior cuff, rhomboid) and wrist flexors and extensors.

Trunk: Do sidebends, extension, and rotation stretching exercises.

Stage 1

Putt	50	3 times/wk
Medium long	0	0 times/wk
Long	0	0 times/wk

Stage 2

Putt	50	3 times/wk
Medium long	20	2 times/wk
Long	0	0 times/wk

Stage 3

Putt	50	3 times/wk
Medium long	40	3 times/wk
Long	0	0 times/wk

Not more than one-third best distance.

Stage 4

Putt	50	3 times/wk
Medium long	50	3 times/wk
Long	10	2 times/wk

Up to one-half best distance.

Stage 5

Putt	50	3 times/wk
Medium long	50	3 times/wk
Long	10	3 times/wk

Stage 6

Putt	50	3 times/wk
Medium long	50	3 times/wk
Long	20	3 times/wk

Play a round of golf in lieu of one practice session per week.

Rehabilitation after Débridement of Irreparable or Massive Rotator Cuff Tears

The rehabilitation program for patients with **"irreparable"** massive rotator cuff tears with arthroscopic subacromial decompression and rotator cuff débridement focuses on **four critical treatment areas:**

- Gradual **attainment of motion** through passive and active-assisted stretching techniques. Full motion should be obtained by 3 to 4 weeks after surgery.
- Gradual restoration of shoulder **strength,** beginning with the rotator cuff and scapulothoracic muscles (Fig. 3–66), then progressing to the deltoid muscles.
- Reestablishment of "balance of muscular forces" at the GH joint to allow arm elevation.
- **The key to restoring active shoulder elevation in these patients is strengthening of the *posterior rotator cuff muscles.***
- Burkhart (2001) reported that weakness of the posterior rotator cuff otherwise "uncouples" the force couple, leading to anterior-superior translation of the humeral head with active arm elevation.

A   **B**

Figure 3–66. Open-chain scapular strengthening with Theraband tubing. *A,* Start. *B,* Finish.

- Restoration of dynamic stability to the GH joint through proprioceptive and neuromuscular training drills.
  - Internal and external rotation rhythmic stabilization drills are done at various degrees of nonpainful arm elevation (see Fig. 3–65).
  - External rotation is strengthened with light isotonic and isometric exercises.
  - Patients should continue their preinjury exercise programs three times a week or more. The fundamental shoulder exercise program is continued (see p. 169).

Shoulder Instability

The GH joint is inherently lax or loose, based on its osseous configuration. It exhibits the greatest amount of motion found in any joint in the body. The shoulder sacrifices stability for mobility and, as a result, is the most common joint dislocated, with over 90% of dislocations occurring anteriorly. "Shoulder instability" is an all encompassing term that includes the entire range of disorders such as dislocation, subluxation, and "pathologic" laxity. To understand the terminology related to shoulder instability, the various terms commonly associated with this condition must be defined. **Translation** is the movement of the humerus with respect to the glenoid articular surface. **Laxity** is the amount of translation that occurs. Some laxity is expected in normal shoulders. In fact, more than a centimeter of posterior laxity is common, especially in athletes. Consequently, **instability must be defined as unwanted translations of the GH joint experienced by the patient.** The ability of the examiner to translate the humerus greater than one cm or on to the rim of the glenoid is not equal to instability. However, if that maneuver reproduces the patient's symptoms, which they may describe as **"slipping"** or **"giving-way"** or **"painful,"** then this is supportive evidence of GH joint instability. Finally, a **shoulder dislocation** is defined as the complete loss of the articulation between the humeral head and the glenoid socket. **Subluxation** refers to a partial loss of the GH joint articulation to the extent that symptoms are produced.

The stability of the GH joint is dependent on its static and dynamic stabilizers. The **static stabilizers,** such as the glenoid labrum and articular congruity, can be affected only by surgical means, not rehabilitation. However, the **dynamic stabilizers,** which primarily consist of the rotator cuff and the coordination between scapular movement and humeral movement, can be dramatically influenced by a proper rehabilitation program. **Strengthening of the musculature around the shoulder is the foundation of all rehabilitation programs for shoulder instability.**

We have already focused on the diagnosis and treatment of overhead athletes who have underlying microinstability that may predispose them to secondary impingement, internal impingement, rotator cuff tendinitis, and/or rotator cuff tears. This section focuses on the diagnosis and treatment of patients with symptomatic anterior, posterior, and multidirectional instability.

Classification of Shoulder Instability

Frequency

Acute
Recurrent
Fixed (chronic)

Cause

Traumatic event (macrotrauma)
Atraumatic event (voluntary, involuntary)

Classification of Shoulder Instability
(*Continued*)

Microtrauma
Congenital
Neuromuscular condition (Erb's palsy, cerebral palsy, seizures)

Direction

Anterior
Posterior
Inferior
Multidirectional

Degree

Dislocation
Subluxation
Microtrauma (transient)

From Warren RF, Craig EV, Altcheck DW: The Unstable Shoulder. Philadelphia, Lippincott-Raven, 1999.

Directional Classification

Anterior Shoulder Instability

Traumatic, acute dislocation (subcoracoid, subglenoid, subclavicular, intrathoracic)

Traumatic, acute subluxation

Recurrent anterior instability
- Chronic recurrent anterior dislocation
- Chronic recurrent anterior subluxation

Fixed (locked) anterior dislocation

Posterior Shoulder Instability

Traumatic, acute dislocation (subacromial, subglenoid, subspinous)

Traumatic, acute subluxation

Recurrent posterior instability
- Recurrent posterior dislocation
- Recurrent posterior subluxation

Voluntary (atraumatic subluxation-dislocation)
- Positional type
- Muscular type

Chronic (locked) dislocation (size of reversed Hill-Sachs lesion)
- <25% of the articular surface
- 25–40% of the articular surface
- <40% of the articular surface

Multidirectional Shoulder Instability

Type I   Global-instability: atraumatic multidirectional instability

Type II   Anterior-inferior instability: acute macrotraumatic episode in the setting of underlying hyperlaxity

Type III   Posterior-inferior instability: repetitive microtraumatic episodes in the setting of underlying hyperlaxity

Type IV   Anterior-posterior instability

From Warren RF, Craig EV, Altcheck DW: The Unstable Shoulder. Philadelphia, Lippincott-Raven, 1999.

Anterior Shoulder Instability

Anterior shoulder instability is the most common type of GH joint instability and can be caused by a traumatic dislocation or repetitive microtrauma resulting in symptomatic episodes of subluxations. Over 90% of shoulder dislocations occur anteriorly, **usually with the arm in abduction and external rotation.** This represents the "weakest position of the glenohumeral joint biomechanically," and is the **"classic position" for anterior instability.**

The **diagnosis of traumatic anterior dislocation** is usually straightforward when one takes a detailed history, including the position of the arm at the time of injury and the mechanism of injury, and performs a detailed physical examination. The mechanism of injury usually involves an indirect levering of the humeral head anteriorly with the shoulder positioned in a combination of abduction and external rotation. Less commonly, the dislocation can be caused by a direct blow to the posterior shoulder with the force directed anteriorly.

Physical Examination
- The affected shoulder usually is held in slight abduction and external rotation, with the forearm cradled by the unaffected arm.
- There may be a palpable fullness in the anterior shoulder.
- Internal rotation and adduction may be limited.
- Evaluation for neurologic injuries is critical before any relocation maneuver is performed. **The axillary nerve is most commonly injured with an anterior dislocation.** This risk increases with patient age, duration of dislocation, and the amount of trauma that caused the dislocation.
- Critical in the evaluation process is a complete radiographic "trauma shoulder series" to rule out concomitant fracture.
- Initial treatment includes a reduction procedure with some form of analgesic control, with radiographs after reduction to confirm successful relocation and a repeat neurologic examination to ensure no nerve injury or entrapment during the reduction.

Recurrent anterior instability is the most common problem after a primary anterior dislocation. The most consistent and significant factor influencing recurrence is **age at primary dislocation,** but in reality, this may be a reflection of the activities more common in a younger population than an older population. **Patients younger than 30 years have an average risk of approximately 70% of recurrent dislocation when treated with a nonsurgical rehabilitation program.** Overall, the average recurrence rate is approximately

50% with nonoperative management. Recurrent instability is diagnosed by history and confirmed with a thorough physical examination with patients demonstrating a positive apprehension sign (see Fig. 3–23) and positive relocation test (see Fig. 3–25). The natural history of recurrent anterior instability is altered if early operative stabilization is performed. In a prospective, randomized study, Kirkley and coworkers (1999) showed a significant difference in the rate of recurrent anterior dislocations in two groups of patients, average age 22 years. **One group was treated with a rehabilitation program and had a redislocation rate of 47%, and the other group was treated with an arthroscopic stabilization procedure and had a redislocation rate of 15% with an average follow-up of two years.**

Nonoperative Treatment

Conservative management of anterior shoulder instability has been associated with a more successful outcome in patients older than 30 years. Younger patients treated conservatively usually require a longer course of immobilization in hopes of achieving a successful outcome. However, it should be recognized that the length of immobilization has been only loosely associated with decreasing the risk of recurrence, with further scientific studies needed to prove its value. **Because recurrence is the most common complication, the goal of the rehabilitation program is to optimize shoulder stability.** Avoidance of any provocative maneuvers and careful muscle strengthening are important components of the rehabilitation program as outlined in the following protocol.

Rehabilitation Protocol
Nonoperative Management of Anterior Shoulder Instability
Bach, Cohen, and Romeo

Phase 1: Weeks 0–2

Restrictions
- Avoid provocative positions of the shoulder that risk recurrent instability
  - External rotation.
  - Abduction.
  - Distraction.

Immobilization
- Sling immobilization—remove for exercises.
- Duration of immobilization is age-dependent based on the theoretical advantage of improved healing of the capsulolabral complex
  - <20 years old—3–4 wk.
  - 20–30 years old—2–3 wk.
  - >30 years old—10 days–2 wk.
  - >40 years old—3–5 days.

Pain Control
- Reduction of pain and discomfort is essential for recovery
  - Medications
    - Narcotics—for 5–7 days following a traumatic dislocation.
    - NSAIDs—to reduce inflammation.
  - Therapeutic modalities
    - Ice, ultrasound, HVGS.
    - Moist heat before therapy, ice at end of session.

Motion: Shoulder
- Begins during phase 1 for patients 30 years and older.
- Follows the protocol as outlined in phase 2.

Motion: Elbow
- Passive—progress to active
  - 0–130 degrees of flexion.
  - Pronation and supination as tolerated.

Muscle Strengthening
- Scapular stabilizer strengthening begins during phase 1 for patients 30 years and older
  - Follows the protocol as outlined in phase 2.
- Grip strengthening.

Phase 2: Weeks 3–4

Criteria for Progression to Phase 2
- Reduced pain and tenderness.
- Adequate immobilization.

Restrictions
- Avoid provocative positions of the shoulder that risk recurrent instability.
- Shoulder motion
  - 140 degrees of forward flexion.
  - 40 degrees of external rotation with the arm at the side.
- Avoid extension—**puts additional stress on anterior structures.**

Immobilization
- Sling—as per criteria outlined in phase 1.

Motion: Shoulder
Goals
- 140 degrees of forward flexion.
- 40 degrees of external rotation with the arm at the side.
Exercises
- Begin with Codman pendulum exercises to promote early motion.
- Passive ROM exercises (see Fig. 3–35).
- Active-assisted ROM exercises (see Fig. 3–34).
- Active ROM exercises.

Rehabilitation Protocol
Nonoperative Management of Anterior Shoulder Instability (Continued)
Bach, Cohen, and Romeo

Muscle Strengthening
- Rotator cuff strengthening
  - Begin with closed-chain isometric strengthening with the elbow flexed to 90 degrees and the arm comfortably at the side (see Fig. 3–36)
    - Internal rotation.
    - External rotation.
    - Forward flexion.
- Strengthening of scapular stabilizers
  - Closed-chain strengthening exercises (see Figs. 3–37 and 3–59)
    - Scapular retraction (rhomboideus, middle trapezius).
    - Scapular protraction (serratus anterior).
    - Scapular depression (latissimus dorsi, trapezius, serratus anterior).
    - Shoulder shrugs (trapezius, levator scapulae).

Phase 3: Weeks 4–8

Criteria for Progression to Phase 3
- Pain-free motion of 140 degrees of forward flexion and 40 degrees of external rotation with the arm at the side.
- Minimal pain or tenderness with strengthening exercises.
- Improvement in strength of rotator cuff and scapular stabilizers.

Restrictions
- Avoid positions that exacerbate instability
  - Abduction–external rotation.
- Shoulder motion
  - 160 degrees of forward flexion.
  - 40 degrees of external rotation with the arm in 30–45 degrees of abduction.

Motion: Shoulder
Goals
- 160 degrees of forward flexion.
- 40 degrees of external rotation with the arm in 30–45 degrees of abduction.

Exercises
- Passive ROM exercises (see Fig. 3–35).
- Active-assisted ROM exercises (see Fig. 3–34).
- Active ROM exercises.

Muscle Strengthening
- Rotator cuff strengthening
  - Closed-chain isometric strengthening with the arm in 35–45 degrees of abduction.
  - Progress to open-chain strengthening with Therabands (see Fig. 3–39A).
    - Exercises performed with the elbow flexed to 90 degrees.
    - Starting position is with the shoulder in the neutral position of 0 degrees of forward flexion, abduction, and external rotation. The arm should be comfortable at the patient's side.

- Exercises are performed through an arc of 45 degrees in each of the five planes of motion.
- Six color-coded bands are available; each provides increasing resistance from 1 to 6 pounds, at increments of 1 pound.
- Progression to the next band occurs usually in 2- to 3-week intervals. Patients are instructed not to progress to the next band if there is any discomfort at the present level.
- Theraband exercises permit concentric and eccentric strengthening of the shoulder muscles and are a form of isotonic exercises (characterized by variable speed and fixed resistance)
  - Internal rotation.
  - External rotation.
  - Abduction.
  - Forward flexion.
- Progress to light isotonic dumbbell exercises
  - Internal rotation.
  - External rotation.
  - Abduction.
  - Forward flexion.
- Strengthening of scapular stabilizers
  - Continue with closed-chain strengthening exercises (see Figs. 3–37 and 3–59).
  - Advance to open chain, isotonic strengthening exercises (see Fig. 3–38).
- Initiate deltoid strengthening in the plane of the scapula to 90 degrees of elevation.

Phase 4: Weeks 8–12

Criteria for Progression to Phase 4
- Pain-free motion of 160 degrees of forward flexion and 40 degrees of external rotation with the arm in 30–45 degrees of abduction.
- Minimal pain or tenderness with strengthening exercises.
- Continued improvement in strength of rotator cuff and scapular stabilizers.
- Satisfactory physical examination.

Goals
- Improve shoulder strength, power, and endurance.
- Improve neuromuscular control and shoulder proprioception.
- Restore full shoulder motion.

Restriction
- Avoid positions that exacerbate instability.

Pain Control
- As outlined in phase 3.

Motion: Shoulder
Goals
- Obtain motion that is at least equal to contralateral side.

continued

Rehabilitation Protocol
Nonoperative Management of Anterior Shoulder Instability *(Continued)*
Bach, Cohen, and Romeo

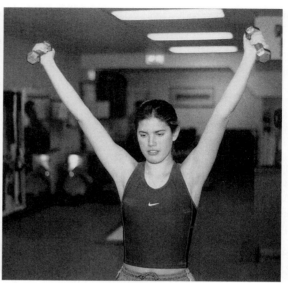

A   B

Figure 3-67. Example of one proprioceptive neuromuscular facilitation pattern. *A,* Start. *B,* Finish.

Exercises
- Utilize passive, active-assisted, and active ROM exercises to obtain motion goals.

Capsular stretching
- Especially posterior capsule (see Fig. 3–48).

Muscle Strengthening
- Continue with rotator cuff, scapular stabilizers, and deltoid strengthening
  - Eight to 12 repetitions, for three sets.

Upper Extremity Endurance Training
- Incorporated endurance training for the upper extremity
  - Upper body ergometer.

Proprioceptive Training
- PNF patterns (Fig. 3–67)

Phase 5: Weeks 12–16

Criteria for Progression to Phase 5
- Pain-free ROM.
- No evidence of recurrent instability.
- Recovery of 70–80% of shoulder strength.
- Satisfactory physical examination.

Goals
- Prepare for gradual return to functional and sporting activities.
- Establish a home exercise maintenance program that is performed at least three times per week for both stretching and strengthening.

Functional Strengthening
- Plyometric exercises (see Fig. 3–40).

Progressive, Systematic Interval Program for Returning to Sports
- Golfers—see p. 195.
- Overhead athletes not before **6 mo**
  - Throwing athletes—see p. 190.
  - Tennis players—see p. 192.

Maximum improvement is expected by 6 mo.

Warning Signs
- Persistent instability.
- Loss of motion.
- Lack of strength progression—especially abduction.
- Continued pain.

Treatment of Complications
- These patients may need to move back to earlier routines.
- May require increased utilization of pain control modalities as outlined above.
- May require surgical intervention
  - Recurrent instability as defined by three or more instability events within a year, or instability that occurs at rest or during sleep. These findings are strong indications for surgical management.

Rehabilitation Protocol
Nonoperative Rehabilitation for Anterior Shoulder Instability
Wilk

The program will vary in length for each individual depending on several factors:
- Severity of injury.
- Acute versus chronic condition.
- ROM/strength status.
- Performance/activity demands.

Phase 1: Acute Motion Phase

Goals
- Reestablish nonpainful ROM.
- Retard muscular atrophy.
- Decrease pain/inflammation.

Note: During the early rehabilitation program, caution must be applied in placing the anterior capsule under stress (i.e., avoid abduction, external rotation) until dynamic joint stability is restored.

Decrease Pain and Inflammation
- Therapeutic modalities (e.g., ice, electrotherapy).
- NSAIDs.
- *Gentle* joint mobilization.

Range of Motion Exercises
- Pendulums.
- Circumduction.
- Rope and pulley
  - Flexion.
  - Abduction to 90 degrees, progress to full ROM.
- L-bar
  - Flexion.
  - Abduction.
  - Internal rotation with arm in scapular plane.
  - External rotation with arm in scapular plane (*progress arm to 90 degrees of abduction as tolerated*).
- Posterior capsular stretching.
- Upper extremity ergometer.

Shoulder hyperextension is contraindicated.

Strengthening Exercises
- Isometrics
  - Flexion.
  - Abduction.
  - Extension.
  - Internal rotation (multiangles).
  - External rotation (scapular plane).
- Weight shifts (closed-chain exercises).

Phase 2: Intermediate Phase

Criteria for Progression to Phase 2
- Full ROM.
- Minimal pain or tenderness.
- "Good" MMT of internal rotation, external rotation, flexion, and abduction.

Goals
- Regain and improve muscular strength.
- Normalize arthrokinematics.
- Improve neuromuscular control of shoulder complex.

Initiate Isotonic Strengthening
- Flexion.
- Abduction to 90 degrees.
- Internal rotation.
- Side-lying external rotation to 45 degrees.
- Shoulder shrugs.
- Extension.
- Horizontal adduction.
- Supraspinatus.
- Biceps.
- Push-ups.

Initiate Eccentric (Surgical Tubing) Exercises at 0 Degrees Abduction
- Internal rotation.
- External rotation.

Normalize Arthrokinematics of the Shoulder Complex
- Continue joint mobilization.
- Patient education of mechanics and activity modification of activity/sport.

Improve Neuromuscular Control of Shoulder Complex
- Initiation of PNF (see Fig. 3–67).
- Rhythmic stabilization drills (see Figs. 3–64 and 3–65).

Continue Use of Modalities (As Needed)
- Ice, electrotherapy modalities.

Phase 3: Advanced Strengthening Phase

Criteria for Progression to Phase 3
- Full nonpainful ROM.
- No palpable tenderness.
- Continued progression of resistive exercises.

Goals
- Improve strength, power, and endurance.
- Improve neuromuscular control.
- Prepare patient/athlete for activity.

Continue Use of Modalities (As Needed)

Continue Posterior Capsular Stretches

Continue Isotonic Strengthening (Progressive Resistance Exercises)

Continue Eccentric Strengthening

Emphasize PNF

Initiate Isokinetics
- Flexion-extension.
- Abduction-adduction.
- Internal-external rotation.
- Horizontal abduction/adduction.

continued

Rehabilitation Protocol
Nonoperative Rehabilitation for Anterior Shoulder Instability *(Continued)*
Wilk

Initiate Plyometric Training
- Surgical tubing.
- Wall push-ups.
- Medicine ball.
- Boxes.

Initiate Military Press
Precaution—avoid excessive stress on anterior capsule.

Phase 4: Return to Activity Phase
Criteria for Progression to Phase 4
- Full ROM.
- No pain or palpable tenderness.
- Satisfactory isokinetic test.
- Satisfactory clinical examination.

Goals
- Maintain optimal level of strength, power, and endurance.
- Progressively increase activity level to prepare patient for full functional return to activity/sport.

Continue All Exercises as in Phase 3

Continue Posterior Capsular Stretches

Initiate Interval Program

Continue Modalities (As Needed)

Follow-up
- Isokinetic test.
- Progress interval program.
- Maintenance of exercise program.

Operative Treatment

Operative stabilization is indicated in patients with irreducible dislocations, displaced tuberosity fractures, and glenoid rim fractures involving 25% or more of the anterior-inferior glenoid rim. **Patients who experience three or more instability events in a year (recurrent) or instability during rest or sleep also are appropriate candidates for surgical management.** A relative indication for surgical intervention is a younger patient, especially an **athlete who desires continued participation in sports** or work activities. **In this population, early surgical intervention will reduce the risk of recurrent instability and allow a return to sport.** The problem with conservative treatment in this patient group is that it is less likely to alter the natural history of the shoulder instability. The athlete may have fewer or no episodes of instability with a conservative treatment program during the "off-season" from her or his sport. However, with the return of the next season, if the instability becomes symptomatic, the athlete will risk losing two seasons, which essentially ends competitive participation, especially for the high-level athlete.

The **traditional open Bankart repair** is the **standard of care** for open stabilization procedures with a **recurrence rate of less than 5%.** Recurrence after arthroscopic stabilization procedures has been highly variable, with early reports suggesting recurrence rates anywhere from 0 to 45%. The higher failure rates are likely the result of poor surgical technique and an accelerated rehabilitation program that ignored the normal biology of tissue repair, which is the same for both operative procedures. **Recent literature has shown a recurrence rate of 8 to 17% after arthroscopic Bankart repairs,** which is related to better surgical technique and more traditional postop-

erative rehabilitation. The advantages of arthroscopic stabilization procedures include cosmetic incisions, less postoperative pain, and earlier recovery of external rotation.

The operative technique chosen depends on which technique the surgeon is most comfortable with. Like arthroscopic rotator cuff repairs, arthroscopic stabilization procedures are technically more challenging and require a clear understanding of the pathoanatomy. Rehabilitation after stabilization procedures is detailed on p. 203. The rehabilitation program is essentially the same for open and arthroscopic techniques because the biology of healing tissue is the same, and the consideration of subscapularis tendon healing is contained within the time-frame of healing for the GH capsulolabral complex.

Complications after Shoulder Stabilization Surgery
Numerous complications may develop after shoulder stabilization surgery for instability and may include:

- Limitation of motion.
- Recurrent instability.
- Inability to return to preinjury level of play in sport.
- Development of osteoarthritis.

The most common complication after shoulder stabilization surgery is loss of motion (especially external rotation).

For these reasons, the goals of rehabilitation after shoulder stabilization are:

1. Maintenance of the integrity of the surgically correct stability.
2. Gradual restoration of full functional ROM.
3. Enhancement of dynamic stability (of muscles surrounding shoulder).
4. Return to full unrestricted activity and sport.

Factors Affecting Rehabilitation after Shoulder Stabilization Procedures

Type of Surgical Procedure

Exposure

Open
Arthroscopic

Type of Procedure
Bankart
Capsular shift, etc.

Method of Fixation

Suture anchors
Bioabsorbable
Sutures

Type of Instability

Anterior
Posterior
Multidirectional

Factors Affecting Rehabilitation after Shoulder Stabilization Procedures *(Continued)*

Tissue Status of Patient

Normal
Hyperelasticity
Hypoelasticity

Patient's Response to Surgery

Dynamic Stabilizers Status

Muscle development
Muscle strength
Dynamic stability
Proprioceptive abilities

Patients Preinjury Activity Status

Athletic versus nonathletic
Overhead thrower versus sedentary
Postoperative goals

Physician's Philosophic Approach

Rehabilitation Protocol
Following an Anterior Surgical Stabilization Procedure
Bach, Cohen, and Romeo

Phase 1: Weeks 0–4

Restrictions
- Shoulder motion
  - 140 degrees of forward flexion.
  - 40 degrees of external rotation
    - Initially with arm at the side.
    - After 10 days, can progress to 40 degrees of external rotation with the arm in increasing amounts of abduction, up to 45 degrees of abduction.
- **Active ROM Only—No Passive ROM or Manipulation by the Therapist**
  - Patients after an open stabilization procedure with a takedown of the subscapularis insertion are restricted from active internal rotation for 4 wk.
- Avoid provocative maneuvers that re-create position of instability (e.g., abduction–external rotation).

Immobilization
- Sling immobilization
  - 4 wk duration—during day and **especially at night.**

Pain Control
- Reduction of pain and discomfort is essential for recovery
  - Medications

- Narcotics—for 7–10 days following surgery.
    - NSAIDs—for patients with persistent discomfort following surgery.
  - Therapeutic modalities
    - Ice, ultrasound, HVGS.
    - Moist heat before therapy, ice at end of session.

Motion: Shoulder
- Goals: **Active ROM exercises only**
  - 140 degrees of forward flexion.
  - 40 degrees of external rotation with arm at the side.
  - After 10 days, can progress to external rotation with the arm abducted—up to 45 degrees of abduction.
  - **No active internal rotation for patients following an open stabilization procedure with removal and subsequent repair of the subscapularis insertion.**
- Exercises
  - Begin with Codman pendulum exercises to promote early motion.
  - Active ROM exercises
    - Passive internal rotation to stomach for those patients restricted from active internal rotation.

continued

Rehabilitation Protocol
Following an Anterior Surgical Stabilization Procedure *(Continued)*
Bach, Cohen, and Romeo

Motion: Elbow
- Passive—progress to active
  - 0–130 degrees of flexion.
  - Pronation and supination as tolerated.

Muscle Strengthening
- Rotator cuff strengthening—within the limits of the active ROM exercises
  - Closed-chain isometric strengthening with the elbow flexed to 90 degrees and the arm at the side (see Fig. 3–36B)
    - Internal rotation
      - No internal rotation strengthening for open stabilization group with removal and subsequent repair of subscapularis insertion before 6 wk.
    - External rotation.
    - Abduction.
    - Forward flexion.
- Grip strengthening.

Phase 2: Weeks 4–8
Criteria for Progression to Phase 2
- Minimal pain and discomfort with active ROM and closed-chain strengthening exercises.
- No sensation or findings of instability with above exercises.

Restrictions
- Shoulder motion: active ROM only
  - 160 degrees of forward flexion.
  - 60 degrees of external rotation.
  - 70 degrees of abduction.
- **Avoid provocative maneuvers that re-create position of instability**
  - *Abduction–external rotation.*
- *Note:* For overhead athletes, the restrictions are less. Although there is a higher risk of recurrent instability, the need for full motion to perform overhead sports requires that most athletes regain motion to within 10 degrees of normal for the affected shoulder by 6–8 wk after surgery.

Immobilization
- Sling—discontinue.

Pain Control
- Medications
  - NSAIDs—for patients with persistent discomfort.
- Therapeutic modalities
  - Ice, ultrasound, HVGS.
  - Moist heat before therapy, ice at end of session.

Motion: Shoulder
- Goals
  - 160 degrees of forward flexion.
  - 50 degrees of external rotation.
  - 70 degrees of abduction.

- Exercises
  - Active ROM exercises.
- *Note:* For overhead athletes, the motion goals should be within 10 degrees of normal for the affected shoulder.

Muscle Strengthening
- Rotator cuff strengthening—within the limits of active ROM exercises
  - Closed-chain isometric strengthening with the elbow flexed to 90 degrees and the arm at the side (see Fig. 3–36B).
    - Internal rotation
      - No internal rotation strengthening for open stabilization group with removal and subsequent repair of subscapularis insertion before 6 wk.
    - External rotation.
    - Abduction.
    - Forward flexion.
  - Progress to light open-chain and isotonic strengthening with Therabands (see Fig. 3–39A)
    - Exercises performed with the elbow flexed to 90 degrees.
    - Starting position is with the shoulder in the neutral position of 0 degrees of forward flexion, abduction, and external rotation.
    - Exercises are performed through an arc of at least 45 degrees in each of the five planes of motion—within the guidelines of allowed motion.
    - Six color-coded bands are available; each provides increasing resistance from 1 to 6 pounds, at increments of one pound.
    - Progression to the next band occurs usually in 2- to 3-wk intervals. Patients are instructed not to progress to the next band if there is any discomfort at the present level.
    - Theraband exercises permit concentric and eccentric strengthening of the shoulder muscles and are a form of isotonic exercises (characterized by variable speed and fixed resistance).
    - Internal rotation
      - Hold internal rotation strengthening until 6 wk for the subscapularis repair group.
    - External rotation.
    - Abduction.
    - Forward flexion.
- Strengthening of scapular stabilizers
  - Closed-chain strengthening exercises (Fig. 3–68; see also Figs. 3–37 and 3–59)
    - Scapular retraction (rhomboideus, middle trapezius).
    - Scapular protraction (serratus anterior).
    - Scapular depression (latissimus dorsi, trapezius, serratus anterior).
    - Shoulder shrugs (trapezius, levator scapulae).

Rehabilitation Protocol
Following an Anterior Surgical Stabilization Procedure (*Continued*)
Bach, Cohen, and Romeo

A

B

Figure 3–68. Closed-chain strengthening of the scapular stabilizers. *A,* Start. *B,* Finish.

Phase 3: Weeks 8–12

Criteria for Progression to Phase 3
- Minimal pain or discomfort with active ROM and muscle strengthening exercises.
- Improvement in strengthening of rotator cuff and scapular stabilizers.
- Satisfactory physical examination.

Goals
- Improve shoulder strength, power, and endurance.
- Improve neuromuscular control and shoulder proprioception.
- Restore full shoulder motion.
- Establish a home exercise maintenance program that is performed at least three times per week for both stretching and strengthening.

Pain Control
- Medications
  - NSAIDs—for patients with persistent discomfort.
  - Subacromial injection: corticosteroid/local anesthetic combination
    - For patients with findings consistent with secondary impingement.
  - GH joint: corticosteroid/local anesthetic combination
    - For patients whose clinical findings are consistent with GH joint pathology.
- Therapeutic modalities
  - Ice, ultrasound, HVGS.
  - Moist heat before therapy, ice at end of session.

Motion: Shoulder

Goals
- Obtain motion that is equal to contralateral side.
- Active ROM exercises.
- Active-assisted ROM exercises (see Fig. 3–34).
- Passive ROM exercises (see Fig. 3–35).
- Capsular stretching (especially posterior capsule [see Fig. 3–48]).

Muscle Strengthening
- Rotator cuff strengthening—three times per week, 8 to 12 repetitions for three sets
  - Continue with advancing theraband strengthening.
  - Progress to light isotonic dumbbell exercises (see Fig. 3–39B).
- Scapular stabilizer strengthening
  - Continue with closed-chain strengthening.
  - Progress to open-chain strengthening (see Figs. 3–38 and 3–39).

Upper Extremity Endurance Training
- Incorporated endurance training for the upper extremity
  - Upper body ergometer.

continued

Rehabilitation Protocol
Following an Anterior Surgical Stabilization Procedure *(Continued)*
Bach, Cohen, and Romeo

Proprioceptive Training
- PNF patterns (see Fig. 3–67).

Functional Strengthening
- Plyometric exercises (see Fig. 3–40).

Progressive, Systematic Interval Program for Returning to Sports
- Golfers—see p. 195.
- Overhead athletes not before 6 mo
  - Throwing athletes—see p. 190.
  - Tennis players—see p. 192.

Maximum improvement is expected by 12 mo; most patients can return to sports and full-duty work status by 6 mo.

Warning Signs
- Persistent instability.
- Loss of motion.
- Lack of strength progression—especially abduction.
- Continued pain.

Treatment of Complications
- These patients may need to move back to earlier routines.
- May require increased utilization of pain control modalities as outlined above.
- May require imaging work-up or repeat surgical intervention.

Rehabilitation Protocol
After Open (Bankart) Anterior Capsulolabral Reconstruction
Wilk

Phase 1: Immediate Postoperative Phase

Goals
- Protect the surgical procedure.
- Minimize the effects of mobilization.
- Diminish pain and inflammation.

Weeks 0–2
- Sling for comfort (1 wk).
- May wear immobilizer for sleep (2 wk)—physician's decision.
- Elbow/hand ROM.
- Gripping exercises.
- Passive ROM and active-assisted ROM (L-bar)
  - Flexion to tolerance.
  - Abduction to tolerance.
  - External and internal rotation in scapular plane.
- Submaximal isometrics.
- Rhythmic stabilization (see p. 183.)
- Cryotherapy, modalities as needed.

Weeks 3–4
- Gradually progress ROM
  - Flexion to 120–140 degrees.
  - External rotation in scapular plane to 35–45 degrees.
  - Internal rotation in scapular plane to 45–60 degrees.
  - Shoulder extension.
- Initiate light isotonics for shoulder musculature
  - Tubing for external and internal rotation.

- Dumbbells; deltoid, supraspinatus, biceps, scapular.
- Continue dynamic stabilization exercises, PNF.
- Initiate self-capsular stretching.

Weeks 5–6
- Progress ROM as tolerated
  - Flexion to 160 degrees (maximum).
  - External and internal rotation at 90 degrees abduction
    - Internal rotation to 75 degrees.
    - External rotation to 70–75 degrees.
  - Shoulder extension to 30–35 degrees.
- Joint mobilization, stretching, etc.
- Continue self-capsular stretching.
- Upper body ergometer arm at 90 degrees abduction.
- Progress all strengthening exercises
  - Continue PNF diagonal patterns (rhythmic stabilization techniques).
  - Continue isotonic strengthening.
  - Dynamic stabilization exercises.

Weeks 6–7
- Progress ROM to
  - External rotation at 90 degrees abduction: 80–85 degrees.
  - External rotation at 90 degrees abduction: 70–75 degrees.
  - Flexion: 165–175 degrees.

Rehabilitation Protocol
After Open (Bankart) Anterior Capsulolabral Reconstruction *(Continued)*
Wilk

Phase 2: Intermediate Phase

Goals
- Re-establish full ROM.
- Normalize arthrokinematics.
- Improve muscular strength.
- Enhance neuromuscular control.

Weeks 8–10
- Progress to full ROM (weeks 7–8).
- Continue all stretching exercises
  - Joint mobilization, capsular stretching, passive and active stretching.
- In overhead athletes, progress external rotation past 90 degrees.
- In nonoverhead athletes, maintain 90-degree external rotation.
- Continue strengthening exercises
  - "Thrower's Ten" Program (for overhead athlete).
  - Isotonic strengthening for entire shoulder complex.
  - PNF manual technique.
  - Neuromuscular control drills.
  - Isokinetic strengthening.

Weeks 10–14
- Continue all flexibility exercises.
- Continue all strengthening exercises.
- May initiate *light* plyometric exercises.
- May initiate *controlled* swimming, golf swings, etc.
- May initiate *light isotonic machine weight* training (weeks 12–14).

Phase 3: Advanced Strengthening Phase (Months 4–6)

Criteria for Progression to Phase 3
- Full ROM.
- No pain or tenderness.
- Satisfactory stability.
- Strength 70–80% of contralateral side.

Goals
- Enhance muscular strength, power, and endurance.
- Improve muscular endurance.
- Maintain mobility.

Weeks 14–20
- Continue all flexibility exercises
  - Self-capsular stretches (anterior, posterior, and inferior).
  - Maintain external rotation flexibility.
- Continue isotonic strengthening program.
- Emphasize muscular balance (external and internal rotation).
- Continue PNF manual resistance.
- May initiate and continue plyometrics.
- Initiate interval throwing program (physician's approval necessary) (see p. 190).

Weeks 20–24
- Continue all exercises listed above.
- Continue and progress all interval sport program (throwing, etc.).

Phase 4: Return to Activity Phase (Months 6–9)

Criteria for Progression to Phase 4
- Full nonpainful ROM.
- Satisfactory stability.
- Satisfactory strength (isokinetics).
- No pain or tenderness.

Goals
- Gradual return to sport activities.
- Maintain strength and mobility of shoulder.

Exercises
- Continue capsular stretching to maintain mobility.
- Continue strengthening program
  - Either "Thrower's Ten" or fundamental shoulder exercise program.
- Return to sport participation (unrestricted).

Rehabilitation Protocol
After Arthroscopic Anterior Shoulder Stabilization
Wilk

Phase 1: Immediate Postoperative Phase—"Restrictive Motion"

Goals
- Protect the anatomic repair.
- Prevent negative effects of immobilization.
- Promote dynamic stability.
- Diminish pain and inflammation.

Weeks 0–2
- No active external rotation or extension or abduction.
- Sling for 2 wk.

continued

Rehabilitation Protocol
After Arthroscopic Anterior Shoulder Stabilization (Continued)
Wilk

- Sleep in immobilizer for 2–4 wk.
- Elbow/hand ROM.
- Hand gripping exercises.
- Passive and gentle active-assisted ROM exercise
  - Flexion to 60 degrees.
  - Elevation in scapular plane to 60 degrees.
  - External and internal rotation with arm in 20 degrees of abduction.
  - External rotation to 5–10 degrees.
  - Internal rotation to 45 degrees.
- Submaximal isometrics for shoulder musculature.
- Cryotherapy, modalities as indicated.

Weeks 3–4
- Discontinue sling.
- May use immobilizer for sleep (physician's decision).
- Continue gentle ROM exercises (passive ROM and active-assisted ROM)
  - Flexion to 90 degrees.
  - Abduction to 75–85 degrees.
  - External rotation in scapular plane to 15–20 degrees.
  - Internal rotation in scapular plane to 55–60 degrees.

Note: Rate of progression based on evaluation of the patient.
- **No active external rotation, extension, or elevation.**
- Continue isometrics and rhythmic stabilization (submaximal).
- Continue use of cryotherapy.

Weeks 5–6
- Gradually improve ROM
  - Flexion to 135–140 degrees.
  - External rotation at 45 degrees abduction: 25–30 degrees.
  - External rotation at 45 degrees abduction: 55–60 degrees.
- May initiate stretching exercises.
- Initiate exercise tubing external and internal rotation (arm at side).
- PNF manual resistance.

Phase 2: Intermediate Phase—Moderate Protection Phase

Goals
- Gradually restore full ROM (week 10).
- Preserve the integrity of the surgical repair.
- Restore muscular strength and balance.

Weeks 7–9
- Gradually progress ROM
  - Flexion to 160 degrees.
  - External rotation at 90 degrees abduction: 70–75 degrees.
  - Internal rotation at 90 degrees abduction: 70–75 degrees.

- Continue to progress isotonic strengthening program.
- Continue PNF strengthening.

Weeks 10–14
- May initiate slightly more aggressive strengthening.
- Progress isotonic strengthening exercises.
- Continue all stretching exercises.
- Progress ROM to functional demands (i.e., overhead athlete).

Phase 3: Minimal Protection Phase

Criteria for Progression to Phase 3
- Full nonpainful ROM.
- Satisfactory stability.
- Muscular strength (good grade or better).
- No pain or tenderness.

Goals
- Establish and maintain full ROM.
- Improve muscular strength, power, and endurance.
- Gradually initiate functional activities.

Weeks 15–18
- Continue all stretching exercises (capsular stretches).
- Continue strengthening exercises
  - "Thrower's Ten" Program or fundamental exercises.
  - PNF manual resistance.
  - Endurance training.
  - Initiate light plyometric program.
  - Restricted sport activities (light swimming, half golf swings).

Weeks 18–21
- Continue all exercise listed earlier.
- Initiate interval sport program (throwing, etc.).

Phase 4: Advanced Strengthening Phase

Criteria for Progression to Phase 4
- Full nonpainful ROM.
- Satisfactory static stability.
- Muscular strength 75–80% of contralateral side.
- No pain or tenderness.

Goals
- Enhance muscular strength, power, and endurance.
- Progress functional activities.
- Maintain shoulder mobility.

Weeks 22–24
- Continue flexibility exercises.
- Continue isotonic strengthening program.
- PNF manual resistance patterns.
- Plyometric strengthening.
- Progress interval sport programs.

Rehabilitation Protocol
After Arthroscopic Anterior Shoulder Stabilization (Continued)
Wilk

Phase 5: Return to Activity Phase (Months 6–9)

Criteria for Progression to Phase 5
- Full functional ROM.
- Satisfactory isokinetic test that fulfills criteria.
- Satisfactory shoulder stability.
- No pain or tenderness.

Goals
- Gradual return to sport activities.
- Maintain strength, mobility, and stability.

Exercises
- Gradually progress sport activities to unrestrictive participation.
- Continue stretching and strengthening program.

Posterior Shoulder Instability

Posterior instability is much less common than anterior instability. Posterior dislocations are most commonly caused by a generalized muscle contraction after a seizure, which can be related to epilepsy, alcohol abuse, or severe electric shock. Patients with a posterior shoulder dislocation hold the arm in adduction and internal rotation. A fullness may be palpable in the posterior shoulder, and **abduction and external rotation may be limited.** A complete radiographic evaluation of the shoulder is required, **especially an axillary lateral view.** If an axillary lateral radiograph cannot be obtained, a CT scan of the GH joint should be done. **In approximately 80% of patients with posterior dislocation of the GH joint, the diagnosis is not made by the initial treating physician because of incomplete radiographic evaluation. This is why *all* shoulder injuries must have an axillary lateral view as part of the radiograph series.**

Posterior instability in athletes commonly results in subluxation, usually because of repetitive microtrauma. For example, an offensive lineman in football may develop this condition because of the forward-flexed and internally rotated shoulder position needed for blocking. On physical examination, patients with posterior instability demonstrate increased posterior translation on posterior draw testing. Symptoms are reproduced when a posteriorly directed force is placed on the patient's arm in the adducted forward-flexed position.

Treatment of Traumatic Posterior Dislocation

Treatment of a traumatic posterior dislocation that is successfully reduced usually **begins with immobilization in a brace that maintains the shoulder in external rotation and neutral to slight extension.** Immobilization is continued for 6 weeks, and then a structured rehabilitation program is followed similar to the one outlined on page 210. Variations may be required depending on the position of immobilization, positions for recurrent instability, freedom of full external rotation, and restriction of internal rotation. **The basic premise of treating an unstable shoulder with physical therapy is to strengthen the dynamic stabilizers (muscles and tendons) while the static stabilizers (including the glenoid labrum) heal.**

Indications for surgical stabilization of a posterior shoulder dislocation include:

- A displaced lesser tuberosity fracture.
- A posterior glenoid rim fracture of more than 25%.
- An impaction fracture of the anterior-superior humeral articular surface (reverse Hill-Sachs lesion) of more than 40%.
- An irreducible dislocation.
- Recurrent posterior dislocations.
- An unstable reduction (usually associated with a reverse Hill-Sachs lesion of 20 to 40%).

Patients with unstable reductions may have pathology similar to that after an anterior dislocation, with avulsion of the capsule and labrum from the posterior glenoid rim. This can be repaired with an open or arthroscopic technique. The rehabilitation protocol after surgical repair of the capsulolabral complex after posterior dislocation is outlined on page 212.

Patients who have symptomatic posterior instability with no history of a traumatic dislocation usually benefit from a rehabilitation program that focuses on strengthening of the dynamic stabilizers. Patients who do not improve after following an organized rehabilitation program for 3 to 6 months may require surgical treatment. These patients usually have a lax posterior capsule, which can be treated with an arthroscopic technique (capsular suture plication, electrothermal capsulorrhaphy [shrinkage]) followed by rehabilitation as outlined on page 211 or with an open posterior stabilization procedure followed by rehabilitation as outlined on page 212.

Rehabilitation Protocol
Non-operative Rehabilitation for Posterior Shoulder Instability
Wilk

This program is designed to return the patient/athlete to their activity/sport as quickly and safely as possible. The program will vary in length for each individual depending on severity of injury, ROM/strength status, and performance/activity demands.

Phase 1: Acute Phase

Goals
- Decrease pain and inflammation.
- Reestablish nonpainful ROM.
- Retard muscle atrophy.

Decrease Pain and Inflammation
- Therapeutic modalities (e.g., ice, heat, electrotherapy).
- NSAIDs.
- Gentle joint mobilization.

Range of Motion Exercises
- Pendulum.
- Rope and pulley.
- L-bar
  - Flexion.
  - Abduction.
  - Horizontal abduction.
  - External rotation.

Strength Exercises
- Isometrics
  - Flexion.
  - Abduction.
  - Extension.
  - External rotation.
- Weight shifts (closed-chain exercises).

Note: Avoid any motion that may place stress on the posterior capsule such as excessive internal rotation, abduction, or horizontal adduction.

Phase 2: Immediate Phase

Criteria for Progression to Phase 2
- Full ROM.
- Minimal pain and tenderness.
- "Good" MMT

Goals
- Regain and improve muscular strength.
- Normal arthrokinematics.
- Improve neuromuscular control of shoulder complex.

Initiate Isotonic Strengthening
- Flexion.
- Abduction to 90 degrees.
- External rotation.
- Internal rotation (from full external rotation to 0 degrees).
- Supraspinatus.
- Extension.
- Horizontal abduction (prone).
- Push-ups.

Initiate Eccentric (Surgical Tubing) Strengthening
- External rotation (from 0 degrees to full external rotation).
- Internal rotation (from full external rotation to 0 degrees).

Normalize Arthrokinematics of Shoulder Complex
- Continue joint mobilization.
- Patient education of mechanics of activity/sport.

Improve Neuromuscular Control of Shoulder Complex
- Initiate PNF.
- Rhythmic stabilization drills.

Continue Use of Modalities (As Needed)
- Ice, electrotherapy modalities.

Phase 3: Advanced Strengthening Phase

Criteria for Progression to Phase 3
- Full nonpainful ROM.
- No palpable tenderness.
- Continued progression of resistive exercises.

Goals
- Improve strength, power, and endurance.
- Improve neuromuscular control.
- Prepare athlete for activity.

Continue Use of Modalities (As Needed)

Continue Anterior Capsule Stretch

Continue Isotonic Strengthening

Continue Eccentric Strengthening

Emphasize PNF (D2 Extension)

Initiate Isokinetics
- Flexion-extension.
- Abduction-adduction.
- Internal and external rotation.
- Horizontal abduction-adduction.

Initiate Plyometric Training
- Surgical tubing.
- Medicine ball.
- Wall push-ups.

Initiate Military Press

Phase 4: Return to Activity Phase

Criteria for Progression to Phase 4
- Full ROM.
- No pain or tenderness.
- Satisfactory clinical examination.
- Satisfactory isokinetic test.

Goals
- Maintain optimal level of strength, power, and endurance.
- Progressively increase activity level to prepare patient/athlete for full functional return to activity/sport.

Continue All Exercises as in Phase 3

Initiate and Progress Interval Program

Rehabilitation Protocol
Posterior Capsular Shift
Wilk

The goal of this rehabilitation program is to return the patient/athlete to activity/sport as quickly and safely as possible while maintaining a stable shoulder. This program is based on shoulder anatomy, biomechanics, and the healing constraints of the surgical procedure.

The posterior capsular shift procedure is one in which the orthopaedic surgeon makes an incision into the ligamentous capsule of the posterior shoulder then pulls the capsule tighter and sutures it together.

Phase 1: Protection Phase (Weeks 0–6)

Precautions
- Postoperative brace in 30–45 degrees abduction, 15 degrees external rotation for 4–6 wk.
- Brace must be worn at all times with the exception of exercise activity and bathing.
- No overhead activity.
- Must sleep in brace.

Goals
- Allow healing of sutured capsule.
- Initiate early protected ROM.
- Retard muscular atrophy.
- Decrease pain and inflammation.

Weeks 0–4
Exercises
- Gripping exercises with putty.
- Active elbow flexion-extension and pronation-supination.
- Active ROM cervical spine.
- Passive ROM progressing to active-assisted ROM.
- Active-assisted ROM
  - External rotation at 30–45 degrees of abduction: 25–30 degrees.
  - Flexion to 90 degrees as tolerated.
  - Internal rotation at 30–45 degrees of abduction (week 3): 15–25 degrees.
- Submaximal shoulder isometrics
  - Flexion.
  - Abduction.
  - Extension.
  - External rotation.

Note: In general all exercises begin with one set of 10 repetitions and should increase by one set of 10 repetitions daily as tolerated to five sets of 10 repetitions.

Cryotherapy: Ice before and after exercises for 20 min. Ice up to 20 min per hour to control pain and swelling.

Criteria for Hospital Discharge
- Passive shoulder ROM 90 degrees flexion and 25 degrees external rotation.
- Minimal pain and swelling.
- "Good" proximal and distal muscle power.

Weeks 4–6
Goals
- Gradual increase in ROM.
- Normalize arthrokinemetrics.
- Improve strength.
- Decrease pain and inflammation.

Range of Motion Exercises
- T-bar active-assisted exercises.
- External rotation from 45–90 degrees of shoulder abduction.
- Shoulder flexion to tolerance.
- Shoulder abduction to 90 degrees.
- Internal rotation at 45 degrees of abduction: 35 degrees.
- Rope and pulley
  - Shoulder abduction to tolerance.
  - Shoulder flexion to 90 degrees.
- All exercises should be performed to tolerance.
- Take to the point of pain and/or tolerance and hold (5 sec).
- *Gentle* self-capsular stretches.

Gentle Joint Mobilization to Reestablish Normal
- Arthrokinetmatics.
- Scapulothoracic joint.
- GH joint—avoid posterior glides.
- SC joint.

Strengthening Exercises
- Active abduction to 90 degrees.
- Active external rotation neutral to 90 degrees.
- Elbow/wrist PRE program.

Conditioning Program For
- Trunk.
- Lower extremities.
- Cardiovascular endurance.

Decrease Pain and Inflammation
- Ice, NSAIDs, modalities.

Brace
- Discontinue 4–6 wk postsurgery per physician's direction.

Phase 2: Intermediate Phase (Weeks 6–12)
Goals
- Full, nonpainful ROM at week 8 (except internal rotation).
- Normalize arthrokinematics.
- Increase strength.
- Improve neuromuscular control.

Weeks 6–9
Range of Motion Exercises
- T-bar active-assisted exercises
  - External rotation to tolerance.
  - Shoulder abduction to tolerance.

continued

Rehabilitation Protocol
Posterior Capsular Shift *(Continued)*
Wilk

- Shoulder flexion to tolerance.
- Rope and pulley: flexion-abduction.

Joint Mobilization
- Continue as above.

Strengthening Exercises
- Tubing for internal and external rotation at 0 degrees abduction.
- Initiate isotonic dumbbell program
  - Shoulder abduction.
  - Shoulder flexion.
  - Latissimus dorsi.
  - Rhomboids.
  - Biceps curl.
  - Triceps kick-out over table.
  - Shoulder shrugs.
  - Push-ups into wall (serratus anterior).

Initiate Neuromuscular Control Exercises for SC Joint

Weeks 10–12

Continue all exercises listed above.

Initiate
- Active-assisted internal rotation 90/90 position.
- Dumbbells supraspinatus.
- Tubing exercises for rhomboids, latissimus dorsi, biceps, and triceps.
- Progressive push-ups.

Phase 3: Dynamic Strengthening Program (Weeks 12–18)

Criteria for Progression to Phase 3
- Full, nonpainful ROM.
- No pain/tenderness.
- Strength 70% contralateral side.

Weeks 13–15
Goals
- Improve strength, power, and endurance.
- Improve neuromuscular control.

Emphasis of Phase 3
- High-speed/high-energy strengthening exercises.
- Eccentric exercises.
- Diagonal patterns.

Exercises
- Continue internal and external rotation tubing exercises at 0 degrees abduction (arm at side).
- Tubing for rhomboids.
- Tubing for latissimus dorsi.
- Tubing for biceps and triceps.
- Continue dumbbell exercise for supraspinatus and deltoid.
- Progressive serratus anterior push-up—anterior flexion.
- Continue trunk and lower extremity strengthening and conditioning exercises.
- Continue self-capsular stretches.

Weeks 16–20
- Continue all exercises as above.
- Emphasis on gradual return to recreational activities.

Phase 4: Return to Activity Phase (Weeks 21–28)

Criteria for Progression to Phase 4
- Full ROM.
- No pain or tenderness.
- Satisfactory clinical examination.
- Satisfactory isokinetic test.

Goal
- Progressively increase activities to prepare patient for unrestricted functional return.

Exercises
- Continue tubing and dumbbell exercises outlined in phase 3.
- Continue ROM exercises.
- Initiate internal programs between 28 and 32 wk (if patient is a recreational athlete).

Rehabilitation Protocol
After Posterior Shoulder Stabilization
Bach, Cohen, and Romeo

Phase 1: Weeks 0–4
Restrictions
- No shoulder motion.

Immobilization
- Use of a gunslinger orthosis for 4 wk.

Pain Control
- Reduction of pain and discomfort is essential for recovery.
- Patients treated with an arthroscopic stabilization procedure experience less postoperative pain than patients treated with an open stabilization procedure
  - Medications

Rehabilitation Protocol
After Posterior Shoulder Stabilization (Continued)
Bach, Cohen, and Romeo

- Narcotics—for 7–10 days following surgery.
- NSAIDs—for patients with persistent discomfort following surgery.
- Therapeutic modalities
  - Ice, ultrasound, HVGS.
  - Moist heat before therapy, ice at end of session.

Motion: Shoulder
- None.

Motion: Elbow
- Passive—progress to active
  - 0–130 degrees of flexion.
  - Pronation and supination as tolerated.

Muscle Strengthening
- Grip strengthening only.

Phase 2: Weeks 4–8

Criteria for Progression to Phase 2
- Adequate immobilization.

Restrictions
- **Shoulder motion: active ROM only**
  - Forward flexion 120 degrees.
  - Abduction 45 degrees.
  - External rotation as tolerated.
  - Internal rotation and adduction to stomach.
- Avoid provocative maneuvers that re-create position of instability
  - Avoid excessive internal rotation.

Immobilization
- Gunslinger—discontinue.

Pain Control
- Medications
  - NSAIDs—for patients with persistent discomfort.
- Therapeutic modalities
  - Ice, ultrasound, HVGS.
  - Moist heat before therapy, ice at end of session.

Shoulder Motion: Active Range of Motion Only
Goals
- Forward flexion 120 degrees.
- Abduction 45 degrees.
- External rotation as tolerated.
- Internal rotation and adduction to stomach.

Exercises
- Active ROM only.

Muscle Strengthening
- Rotator cuff strengthening.
- Closed-chain isometric strengthening with the elbow flexed to 90 degrees and the arm at the side (see Fig. 3–36)
  - Forward flexion.
  - External rotation.
  - Internal rotation.

- Abduction.
- Adduction.
- Strengthening of scapular stabilizers
  - Closed-chain strengthening exercises (see Figs. 3–37, 3–59, and 3–68).
  - Scapular retraction (rhomboideus, middle trapezius).
  - Scapular protraction (serratus anterior).
  - Scapular depression (latissimus dorsi, trapezius, serratus anterior).
  - Shoulder shrugs (trapezius, levator scapulae).

Phase 3: Weeks 8–12

Criteria for Progression to Phase 3
- Minimal pain and discomfort with active ROM and closed-chain strengthening exercises.
- No sensation or findings of instability with above exercises.

Restrictions
- Shoulder motion: active and active-assisted motion exercises
  - 160 degrees of forward flexion.
  - Full external rotation.
  - 70 degrees of abduction.
  - Internal rotation and adduction to stomach.

Pain Control
- Medications
  - NSAIDs—for patients with persistent discomfort.
- Therapeutic modalities
  - Ice, ultrasound, HVGS.
  - Moist heat before therapy, ice at end of session.

Motion: Shoulder
Goals
- 160 degrees of forward flexion.
- Full external rotation.
- 70 degrees of abduction.
- Internal rotation and adduction to stomach.

Exercises
- Active ROM exercises.
- Active-assisted ROM exercises (see Fig. 3–34).

Muscle Strengthening
- Rotator cuff strengthening–three times per week, 8 to 12 repetitions for three sets
  - Continue with closed-chain isometric strengthening.
  - Progress to open-chain strengthening with Thera-bands (see Fig. 3–39A)
    - Exercises performed with the elbow flexed to 90 degrees.
    - Starting position is with the shoulder in the neutral position of 0 degrees of forward flexion, abduction, and external rotation.

continued

Rehabilitation Protocol
After Posterior Shoulder Stabilization (Continued)
Bach, Cohen, and Romeo

- Exercises are performed through an arc of 45 degrees in each of the five planes of motion.
- Six color-coded bands are available; each provides increasing resistance from 1 to 6 pounds, at increments of 1 pound.
- Progression to the next band occurs usually in 2- to 3-wk intervals. Patients are instructed not to progress to the next band if there is any discomfort at the present level.
- Theraband exercises permit concentric and eccentric strengthening of the shoulder muscles and are a form of isotonic exercises (characterized by variable speed and fixed resistance)
  - Internal rotation.
  - External rotation.
  - Abduction.
  - Forward flexion.
- Progress to light isotonic dumbbell exercises
  - Internal rotation (see Fig. 3–39B).
  - External rotation (see Fig. 3–39C).
  - Abduction.
  - Forward flexion.
- Strengthening of scapular stabilizers
  - Continue with closed-chain strengthening exercises.
  - Advance to open-chain isotonic strengthening exercises (see Figs. 3–38 and 3–66).

Phase 4: Months 3–6

Criteria for Progression to Phase 4
- Minimal pain or discomfort with active ROM and muscle strengthening exercises.
- Improvement in strengthening of rotator cuff and scapular stabilizers.
- Satisfactory physical examination.

Goals
- Improve shoulder strength, power, and endurance.
- Improve neuromuscular control and shoulder proprioception.
- Restore full shoulder motion.
- Establish a home exercise maintenance program that is performed at least three times per week for both stretching and strengthening.

Pain Control
- Medications
  - NSAIDs—for patients with persistent discomfort.
  - Subacromial injection: corticosteroid/local anesthetic combination for patients with findings consistent with secondary impingement.
  - GH joint: corticosteroid/local anesthetic combination for patients whose clinical findings are consistent with GH joint pathology.
- Therapeutic modalities
  - Ice, ultrasound, HVGS.
  - Moist heat before therapy, ice at end of session.

Motion: Shoulder
Goals
- Obtain motion that is equal to contralateral side.
- Active ROM exercises.
- Active-assisted ROM exercises (see Fig. 3–34).
- Passive ROM exercises (see Fig. 3–35).
- Capsular stretching (especially posterior capsule [see Fig. 3–48]).

Muscle Strengthening
- Rotator cuff and scapular stabilizer strengthening as outlined above
  - Three times per week, 8 to 12 repetitions for three sets.

Upper Extremity Endurance Training
- Incorporated endurance training for the upper extremity
  - Upper body ergometer.

Proprioceptive Training
- PNF patterns (see Fig. 3–67).

Functional Strengthening
- Plyometric exercises (see Fig. 3–40).

Progressive, Systematic Interval Program for Returning to Sports
- Golfers—see p. 195.
- Overhead athletes not before 6 mo
  - Throwing athletes—see p. 190.
  - Tennis players—see p. 192.

Maximum improvement is expected by 12 mo.

Warning Signs
- **Persistent instability.**
- **Loss of motion.**
- **Lack of strength progression—especially abduction.**
- **Continued pain.**

Treatment of Complications
- **These patients may need to move back to earlier routines.**
- **May require increased utilization of pain control modalities as outlined above.**
- **May require imaging work-up or repeat surgical intervention.**

Multidirectional Instability

Multidirectional shoulder instability is not the result of a traumatic injury, but is associated with hyperlaxity of the GH joint capsule in association with rotator cuff weakness. Multidirectional shoulder instability can be simply defined as symptomatic instability in more than one direction. Patients may have a history of laxity in other joints, demonstrated by frequent ankle sprains or recurrent patellar dislocations. Physical examination often finds generalized joint laxity, **but the key to the diagnosis is the reproduction of symptoms with unwanted GH joint translation.** Patients demonstrate increased laxity in multiple directions and have a positive sulcus sign or varying degrees of inferior translation of the GH joint.

Treatment

Multidirectional instability is treated conservatively with a rehabilitation program focused on strengthening of the rotator cuff, the scapular stabilizers, and the deltoid mus-

cles. Surgical stabilization is considered if an extensive trial of rehabilitation for at least 6 months fails to relieve symptoms. If conservative treatment fails, an open inferior capsular shift from an anterior approach is recommended. The goal of this procedure is to balance tension on all sides of the GH joint and surgically reduce capsular volume. The postoperative rehabilitation protocol is outlined on this page. Arthroscopic treatment for multidirectional instability is currently evolving. Two techniques for reducing capsular volume with promising results are suture capsular plication and electrothermal capsulorrhaphy (shrinkage). The postoperative rehabilitation protocol is outlined on page 217.

Rehabilitation Protocol
After Open Inferior Capsular Shift for Multidirectional Instability
Bach, Cohen, and Romeo

Phase 1: Weeks 0– 6

Restriction
- Shoulder motion: none for 6 wk.

Immobilization
- Sling or gunslinger orthosis
  - 6 wk—during day and at night.

Pain Control
- Reduction of pain and discomfort is essential for recovery
  - Medications
    - Narcotics—for 7–10 days following surgery.
    - NSAIDs—for patients with persistent discomfort following surgery.
  - Therapeutic modalities
    - Ice, ultrasound, HVGS.
    - Moist heat before therapy, ice at end of session.

Motion: Shoulder
- None.

Motion: Elbow
- Passive—progress to active
  - 0 to 130 degrees of flexion.
  - Pronation and supination as tolerated.

Muscle Strengthening
- Rotator cuff strengthening
  - Closed-chain isometric strengthening with the elbow flexed to 90 degrees and the arm at the side in brace (see Fig. 3–36)
    - External rotation.
    - Abduction.
    - Forward flexion.
- Grip strengthening.

Phase 2: Weeks 7–12

Criteria for Progression to Phase 2
- Minimal pain or discomfort with ROM and closed-chain strengthening exercises.
- No sensation or findings of instability with these maneuvers.

- Satisfactory physical examination.

Restrictions
- Shoulder motion: active ROM only
  - 140 degrees of forward flexion.
  - 40 degrees of external rotation.
  - 70 degrees of abduction.
  - Internal rotation to stomach.
- Avoid positions that re-create instability.

Pain Control
- Medications
  - NSAIDs—for patients with persistent discomfort.
- Therapeutic modalities
  - Ice, ultrasound, HVGS.
  - Moist heat before therapy, ice at end of session.

Motion: Shoulder
- Goals
  - 140 degrees of forward flexion.
  - 40 degrees of external rotation.
  - 70 degrees of abduction.
  - Internal rotation to stomach.
- Exercises
  - Active ROM exercises.

Muscle Strengthening
- Rotator cuff strengthening–three times per week, 8 to 12 repetitions for three sets
  - Continue with closed-chain isometric strengthening.
  - Progress to open-chain strengthening with Therabands (see Fig. 3–39A)
    - Exercises performed with the elbow flexed to 90 degrees.
    - Starting position is with the shoulder in the neutral position of 0 degrees of forward flexion, abduction, and external rotation.
    - Exercises are performed through an arc of 45 degrees in each of the five planes of motion.
    - Six color-coded bands are available; each provides increasing resistance from 1 to 6 pounds, at increments of one pound.

continued

Rehabilitation Protocol
After Open Inferior Capsular Shift for Multidirectional Instability (Continued)
Bach, Cohen, and Romeo

- Progression to the next band occurs usually in 2 to 3-wk intervals. Patients are instructed not to progress to the next band if there is any discomfort at the present level.
- Theraband exercises permit concentric and eccentric strengthening of the shoulder muscles and are a form of isotonic exercises (characterized by variable speed and fixed resistance)
  - Internal rotation.
  - External rotation.
  - Abduction.
  - Forward flexion.
- Progress to light isotonic dumbbell exercises (see Fig. 3–39B and C)
  - Internal rotation.
  - External rotation.
  - Abduction.
  - Forward flexion.
- Strengthening of scapular stabilizers
  - Closed-chain strengthening exercises (see Figs. 3–37, 3–59, and 3–68)
    - Scapular retraction (rhomboideus, middle trapezius).
    - Scapular protraction (serratus anterior).
    - Scapular depression (latissimus dorsi, trapezius, serratus anterior).
    - Shoulder shrugs (trapezius, levator scapulae).
  - Progress to open-chain strengthening (Fig. 3–69; see also Figs. 3–38 and 3–59).

Phase 3: Months 3–6

Criteria for Progression to Phase 3
- Minimal pain or discomfort with active ROM and muscle strengthening exercises.
- Improvement in strengthening of rotator cuff and scapular stabilizers.
- Satisfactory physical examination.

Figure 3–69. Open-chain strengthening of the scapular stabilizers using Theraband tubing.

Goals
- Improve shoulder complex strength, power, and endurance.
- Improve neuromuscular control and shoulder proprioception.
- Restore full shoulder motion.
- Establish a home exercise maintenance program that is performed at least three times per week for both stretching and strengthening.

Pain Control
- Medications
  - NSAIDs—for patients with persistent discomfort.
  - Subacromial injection: corticosteroid/local anesthetic combination
    - For patients with findings consistent with secondary impingement
  - GH joint: corticosteroid/local anesthetic combination
    - For patients whose clinical findings are consistent with GH joint pathology
- Therapeutic modalities
  - Ice, ultrasound, HVGS.
  - Moist heat before therapy, ice at end of session.

Motion: Shoulder
- Goals
  - Obtain motion that is equal to contralateral side.
  - Active ROM exercises.
  - Active-assisted ROM exercises (see Fig. 3–34).
  - Passive ROM exercises (see Fig. 3–35).
  - Capsular stretching for selective areas of shoulder to "balance" the laxity (do not aim for full ROM).

Muscle Strengthening
- Rotator cuff and scapular stabilizer strengthening as outlined above
  - Three times per week, 8 to 12 repetitions for three sets.
- Deltoid strengthening (Fig. 3–70; see also Fig. 3–58).

Upper Extremity Endurance Training
- Incorporated endurance training for the upper extremity
  - Upper body ergometer.

Proprioceptive Training
- PNF patterns (see Fig. 3–67).

Functional Strengthening
- Plyometric exercises (see Fig. 3–40).

Progressive, Systematic Interval Program for Returning to Sports
- Golfers— see p. 195.
- Overhead athletes not before **6 mo**
  - Throwing athletes— see p. 190.
  - Tennis players— see p. 192.

Maximum improvement is expected by 12 mo.

Rehabilitation Protocol
After Open Inferior Capsular Shift for Multidirectional Instability *(Continued)*
Bach, Cohen, and Romeo

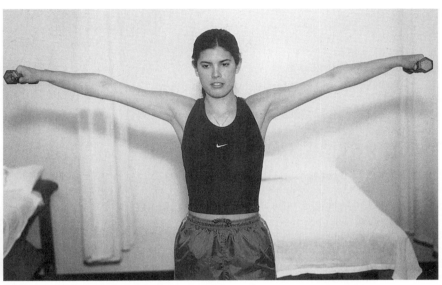

A   **B**

Figure 3–70. Isotonic deltoid strengthening with light dumbbells. *A,* Start. *B,* Finish.

Warning Signs
- Persistent instability after surgery.
- Development of instability symptoms from 6 to 12 mo suggests a failure to reestablish the stability of the GH joint.
- Loss of motion.
- Lack of strength progression—especially abduction.
- Continued pain.

Treatment of Complications
- These patients may need to move back to earlier routines.
- May require increased utilization of pain control modalities as outlined above.
- May require imaging work-up or repeat surgical intervention.

Rehabilitation Protocol
After Thermal Capsulorrhaphy for Multidirectional Instability
Bach, Cohen, and Romeo

Phase 1: Weeks 0–6

Restrictions
- Strict shoulder immobilization for 6 wk
  - Sling or gunslinger orthosis, depending on degree of instability.

Pain Control
- Reduction of pain and discomfort is essential for recovery
  - Medications
    - Narcotics—for 7–10 days following surgery.
    - NSAIDs—for patients with persistent discomfort following surgery.
  - Therapeutic modalities
    - Ice, ultrasound, HVGS.
    - Moist heat before therapy, ice at end of session.

Motion: Shoulder
- None.

Motion: Elbow
- Passive—progress to active.
- 0–130 degrees of flexion.
- Pronation and supination as tolerated.

continued

Rehabilitation Protocol
After Thermal Capsulorrhaphy for Multidirectional Instability *(Continued)*
Bach, Cohen, and Romeo

Muscle Strengthening
- Grip strengthening.

Phase 2: Weeks 6–12
Criteria for Progression to Phase 2
- Adequate immobilization.

Restrictions
- Shoulder motion: active ROM only
  - 140 degrees of forward flexion.
  - 40 degrees of external rotation with arm at the side.
  - 60 degrees of abduction.

Immobilization
- Sling or gunslinger orthosis at night.

Pain Control
- Medications
  - NSAIDs—for patients with persistent discomfort.
- Therapeutic modalities
  - Ice, ultrasound, HVGS.
  - Moist heat before therapy, ice at end of session.

Motion: Shoulder
Goals
- 140 degrees of forward flexion.
- 40 degrees of external rotation with arm at the side.
- 60 degrees of abduction.

Exercises
- Active ROM exercises.

Muscle Strengthening
- Rotator cuff strengthening
  - Closed-chain isometric strengthening with the elbow flexed to 90 degrees and the arm at the side (see Fig. 3–36)
    - Internal rotation.
    - External rotation.
    - Abduction.
    - Forward flexion.

Phase 3: Months 3–6
Criteria for Progression to Phase 2
- Minimal pain or discomfort with active ROM and closed-chain strengthening exercises.
- No sensation or findings of instability with these maneuvers.
- Satisfactory physical examination.

Restrictions
- Shoulder motion
  - 160 degrees of forward flexion.
  - External rotation as tolerated with arm at side.
  - 90 degrees of abduction.
- Avoid extreme positions that may lead to instability.

Pain Control
- Medications
  - NSAIDs—for patients with persistent discomfort.
  - Subacromial injection: corticosteroid/local anesthetic combination
    - For patients with findings consistent with secondary impingement.
  - GH joint: corticosteroid/local anesthetic combination
    - For patients whose clinical findings are consistent with GH joint pathology.
- Therapeutic modalities
  - Ice, ultrasound, HVGS.
  - Moist heat before therapy, ice at end of session.

Motion: Shoulder
Goals
- 160 degrees of forward flexion.
- External rotation as tolerated with arm at side.
- 90 degrees of abduction.
- *Note:* The goal is a functional ROM without symptoms of instability, *not* full ROM.

Exercises
- Active ROM exercises.
- Active-assisted ROM exercises (see Fig. 3–34).
- Passive ROM exercises (see Fig. 3–35).

Muscle Strengthening
- Rotator cuff strengthening—three times per week, 8–12 repetitions for three sets
  - Continue with closed-chain isometric strengthening.
  - Progress to open-chain strengthening with Therabands (see Fig. 3–39A)
    - Exercises performed with the elbow flexed to 90 degrees.
    - Starting position is with the shoulder in the neutral position of 0 degrees of forward flexion, abduction, and external rotation.
    - Exercises are performed through an arc of 45 degrees in each of the five planes of motion.
    - Six color-coded bands are available; each provides increasing resistance from 1 to 6 pounds, at increments of one pound.
    - Progression to the next band occurs usually in 2 to 3-wk intervals. Patients are instructed not to progress to the next band if there is any discomfort at the present level.
    - Theraband exercises permit concentric and eccentric strengthening of the shoulder muscles and are a form of isotonic exercises (characterized by variable speed and fixed resistance)
      - Internal rotation.
      - External rotation.

Rehabilitation Protocol
After Thermal Capsulorrhaphy for Multidirectional Instability *(Continued)*
Bach, Cohen, and Romeo

- Abduction.
- Forward flexion.
- Progress to light isotonic dumbbell exercises (see Fig. 3–39B)
  - Internal rotation.
  - External rotation.
  - Abduction.
  - Forward flexion.
- Strengthening of scapular stabilizers
  - Closed-chain strengthening exercises (see Figs. 3–37, 3–59, and 3–68)
    - Scapular retraction (rhomboideus, middle trapezius).
    - Scapular protraction (serratus anterior).
    - Scapular depression (latissimus dorsi, trapezius, serratus anterior).
    - Shoulder shrugs (trapezius, levator scapulae).
  - Progress to open-chain strengthening (see Figs. 3–38 and 3–69).
- Deltoid strengthening (see Figs. 3–58 and 3–70).

Phase 4: Months 6–12

Criteria for Progression to Phase 4
- Minimal pain or discomfort with active ROM and muscle strengthening exercises.
- Improvement in strengthening of rotator cuff and scapular stabilizers.
- Satisfactory physical examination.

Goals
- Improve shoulder complex strength, power, and endurance.
- Improve neuromuscular control and shoulder proprioception.
- Restore functional range of shoulder motion.
- Establish a home exercise maintenance program that is performed at least three times per week for both stretching and strengthening.

Pain Control
- Medications
  - NSAIDs—for patients with persistent discomfort.
  - Subacromial injection: corticosteroid/local anesthetic combination
    - For patients with findings consistent with secondary impingement.
  - GH joint corticosteroid/local anesthetic combination
    - For patients whose clinical findings are consistent with GH joint pathology.
- Therapeutic modalities
  - Ice, ultrasound, HVGS.
  - Moist heat before therapy, ice at end of session.

Motion: Shoulder
Goals
- Obtain functional ROM without symptoms of instability; usually 10–20 degrees less motion than opposite side.

Exercises
- Active ROM exercises.
- Active-assisted ROM exercises (see Fig. 3–34).
- Passive ROM exercises (see Fig. 3–35).
- Capsular stretching
  - Especially posterior capsule (see Fig. 3–48).

Muscle Strengthening
- Rotator cuff, deltoid and scapular stabilizer strengthening as outlined above
  - Three times per week, 8–12 repetitions for three sets.

Upper Extremity Endurance Training
- Incorporated endurance training for the upper extremity
  - Upper body ergometer.

Proprioceptive Training
- PNF patterns (see Fig. 3–67).

Functional Strengthening
- Plyometric exercises (see Fig. 3–40).

Progressive, Systematic Interval Program for Returning to Sports
- Throwing athletes—see p. 190.
- Tennis players—see p. 192.
- Golfers— see p. 195.

Maximum improvement is expected by 12 mo.

Warning Signs
- Persistent instability after surgery.
- Development of instability symptoms from 6 to 12 mo suggests a failure to reestablish the stability of the GH joint.
- Loss of motion.
- Lack of strength progression—especially abduction.
- Continued pain.

Treatment of Complications
- These patients may need to move back to earlier routines.
- May require increased utilization of pain control modalities as outlined above.
- May require imaging work-up or repeat surgical intervention.

Rehabilitation Protocol
An Accelerated Rehabilitation Program after Anterior Capsular Shift–Acquired Instability in Overhead Athletes
Wilk

This rehabilitation program's goal is to return the patient/athlete to the activity/sport as quickly and safely as possible, while maintaining a stable shoulder. The program is based on muscle physiology, biomechanics, anatomy, and the healing process after surgery for a capsular shift.

The capsular-shift procedure is one in which the orthopaedic surgeon makes an incision into the ligamentous capsule of the shoulder, pulls the capsule tighter, and then sutures the capsule together.

The ultimate goal is a functional shoulder and a return to presurgery functional level.

Phase 1: Protection Phase (Weeks 0–6)

Goals
- Allow healing of sutured capsule.
- Begin early protected ROM.
- Retard muscular atrophy.
- Decrease pain and inflammation.

Weeks 0–2

Precautions
- Sleep in immobilizer for 2 wk.
- No overhead activities for 4–6 wk.
- Wean from immobilizer and into sling as soon as possible (orthopaedist or therapist will tell you when).

Exercises
- Gripping exercises.
- Elbow flexion-extension and pronation-supination.
- Pendulum exercises (nonweighted).
- Rope and pulley active-assisted exercises
  - Shoulder flexion to 90 degrees.
  - Shoulder abduction to 60 degrees.
- L-bar exercises
  - External rotation to 15–20 degrees with arm in scapular plane.
  - Shoulder flexion-extension to tolerance.
- Active ROM cervical spine.
- Isometrics
  - Flexors, extensors, external and internal rotation, abduction.

Criteria for Hospital Discharge
- Shoulder ROM (active-assisted ROM) flexion 90 degrees; abduction 45 degrees; external rotation 40 degrees.
- Minimal pain and swelling.
- "Good" proximal and distal muscle power.

Weeks 2–4

Goals
- Gradual increase in ROM.
- Normalize arthrokinematics.
- Improve strength.
- Decrease pain and inflammation.

Range of Motion Exercises
- L-bar active-assisted exercises.
- External rotation at 45 degrees abducted to 45 degrees.
- Internal rotation at 45 degrees abducted to 45 degrees.
- Shoulder flexion-extension to tolerance.
- Shoulder abduction to tolerance.
- Shoulder horizontal abduction-adduction.
- Rope and pulley extension-flexion
  - All exercises performed to tolerance.
  - Take to point of pain or resistance or both and hold.
  - *Gentle* self-capsular stretches.

Gentle Joint Mobilization to Reestablish Normal Arthrokinematics to
- Scapulothoracic joint.
- GH joint.
- SC joint.

Strengthening Exercises
- Isometrics.
- May initiate tubing for external and internal rotation at 0 degrees of shoulder abduction.

Conditioning Program For
- Trunk.
- Lower extremities.
- Cardiovascular.

Decrease Pain and Inflammation
- Ice, NSAIDs, modalities.

Weeks 4–5
- Active-assisted ROM flexion to tolerance (approximately 145 degrees).
- Internal and external rotation at 90 degrees abduction to tolerance.
- Initiate isotonic (light weight) strengthening.
- Gentle joint mobilization (grade III).

Week 6
- Active-assisted ROM; continue all stretching exercises.
- Progress external and internal rotation at 90 degrees abduction.
- External and internal rotation at 90 degrees abduction: 75 degrees.
- Internal and external rotation at 90 degrees abduction: 75 degrees.
- Flexion to 165–170 degrees.
- Extension to 30 degrees.

Phase 2: Intermediate Phase (Weeks 7–12)

Goals
- Full nonpainful ROM at week 8.
- Normalize arthrokinematics.
- Increase strength.
- Improve neuromuscular control.

Rehabilitation Protocol
An Accelerated Rehabilitation Program after Anterior Capsular Shift–Acquired Instability in Overhead Athletes *(Continued)*
Wilk

Weeks 7–9

Range of Motion Exercises
- L-bar active-assisted exercises.
- Continue all exercises listed above.
- Gradually increase ROM to full ROM week 8
  - External rotation at 90 degrees abduction: 85–90 degrees.
  - Internal rotation at 90 degrees abduction: 70–75 degrees.
- Continue self-capsular stretches.
- Continue joint mobilization.

Strengthening Exercises
- Initiate isotonic dumbbell program
  - Side-lying external rotation
  - Side-lying internal rotation.
  - Shoulder abduction.
  - Supraspinatus.
  - Latissimus dorsi.
  - Rhomboids.
  - Biceps curls.
  - Triceps curls.
  - Shoulder shrugs.
  - Push-ups into chair (serratus anterior).
- Continue tubing at 0 degrees and at 90 degrees abduction for external and internal rotation.

Initiate Neuromuscular Control Exercises for Scapulothoracic Joint

Weeks 10–12
- Continue all exercises listed above.
- Initiate tubing exercises for rhomboids, latissimus dorsi, biceps, and triceps.
- Initiate aggressive stretching and joint mobilization, if needed.
- Progressive ROM for overhead thrower to functional ROM.

Phase 3: Dynamic Strengthening Phase (Weeks 12–20)

Advanced Strengthening Phase (weeks 13–16)

Criteria for Progression to Phase 3
- Full nonpainful ROM.
- No pain or tenderness.
- Strength 70% or better compared with contralateral side.
- Satisfactory shoulder joint stability.

Goals
- Improve strength, power, and endurance.
- Improve neuromuscular control.
- Maintain shoulder mobility.
- Prepare athlete to begin to throw.

Emphasis
- High-speed, high-energy strengthening exercises.
- Eccentric exercises.

- Diagonal patterns.
- Functional positions of stretches and strengthening.

Exercises
- Continue self-capsular stretches (very important).
- "Thrower's Ten" exercises (p. 165).
  - Tubing exercises in 90/90 position for internal and external rotation (slow set, fast sets).
  - Isotonics for
    - Rhomboids.
    - Latissimus dorsi.
    - Biceps.
    - Diagonal patterns D2 extension.
    - Diagonal patterns D2 flexion.
  - Continue dumbbell exercises for supraspinatus and deltoid.
  - Continue serratus anterior strengthening exercises, push-ups floor.
  - Continue all isotonic strengthening.
- Continue trunk–lower extremity strengthening exercises.
- Continue neuromuscular exercises.
- Initiate plyometric training program.

Weeks 17–20
- Initiate interval sport programs.
- Continue all exercises.
- Progress plyometrics for shoulder
  - External rotation at 90 degrees abduction.
  - Internal rotation at 90 degrees abduction.
  - D2 extension plyometrics.
  - Biceps plyometrics.
  - Serratus anterior plyometrics.

Phase 4: Throwing Phase (Weeks 20–26)

Criteria for Progression to Phase 4
- Full ROM.
- No pain or tenderness.
- Isokinetic test that fulfills criteria to throw.
- Satisfactory clinical examination.

Goals
- Progressively increase activities to prepare patient for full functional return.

Exercise
- Progress interval throwing program.
- Continue "Thrower's Ten" exercises.
- Continue plyometric five exercises.
- Continue all flexibility exercises.

Interval Throwing Program
- Interval throwing program phase 2, 22nd wk.

Return to Sports (Weeks 26–30)

Rehabilitation Protocol
Regular Rehabilitation after an Anterior Capsular Shift for General Orthopaedic Patients
Wilk

This rehabilitation program's goal is to return the patient/athlete to the activity/sport as quickly and safely as possible, while maintaining a stable shoulder. The program is based on muscle physiology, biomechanics, anatomy, and the healing process after surgery for a capsular shift.

The capsular shift procedure is one in which the orthopaedic surgeon makes an incision into the ligamentous capsule of the shoulder, pulls the capsule tighter, and then sutures the capsule together.

The ultimate goal is a functional shoulder and a pain-free return to presurgery functional level.

Compliance with the rehabilitation program is critical to the patient's ultimate outcome.

Note: This protocol progresses more slowly than that for the overhead athlete because of assumed inadequate capsular structures and relatively poor dynamic stabilizers.

Phase 1: Protection Phase (Weeks 0–6)
Goals
- Allow healing of sutured capsule.
- Begin early protected and restricted ROM.
- Retard muscular atrophy and enhance dynamic stability.
- Decrease pain and inflammation
  - Brace: patients with bidirectional instability are placed in sling for 4–6 wk.
  - Patients with multidirectional instability are placed in abduction brace for 4–6 wk. **Physician will make determination.**

Weeks 0–2
Precautions
- Sleep in immobilizer for 4 wk.
- No overhead activities for 6–8 wk.
- Compliance with rehabilitation program is critical.

Exercises
- Gripping exercises with putty.
- Elbow flexion-extension and pronation-supination.
- Pendulum exercises (nonweighted).
- Rope and pulley active-assisted exercises
  - Shoulder flexion to 90 degrees.
  - Shoulder elevation in scapular plane to 60 degrees.
- L-bar exercises
  - External rotation to 15 degrees with arm abducted at 30 degrees.
  - No shoulder abduction or extension.
- Active ROM cervical spine.
- Isometrics
  - Flexors, extensors, external and internal rotation, and abduction.

Criteria for Hospital Discharge
- Shoulder ROM (active-assisted ROM): flexion 90 degrees; abduction 45 degrees; external rotation 20 degrees.
- Minimal pain and swelling.
- "Good" proximal and distal muscle power.

Weeks 2–4
Goals
- Gradual increase in ROM.
- Normalize arthrokinematics.
- Improve strength.
- Decrease pain and inflammation.

Range of Motion Exercises
- L-bar active-assisted exercises, gentle passive ROM exercises
  - External rotation to 25–30 degrees in scapular plane.
  - Internal rotation to 30–35 degrees in scapular plane.
  - Shoulder flexion to 105–115 degrees.
  - Shoulder elevation in scapular plane to 115 degrees.
  - Rope and pulley flexion.
- All exercises performed to tolerance and therapist/physician motion guidelines.
- Take to point of pain or resistance or both and hold.
- *Gentle* self-capsular stretches.

Gentle Joint Mobilization to Reestablish Normal Arthrokinematics To
- Scapulothoracic joint.
- GH joint.
- SC joint.

Strengthening Exercises
- Isometrics.
- Rhythmic stabilization exercises.
- May initiate tubing for external and internal rotation at 0 degrees.

Conditioning Program For
- Trunk.
- Lower extremities.
- Cardiovascular.

Decrease Pain and Inflammation
- Ice, NSAIDs, modalities.

Weeks 4–6
- Continue all exercises listed above.
- Range of motion exercises
  - L-bar active-assisted exercises
    - External rotation at 45 degrees of shoulder abduction: 25–35 degrees.
    - Continue all others to tolerance (based on end feel).

Rehabilitation Protocol
Regular Rehabilitation after an Anterior Capsular Shift for General Orthopaedic Patients (Continued)
Wilk

- Continue stabilization exercises
  - PNF with rhythmic stabilization, neuromuscular exercises.

Phase 2: Intermediate Phase (Weeks 6–12)
Goals
- Full nonpainful ROM at weeks 10–12.
- Normalize arthrokinematics.
- Increase strength.
- Improve neuromuscular control.

Weeks 6–8
Range of Motion Exercises
- L-bar active-assisted exercises at 90 degrees abduction.
- Continue all exercises listed above.
- Gradually increase ROM to full ROM, week 12.
- Continue joint mobilization.
- May initiate internal and external rotation ROM at 90 degrees of abduction.

Strengthening Exercises
- Initiate isotonic dumbbell program
  - Side-lying external rotation.
  - Side-lying internal rotation.
  - Shoulder abduction.
  - Supraspinatus.
  - Latissimus dorsi.
  - Rhomboids.
  - Biceps curls.
  - Triceps curls.
  - Shoulder shrugs.
  - Push-ups into chair (serratus anterior).
- Continue tubing at 0 degrees for external and internal rotation.
- Continue stabilization exercises for GH joint.

Initiate Neuromuscular Control Exercises for SC Joint.
Weeks 8–10
- Continue all exercises listed above; emphasis on neuro-muscular control drills, PNF stabilization drills, and scapular strengthening.
- Initiate tubing exercises for rhomboids, latissimus dorsi, biceps, and triceps.
- Progress ROM to full ROM
  - External rotation at 90 degrees abduction: 80–85 degrees.
  - Internal rotation at 90 degrees abduction: 70–75 degrees.
  - Flexion to 165–170 degrees.

Phase 3: Dynamic Strengthening Phase (Weeks 12–20)—Advanced Strengthening Phase

Note: Aggressive strengthening or stretching program based on type of patient. Therapist and/or physician will determine.

Weeks 12–17
Criteria for Progression to Phase 3
- Full nonpainful ROM. **Patient must fulfill this criterion before progressing to this phase.**
- No pain or tenderness.
- Strength 70% or better compared with contralateral side.

Goals
- Improve strength, power, and endurance.
- Improve neuromuscular control.
- Prepare athletic patient for gradual return to sports.

Emphasis
- Dynamic stabilization exercises.
- Eccentric exercises.
- Diagonal patterns, functional movements.

Exercises
- Fundamental shoulder exercises
  - Emphasis: neuromuscular control drills, PNF rhythmic stabilization, rotator cuff strengthening, scapular strengthening.
- Continue tubing exercises for internal and external rotation at 0 degrees abduction (arm at side).
- Continue isotonics for
  - Rhomboids.
  - Latissimus dorsi.
  - Biceps.
  - Diagonal patterns D2 extension.
  - Diagonal patterns D2 flexion.
- Continue dumbbell exercises for supraspinatus and deltoid.
- Continue serratus anterior strengthening exercises, push-ups floor.
- Continue trunk and lower extremity strengthening exercises.
- Continue neuromuscular exercises.
- Continue self-capsular exercises.

Weeks 17–20
- Continue all exercises.
- Emphasis on gradual return to recreational activities.

Phase 4: Return to Activity (Weeks 20–28)

Criteria for Progression to Phase 4
- Full ROM.
- No pain or tenderness.
- Isokinetic test that fulfills criteria.
- Satisfactory clinical examination.

Goals
- Progressively increase activities to prepare patient for full functional return.

continued

Rehabilitation Protocol
Regular Rehabilitation after an Anterior Capsular Shift for General Orthopaedic Patients (Continued)
Wilk

Exercises
- Initiate interval sports programs (if patient is a recreational athlete).
- Continue tubing exercises as listed in phase 3.

- Continue all strengthening exercises.
- Continue ROM exercises.

Rehabilitation Protocol
After Thermal-Assisted Capsulorraphy for Atraumatic Congenital Instability
Wilk

Phase 1: Protection Phase (Weeks 0–8)

Goals
- Allow healing of tightened capsule.
- Begin early protected motion of the elbow, wrist, and hand.
- Decrease pain and inflammation.

Weeks 0–2

Precautions
- Sleep in immobilizer/sling for 14 days.
- No overhead activities for 12 wk.
- Avoid abduction, flexion, and external rotation.

Exercises
- Gripping exercises with putty.
- Elbow flexion-extension and pronation-supination.
- Active ROM cervical spine.
- After 10 days, active abduction may be allowed, but is not to exceed 90 degrees.

Weeks 3–4

Goals
- Gradual increase in ROM.
- Normalize arthrokinematics.
- Improve strength.
- Decrease pain and inflammation.

Range of Motion Exercises
- Active-assisted exercises (pulley and L-bar)
  - Forward flexion to 90 degrees.
  - Abduction to 90 degrees.
  - External rotation to 45 degrees at 0 degrees and 90 degrees of abduction.
  - Extension to 20 degrees.

Strengthening Exercises
- Isometrics initiated in all planes to tolerance.
- PREs to elbow and wrist.
- Scapular strengthening.

Conditioning Program For
- Trunk.
- Lower extremities.
- Cardiovascular.

Decrease Pain and Inflammation
- Ice, NSAIDs, modalities.

Weeks 4–6

Goal
- Gradual increase to full ROM.

Range of Motion Exercises
- L-bar active-assisted exercises
  - External rotation to tolerance at 0, 45, and 90 degrees of abduction.
  - Internal rotation to tolerance at 0, 45, and 90 degrees of abduction.

Strengthening Exercises
- Continue with exercises above.
- PNF.
- Scapular strengthening.
- Therapeutic tubing initiated.

Gentle Mobilization to Reestablish Normal Arthokinematics To
- Scapulothoracic joint.
- GH joint.
- SC joint.

Phase 2: Intermediate Phase (Weeks 6–12)

Goals
- Full nonpainful ROM at weeks 10–12.
- Normalize arthrokinematics.
- Increase strength.
- Improve neuromuscular control.

Rehabilitation Protocol
After Thermal-Assisted Capsulorraphy for Atraumatic Congenital Instability
(Continued)
Wilk

Weeks 6–8
Range of Motion Exercises
- L-bar active-assisted exercises at 90 degrees abduction.
- Initiate self-capsular stretches.
- Continue joint mobilization.
- Gradually increase to full ROM by week 12.

Strengthening Exercises
- Continue all exercises listed above.
- Initiate isotonic dumbbell and tubing program
  - Side-lying external rotation.
  - Side-lying internal rotation.
  - Shoulder abduction.
  - Supraspinatus.
  - Latissimus dorsi.
  - Rhomboids.
  - Biceps curl.
  - Triceps curl.
  - Shoulder shrugs.
  - Push-ups.
- Continue neuromuscular control exercises for scapulothoracic joint.

Weeks 8–12
- Continue with all exercises listed above.
- Continue with joint mobilizations and self-capsular stretches.

Phase 3: Dynamic Strengthening Phase (Weeks 12–20)—Advanced Strengthening Phase

Criteria for Progression to Phase 3
- Full nonpainful ROM.
- No pain or tenderness.
- Strength 70% or greater compared with contralateral side.

Goals
- Improve strength, power, and endurance.
- Improve neuromuscular control.
- Prepare the athlete to begin to throw.

Emphasis
- High-speed, high-energy strengthening exercises.
- Eccentric exercises.
- Diagonal patterns.

Exercises
- "Thrower's Ten" exercises (p. 165).
- Continue tubing exercises for external and internal rotation.
- Tubing for rhomboids.
- Tubing for latissimus dorsi.
- Tubing for biceps.
- Tubing for diagonal patterns D2 extension.
- Tubing for diagonal patterns D2 flexion.
- Continue dumbbell exercises for supraspinatus and deltoid.
- Continue serratus anterior strengthening exercises push-ups floor.
- Continue trunk and lower extremity strengthening exercises.
- Continue neuromuscular exercises.
- Continue self-capsular stretches.
- Gradual return to recreational activities.

Phase 4: Return to Activity (Weeks 20–28)

Criteria for Progression to Phase 4
- Full ROM.
- No pain or tenderness.
- Isokinetic test that fulfills criteria.
- Satisfactory clinical examination.

Goals
- Progressively increase activities to prepare patient for full functional return.

Exercises
- Initiate interval throwing program.
- Continue tubing exercises as listed in phase 3.
- Continue ROM exercises.

Initiate interval throwing program between weeks 22 and 28.

Rehabilitation Protocol
After Thermal-Assisted Anterior Capsulorrhaphy in Overhead Athletes
Wilk

Note: This procedure is designed to arthroscopically remove the capsular hypermobility seen in overhead athletes without the potential loss of motion after an open capsular shift.

Phase 1: Protection Phase (Day 1–Week 6)
Goals
- Allow soft tissue healing.
- Diminish pain and inflammation.

continued

Rehabilitation Protocol
After Thermal-Assisted Anterior Capsulorrhaphy in Overhead Athletes *(Continued)*
Wilk

- Initiate protected motion.
- Retard muscular atrophy.

Weeks 0–2
- Sling use for 7–10 days.
- Sleep in sling/brace for 7 days.

Exercises
- Hand-gripping exercises.
- Elbow and wrist ROM exercises.
- Active ROM cervical spine.
- Passive and active-assisted ROM exercises
  - Elevation to 75–90 degrees.
  - Internal rotation in scapular plane: 45 degrees by 2 wk.
  - External rotation in scapular plane: 25 degrees by 2 wk.
- Rope and pulley (flexion) active-assisted ROM.
- Cryotherapy to control pain.
- Submaximal isometrics.
- Rhythmic stabilization exercises at 7 days.
- Proprioception and neuromuscular control drills.

Weeks 3–4
Range of Motion Exercises (Active-Assisted ROM, Passive ROM, Active ROM)
- Elevation to 125–135 degrees.
- Internal rotation in scapular plane, full motion.
- External rotation in scapular plane: 45–50 degrees by week 4.
- At week 4, begin external and internal rotation at 90 degrees abduction.

Strengthening Exercises
- Initiate *light* isotonic program.
- External and internal rotation exercise tubing (0 degrees abduction).
- Continue dynamic stabilization drills.
- Scapular strengthening exercises.
- Biceps/triceps strengthening.
- PNF D2 flexion-extension manual resistance.

Pain Control
- Continue use of cryotherapy and modalities as needed.

Weeks 5–6
- Continue all exercises listed above.
- Progress ROM to
  - Elevation to 145–160 degrees by week 6.
  - External rotation at 90 degrees abduction: (75–80 degrees).
  - Internal rotation at 90 degrees abduction: (65–70 degrees).
- Initiate "Thrower's Ten" strengthening program.

Phase 2: Intermediate Phase (Weeks 7–12)
Goals
- Restore full ROM (week 7).
- Restore functional ROM (weeks 10–11).

- Normalize arthrokinematics.
- Improve dynamic stability, muscular strength.

Weeks 7–8
- Progress ROM to
  - Elevation to 180 degrees.
  - External rotation at 90 degrees abduction: 90–100 degrees by week 8.
  - Internal rotation at 90 degrees abduction: 70–75 degrees.
- Continue stretching program.
- Strengthening exercises
  - Continue "Thrower's Ten" program.
  - Continue manual resistance, dynamic stabilization drills.
  - Initiate plyometrics (two-handed drills).

Weeks 9–12
- Progress ROM to the overhead athlete's demands
  - Gradual progression from weeks 9 to 12.
- Strengthening exercises
  - Progress isotonic program.
  - May initiate more aggressive strengthening
    - Push-ups.
    - Shoulder press.
    - Bench-press.
    - Pull-downs.
    - Single-arm plyometrics.

Phase 3: Advanced Activity and Strengthening Phase (Weeks 13–20)
Criteria for Progression to Phase 3
- Full ROM.
- No pain or tenderness.
- Muscular strength 80% of contralateral side.

Goals
- Improve strength, power, and endurance.
- Enhance neuromuscular control.
- Functional activities.

Weeks 13–16
- Continue all stretching exercises
  - Self-capsular stretches, active ROM passive stretching.
- Continue all strengthening exercises
  - Isotonics.
  - Plyometrics.
  - Neuromuscular control, dynamic stabilization drills.
- Initiate interval sport program (throwing, tennis, swimming, etc.).

Weeks 16–20
- Progress all exercises listed above.
- May resume normal training program.

Rehabilitation Protocol
**After Thermal-Assisted Anterior Capsulorrhaphy in Overhead
Athletes** (Continued)
Wilk

- Continue specific strengthening exercises.
- Progress interval program (throwing program in phase 2).

Phase 4: Return to Activity Phase (Weeks 22–26)

Criteria for Progression to Phase 4
- Full functional ROM.
- No pain or tenderness.
- Satisfactory muscular strength (isokinetic test).
- Satisfactory clinical examination.

Goals
- Gradual return to unrestricted activities.
- Maintain static and dynamic stability of shoulder joint.

Exercises
- Continue maintenance for ROM.
- Continue strengthening exercises.
- Gradual return to competition.

Frozen Shoulder (Adhesive Capsulitis)

Codman introduced the term "frozen shoulder" in 1934 to describe patients who had a painful loss of shoulder motion with normal radiographic studies. In 1946, Neviaser named the condition "adhesive capsulitis" based on the radiographic appearance with arthrography, which suggested "adhesions" of the capsule of the GH joint limiting overall joint space volume. **Patients with adhesive capsulitis have a painful restriction of** *both* **active and passive GH joint motion in all planes, or a global loss of GH joint motion.**

This condition most commonly occurs in patients 40 to 60 years of age, with a higher incidence in females. The onset of an "idiopathic" frozen shoulder has been associated with extended immobilization, relatively mild trauma (e.g., strain or contusion), and surgical trauma, especially breast or chest wall procedures. Adhesive capsulitis is associated with medical conditions such as diabetes, hyperthyroidism, ischemic heart disease, inflammatory arthritis, and cervical spondylosis. **The most significant association is with insulin-dependent diabetes.** Bilateral disease occurs in approximately 10% of patients, but can be as high as 40% in patients with a history of insulin-dependent diabetes.

Adhesive capsulitis is classically characterized by three stages. The length of each stage is variable, but typically the first stage lasts for 3 to 6 months, the second stage from 3 to 18 months, and the final stage from 3 to 6 months.

The **first stage is the "freezing" phase,** characterized by the onset of an aching pain in the shoulder. The pain is usually more severe at night and with activities, and may be associated with a sense of discomfort that radiates down the arm. Often, a specific traumatic event is difficult for the patient to recall. As symptoms progress, there are fewer arm positions that are comfortable. Most patients will position the arm in adduction and internal rotation. This position represents the "neutral isometric

position of relaxed tension for the inflamed glenohumeral capsule, biceps, and rotator cuff." Unfortunately, many of these patients are initially treated with immobilization, which only worsens the "freezing" process.

The second stage is the progressive stiffness or "frozen" phase. Pain at rest usually diminishes during this stage, leaving the patient with a shoulder that has restricted motion in all planes. Activities of daily living become severely restricted. Patients complain about their inability to reach into the back pocket, fasten the bra, comb the hair, or wash the opposite shoulder. When performing these activities, a sharp, acute discomfort can occur as the patient reaches the restraint of the tight capsule. Pain at night is a common complaint and is not easily treated with medications or physical modalities. This stage can last from 3 to 18 months.

The final stage is the resolution or "thawing" phase. This stage is characterized by a slow recovery of motion. Aggressive treatment with physical therapy, closed manipulation, or surgical release may accelerate recovery, moving the patient from the frozen stage into the thawing phase, as long as ROM activities are practiced daily.

The **diagnosis of adhesive capsulitis** may be suggested by a careful history and physical examination. The history should focus on the onset and duration of symptoms, a description of any antecedent trauma, and any associated medical conditions. The findings on the physical examination vary depending on the stage at which the patient presents for treatment. **In general, a global loss of active** *and* **passive motion is present; the loss of external rotation with the arm at the patient's side is a hallmark of this condition. The loss of** *passive* **external rotation is the single most important finding on physical examination and helps to differentiate the diagnosis from a rotator cuff problem because problems of the rotator cuff generally do not result in a loss of** *passive* **external rotation.** The diagnosis of a frozen shoulder is confirmed when radiographic studies are normal. Posteri-

Table 3–6

Differential Diagnoses for Shoulder Stiffness

Extrinsic Causes

Neurologic

Parkinson's disease

Automatic dystrophy (RSD)

Intradural lesions

Neural compression

   Cervical disc disease

   Neurofibromata

Foraminal stenosis

Neurologic amyotrophy

Hemiplegia

Head trauma

Muscular

Poliomyositis

Cardiovascular

Myocardial infarction

Thoracic outlet syndrome

Cerebral hemorrhage

Infections

Chronic bronchitis

Pulmonary tuberculosis

Metabolic

Diabetes mellitus

Thyroid disease

Progressive systemic sclerosis

   (scleroderma)

Paget's disease

Inflammatory

Rheumatologic disorders

   (see Table 20–1)

Polymyalgia rheumatica

Trauma

Surgery

   Axillary node dissection,

   sternotomy, thoracotomy

Fractures

   Cervical spine, ribs, elbow,

   hand, etc.

Medications

Isoniazid, phenobarbitone

Congenital

Klippel-Feil

Sprengel's deformity

Glenoid dysplasia

Atresia

Contractures

   Pectoralis major

   Axillary fold

Behavioral

Depression

Hysterical paralysis

Referred Pain

Diaphragmatic irritation

Neoplastic

Pancoast tumor

Lung carcinoma

Metastatic disease

Intrinsic Causes

Bursitis

Subacromial

Calcific tendinitis

Snapping scapula

Biceps Tendon

Tenosynovitis

Partial or complete tears

SLAP lesions

Rotator Cuff

Impingement syndrome

Partial rotator cuff tears

Complete rotator cuff tears

Trauma

Fractures

   Glenoid

   Proximal humerus

Surgery

   Postoperative shoulder, breast,

   head, neck, chest

Gastrointestinal disorders

   Esophoglis

   Ulcers

   Cholecystitis

Instability—Glenohumeral

Recurrent dislocation anterior

and posterior

Chronic dislocation

Arthritides

Glenohumeral and

acromiaclavicular

   Osteoarthritis

   Rheumatoid

   Psoriatic

   Infectious

   Neuropathic

Miscellaneous

Avascular necrosis

Hemarthrasis

Osteochondromatosis

Suprascapular nerve palsy

RSD, reflex sympathetic dystrophy; SLAP, superior labrum from anterior to posterior.

From Rockwood CA, Matsen FA: The Shoulder. Philadelpha, WB Saunders, 1990.

---

orly dislocated shoulders also lack external rotation and abduction, but the axillary lateral x-ray reveals a dislocated humeral head. The differential diagnoses for shoulder stiffness are listed in Table 3–6. The physician should also be aware of possible underlying disorders that may have caused the adhesive capsulitis (e.g., a painful rotator cuff tear that caused the patient to stop using the arm).

Treatment

Even though adhesive capsulitis is believed to be a "self-limiting" process, it can be severely disabling for months to years and, as a result, requires aggressive treatment once the diagnosis is made. Initial treatment should include an aggressive physical therapy program to help regain shoulder motion. For patients in the initial painful or freezing phase, pain relief may be obtained with a course of anti-inflammatory medications, the judicious use of GH joint corticosteroid injections, or therapeutic modality treatments. Intra-articular corticosteroid injections may help to abort the abnormal inflammatory process often associated with this condition. The rehabilitation program for adhesive capsulitis is outlined on page 229. An algorithm for the treatment of shoulder stiffness is shown in Figure 3–71.

Operative intervention is indicated in patients who show no improvement after a 3-month course of aggressive management that includes medications, corticosteroid injection, and physical therapy. In patients who do not have a history of diabetes, our initial intervention is a manipulation under anesthesia followed by outpatient physical therapy as outlined on page 229. Patients with a history of diabetes in whom conservative management fails and patients who fail to regain shoulder motion after manipulation are treated with an arthroscopic surgical release followed by physical therapy.

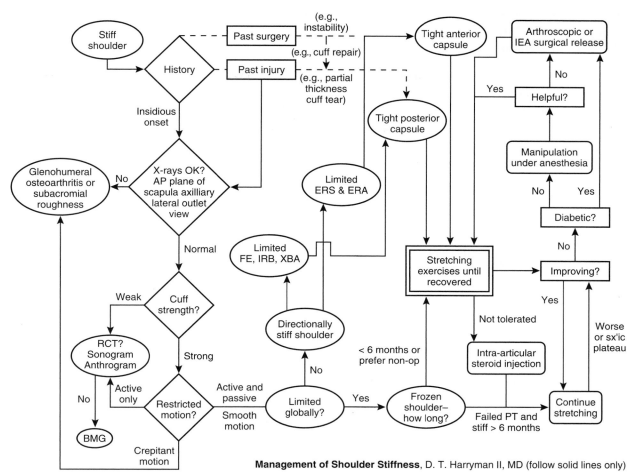

Figure 3–71. Treatment algorithm for patients with a stiff shoulder. AP, anterior-posterior; BMG, below medium grade; ERA, external rotation abduction; ERS, external rotation supine; FE, forward elevation; IRB, internal rotation back; PT, physical therapy; RCT, rotator cuff tissue; sx'ic, symptomatic; XBA, external rotation line on back. (From Rockwood CA Jr, Matsen FA III: The Shoulder, 2nd ed. Philadelphia, WB Saunders, 1988.)

Rehabilitation Protocol
Frozen Shoulder (Adhesive Capsulitis)
Bach, Cohen, and Romeo

Phase 1: Weeks 0–8

Goals
- Relieve pain.
- Restore motion.

Restrictions
- None.

Immobilization
- None.

Pain Control
- Reduction of pain and discomfort is essential for recovery
  - Medications
    - NSAIDs—first-line medications for pain control.
    - GH joint injection: corticosteroid/local anesthetic combination.
    - Oral steroid taper—for patients with refractive or symptomatic frozen shoulder (Pearsall and Speer, 1998)

continued

Rehabilitation Protocol
Frozen Shoulder (Adhesive Capsulitis) *(Continued)*
Bach, Cohen, and Romeo

- Because of potential side effects of oral steroids, patients must be thoroughly questioned about their past medical history.
- Therapeutic modalities
  - Ice, ultrasound, HVGS.
  - Moist heat before therapy, ice at end of session.

Motion: Shoulder
Goals
- Controlled, aggressive ROM exercises.
- Focus is on stretching at ROM limits.
- No restrictions on range, but therapist and patient have to communicate to avoid injuries.

Exercises
- Initially focus on forward flexion and external and internal rotation with the arm at the side, and the elbow at 90 degrees.
- Active ROM exercises.
- Active-assisted ROM exercises (see Fig. 3–34).
- Passive ROM exercises (see Fig. 3–35).
- A home exercise program should be instituted from the beginning
  - Patients should perform their ROM exercises three to five times per day.
  - A sustained stretch, of 15–30 sec, at the end ROMs should be part of all ROM routines.

Phase 2: Weeks 8–16
Criteria for Progression to Phase 2
- Improvement in shoulder discomfort.
- Improvement of shoulder motion.
- Satisfactory physical examination.

Goals
- Improve shoulder motion in all planes.
- Improve strength and endurance of rotator cuff and scapular stabilizers.

Pain Control
- Reduction of pain and discomfort is essential for recovery
  - Medications
    - NSAIDs—first-line medications for pain control.
    - GH joint injection: corticosteroid/local anesthetic combination.
    - Oral steroid taper—for patients with refractive or symptomatic frozen shoulder (Pearsall and Speer, 1998)
      - Because of potential side effects of oral steroids, patients must be thoroughly questioned about their past medical history.
  - Therapeutic modalities
    - Ice, ultrasound, HVGS.
    - Moist heat before therapy, ice at end of session.

Motion: Shoulder
Goals
- 140 degrees of forward flexion.
- 45 degrees of external rotation.
- Internal rotation to twelfth thoracic spinous process.

Exercises
- Active ROM exercises.
- Active-assisted ROM exercises (see Fig. 3–34).
- Passive ROM exercises (see Fig. 3–35).

Muscle Strengthening
- Rotator cuff strengthening—three times per week, 8 to 12 repetitions for three sets
  - Closed-chain isometric strengthening with the elbow flexed to 90 degrees and the arm at the side. (see Fig. 3–36)
    - Internal rotation.
    - External rotation.
    - Abduction.
    - Forward flexion.
  - Progress to open-chain strengthening with Therabands (see Fig. 3–39A)
    - Exercises performed with the elbow flexed to 90 degrees.
    - Starting position is with the shoulder in the neutral position of 0 degrees of forward flexion, abduction, and external rotation.
    - Exercises are performed through an arc of 45 degrees in each of the five planes of motion.
    - Six color-coded bands are available; each provides increasing resistance from 1 to 6 pounds, at increments of one pound.
    - Progression to the next band occurs usually in 2- to 3-wk intervals. Patients are instructed not to progress to the next band if there is any discomfort at the present level.
    - Theraband exercises permit concentric and eccentric strengthening of the shoulder muscles and are a form of isotonic exercises (characterized by variable speed and fixed resistance)
      - Internal rotation.
      - External rotation.
      - Abduction.
      - Forward flexion.
  - Progress to light isotonic dumbbell exercises
    - Internal rotation (see Fig. 3–39B).
    - External rotation (see Fig. 3–39C).
    - Abduction.
    - Forward flexion.
- Strengthening of scapular stabilizers
  - Closed-chain strengthening exercises (see Figs. 3–37, 3–59, and 3–68)
    - Scapular retraction (rhomboideus, middle trapezius).
    - Scapular protraction (serratus anterior).

Rehabilitation Protocol
Frozen Shoulder (Adhesive Capsulitis) *(Continued)*
Bach, Cohen, and Romeo

- Scapular depression (latissimus dorsi, trapezius, serratus anterior).
- Shoulder shrugs (trapezius, levator scapulae).
- Progress to open-chain strengthening (see Figs. 3–38 and 3–69).
- Deltoid strengthening (see Figs. 3–58 and 3–70).

Phase 3: Months 4 and Beyond

Criteria for Progression to Phase 4
- Significant functional recovery of shoulder motion
  - Successful participation in activities of daily living.
- Resolution of painful shoulder.
- Satisfactory physical examination.

Goals
- Home maintenance exercise program
  - ROM exercises two times a day.
  - Rotator cuff strengthening three times a week.
  - Scapular stabilizer strengthening three times a week.

Maximum improvement by 6–9 mo after initiation of treatment program.

Warning Signs
- Loss of motion.
- Continued pain.

Treatment of Complications
- These patients may need to move back to earlier routines.
- May require increased utilization of pain control modalities as outlined above.
- If loss of motion is persistent and pain continues, patients may require surgical intervention
  - Manipulation under anesthesia.
  - Arthroscopic release.

Rehabilitation after Shoulder Arthroplasty (Replacement)

Shoulder arthroplasty is one of the few surgical procedures involving the shoulder that require the patient to spend time in the hospital after surgery. As a result, a supervised rehabilitation program is started during the hospitalization on the first day after surgery to begin mobilization of the reconstructed shoulder joint. Rehabilitation after shoulder arthroplasty follows the normal sequence of allowing time for tissue healing, joint mobilization, and finally, muscle strengthening and function.

The ability to begin the rehabilitation process so soon after surgery is the direct result of improvements in the surgical approach to the GH joint. Earlier approaches required release of the deltoid origin to expose the shoulder for prosthetic replacement. This necessitated a more conservative, delayed rehabilitation program to avoid postoperative detachment of the deltoid repair. At present, the only muscle violated during the surgical exposure is the subscapularis muscle, and the rehabilitation protocol must be mindful of the time required for the subscapularis tendon to heal. **The amount of external rotation and active internal rotation that the patient can perform in the first 4 to 6 weeks is limited to motion parameters that can be achieved at the time of surgery.** The goal of rehabilitation is to establish a range of motion that will allow a functional recovery.

Long-term function and rehabilitation progression are affected by the presence or absence of good functional rotator cuff tissue (RTC). Postoperative rehabilitation protocols often are divided into RTC-deficient and RTC-intact groups.

Rehabilitation Protocol
After Shoulder Arthroplasty
Bach, Cohen, and Romeo

Phase 1: Weeks 0–6

Restrictions
- Shoulder motion
  - Week 1
    - 120 degrees of forward flexion.

- 20 degrees of external rotation with the arm at the side.
- 75 degrees of abduction with 0 degrees of rotation.

continued

Rehabilitation Protocol
After Shoulder Arthroplasty *(Continued)*
Bach, Cohen, and Romeo

- Week 2
  - 140 degrees of forward flexion.
  - 40 degrees of external rotation with the arm at the side.
  - 75 degrees of abduction with 0 degrees of rotation.
- No active internal rotation.
- No backward extension.

Immobilization
- Sling
  - After 7–10 days, sling used for comfort only.

Pain Control
- Reduction of pain and discomfort is essential for recovery
  - Medications
    - Narcotics—for 7–10 days following surgery.
    - NSAIDs—for patients with persistent discomfort following surgery.
  - Therapeutic modalities
    - Ice, ultrasound, HVGS.
    - Moist heat before therapy, ice at end of session.

Motion: Shoulder
- Goals
  - 140 degrees of forward flexion.
  - 40 degrees of external rotation.
  - 75 degrees of abduction.
- Exercises
  - Begin with Codman pendulum exercises to promote early motion.
  - Passive ROM exercises (see Fig. 3–35).
  - Capsular stretching for anterior, posterior, and inferior capsule, by using the opposite arm to assist with motion (see Fig. 3–49).
  - Active-assisted motion exercises (see Fig. 3–34)
    - Shoulder flexion.
    - Shoulder extension.
    - Internal and external rotation.
  - Progress to active ROM exercises.

Motion: Elbow
- Passive—progress to active
  - 0 to 130 degrees.
  - Pronation and supination as tolerated.

Muscle Strengthening
- Grip strengthening only.

Phase 2: Weeks 6–12
Criteria for Progression to Phase 2
- Minimal pain and tenderness.
- Nearly complete motion.
- Intact subscapularis without evidence of tendon pain on resisted internal rotation.

Restrictions
- Increase ROM goals
  - 160 degrees of forward flexion.
  - 60 degrees of external rotation with the arm at the side.
  - 90 degrees of abduction with 40 degrees of internal and external rotation.

Immobilization
- None.

Pain Control
- NSAIDs—for patients with persistent discomfort following surgery.
- Therapeutic modalities
  - Ice, ultrasound, HVGS.
  - Moist heat before therapy, ice at end of session.

Motion: Shoulder
- Goals
  - 160 degrees of forward flexion.
  - 60 degrees of external rotation with the arm at the side.
  - 90 degrees of abduction with 40 degrees of internal and external rotation.
- Exercises
  - Increase active ROM in all directions.
  - Focus on passive stretching at end ranges to maintain shoulder flexibility (see Fig. 3–35).
  - Utilize joint mobilization techniques for capsular restrictions, especially the posterior capsule (see Fig. 3–48).

Muscle Strengthening
- Rotator cuff strengthening: Only three times per week to avoid rotator cuff tendinitis, which will occur with overtraining
  - Begin with closed-chain isometric strengthening (see Fig. 3–36)
    - External rotation.
    - Abduction.
  - Progress to open-chain strengthening with Therabands (see Fig. 3–39A)
    - Exercises performed with the elbow flexed to 90 degrees.
    - Starting position is with the shoulder in the neutral position of 0 degrees of forward flexion, abduction, and external rotation.
    - Exercises are performed through an arc of 45 degrees in each of the five planes of motion.
    - Six color-coded bands are available; each provides increasing resistance from 1 to 6 pounds, at increments of one pound.
    - Progression to the next band occurs usually in 2- to 3-week intervals. Patients are instructed not to progress to the next band if there is any discomfort at the present level.

Rehabilitation Protocol
After Shoulder Arthroplasty (Continued)
Bach, Cohen, and Romeo

- Theraband exercises permit concentric and eccentric strengthening of the shoulder muscles and are a form of isotonic exercises (characterized by variable speed and fixed resistance)
  - External rotation.
  - Abduction.
  - Forward flexion.
  - Progress to light isotonic dumbbell exercises
    - External rotation (see Fig. 3–39C).
    - Abduction.
    - Forward flexion.
- Scapular stabilizer strengthening
  - Closed-chain strengthening exercises (see Figs. 3–37, 3–59, and 3–68)
    - Scapular retraction (rhomboideus, middle trapezius).
    - Scapular protraction (serratus anterior).
    - Scapular depression (latissimus dorsi, trapezius, serratus anterior).
    - Shoulder shrugs (trapezius, levator scapulae).

Phase 3: Months 3–12
Criteria for Progression to Phase 3
- Full painless ROM.
- Satisfactory physical examination.

Goals
- Improve shoulder strength, power, and endurance.
- Improve neuromuscular control and shoulder proprioception.
- Prepare for gradual return to functional activities.
- Home maintenance exercise program
  - ROM exercises two times a day.
  - Rotator cuff strengthening three times a week.
  - Scapular stabilizer strengthening three times a week.

Motion
- Achieve motion equal to contralateral side.
- Utilize both active and passive ROM exercises to maintain motion.

Muscle Strengthening
- Shoulder
  - Begin internal rotation and extension strengthening
    - First closed-chain isometric strengthening and advance to Theraband and light weight isotonic strengthening.
- Scapular stabilizers
  - Progress to open- and closed-chain strengthening (see Figs. 3–38, 3–59, and 3–69).
- Deltoid strengthening (see Figs. 3–58 and 3–70).
- Eight to 12 repetitions for each exercise, for three sets.
- Strengthening only three times per week to avoid rotator cuff tendinitis.

Functional Strengthening
- Plyometric exercises (see Fig. 3–40).

Maximum improvement by 12–18 mo.

Warning Signs
- Loss of motion.
- Continued pain.

Treatment of Complications
- **These patients may need to move back to earlier routines.**
- **May require increased use of pain control modalities as outlined above.**

Rehabilitation Protocol
After Total Shoulder Arthroplasty (in a Rotator Cuff Tissue–Deficient Group)
Wilk

The goal of the rehabilitation process is to provide greater joint stability to the patient, while decreasing pain and improving functional status. The goal of the tissue-deficient group (bone loss, muscle loss) is joint stability and less joint mobility. The key to the success of the rehabilitation following shoulder replacement is compliance to your exercise program.

Phase 1: Immediate Motion Phase (Weeks 0–4)
Goals
- Increase passive ROM.
- Decrease shoulder pain.
- Retard muscular atrophy.

continued

Rehabilitation Protocol
After Total Shoulder Arthroplasty (in a Rotator Cuff Tissue–Deficient Group) *(Continued)*
Wilk

Exercises
- Continuous passive motion.
- Passive ROM
  - Flexion 0–90 degrees.
  - External rotation at 30 degrees abduction: 0–20 degrees.
  - Internal rotation at 30 degrees abduction: 0–30 degrees.
- Pendulum exercises.
- Elbow and Wrist ROM.
- Gripping exercises.
- Isometrics
  - Abductors.
  - External and internal rotation.
- Ropes and pulley (second week).
- Active-assisted motion exercises (when able).

Phase 2: Active Motion Phase (Weeks 5–8)
Goals
- Improve shoulder strength.
- Improve ROM.
- Decrease pain and inflammation.
- Increase functional activities.

Exercises
- Active-assisted ROM exercises with L-bar (begin weeks 2–3, or when tolerable)
  - Flexion.
  - External rotation.
  - Internal rotation.
- Rope and pulley
  - Flexion.
- Pendulum exercises.
- Active ROM exercises
  - Seated flexion (short arc 45–90 degrees).
  - Supine flexion (full available range).
- Seated abduction 0–90 degrees.
- Exercise tubing internal and external rotation (weeks 4–6).
- Dumbbell biceps and triceps.
- Gentle joint mobilization (weeks 6–8).

Phase 3: Strengthening Phase (Weeks 8–12)
Criteria for Progression to Phase 3
- Passive ROM: flexion 0–120 degrees.
  - External rotation at 90 degrees abduction: 30–40 degrees.
  - Internal rotation at 90 degrees abduction: 45–55 degrees.
- Strength level $^4/_5$ for external and internal rotation and abduction.
- *Note:* Some patients will never enter this phase.

Goals
- Improve strength of shoulder musculature.
- Improve and gradually increase functional activities.

Exercises
- Exercise tubing
  - External rotation.
  - Internal rotation.
- Dumbbell strengthening
  - Abduction.
  - Supraspinatus.
  - Flexion.
- Stretching exercise.
- L-bar stretches
  - Flexion.
  - External rotation.
  - Internal rotation.

Biceps Tendon Disorders

Important Rehabilitation Points
- **The long head of the biceps functions as a secondary humeral head depressor and stabilizer.**
- In many overhead sports, the biceps aids acceleration and deceleration of the arm.
- Bicipital problems in athletes usually occur in conjunction with other shoulder disorders (rotator cuff pathology, GH joint instability).
- For this reason, a thorough evaluation of the remainder of the shoulder should be done if a biceps disorder is found (e.g., biceps tendinitis).
- As the long head of the biceps tendon courses from its attachment to the superior glenoid labrum, it exits the GH joint and proceeds through the rotator cuff interval beneath the coracohumeral ligament. It then enters the bicipital groove where it is restrained by the transverse humeral ligament (Fig. 3–72).

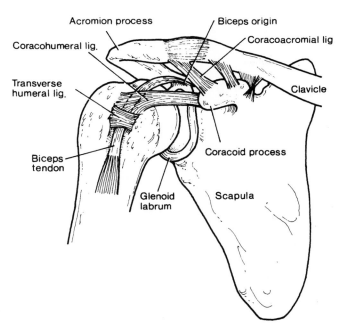

Figure 3–72. Anterior aspect of the right shoulder showing the tendon of the long head of the biceps muscle and its relationships. (From Andrews JR, Zarins B, Wilk KE: Injuries in Baseball. Philadelphia, Lippincott-Raven, 1997, p. 112.)

- Synder (1990) introduced the term **"SLAP lesion"** to characterize injuries to the superior labrum at the biceps origin. There are four patterns of injury in this classification system (Table 3–7). The SLAP eponym came from the lesions beginning posterior to the biceps anchor and extending anteriorly (superior labrum from anterior to posterior lesion or **SLAP** lesion).
- See Figure 3–73 for intraoperative (arthroscopic appearance) of SLAP lesions.
- The most common complaints with SLAP lesions are catching, popping, locking, or grinding of

Table 3-7

Classification of Superior Labrum from Anterior to Posterior (SLAP) Lesions

Type	Characteristics
Type 1 SLAP	Degenerative fraying of the superior labrum but the biceps attachment to the labrum is intact. The biceps anchor is intact (see Fig. 3–73A).
Type 2 SLAP	The biceps anchor has pulled away from the glenoid attachment (see Fig. 3–73B).
Type 3 SLAP	Involve a bucket-handle tear of the superior labrum with an intact biceps anchor (see Fig. 3–73C).
Type 4 SLAP	Similar to type 3 tears but the tear also extends into the biceps tendon (see Fig. 3–73D). The torn biceps tendon and labrum are displaced into the joint.
Complex SLAP	A combination of two or more SLAP types, usually 2 and 3 or 2 and 4.

the shoulder. This typically occurs with overhead activities.
- Traction and compression are the most common injuries that lead to SLAP lesions. A sudden pull occurs in many instances, such as grabbing an object in an attempt to avoid a fall.
- The diagnostic examinations for SLAP lesions are reviewed on page 134 (e.g., Speed test, Yergason test).

Operative Treatment—SLAP Lesions

- Concomitant GH joint pathology must also be treated.
- **Type 1 lesion**—The superior labrum is débrided back to a stable rim with a motorized shaver to prevent subsequent mechanical catching.
- **Type 2 lesion**—The lesion is repaired with staples, tacks, or various suture anchors.
- **Type 3 lesions,** with a bucket-handle tear, are carefully probed to ensure a stable biceps anchor and remaining labrum. The torn fragment is then resected, leaving a smooth transition zone.
- **Type 4 lesions**—Treatment is based on the extent of tearing in the biceps tendon. If the torn segment composes less than 30% of the tendon, then the detached labral and biceps tissue can be resected. If more than 30% is involved then
  - *In an older patient* with biceps pain, the labrum is débrided and tenodesis of the biceps is done.
  - *In a younger patient,* the tendon is preserved (arthroscopic suture repair).

Rehabilitation Considerations

- Types 2 and 4 repairs have a more conservative rehabilitation regimen. A sling is used for 3 weeks with elbow, wrist, and hand exercises.
- Pendulum exercises are begun after 1 week.
- External rotation beyond neutral and extension of the arm behind the body with the elbows extended are **avoided** for at least 4 weeks.
- Protected biceps strengthening is begun, but no stressful biceps activity is allowed for 3 months.

Biceps Rupture (Complete Long Head Tears)

- Treatment of complete long head tears is individualized.
- Most patients who are willing to accept the cosmetic deformity ("Popeye" arm) and minimal functional deficit are treated nonoperatively.
- Young, athletic individuals who perform tasks or lifting that requires supination strength may be offered a biceps tenodesis and arthroscopic subacromial decompression.

Figure 3–73. SLAP lesions. *A,* Type 1. *B,* Type 2. *C,* Type 3. *D,* Type 4. (*A–D,* From Warren RR, Craig EV, Altchek DW: The Unstable Shoulder. Philadelphia, Lippincott-Raven, 1999.)

Rehabilitation Protocol
After Arthrosopic Repair of Type 2 SLAP Lesions
Wilk

Phase 1: Immediate Postoperative Phase— "Restrictive Motion" (Day 1–Week 6)

Goals
- Protect the anatomic repair.
- Prevent negative effects of immobilization.

- Promote dynamic stability.
- Diminish pain and inflammation.

Weeks 0–2
- Sling for 4 wk.
- Sleep in immobilizer for 4 wk.

Rehabilitation Protocol
After Arthrosopic Repair of Type 2 SLAP Lesions *(Continued)*
Wilk

- Elbow and hand ROM.
- Hand-gripping exercises.
- Passive and gentle active-assisted ROM exercise
  - Flexion to 60 degrees (week 2: flexion to 75 degrees).
  - Elevation in scapular plane to 60 degrees.
  - External and internal rotation with arm in scapular plane.
  - External rotation to 10–15 degrees.
  - Internal rotation to 45 degrees.
  - *Note:* **No active external rotation or extension or abduction.**
- Submaximal isometrics for shoulder musculature.
- **NO isolated biceps contractions.**
- Cryotherapy, modalities as indicated.

Weeks 3–4
- Discontinue use of sling at 4 wk.
- Sleep in immobilizer until week 4.
- Continue gentle ROM exercises (passive ROM and active-assisted ROM)
  - Flexion to 90 degrees.
  - Abduction to 75–85 degrees.
  - External rotation in scapular plane to 25–30 degrees.
  - Internal rotation in scapular plane to 55–60 degrees.
  - *Note:* **Rate of progression based on evaluation of the patient.**
- No active external rotation, extension, or elevation.
- Initiate rhythmic stabilization drills.
- Initiate proprioception training.
- Tubing external and internal rotation at 0 degrees abduction.
- Continue isometrics.
- Continue use of cryotherapy.

Weeks 5–6
- Gradually improve ROM.
  - Flexion to 145 degrees.
  - External rotation at 45 degrees abduction: 45–50 degrees.
  - Internal rotation at 45 degrees abduction: 55–60 degrees.
- May initiate stretching exercises.
- May initiate light (easy) ROM at 90 degrees abduction.
- Continue tubing external and internal rotation (arm at side).
- PNF manual resistance.
- Initiate active shoulder abduction (without resistance).
- Initiate full can exercise (weight of arm).
- Initiate prone rowing, prone horizontal abduction.
- NO biceps strengthening.

Phase 2: Intermediate Phase—Moderate Protection Phase (Weeks 7–14)
Goals
- Gradually restore full ROM (week 10).
- Preserve the integrity of the surgical repair.
- Restore muscular strength and balance.

Weeks 7–9
- Gradually progress ROM
  - Flexion to 180 degrees.
  - External rotation at 90 degrees abduction: 90–95 degrees.
  - Internal rotation at 90 degrees abduction: 70–75 degrees.
- Continue to progress isotonic strengthening program.
- Continue PNF strengthening.
- Initiate "Thrower's Ten" program.

Weeks 10–12
- May initiate slightly more aggressive strengthening.
- Progress external rotation to thrower's motion
  - External rotation at 90 degrees abduction: 110–115 in throwers (weeks 10–12).
- Progress isotonic strengthening exercises.
- Continue all stretching exercises. **Progress ROM to functional demands (i.e., overhead athlete).**
- Continue all strengthening exercises.

Phase 3: Minimal Protection Phase (Weeks 14–20)
Criteria for Progression to Phase 3
- Full nonpainful ROM.
- Satisfactory stability.
- Muscular strength (good grade or better).
- No pain or tenderness.

Goals
- Establish and maintain full ROM.
- Improve muscular strength, power, and endurance.
- Gradually initiate functional activities.

Weeks 14–16
- Continue all stretching exercises (capsular stretches).
- Maintain thrower's motion (especially external rotation).
- Continue strengthening exercises
  - "Thrower's Ten" program or fundamental exercises.
  - PNF manual resistance.
  - Endurance training.
  - Initiate light plyometric program.
  - Restricted sport activities (light swimming, half golf swings).

Weeks 16–20
- Continue all exercises listed above.
- Continue all stretching.
- Continue "Thrower's Ten" program.

continued

Rehabilitation Protocol
After Arthrosopic Repair of Type 2 SLAP Lesions (Continued)
Wilk

- Continue plyometric program.
- Initiate interval sport program (e.g., throwing). **See interval throwing program.**

Phase 4: Advanced Strengthening Phase (Weeks 20–26)

Criteria for Progression to Phase 4
- Full nonpainful ROM.
- Satisfactory static stability.
- Muscular strength 75–80% of contralateral side.
- No pain or tenderness.

Goals
- Enhanced muscular strength, power, and endurance.
- Progress functional activities.
- Maintain shoulder mobility.

Weeks 20–26
- Continue flexibility exercises.
- Continue isotonic strengthening program.

- PNF manual resistance patterns.
- Plyometric strengthening.
- Progress interval sport programs.

Phase 5: Return to Activity Phase (Months 6–9)

Criteria for Progression to Phase 5
- Full functional ROM.
- Muscular performance isokinetic (fulfills criteria).
- Satisfactory shoulder stability.
- No pain or tenderness.

Goals
- Gradual return to sport activities.
- Maintain strength, mobility, and stability.

Exercises
- Gradually progress sport activities to unrestrictive participation.
- Continue stretching and strengthening program.

Rehabilitation Protocol
After Arthroscopic Débridement of Type 1 or 3 SLAP Lesion and/or Partial Rotator Cuff Débridement (Not a Rotator Cuff Repair)
Wilk

This rehabilitation program's goal is to return the patient/athlete to activity/sport as quickly and safely as possible.

This program is based on muscle physiology, biomechanics, anatomy, and healing response.

Phase 1: Motion Phase (Days 1–10)

Goals
- Reestablish nonpainful ROM.
- Retard muscular atrophy.
- Decrease pain and inflammation.

Range of Motion
- Pendulum exercise.
- Rope and pulley.
- L-bar exercises
  - Flexion-extension.
  - Abduction-adduction.
  - External and internal rotation (begin at 0 degrees abduction progress to 45 degrees abduction, then 90 degrees abduction).
- Self-stretches (capsular stretches).

Exercises
- Isometrics *Note:* **No Biceps** isometrics for 5–7 days postoperative.

- May initiate tubing for external and internal rotation at 0 degrees abduction late phase (usually 7–10 days postoperative).

Decrease Pain and Inflammation
- Ice, NSAIDs, modalities.

Phase 2: Intermediate Phase (Weeks 2–4)

Criteria for Progression to Phase 2
- Full ROM.
- Minimal pain and tenderness.
- "Good" MMT of internal and external rotation and flexion.

Goals
- Regain and improve muscular strength.
- Normalize arthokinematics.
- Improve neuromuscular control of shoulder complex.

Week 2
Exercises
- Initiate isotonic program with dumbbells
  - Shoulder musculature.
  - Scapulothoracic.
  - Tubing external and internal rotation at 0 degrees abduction.

Rehabilitation Protocol
After Arthroscopic Débridement of Type 1 or 3 SLAP Lesion and/or Partial Rotator Cuff Débridement (Not a Rotator Cuff Repair) *(Continued)*
Wilk

- Side-lying external rotation.
- Prone rowing external rotation.
- PNF manual resistance with dynamic stabilization.
- Normalize arthrokinematics of shoulder complex
  - Joint mobilization.
  - Continue stretching of shoulder (external and internal rotation at 90 degrees abduction).
- Initiate neuromuscular control exercises.
- Initiate proprioception training.
- Initiate trunk exercises.
- Initiate upper extremity endurance exercises.

Decrease Pain and Inflammation
- Continue use of modalities, ice, as needed.

Week 3

Exercises
- "Thrower's Ten" program.
- Emphasis rotator cuff and scapular strengthening.
- Dynamic stabilization drills.

Phase 3: Dynamic Strengthening Phase— Advanced Strengthening Phase (Weeks 5–6)

Criteria for Progression to Phase 3
- Full nonpainful ROM.
- No pain or tenderness.
- Strength 70% compared with contralateral side.

Goals
- Improve strength, power, and endurance.
- Improve neuromuscular control.
- Prepare athlete to begin to throw, etc.

Exercises
- Continue "Thrower's Ten" program.
- Continue dumbbell strengthening (supraspinatus, deltoid).

- Initiate tubing exercises in the 90/90 position for external and internal rotation (slow/fast sets).
- Exercises for scapulothoracic musculature.
- Tubing exercises for biceps.
- Initiate plyometrics (two-hand drills progress to one-hand drills).
- Diagonal patterns (PNF).
- Initiate isokinetic strengthening.
- Continue endurance exercises: neuromuscular control exercises.
- Continue proprioception exercises.

Phase 4: Return to Activity Phase (Week 7 And Beyond)

Criteria for Progression to Phase 4
- Full ROM.
- No pain or tenderness.
- Isokinetic test that fulfills criteria to throw.
- Satisfactory clinical examination.

Goal
- Progressively increase activities to prepare patient for full functional return.

Exercises
- Initiate interval sport program (e.g., throwing, tennis).
- Continue all exercises as in phase 3 (throw and train on same day), (lower extremity and ROM on opposite days).
- Progress interval program.

Follow-up Visits
- Isokinetic tests.
- Clinical examination.

Rehabilitation Protocol
After Proximal Biceps Tendon Repair (Complete Rupture of Long Head of the Biceps)
Wilk

- Shoulder brace/immobilizer for 4 wk.
- Pendulums.
- Active-assisted ROM elbow 0–145 degrees with gentle ROM into extension.
- Shoulder isometrics for 10–14 days.
- Shoulder active-assisted ROM L-bar external and internal rotation in scapular plane.
- Shoulder passive ROM: flexion, external and internal rotation.

4 Weeks
- Light shoulder PREs.

8 Weeks
- Progress to isotonic program
  - Bench press.
  - Shoulder press.

Rehabilitation Protocol
After Distal Biceps Tendon Repair (at the Elbow)
Wilk

Immobilization

- Posterior splint, elbow immobilization at 90 degrees for 5–7 days.

Brace

- Elbow placed in hinged ROM brace at 5–7 days postoperative. ROM set 45 degrees to full flexion.
- Gradually increase elbow ROM in brace.

Range of Motion Progression

Week 2	45 degrees to full elbow flexion.
Week 3	45 degrees to full flexion.
Week 4	30 degrees to full elbow flexion.
Week 5	20 degrees to full elbow flexion.
Week 6	10 degrees to full elbow flexion; full supination-pronation.
Week 8	Full ROM of elbow; full supination-pronation.

Range of Motion Exercises

Weeks 2–3	Passive ROM for elbow flexion and supination; active-assisted ROM for elbow extension and pronation.
Weeks 3–4	Initiate active-assisted ROM elbow flexion.
Week 4	Active ROM elbow flexion.

Strengthening Program

Week 1	Isometrics for triceps and shoulder muscles.
Week 2	Isometrics (submaximal biceps curls).
Week 3–4	Active ROM, no resistance applied.
Week 8	PRE program is initiated for elbow flexion and supination-pronation.

- Begin with one pound and gradually increase.
- Program shoulder strengthening program
  - Weeks 12–14: May initiate light weight training such as bench press and shoulder press.

Interval training programs for return to throwing, tennis, golf after shoulder injury. Please see sections for all interval throwing programs.

Acromioclavicular Joint Injury

Rehabilitation Rationale

Anatomy

The acromioclavicular (AC) joint is a diarthrodial joint with a fibrocartilaginous intra-articular disc. Two significant ligamentous structures are associated with the joint: the AC ligaments, which provide horizontal stability (Fig. 3–74), and the coracoclavicular ligaments, which are the main supensory ligament of the upper extremity, providing vertical stability to the joint.

Recent studies show that only 5 to 8 degrees of motion of the AC joint is possible in any plane.

The most common mechanism of injury of the AC joint is a direct force from a fall on the point of the shoulder (Fig. 3–75).

Rockwood (1990) classifies AC joint injuries into six types (Fig. 3–76).

- Type I
  - Mild sprain of the AC ligament.
  - No disruption of AC or coracoclavicular ligaments.
- Type II
  - Disruption of AC joint.
  - AC joint wider because of disruption (<4 mm or 40% difference).
  - Sprained but *intact* coracoclavicular ligaments with coracoclavicular space essentially the same as the normal shoulder on radiographs.
  - Downward force (weight) may disrupt AC ligament, but *not* the coracoacromial ligament.
- Type III
  - Coracoclavicular and AC ligaments disrupted.
  - Shoulder complex displaced inferiorly.
  - Coracoclavicular interspace 25 to 100% greater than in normal shoulder, or 4 mm distance (especially with weights applied).
- Type IV
  - Clavicle is displaced posteriorly through fibers of trapezius.
  - AC ligament and coracoclavicular ligaments disrupted.
  - Deltoid and trapezius muscles detached from distal clavicle.

Figure 3–74. Anatomic diagram of a normal AC joint shows the AC and coracoclavicular (CC) ligaments that are often injured when an athlete sustains an AC injury. (From Bach BR, Van Fleet TA, Novak PJ: Acromioclavicular injuries: controversies in treatment. Physician Sports Med 20[12]: 87–95, 1992.)

Figure 3–75. The most common mechanism of AC joint injury is a direct force that occurs from a fall on the point of the shoulder.

Figure 3–76. Diagnosis of AC joint injuries includes classification according to extent of ligament damage. Type I sprains involve a partial disruption of the AC ligament and capsule; type II sprains entail a ruptured AC ligament and capsule with incomplete injury to the coracoclavicular (CC) ligament; type III separations exhibit complete tearing of the AC and CC ligaments; type IV injuries involve clavicular displacement posteriorly into or through the trapezius muscles; type V injuries are severe type III injuries with a greater CC interval; and type VI injuries entail displacement of the clavicle inferior to the coracoid process. (From Bach BR, Van Fleet TA, Novak PJ: Acromioclavicular injuries: controversies in treatment. Physician Sports Med 20[12]:87–95, 1992.)

- Type V
  - Vertical separation of clavicle is greatly separated from scapula over a type III injury (100 to 300% more than normal shoulder).
- Type VI
  - Clavicle is dislocated inferiorly under the coracoid process.

Types I and II injuries are treated conservatively, as are type III injuries in nonactive, nonlaboring patients. Most types IV, V, and VI injuries require open reduction and internal fixation, as do type III injuries in more active individuals.

Rehabilitation Protocol
Acromioclavicular Joint Injuries
Rockwood and Matsen

Type 1 Injury

Day 1
- Apply ice to shoulder for 24–48 hr.
- Fit sling for comfort up to 7 days.
- Perform active ROM for fingers, wrist, elbow every 3–4 hr.
- Gently maintain normal ROM with rest in sling as needed.
- Begin pendulum exercises on day 2 or 3.

Days 7–10
- Symptoms typically subside.
- Discontinue sling.
- Do not permit any heavy lifting, stresses, or contact sports until full painless ROM and no point tenderness over AC joint (usually at 2 wk).

Type 2 Injury

Day 1
- Apply ice for 24–48 hr.
- Fit sling for comfort for 1–2 wk.

Day 7
- Begin gentle ROM exercises of shoulder and allow use of arm for dressing, eating, and activities of daily living.

- Discard sling at 7–14 days.
- Do not permit any heavy lifting, pushing, pulling, or contact sports for at least 6 wk.

Type 3 Injury

Nonoperative treatment indicated for inactive and nonlaboring patients.

Day 1
- Discuss "bump" remaining on shoulder, natural history, surgical risks, and recurrence.
- Apply ice for 24 hr.
- Prescribe mild analgesics for several days.
- Place in a sling.
- Begin performing activities of daily living at 3–4 days.
- Slowly progress to functional ROM with gentle passive ROM exercises at about 7 days.
- Patient typically has full ROM at 2–3 wk with gentle ROM exercises.

Rehabilitation Protocol
After Acromioclavicular Joint Stabilization Using Biodegradable Material
Wilk

Phase 1: Motion Phase (Weeks 0–2)

Goals
- Reestablish full nonpainful ROM.
- Retard muscular atrophy.
- Decrease pain and inflammation.

Range of Motion Exercises
- T-bar active-assisted ROM exercises
  - Flexion to tolerance.
  - External and internal rotation (begin at 0 degrees abduction, progress to 45 degrees abduction, then to 90 degrees abduction).
- Rope and pulley flexion.

- Pendulum exercises.
- Self-capsular stretches.

Note: **Restrict horizontal abduction and adduction.**

Strengthening Exercises
- Isometrics.
- External and internal rotation, abduction, extension, biceps, triceps.

Note: **No resisted shoulder flexion.**

- Initiate external and internal rotation with exercise tubing at 0 degrees abduction when pain free.

Rehabilitation Protocol
After Acromioclavicular Joint Stabilization Using Biodegradable Material *(Continued)*
Wilk

Decrease Pain and Inflammation
- Ice, NSAIDs, modalities.

Phase 2: Intermediate Phase (Weeks 2–8)

Criteria for Progression to Phase 2
- Full nonpainful ROM.
- Minimal pain and tenderness.
- Stable AC joint on clinical examination.
- Good (grade $^4/_5$) MMT of external and internal rotation and abduction.

Goals
- Regain and improve muscular strength.
- Normalize arthrokinematics.
- Improve neuromuscular control of shoulder complex.

Week 3
Range of Motion Exercises
- Continue active-assisted ROM with T-bar.
- Continue self-capsular stretches.

Strengthening Exercises
- Initiate isotonic strengthening (light resistance)
  - Shoulder abduction.
  - Shoulder extension.
  - Shoulder external and internal rotation.
  - Biceps and triceps.
  - Scapular musculature

Note: **Restricted shoulder resistance flexion prohibited.**

- Initiate neuromuscular control exercises (PNF).
- Initiate manual resistance.

Pain Control
- Continue use of modalities, ice as needed.

Week 6
Range of Motion Exercises
- Continue stretching program.

Strengthening Exercises
- Continue all strengthening exercise listed above.
- Initiate *light* resistance shoulder flexion.
- Initiate upper extremity endurance exercises.
- Initiate *light* isotonic resistance progression

NO shoulder press or bench press or pectoralis deck or pullovers.

- Rhythmic stabilization exercise for shoulder flexion-extension.

Phase 3: Dynamic Strengthening Phase (Weeks 8–16)

Criteria for Progression to Phase 3
- Full nonpainful ROM.
- No pain or tenderness.
- Strength 70% of contralateral side.

Goals
- Improve strength, power, and endurance.
- Improve neuromuscular control and dynamic stability to the AC joint.
- Prepare athlete for overhead motion.

Strengthening Exercises
- Continue isotonic strengthening exercises
  - Initiate light bench press, shoulder press (progress weight slowly).
  - Continue with resistance exercises for
    - Shoulder abduction.
    - Shoulder external and internal rotation.
    - Shoulder flexion.
    - Latissimus dorsi (rowing, pull-downs).
    - Biceps and triceps.
  - Initiate tubing PNF patterns.
  - Initiate external and internal rotation at 90 degrees abduction.
  - Scapular strengthening (four directions)
    - Emphasis on scapular retractors, elevators.
  - Neuromuscular control exercises for GH and scapulothoracic joints
    - Rhythmic stabilization
      - Shoulder flexion-extension.
      - Shoulder external and internal rotation (90/90).
      - Shoulder abduction-adduction.
      - PNF D2 patterns.
      - Scapular retraction-protraction.
      - Scapular elevation-depression.
    - Program to plyometric upper extremity exercises.
- Continue stretching to maintain mobility.

Phase 4: Return to Activity Phase (Weeks 16 and Beyond)

Criteria for Progression to Phase 4
- Full nonpainful ROM.
- No pain or tenderness.
- Isokinetic test that fulfills criteria (shoulder flexion-extension, abduction-adduction).
- Satisfactory clinical examination.

Goal
- Progressively increase activities to prepare patient/athlete to full functional return.

Exercises
- Initiate interval sports program.
- Continue all exercises listed in phase 3.
- Progress resistance exercise levels and stretching.

Scapular Dyskinesis

W. Ben Kibler, MD, and John McMullen, MS, ATC

Background

The scapula plays many roles in normal shoulder function. It is a stable socket for the normal ball-and-socket kinematics. It retracts and protracts in cocking and follow-through movements, elevates with arm abduction, provides a stable base of origin for shoulder muscles, and is an important link in the proximal-to-distal activation sequences of the kinetic chains of overhead activity. These roles depend on proper scapular motion and position.

Alterations in scapular motion and position are termed "scapular dyskinesis" and are present in 67 to 100% of shoulder injuries.

Scapular rehabilitation is a key component of shoulder rehabilitation and should be instituted early in shoulder rehabilitation—frequently while the shoulder injury is healing.

The scapular dyskinesis protocol we use approaches rehabilitation of the scapula from a proximal-to-distal perspective. It uses muscle activation patterns to achieve this by facilitation through complementary trunk and hip movement. Lower extremity and trunk activation establishes the normal kinetic chain sequences that yield the desired scapular motion. Once scapular motion is normalized, these kinetic chain movement patterns are the framework for exercises to strengthen the scapular musculature. Closed–kinetic chain (CKC) exercises begin in the early or acute phase to stimulate cocontractions of rotator cuff and scapular musculature and promote scapulohumeral control and GH joint stability.

The distal area is an intrinsic load to the scapula, with the magnitude of the load depending on elbow flexion-extension and arm position. Function, rather than time, determines a patient's progress through the stages of the protocol. In this proximal-to-distal perspective, arm motion and strengthening activities are dependent on scapular control. A prerequisite for the addition of arm motion in the scapular program is appropriate, controlled scapular motion. Therefore, the movement pattern of the scapula determines the plane and degree of arm elevation or rotation in an exercise. If a scapular compensation presents on the introduction of a new arm position, new arm motion, or new load to the scapula, the arm position or motion should be changed to ensure the resulting scapular motion is appropriate. Hip and trunk motion should be used as necessary to facilitate appropriate scapular motion. These facilitating motions may be decreased as scapular control increases.

Rehabilitation Protocol
Scapular Dyskinesis
Kibler and McMullen

Acute Phase (Usually 0–3 Weeks)

- Initially, avoid painful arm movement and establish scapular motion.
- Begin soft tissue mobilization, electrical modalities, ultrasound, and assisted stretching, if muscular inflexibility is limiting motion. The pectoralis minor, levator scapulae, upper trapezius, latissimus dorsi, infraspinatus, and teres minor are frequently inflexible as a result of the injury process.
- Use modalities and active, active-assisted passive, and PNF stretching techniques for these areas.
- Begin upper extremity weight shifts, wobble board exercises, scapular clock (Fig. 3–77), rhythmic ball stabilization and weight-bearing isometric extension (Fig. 3–78) to promote safe cocontractions.
- Use these CKC exercises in various planes and levels of elevation, but coordinate them with appropriate scapular positioning.
- Initiate scapular motion exercises without arm elevation.
- Use trunk flexion and forward rotation to facilitate scapular protraction and active trunk extension, backward rotation and hip extension to facilitate scapular retraction. These postural changes require that the patient

Figure 3–77. Scapular clock exercise. The patient reciprocally moves the scapula in a closed–kinetic chain (CKC) position.

Rehabilitation Protocol
Scapular Dyskinesis *(Continued)*
Kibler and McMullen

Figure 3–78. Weight-bearing isometric shoulder extension. Axial load with extension muscle activation stimulates thoracic extension and lower trapezius activation.

assume a contralateral side-foot-forward stance and actively shift body weight forward for protraction and backward for retraction (Fig. 3–79). Patients who are unable to drive the trunk motion with the hips from this stance may actively stride forward and back with each reciprocal motion.

Figure 3–79. Stance for scapular motion exercises.

- Include arm motion with scapular motion exercises because the scapular motion improves to reestablish scapulohumeral coupling patterns. Keep the arm close to the body initially to minimize the intrinsic load.
- Emphasize lower abdominal and hip extensor exercises from the standing position. These muscle groups help stabilize the core and are instrumental in establishing thoracic posture.

Full active scapular motion is often limited by muscular inflexibility and myofascial restrictions. These soft tissue limitations must be alleviated for successful scapular rehabilitation. The pain and restriction of motion associated with these conditions limits progression through rehabilitation and leads to muscular compensation patterns, impingement, and possible GH joint injury.

Recovery Phase (3–8 weeks)

Proximal stability and muscular activation are imperative for appropriate scapular motion and strengthening. Strengthening is dependent on motion, and motion is dependent on posture.

- Continue to emphasize lower abdominal and hip extensor exercises along with flexibility exercises for the scapular stabilizers.
- Increase the loads on CKC exercises such as wall push-ups, table push-ups, and modified prone push-ups.
- Also, increase the level of arm elevation in CKC exercises as scapular control improves.

Position the patient for CKC exercises by placing the hand on a table, wall, or other object and then moving the body relative to the fixed hand to define the plane and degree of elevation. This method assures appropriate scapular position relative to the position of the arm. If the normal scapular positioning cannot be achieved in this manner, the arm position requires adjustment.

- Add arm elevation and rotation patterns to scapular motion exercises, as able (Fig. 3–80). Use diagonal patterns, scapular plane, and flexion. Progress toward active abduction. If intrinsic loads are too great with the introduction of active elevation, use axially loaded exercises as a transition to open–kinetic chain (OKC) exercises. In these exercises, the patient applies a moderate load through the upper extremity, as in the CKC exercises, but also slides the arm into elevation. Wall slides (Fig. 3–81) and table slides are examples. Incorporate trunk and hip motion with these exercises.
- Begin tubing exercises using hip and trunk extension with retraction and hip and trunk flexion with protraction (Fig. 3–82). Use various angles of pull and planes of motion. Deemphasize upward pull until upper trapezius dominance is eliminated.
- As scapulohumeral coupling and control are achieved, dumbbell punches may be introduced. Use complemen-

continued

Rehabilitation Protocol
Scapular Dyskinesis (Continued)
Kibler and McMullen

Figure 3–80. Progression of arm motion with scapular motion exercise patterns.

Figure 3–82. Tubing pulls incorporating trunk and hip extension.

tary strides to incorporate the kinetic chain contribution and reciprocal motions (Fig. 3–83). Vary the height of punches while maintaining scapular control.

• Use lunges with dumbbell reaches to emphasize kinetic chain timing and coordination (Fig. 3–84). Vary the level of arm elevation, amount of external rotation, and degree of elbow flexion in the standing, or return, posi-

tion to increase the functional demand on the scapular muscles. Vary the direction of the lunge to vary the plane of emphasis for the scapular motion. Avoid scapular compensations such as "winging" or "shrugging." If compensations occur, reduce the load until there is appropriate scapular motion and scapulothoracic congruency with the exercise.

Figure 3–81. Wall slides. While maintaining an axial load, the patient slides the hand in a prescribed pattern.

Figure 3–83. Dumbbell punches with a stride.

Rehabilitation Protocol
Scapular Dyskinesis *(Continued)*
Kibler and McMullen

Figure 3–84. Lunge and reach. The return or standing position may be with the hands at the shoulders and the elbows pointing down or may include arm elevation, depending on the stage of recovery.

Functional Phase (6–10 Weeks)

- When there is good scapular control and motion throughout the range of shoulder elevation, initiate plyometric exercises such as medicine ball toss and catch (Fig. 3–85) and tubing plyometrics.
- Continue to include kinetic chain activation. Move to various planes as scapular control improves.
- Slow, resisted sport-skill movements, such as the throwing motion, are good activities to promote kinetic chain stabilization while dynamically loading the scapular muscles.
- Overhead dumbbell presses and punches, in various planes, are advanced exercises requiring good scapular control through a full and loaded GH joint ROM (Fig. 3–86).

- The lunge-and-reach series can be progressed to overhead reaches in the return position.
- Progressively add external resistance to exercises introduced earlier in the program. The volume of work becomes a progression as do the difficulty of the exercise and the amount of resistance.
- Challenging lower extremity stability using wobble boards, trampoline, slide boards, and the like also increases the load on the scapular musculature without sacrificing the functional movements.

Figure 3–85. Medicine ball plyometric exercise.

Figure 3–86. Overhead dumbbell press.

Physical Findings in Common Conditions of the Shoulder and Upper Arm

Impingement Syndrome

Hawkins impingement test abnormal.
Neer impingement sign often present.
Supraspinatus resistance testing often painful.
Painful arc of abduction often present.
Subacromial bursa tender (variable).

Rotator Cuff Tear

Supraspinatus resistance painful and usually weak.
Hawkins impingement reinforcement test abnormal.
Neer impingement sign often present.
Painful arc of abduction present.
Supraspinatus atrophy present (more severe cases).
Infraspinatus resistance painful and possibly weak (more severe cases).
Loss of active motion, particularly abduction (variable).
Drop-arm sign present (only in more severe cases).
Loss of active external rotation (massive tears).
After injection into the subacromial space (lidocaine test), pain often improves but weakness of rotator cuff remains.

Anterior Instability (Recurrent Subluxation or Dislocation)

Apprehension in response to apprehension test.
Reduction of apprehension in response to relocation test.
Increased anterior laxity to passive testing (drawer test, load-and-shift test).
Signs of axillary nerve injury (occasionally) (deltoid weakness and numbness over lateral shoulder).
Signs of musculocutaneous nerve injury (rarely) (biceps weakness and numbness over lateral forearm).

Posterior Instability (Recurrent Subluxation or Dislocation)

Increased posterior laxity to passive testing (posterior drawer test, load-and-shift test).
Mildly abnormal sulcus test (variable).
Symptoms reproduced by jerk test or circumduction test (variable).
Voluntary dislocation or subluxation possible (occasionally).

Multidirectional Instability

Abnormal sulcus sign.
Increased anterior and/or posterior laxity to passive testing (drawer test, load-and-shift test).
Additional signs of anterior posterior instability depending on predominant direction of symptomatic episodes.
Ability to voluntarily dislocate (occasionally).
Often generalized ligamentous laxity noted (thumb to wrist, elbow hyperextension).

Acromioclavicular Joint Injury

Tenderness of AC joint.
Localized swelling in AC joint.
Usually a direct blow to the point of the shoulder (e.g., a fall or football hit).
Increase in prominence of distal clavicle (variable, depending on severity of injury).
Tenderness of coracoclavicular ligaments (more severe injuries).
Pain with cross-chest adduction (see Fig. 3–32).

Rarely, distal clavicle displaced posteriorly (type IV injuries).
O'Brien test produces pain on top of shoulder (variable).

Biceps Tendinitis

Biceps tendon tender.
Speed test painful.
Yergason test painful (occasionally).
Biceps instability test abnormal (occasionally, if biceps tendon unstable).
Look for signs of concomitant rotator cuff pathology (variable) if biceps (a secondary humeral head depressor) is "trying to help" a weakened rotator cuff.

Suprascapular Nerve Compression or Injury

Supraspinatus and infraspinatus weakness and atrophy (if compression prior to innervation of supraspinatus).
Infraspinatus weakness and atrophy alone (if compression at the spinoglenoid notch).

Rheumatoid Arthritis

Local warmth and swelling.
Muscle atrophy often present.
Signs of rheumatoid involvement at other joints.

Thoracic Outlet Syndrome

Symptoms reproduced by Roos test, Wright maneuver, Adson test, or hyperabduction test (variable).
Diminution of pulse with Adson test, Wright maneuver, Halsted test, or hyperabduction test (variable).

Adhesive Capsulitis (Frozen Shoulder)

Generalized decrease in both active (patient lifts arm) and passive (examiner lifts arm) ROM, including forward flexion, abduction, internal rotation, and external rotation.
Pain elicited by passive ROM or any passive manipulation that stresses the limits of the patient's reduced motion.
Generalized weakness or atrophy (variable).

Stinger Syndrome (Burners)

Tenderness over brachial plexus.
Weakness in muscles innervated by involved portion of the plexus (deltoid most commonly involved, elbow flexors second most commonly involved).

Referred Pain from Cervical Radiculopathy

Motor, sensory, or reflex changes noted (radicular).
Spurling test of neck positive (variable).
Symptoms of findings distal to the elbow (e.g., hand numbness in C_6 distribution).
Provocative tests of the shoulder normal.

Weight-lifters Osteolysis of the AC Joint

Point tender at the AC joint.
History of repetitive weight-lifting.
Irregularity, narrowing of the AC joint noted on radiographs.
Usually no trauma history.
Positive cross-chest adduction sign.

Modified from Reider B: The Orthopaedic Physical Examination. Philadelphia, WB Saunders, 1999.

Bibliography

Bach BR Jr: Personal communication, Nov. 1999.

Bahr R, Craig EV, Engbresten L: The clinical presentation of shoulder instability including on-the-field management. Clin Sports Med 14:761–776, 1995.

Blom S, Dhalback LO: Nerve injuries in dislocations of the shoulder joint and fractures of the neck of the humerus. Acta Chir Scand 136:461–466, 1970.

Burkhart SS: Arthroscopic treatment of massive rotator cuff tears. Clin Orthop 390:107–118, 2001.

Codman EA: The Shoulder: Rupture of the Supra-spinatus Tendon and Other Lesions in or about the Subacromial Bursa. Boston, Thomas Todd, 1934.

Cofield RH, Boardman ND, Bengtson KA, et al: Rehabilitation after total shoulder arthroplasty. J Arthroplasty 16(4):483–486, 2001.

Dines DM, Levinson M: The conservative management of the unstable shoulder including rehabilitation. Clin Sports Med 14:797–816, 1995.

Frieman BG, Albert TJ, Fenlin JM Jr: Rotator cuff disease: a review of diagnosis, pathophysiology, and current trends in treatment. Arch Phys Med Rehabil 75:604–609, 1994.

Gross ML, Distefano MC: Anterior release test: a new test for shoulder instability. Clin Orthop 339:105–108, 1997.

Gusmer PB, Potter HG: Imaging of shoulder instability. Clin Sports Med 14:777–795, 1995.

Harryman DT II, Lazarus MD, Rozencwaig R: The stiff shoulder. In Rockwood CA Jr, Matsen FA III (eds): The Shoulder, 2nd ed. Philadelphia, WB Saunders, 1998, pp. 1064–1112.

Hawkins RJ, Montadi NG: Clinical evaluation of shoulder instability. Clin J Sports Med 1:59–64, 1991.

Hill AV: The mechanics of voluntary muscle. Lancet 2:947–951, 1951.

Host HH: Scapular taping in the treatment of anterior shoulder impingement. Phys Ther 75:803–811, 1995.

Kibler WB: Shoulder rehabilitation: principles and practice. Med Sci Sports Exerc 30:S40–S50, 1998.

Kibler WB: Normal shoulder mechanics and function. In Springfield DS (ed): Instructional Course Lectures, vol. 46. Rosemont, Ill, American Academy of Orthopaedic Surgeons, 1997, pp. 39–42.

Kibler WB, Garrett WE Jr: Pathophysiologic alterations in shoulder injury. In Springfield DS (ed): Instructional Course Lectures, vol. 46. Rosemont, Ill, American Academy of Orthopaedic Surgeons, 1997, pp. 3–6.

Kibler WB, Livingston B, Chandler TJ: Shoulder rehabilitation: clinical application, evaluation, and rehabilitation protocols. In Springfield DS (ed): Instructional Course Lectures, vol. 46. Rosemont, Ill, American Academy of Orthopaedic Surgeons, 1997, pp. 43–51.

Kibler WB, Livingston B, Chandler TJ: Current concepts in shoulder rehabilitation. Adv Oper Orthop 3:249–301, 1996.

Kim SH, Ha KI, Ahn JH, Choi HJ: Biceps local test II: a clinical test for SLAP lesions of the shoulder. Arthroplasty 17(2):160–164, 2001.

Kirkley A, Griffin S, Richards C, et al: Prospective randomized clinical trial comparing effectiveness of immediate arthroscopic stabilization versus immobilization and rehabilitation in first traumatic anterior dislocations of the shoulder. Arthroscopy 15:507–514, 1999.

Lehman C, Cuomo F, Kummer FJ, Zuckerman JD: The incidence of full thickness rotator cuff tears in a large cadaveric population. Bull Hosp Jt Dis 54:30–31, 1995.

Liu SH, Henry MH, Nuccion SL: A prospective evaluation of a new physical examination in predicting glenoid labral tears. Am J Sports Med 24(6):721–725, 1996.

Matsen FA III, Thomas SC, Rockwood CA Jr, Wirth MA: Glenohumeral instability. In Rockwood CA Jr, Matsen FA III (ed): The Shoulder, 2nd ed. Philadelphia, WB Saunders, 1998, pp. 611–754.

Morrey BF, Eiji I, Kai-nan A: Biomechanics of the shoulder. In Rockwood CA Jr, Matsen FA III (ed): The Shoulder, 2nd ed. Philadelphia, WB Saunders, 1998, pp. 233–276.

Neer CS II: Anterior acromioplasty for the chronic impingement syndrome in the shoulder. J Bone Joint Surg 54A:41–50, 1972.

Neviaser RJ, Neviaser TJ: Observations on impingement. Clin Orthop 254:60–63, Review 1990.

Nichols TR: A biomechanical perspective on spinal mechanisms of coordinated muscular action. Acta Anat 15:1–13, 1994.

Pearsall AW, Speer KP: Frozen shoulder syndrome: diagnostic and treatment strategies in the primary care setting. Med Sci Sports Exerc 30:S33–S39, 1998.

Poppen NK, Walker PS: Forces at the glenohumeral joint in abduction. Clin Orthop 135:165–170, 1978.

Post M, Silver R, Singh M: Rotator cuff tear. Clin Orthop 173:78–91, 1983.

Rockwood CA, Matsen FA: The Shoulder. Philadelphia, WB Saunders, 1990.

Romeo AA: Personal communication, Oct. 1999.

Romeo AA, Hang DW, Bach BR Jr, Shott S: Repair of full thickness rotator cuff tears. Gender, age, and other factors affecting outcome. Clin Orthop 367:243–255, 1999.

Schmitt L, Snyder-Mackler L: Role of scapular stabilizers in etiology and treatment of impingement syndrome. J Orthop Sports Phys Ther 29:31–38, 1999.

Shelbourne KD, Nitz P: Accelerated rehabilitation after anterior cruciate ligament reconstruction. Am J Sports Med 18:192–199, 1990.

Snyder SJ, Karzel RP, Del Pizzo W, Ferkel RD, Friedman MJ: SLAP lesions of the shoulder. Arthroscopy 6(4):274–279, 1990.

Speer KP, Cavanaugh JT, Warren RF: A role for hydrotherapy in shoulder rehabilitation. Am J Sports Med 21:850–853, 1993.

Speer KP, Garret WE Jr: Muscular control of motion and stability about the pectoral girdle. In Matsen FA III, Fu FH, Hawkins RJ (eds): The Shoulder: A Balance of Mobility and Stability. Rosemont, Ill, American Academy of Orthopaedic Surgeons, 1993, pp. 159–172.

Stollsteimer GT, Savoie FH: Arthrosopic rotator cuff repair: current indications, limitations, techniques, and results. In Cannon WD Jr (ed): Instructional Course Lectures, vol. 47. Rosemont, Ill, American Academy of Orthopaedic Surgeons, 1998, pp. 59–65.

Tauro JC: Arthroscopic rotator cuff repair: analysis of technique and results at 2 and 3 year follow-up. Arthroscopy 14:45–51, 1998.

Tibone JE, Bradely JP: The treatment of posterior subluxation in athletes. Clin Orthop 29:1124–1137, 1993.

Warren RF, Craig EV, Altcheck DW: The Unstable Shoulder. Philadelphia, Lippincott-Raven, 1999.

Wilk KE, Meister K, Andrews JR: Current concepts in the rehabilitation of the overhead throwing athlete. Am J Sports Med 30(1):136–151, Review 2002.

Wilk KE, Andrews JR, Crockett HC: Rehabilitation after rotator cuff surgery: techniques in shoulder and elbow. Am J Acad Orthop Surg 5(3):130–140, 1997.

Wilk KE, Arrigo C: Current concepts in the rehabilitation of the athletic shoulder. J Orthop Sports Phys Ther 18:365–378, 1993.

Wilk KE, Crockett HC, Andrews JR: Rehabilitation after rotator cuff surgery. Tech Shoulder Elbow Surg 1(2):128–144, 2000.

Wirth MA, Basamania C, Rockwood CA Jr: Nonoperative management of full-thickness tears of the rotator cuff. Orthop Clin North Am 28:59–66, 1997.

Yamaguchi K, Flatow EL: Management of multidirectional instability. Clin Sports Med 14:885–902, 1995.

Yocum LA, Conway JE: Rotator cuff tear: clinical assessment and treatment. In Jobe FW (ed): Operative Techniques in Upper Extremity Sports Injuries. St. Louis, Mosby, 1996, pp. 223–245.

Zasler ND: AAOS annual meeting: Specialty Society Day. Anaheim, Feb. 7, 1999.

Chapter 4
Knee Injuries

Michael D'Amato, MD, and Bernard R. Bach Jr., MD

The Painful Knee: Evaluation, Examination, and Imaging

Shawn Bonsell, MD, and Robert W. Jackson, MD

The most effective tools for diagnosis of knee conditions are a thorough history and a careful physical examination. The use of a standardized form (see p. 263) for every knee evaluation helps ensure that all aspects of the history and examination are included and that the evaluation proceeds in a logical, systematic fashion.

History Taking

The history of a patient's knee problem provides more information leading to a correct and full diagnosis than any other aspect of the evaluation. Most experienced knee surgeons can narrow the diagnosis to one or two possibilities based on the history alone. Many etiologies of knee pain may be ruled out by history (e.g., history of gradual insidious onset of anterior knee pain with no acute injury, popping, or instability makes an anterior cruciate ligament [ACL] tear highly unlikely). A detailed, thorough history and physical examination compare with a cursory examination and MRI, much like a rifle compares with a shotgun. Over-reliance on radiographic imaging is prevalent today and should be avoided.

If the knee problem is due to a single, specific injury, the possible knee pathology is limited to a distinct group of injuries (e.g., meniscal, ligamentous, fracture, tendon rupture, etc.). Insidious, nontraumatic onset of knee pain is more indicative of an overuse injury, an inflammatory

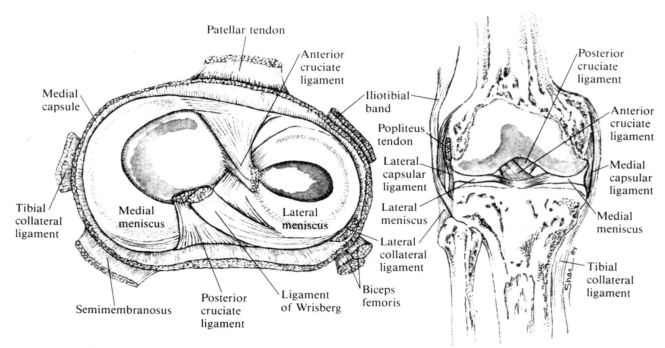

Anatomy of the knee. *Left:* Top view showing the plateau of the tibia. *Right:* Front view (with patella removed). (From Underwood DL, Chabon S: Sports injuries to the knee: A practical approach. PA Outlook (July–Aug.):89–96, 1984.

syndrome, or an arthritic etiology rather than an acute ligamentous or meniscal injury.

Determining whether the cause of knee pain is an **acute, traumatic** injury or one of **gradual, insidious** onset points to different subsets of etiologies (e.g., ligament tear vs. inflammatory origin).

A thorough physical examination includes documentation of a number of factors.

- *Chief complaint.* It is important to ask *how this began* and to determine if the chief complaint is swelling, locking, popping, instability, or joint line pain.
- *Bilaterality.* This usually suggests a nontraumatic, insidious onset of knee pain.
- *Duration and onset of symptoms.* It is important to determine whether the patient's pain is improving or worsening. The patient may have one episode of knee pain, which has never gotten better, or the pain may be intermittent or aggravated by specific activities.
- *Knee symptoms (acute or chronic).* In *acute, traumatic* injuries, it is important to understand the *mechanism* of knee injury. What was the patient doing at the time the knee was hurt? Was there a direct force applied to the knee by another object, such as another player's body? If so, where did the force strike the knee and what position was the knee forced into (valgus, varus, hyperextended)? Was the patient struck in the lateral aspect of the knee with a valgus-type injury? Was this a contact or noncontact injury that occurred while cutting, twisting, or pivoting? Did the patient feel or hear a pop? Is there immedi-

ate swelling of the knee? Did the swelling occur *within the first 2 hours* (which is more indicative of an acute hemarthrosis) or *within the next 24 hours* (indicating a probable inflammatory effusion)? Was the patient able to continue playing?

- *Age, sex, and activity level.* Certain knee problems are more common in certain age groups and among men or women (e.g., anterior knee pain or patellofemoral knee pain is most common in young, athletic females).

Approximately 75% of knee injuries in which the patient suffered the triad of: 1) an **acute blow** or twisting or cutting injury, 2) an **immediate effusion** of the knee and 3) the **inability to continue play** are ACL injuries. This information in the history would lead to a correct diagnosis of ACL injury before the physican's examination 75% of the time.

Has the patient had antecedent symptoms before the acute injury or previous surgeries to the knee? Is the patient having any difficulties with ambulation now, including *locking, popping, giving out,* or *instability, clicking,* or *continued swelling?* Did the patient feel the sensation of the kneecap going back into place as the knee was straightened (suggesting acute patellar dislocation that reduced by simple knee extension)?

For patient with *chronic* symptoms, it is important to rule out systemic illness as the etiology of the knee pain. Infectious, neurologic, vascular, neoplastic, inflammatory, and arthritic causes all must be considered. Inquiries about other areas of the body may be helpful (e.g., multiple-joint pain). Did the patient have antecedent fever, chills, weight loss, or upper respiratory infection or sexually transmitted disease?

Nontraumatic (Often Chronic) Causes of Knee Pain

Overuse injuries

- Tendinitis
- Bursitis
- Stress fracture

Septic arthritis (EMERGENCY!)

Gonococcal arthritis

Rheumatoid arthritis

Rheumatic fever

Juvenile arthritis

Polymyalgia rheumatica

Crystal-induced disease

- Gout/pseudogout

Charcot joint

Osteochondritis dissecans (OCD)

Reflex sympathetic dystrophy (RSD)

Seronegative spondyloarthropathy

- Ankylosing spondylitis
- Reiter's syndrome
- Psoriatic spondylitis
- Inflammatory bowel disease

Collagen vascular disease

- Scleroderma
- Polymyositis
- Polyarteritis nodosa
- Mixed connective tissue disease

Lyme disease

Tuberculosis

Viral synovitis

Fungal infection

Neoplasm (benign or malignant)

Detailed Analysis of Symptom Complex

Each patient should be questioned about the presence of popping, locking, catching, instability episodes, swelling, stiffness, night pain, difficulty with weight-bearing activities, ambulation, stair climbing, getting in and out of a chair, deep squatting, or kneeling. Has the patient noted a limp?

- *Popping.* Popping is so common that it is practically useless in terms of making a specific diagnosis. Painful popping is more likely to be of significance than nonpainful popping, but all types of injuries can create popping in and around knee joints.
- *Giving way.* A sudden weakness in the leg that causes the leg to go into mild hyperextension or flexion is often a muscular phenomenon, such as a weak quadriceps. If the patient describes a true joint subluxation with bones going out of place, this may indicate a ligamentous tear (usually the ACL) and/or patellar instability (subluxation).
- *Locking.* Locking is a very useful sign if the patient says that the knee locks for a relatively long time and has to be passively moved in a certain way to regain motion or extension. Locking is typically indicative of a meniscal injury or loose body within the joint. A "locked" knee typically still has flexion, but the patient has difficulty getting the last 5 to 20 degrees of full extension.

- *Catching.* Many patients describe catching as a transient phenomenon that does not require a specific maneuver to correct. Catching is more typical with either an extensor mechanism disorder (e.g., maltracking of the patella) or a small meniscal tear.
- *Exacerbating and relieving factors of the knee pain.* These include treatment modalities that have improved the pain (e.g., physical therapy, cortisone injections, medications, and splinting or bracing) as well as what makes the symptoms worse (e.g., walking, running, athletic activity, stair climbing, or job activities). Is the pain worse in the morning when the patient gets out of bed and does it abate during the day, or is it worse after prolonged ambulation or is it weather related? Does the knee pain affect activities of daily living and the quality of life? Has the patient noticed a limp or had to walk with a cane or crutches? On a scale of 0 to 10, with the worst pain they have ever experienced being a 10, what does their daily pain rate?

The history also must document any previous diagnoses, injuries, or knee surgeries and any medical problems, medications, or drug allergies. For example, the treating physician should know if a patient has already undergone a medial meniscectomy, because the radiologist will often transcribe this signal void from excision as a medial meniscal tear. Once a thorough history has been obtained, it is helpful to have patients reiterate their current and most troublesome knee symptoms (pain, swelling, instability, stiffness, locking).

As a transition into the physical examination, the patient should point to the area of most trouble. This location is documented as **anterior** (quadriceps, patella, patellar retinaculum, patellar tendon), **lateral** (lateral joint line, lateral femoral condyle, lateral tibial plateau), **medial** (medial joint line, medial femoral condyle, medial plateau), or **posterior** (popliteal fossa, posteromedial or posterolateral joint line).

Physical Examination

A thorough knee examination begins with a relaxed and comfortable patient. Both knees should be examined simultaneously to allow inspection for asymmetry.

Examination of the Entire Extremity

Before actually examining the knee, the physician should inspect the entire extremity with the knee evident and both shoes and socks off. The patient's gait should be observed. Sometimes, it is helpful to observe the patient's gait when he or she is not aware he or she is being watched by the examiner (possible secondary gain issues).

With the patient standing, the weight-bearing alignment of the knee should be evaluated, documenting varus, valgus, or normal alignment; any recurvatum deformity,

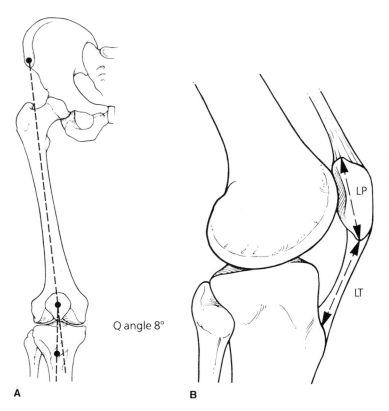

Q angle 8°

A   B

Figure 4–1. *A,* The **Q-angle** (quadriceps) is an angle formed between lines drawn from the anterior superior iliac spine of the pelvis to the middle of the patella and a line drawn from the middle of the patella to the tibial tubercle. The angle is measured with the knee in full extension. An angle greater than 20 degrees is abnormal and is often associated with lateral tracking or instability of the patella. *B,* **Insall's technique for measuring patella alta** and the like. The ratio of the patellar tendon length (LT) is divided by the length of the patella (LP). A 1.2:1 ratio indicates a normal extensor mechanism. A ratio greater than 1.2:1 indicates patella alta (long patellar tendon). This is often associated with anterior knee pain, patellar malalignment, and instability. In patella alta, the "high" patella does not properly engage in the trochlear groove. (*A* and *B,* From Sebastianelli WJ: Anterior knee pain: sorting through a complex differential. J Musculoskel Med 10[7]:55–66, 1993. Artist: William Westwood.)

internal or external rotation of the leg (tibial torsion, femoral anteversion); the Q-angle of the patellofemoral joint and any patella alta, patella baja, or squinting of the patella (Fig. 4–1). Evaluation of the biomechanical alignment of the entire limb includes noting any pes planus deformity that increases the Q-angle at the knee (Fig. 4–2). The skin should be examined for any abnormalities,

such as altered appearance (shiny), temperature (hot or cold), sensation (hyperesthetic or hypoesthetic), or sweating that may indicate RSD. Popliteal, dorsalis pedis, and posterior tibial pulses should be documented, as well as function of the sensory and motor (peroneal and tibial) nerves. Examination of the asymptomatic limb is helpful for comparison with the symptomatic side.

Sometimes, knee pain is referred pain from the hip (anterior thigh pain), and this should be ruled out as a source of pain. In **pediatric patients,** failure to examine the hip to rule out referred pain to the knee may lead to a missed diagnosis of Legg-Calve-Perthes, slipped capital femoral epiphysis, hip fracture, or septic hip.

Detailed Inspection of the Knee

- *Visual inspection of the knee.* The presence of effusion, discoloration, ecchymosis, or previous surgical incisions should be documented. Swelling should be described as generalized (intra-articular) or localized (bursal, such as prepatellar bursitis or pes anserinus bursitis). The circumferential size of the quadriceps should be compared with that of the uninvolved leg, and the circumferences of the thigh and calf of both legs are measured from a fixed and measured point above and below the tibial tuberosity.
- *Palpation of the knee.* In a systematic fashion, all aspects of the knee are checked for areas of point tenderness to palpation: medial and lateral joint line,

Figure 4–2. Genu valgum (severe) at the knee exacerbated by underlying pes planus, contributing to an increased Q-angle.

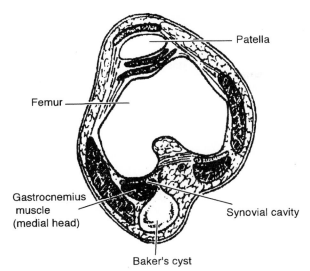

Figure 4–3. Cross-section of the knee showing a posterior location for a Baker's cyst. (From Black KP, Skrzynski MC: Arthroscopy in knee diagnosis and surgery: an update. J Musculo Med 10[2]79–94, 1993.)

medial and lateral collateral ligaments, patellofemoral joint, patellar tendon, inferior and superior poles of the patella, tibial tubercle, Gerdy's tubercle, iliotibial band insertion laterally, pes anserinus insertion (Voshell or pes anserinus bursitis), and posterior politeal fossa (Baker cyst) (Fig. 4–3). The integrity of the quadriceps and patellar tendon is evaluated by having the patient perform a straight-leg raise (SLR).

- *Range of motion (ROM) of the knee (active and passive).* Active ROM is tested by having the patient move the leg to full extension and then to perform

an SLR against gravity. The patient then moves the knee into full flexion, and this is compared with flexion of the contralateral knee. If there is restriction in active ROM, passive ROM should be checked.

Tracking of the patella is observed through full knee ROM, and the presence of a J-sign or maltracking is documented (see p. 324).

The **patellar apprehension test** documents pain or anxiety with lateral displacement and compression of the patella, indicating patellar instability or subluxation (Fig. 4–4). Other tests for patellar mobility, patellar tilt, and patellar glide are described in the section on patellofemoral disorders (see pp. 325–326).

Knee Ligament Examination

Several **stress testing maneuvers** are used for ligamentous and patellar examination (Table 4–1). Valgus stress should be applied to the **medial collateral ligament (MCL)** and medial capsule with the knee at 0 and 30 degrees of flexion and the amount of opening of the medial joint line on valgus stressing is recorded (Fig. 4–5). Opening of the medial joint line at 30 degrees of flexion implied a grade II or III MCL tear (see p. 309). Opening at 0 degrees of flexion implies a more severe injury of the MCL, with concomitant pathology such as an ACL injury.

The **lateral collateral ligament (LCL)** and lateral capsule are stressed with a varus force with the knee in the same positions, and the amount of opening is recorded (Fig. 4–6). The **posterior cruciate ligament (PCL)** is checked for a posterior drawer sign with the knee at 90 degrees (Fig. 4–7) and for a positive posterior sag (Fig. 4–8).

A

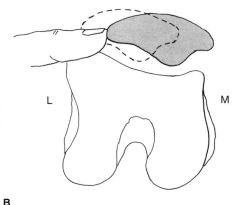

B

Figure 4–4. *A,* Patellar apprehension test looks for anxiety or pain when the examiner performs lateral displacement or compression of the patella. A positive test indicates underlying patella instability or subluxation. *B,* Lateral displacement of the patella, causing pain or anxiety.

Table 4-1

Ligamentous Testing of the Knee

Test	Purpose	Method	Results
Lachman test	ACL insufficiency	Patient is supine, with knee in 20 degrees of flexion. Examiner stands on side of injured knee and pulls the tibia anteriorly.	A "give" reaction or mushy end point indicates ACL disruption Most sensitive ACL test.
Anterior drawer test	ACL insufficiency	Patient is supine with knee flexed to 90 degrees. Examiner attempts to pull tibia from its anatomic position to a displaced anterior position.	Result is positive if tibia can be anteriorly displaced on the femur.
Posterior drawer test	PCL insufficiency	Patient is supine with knee flexed to 90 degrees. Examiner attempts to posteriorly displace the tibia on the femur by pushing tibia posteriorly.	In PCL insufficiency, there is posterior sagging of the tibia.
Varus/valgus stress test	Medial and lateral collateral ligamentous stability; evaluate for possible growth plate injury in the skeletally immature patient.	Patient is positioned with the knee first in full extension and then in 30 degrees of flexion. Standing on the side of the injured leg, the examiner applies varus and valgus stress to the knee in both the extended and the 30-degree flexed positions. The degree of joint opening is compared with that in the uninvolved side.	Grade I collateral ligament sprains often have tenderness with little or no joint opening. Grade III opening of greater than 15 mm suggests ligament disruption. Stress radiographs of growth plate injuries show opening or gapping of the affected growth plate.
Pivot shift test	ACL insufficiency (assesses anterior displacement of the lateral tibial plateau on the lateral femoral condyle)	Knee is positioned in 30 degrees of flexion. Examiner places one hand under the heel and the other on the lateral aspect of the proximal tibia, then applies valgus stress. The knee is then brought into extension.	In ACL disruption, the lateral tibial plateau is in the anatomic position when the knee is flexed and subluxes anteriorly during extension.
Reverse pivot shift test	PCL insufficiency	Knee is positioned in 30 degrees of flexion. Test is done as for the pivot shift test.	In PCL and posterolateral insufficiency, the lateral tibial plateau is reduced with the knee in extension and, during flexion, falls posteriorly and rotates with respect to the medial tibial plateau. Straight posterior laxity with isolated PCL injury allows posterior displacement of the tibia on the femur but prevents a reverse pivot shift.
Quadriceps active drawer test	Posterior instability	Knees positioned in 90 degrees of flexion. Examiner places posterior pressure on the tibia, then asks the patient to actively fire the quadriceps by trying to slide the heel forward.	In posterior laxity, the quadriceps draws the tibia forward.

ACL, anterior cruciate ligament; PCL, posterior cruciate ligament.
From Meislin RJ: Managing collateral ligament tears of the knee. J Musculoskel Med 24:11, 1996.

The **ACL** is checked with a **Lachman test** with the knee in 30 degrees of flexion (Fig. 4–9A). An **anterior drawer test** (see Fig. 4–9B) can also be done with the knee in 90 degrees of flexion.

The most sensitive test for an ACL tear is a Lachman test with a relaxed patient and relaxed lower extremity.

With very cooperative patients, a **pivot shift test** (see Fig. 4–9C) can be done, but this is painful and requires significant cooperation. Thus, this should be the last attempted maneuver in the examination because the pain is not tolerated by most patients and may inhibit further examination.

Meniscal Evaluation

The most common **meniscal tests** are those described by McMurray and Apley. **McMurray's test** (Fig. 4–10) is done with the knee flexed as far as possible and

Figure 4–5. Valgus stress testing of the medial collateral ligament (MCL) at 0 degrees of knee flexion (*A* and *B*) and 30 degrees of knee flexion (*C* and *D*). Medial opening at 0 degrees of knee flexion indicates more injury (e.g., anterior cruciate ligament or capsule) than just an isolated MCL tear. (*B*, From Meislin RJ: Managing collateral ligament tears of the knee. Physician Sports Med 24:90–96, 1996; *D*, from Laprade RF, Wentorff F: Acute knee injuries. Physician Sports Med 27:107–111, 1999.)

with the foot and tibia either externally rotated (to test the medial meniscus) or internally rotated (to test the lateral meniscus). While the tibia is held in the appropriate position, the knee is brought from the position of acute flexion into extension. The classic finding is a painful pop along the appropriate joint line, palpable or audible to the examiner. In some knees, significant pain may be elicited over the appropriate joint line without a true popping.

The **Apley compression test** (Fig. 4–11) is done with the patient prone and the knee flexed to 90 degrees. The examiner pushes downward on the sole of the patient's foot toward the examination table. This com-

presses the menisci between the tibia and the femur. Then, with the tibia in external rotation (for the medial meniscus) or internal rotation (for the lateral meniscus), the knee is moved through a full ROM while compression is maintained. A positive response is pain over the joint line being tested.

Flexibility of the hamstrings and quadriceps and Ober's test should be documented on the examination as well (see section on patellofemoral disorders, p. 324).

Aspiration of the Knee

In patients with a tense, painful hemarthrosis, aspiration of the knee provides significant pain relief. Studies

A   **B**

C   **D**

Figure 4–6. Lateral collateral ligament (LCL) testing by applying a varus force to the knee at 0 degrees of knee flexion (*A* and *B*) and 30 degrees of knee flexion (*C* and *D*). (*B*, From Meislin RJ: Managing collateral ligament tears of the knee. Physician Sports Med 24:90–96, 1996; *D*, from Laprade RF, Wentorff F: Acute knee injuries. Physician Sports Med 27:107–111, 1999.)

have also documented that large effusions (>40 ml of fluid) provide an inhibitory feedback mechanism for the quadriceps and essentially shut down its function. Aspiration of the knee joint is useful for obtaining blood and serous fluid to be examined for infection or crystals. Knee aspirate (excluding traumatic hemarthrosis) is sent to the laboratory for

- Cell count and differential cell count (purple-top tube).

- Cultures (Gram's stain, aerobic, anaerobic, acid-fast bacilli [AFB]/fungal).
- Crystals (green-top tube). Gout is negatively birefringent under polarized light, with needle-shaped crystals; pseudogout (chondrocalinosis) is positively birefringent under polarized light, and is pleomorphic in appearance. Some literature suggests that glucose, clot, and viscosity should also be tested.

Knee Aspirate

Finding	Normal Knee	Septic Arthritis	Rheumatoid Arthritis	Degenerative Joint Disease
Appearance	Clear	Turbid (cannot read a newspaper through test tube)	Cloudy	Clear
Cell count/mm³	200	Usually > 50,000*	2000–50,000	2000
Differentiated cell count	Monos	Polys	50/50	Monos
Glucose	Within 60% or more of serum glucose	Very Low	Low	Normal

* > 50,000 WBCs shows infected joint and requires emergent washout (debridement and irrigation) of the joint.

A   **B**

Figure 4–7. *A,* **Posterior drawer test for the posterior cruciate ligament (PCL).** The examiner pushes posteriorly on the tibia with the knee relaxed and bent at a 90-degree angle. Increased laxity as compared to the unaffected limb indicates a probable PCL tear. Compare with the unaffected limb. Laxity is measured by the relationship of the medial tibial plateau to the medial femoral condyle. *B,* Posterior drawer test for PCL injury is done with the patient supine, the knee flexed 90 degrees, and the quadriceps and hamstring muscles completely relaxed. The examiner holds the tibia in neutral position by sitting on the patient's foot. The examiner gently pushes the proximal tibia posteriorly to assess PCL integrity. Excursion and a soft endpoint, when compared with the opposite side, suggest an injury. (*B* and *C,* From Laprade RF, Wentorf F: Acute knee injuries: on-the-field and sideline evaluation. Physician Sports Med 27[10]:107–111, 1999.)

Fat droplets noted in the aspirate after an acute injury indicate a bony injury (fracture) with communication of the marrow cavity with the interior of the joint. Fat droplets in the knee aspirate can typically be seen when the aspirate is squirted into a metal or plastic basin.

Installation of 1% lidocaine into the knee during aspiration of blood or fluid may also allow a better ligamentous evaluation after the patient's comfort level has improved.

Technique of Knee Aspiration and Cortisone Injection (Brotzman)

- Sterile preparation of knee with povidone-iodine (Betadine) or alcohol (Fig. 4–12).
- Patient lying flat on back with knee straight, relaxed, and well supported.
- A lateral suprapatellar approach is probably safest and easiest.
- Site is numbed with 5 to 10 ml of 1% lidocaine using a 1.5-inch, 25-gauge needle, using sterile technique (see figure 4–12 for landmarks).
- After 2 minutes to allow anesthetic to produce "numbing," an 18- or 20-gauge spinal needle (which is attached a 20-ml or larger syringe) is inserted through the "numb" track of the 25-gauge needle using sterile technique.
- Placing a thumb on the medial side of the relaxed patella and pushing the patella laterally identifies the interval for needle insertion (for both the 25-gauge and the spinal needle). This interval is between the lateral patellar edge and the lateral

femoral condyle. The horizontal needle insertion should be at the superior aspect of the patella to take advantage of the large, fluid-filled suprapatellar pouch that extends superiorly (proximally) from the patella.

- As much fluid as possible is aspirated through the spinal needle, maintaining sterility.
- Leaving the spinal needle in place and without contaminating the needle hub, the examiner removes the syringe and attaches a 5-ml syringe containing cortisone to the needle. The cortisone is injected and the needle is removed.
- Pressure is maintained on the injection site for 5 minutes after the needle is removed.
- The patient is advised to rest, elevate the limb, and apply ice to the area. Pain medication may be required for 2 or 3 days.

Imaging

Radiographic imaging of the knee should be used to confirm or refute the clinical diagnosis already made from the history and physical examination. In patients with **acute trauma, anteroposterior (AP), lateral,** and **sunrise views** of the knee are usually sufficient to rule out displaced fractures. In patients with **chronic pain standing AP (weight bearing), lateral, tunnel** (to rule out OCD lesions), and **sunrise views** are appropriate. Imaging of the contralateral, asymptomatic knee may also help appreciate differences in joint space width, bone density, physeal fractures, soft tissue swelling, and osteophyte formation.

Figure 4–8. *A,* **Posterior sag test for the PCL.** *B,* In the Godfrey test, the tibia sags posteriorly when the hip and knee are flexed at 90 degrees, indicating PCL damage. Gravity causes the proximal tibia to sag posteriorly and the normal contour of the bone is lost. *C,* To rule out associated injuries of the posterolateral corner (arcuate complex) and posteromedial corner, the physician evaluates axial rotation. An assistant stabilizes the patient's femurs while the physician externally rotates the tibias. The test is positive if the injured side demonstrates a greater degree of tibial rotation. *D,* In Loomer's variation on the posterolateral drawer test, the patient lies supine. With the patient's hips and knees in 90 degrees of flexion and the knees together, the examiner grasps and maximally externally rotates the patient's feet. Excessive external rotation in one extremity marks a positive test and is easily seen. The examiner will also note mild posterior displacement or sag of the tibia. (*B,* From Allen AA, Harner CD: When your patient injures the posterior cruciate ligament. J Musculoskel Med 13[2]:44, 1996. Artist: Charles H. Boyter. *C,* from Meislin RJ: Managing collateral ligament tears of the knee. Physician Sports Med 24[3]:90–96,1996; *D,* from Swain RA, Wilson FD: Diagnosing posterolateral rotatory knee instability. Physician Sports Med 21[4]:62–71, 1993.)

A

B

C

Figure 4–9. *A,* **The Lachman test** is the most sensitive maneuver for detecting instability of the ACL. With the patient's knee in 20 to 30 degrees of flexion, the physician stabilizes the femur with one hand and applies an anteriorly directed force to the proximal tibia with the other hand. Increased anterior translation of the tibia (compared with the uninvolved knee) or a soft endpoint, indicates ACL disruption. *B,* Anterior drawer test. The patient lies supine with the knee bent at 90 degrees. The examiner places the patient's thigh over the foot to anchor and pulls forward on the relaxed tibia and assesses the anterior translation and quality of the endpoint. *C,* For the pivot shift test, internal rotation and valgus forces are applied to the nearly fully extended (straight) knee (*top*). If the ACL is torn, the tibia will sublux slightly anterolaterally. As the knee is then flexed to about 40 degrees (*bottom*), the iliotibial band changes from a knee extensor to a flexor and reduces the subluxed tibia, sometimes with an audible clunk—a positive test for an ACL tear. A positive test should not be repeated because of risk to the meniscus. (*A,* From Cameron ML, Mizuno Y, Cosgarea AJ: Diagnosing and managing ACL injuries. J Musculoskel Med 17:47–53, 2000. Artist: Robert Marguiles. *C,* from Rey JM: A proposed natural history of symptomatic ACL knee injuries. Clin Sports Med 7:697–709, 1988.)

In all patients older than 30 years, a **bilateral weight-bearing AP** view should be obtained to look for joint line narrowing indicative of arthritis. Pediatric patients (<20 years old) should have a tunnel view as part of the routine radiographic series to evaluate otherwise occult OCD lesions.

MRI generally is not needed in the routine evaluation of the knee, but may be helpful for evaluation of tumors around the knee. When soft tissue masses are identified or bone involvement is seen on radiographs, MRI can help determine their extent. After acute trauma when the knee

is too painful or swollen for an accurate examination and immediate diagnosis is necessary, MRI is helpful to distinguish between a bone bruise, an articular cartilage injury, and a meniscal tear. It is also effective in determining the extent of possible osteomyelitis or avascular necrosis.

The decision to use MRI or arthroscopy or both probably is best made by the orthopaedic surgeon rather than the referring primary care physician, because MRI may not be necessary if arthroscopy seems warranted (e.g., locked knee, hemarthrosis with an ACL tear, symptomatic

Figure 4–10. McMurray test. Flex the knee maximally. Externally rotate the foot (for medial meniscus) and passively extend the knee, looking for a click or pain medially. (From Hunter-Griffin LY (ed.): Athletic Training and Sports Medicine, 2nd ed. American Academy of Orthopaedic Surgeons, Rosemont, Illinois, 1994.)

loose body, etc.). Several factors should be considered in making this decision. MRI is a noninvasive diagnostic tool. Arthroscopy is invasive, but not only does it confirm or modify the clinical diagnosis, it also has therapeutic capabilities. MRI is expensive and should be used judiciously. It is not required before every arthroscopic examination. In general, a working diagnosis should be made from the history, physical examination, and plain radiographs before arthroscopic examination, and the findings at arthroscopic examination should confirm this diagnosis.

CT is helpful for evaluation for complex, intra-articular fractures, such as tibial plateau fractures, and to characterize bone tumors around the knee.

Arteriograms are helpful when ischemia or claudication may be causing pain around the knee and to rule out vascular injury with acute knee dislocations.

Primary Care Physician Pearls for History and Examination of the Knee

- **Immediate bloody effusion** after acute injury most commonly occurs with intra-articular ligament tears (ACL and PCL, not extraarticular MCL or LCL), fractures about the knee, quadriceps rupture, patellar dislocations (torn medial retinaculum), or peripheral meniscal tears (bleeding from the perimeniscal capillary plexus).
- **Locking** of the knee in flexion with difficulty working it back into full extension is almost pathognomonic for a meniscal tear (often bucket-handle). A dislocated (or subluxed) patella or intra-articular loose body or detached OCD lesion are other likely causes of locking. True locking is almost always an indication for operative intervention (arthroscopy).
- **Gradual onset of anterior knee pain** in young female athletes (patellofemoral pain) is common. This is typically exacerbated by activities involving deep knee flexion (squatting, kneeling, stairs, running, chair to stand). Knee flexion increases patellofemoral joint reaction forces (PFJRFs) (see section on patellofemoral disorders, p. 320).
- **Instability or giving way** of the knee usually is indicative of ligamentous tear (ACL) or quadriceps atrophy (usually postoperative or after chronic effusion or knee injury causing inhibitory feedback to the quadriceps).
- **Pes anserinus bursitis** or **Voshell's bursitis** is a commonly missed cause of **medial** knee pain. Tenderness or inflammation are typically medial, but two to three fingerbreadths below the medial joint line at the pes anserinus tendon insertion.
- The ability to perform an SLR, indicating an intact extensor mechanism, is important in determining whether operative (inability to perform SLR) or nonoperative (ability to perform SLR) treatment of the extensor mechanism is indicated. An inability to perform SLR in a patient with patellar fracture is an indication for operative fixation of a displaced fracture (see Patella Fractures section).
- **Chondromalacia** is a pathologic description of fissuring and changes in the articular cartilage of the knee (such as in the patella or weight-bearing knee surfaces). Anterior knee pain or patellofemoral joint pain or subluxation is the correct description of findings on physical examination. Using the term "chondromalacia" is incorrect unless the examiner is viewing the articular cartilage during arthroscopic intra-articular examination.

KNEE EXAMINATION

DATE: _____ PATIENT NAME: _____ AGE: _____

	Acct. # _____ Date of Birth _____					NEW C/O ☐
						F/U ☐
VITALS:	BP	Pulse	Temperature	Weight	Height	POST-OP ☐

GENERAL APPEARANCE	CC	ESTABLISHED PATIENT NEW C/O ☐

R   L   Bilateral

GENERAL APPEARANCE

- ☐ NAD
- ☐ ASA
- ☐ Obese
- ☐ Normal Weight
- ☐ O x 3
- ☐ Oriented times

_____

☐ # OF WEEKS POST-OP

REVIEW OF SYSTEMS:

CHANGES IN INTERIM:

YES ☐
_____
_____
_____
_____
_____

NO ☐

Exacerbating Activities:
_____ Stairs
_____ Squatting
_____ Standing
_____ Kneeling
_____ Twisting
_____ Running
_____ Night
Other _____
_____
_____
_____

X-rays on Return:

Relieving Factors:
_____ Ice
_____ NSAIDS
_____ Rest
Other _____
_____
_____
_____

Subjective	Acute Trauma ☐	Insidious Onset ☐	Chronic ☐	Other ☐

Symptoms	Popping ☐	Catching ☐	Stiff ☐	Worsening ☐
	Locking ☐	Swelling ☐	Limping ☐	Improving ☐
	Unstable ☐	Warmth ☐	Night Pain ☐	Movie Theater Sign ☐

INITIALS:	Page 1 of 3

Knee encounter form—Brotzman

KNEE EXAMINATION

DATE: _____   PATIENT NAME: _____   AGE: _____

_____   _____

Location of Symptoms		

☐ Anterior   ☐ Medial   ☐ Posterior   ☐ Pes Anserinus

☐ Patellofemoral   ☐ Lateral   ☐ Diffuse   ☐ Tibial Tubercle

Referred From: ☐ Prepatellar Bursa   ☐ Other _____

_____

Swelling at Time of Injury   None ☐   Swollen within 2 hours ☐   Swollen > 2 hours ☐   Bruising ☐

Exam

Effusion: None   1   2   3

ROM: _____   * Extension/full

_____   * Flexion/full

Hip Exam: Normal ☐   Pain on Internal Rotation ☐

Aspirated Knee ☐   Blood _____ Purulent Material   Serous _____ _____ cc

Patello-femoral

Patellar Mobility: ☐ Tight   ☐ Normal   ☐ Excess.

Patellar Maltracking ☐
Q-Angle Increased ☐
Pes Planus ☐
VMO Atrophy ☐
Crepitance ☐
Positive Apprehension Test ☐

↑ _____ Medial or _____ Lateral Guide (check one)

Flexibility: Quad   Ober's ☐   Hamstring ☐

Positive Patellat Tilt ☐   Palpable Plica ☐

General Ligamentous Laxity ☐

Lateral Patellar Subluxation ☐

J-sign ☐   Leg Lift: Can Do ☐   Cannot Do ☐

Pulses of Foot: Two ☐   One ☐   Absent ☐

X-Rays: ☐ Normal   ☐ No Fracture

Arthritis: ☐ Mild   ☐ Moderate   ☐ Severe

Joint Line

Tender:
MedialJoint Line ☐
Lateral Joint Line ☐
Patellofemoral ☐
Posterior ☐

☐ Mild Tenderness

☐ Moderate Tenderness

☐ Severe Tenderness

☐ Medial Joint Line
☐ Lateral Joint Line
☐ Tricompartmental
☐ Patellofemoral
☐ Other _____

MRI Results _____
_____
_____

Other Three Extremities:

• Alignment   OK ☐
Other: _____

• ROM   OK ☐
Other: _____

• Stability   OK ☐
Other: _____

• Strength/Tone   OK ☐
Other: _____

INITIALS: _____   Page 2 of 3

KNEE EXAMINATION

DATE: _____   PATIENT NAME: _____   AGE: _____

Diagnosis: _____

Meniscus	McMurray's Sign:	Diagnosis:	**ACL**	☐	**PCL**	☐

McMurray's Sign:
Positive ☐   Negative ☐
Pain on McMurray's ☐
Medial ☐   Lateral ☐

Diagnosis: **ACL** ☐   **PCL** ☐
Medial Meniscal Tear   Lateral Meniscal Tear
MCL Injury   Internal Derangement

Ligaments

ACL (Stability)

Lachman's Sign:
Positive ☐   Negative ☐
Mushy ☐   Cannot Relax ☐
Pivot Shift:
Positive ☐   Negative ☐
Anterior Drawer:
Positive ☐   Negative ☐

PLAN:
1. NSAID _____
2. PT _____
3. Rest
4. MRI ☐   BONE SCAN ☐   CT ☐
5. Injection today ☐   Follow up Injection
6. Surgery _____
7. Palumbo ☐   8. McConnell ☐   9. Orthotics ☐
10. ☐   Low Impact/↓PFJRFs
    ☐   Activity Modification   Other: _____
    ☐   Conservative Measures   _____
    ☐   Observation   _____

Collateral Ligaments

MCL   At 0°   Stable 1 2 3
       At 30°   Stable 1 2 3
LCL   At 0°   Stable 1 2 3
       At 30°   Stable 1 2 3

PCL

Posterior Drawer:
Positive ☐   Negative ☐

Posterior Sag:
Positive ☐   Negative ☐

Quadriceps Girth: L is _____ centimeters   Symmetric ☐
                     R is _____ centimeters   Atrophy

Standing Alignment   ☐ Genu Valgum   ☐ Genu Varum   ☐ Normal   ☐ Recurvatum

Gait	Limp ☐ Normal Gait ☐ Other _____

Skin	Normal ☐ Shiny ☐ Warm ☐ Bruised ☐ Erythematous ☐

Work Status

Work Duty:
Full ☐
Light ☐
None ☐
Clerical ☐

Restrictions:
No Squatting ☐
No Bending ☐
No Lifting Over ☐ lbs.
No Ladders   Other _____

No Climbing ☐
No Pulling ☐
No Pushing ☐

Length of Restrictions:
Until Next Office Visit ☐
_____ Weeks
_____ Months
_____ Pending

☐   Return Visit: 1 2 3 4 5 6 7 8 9 10 11 12 Weeks ☐   Months ☐
We discussed with this patient the natural history of this problem and surgical versus
nonsurgical treatment, as well as what he/she can expect to gain from surgery. We
have also discussed the risks, benefits, and possible complications of surgery at length.

INITIALS:	Page 3 of 3

Figure 4–11. Appley compression test (meniscal test). The prone knee is flexed to 90 degrees. The knee is compressed (pushed downward) while the knee is alternately externally and internally rotated at the foot. Medial pain on external rotation suggests a medial meniscal tear. Lateral pain on internal rotation suggests a probable lateral meniscal tear.

Figure 4–12. Knee injection and aspiration. A lateral approach into the swollen distended suprapatellar pouch (bursa) is used for knee aspiration. (From Goss JA, Adams RF: Local injection of corticosteroids in rheumatic diseases. J Musculoskel Med 10[3]:83–92, 1993. Artist: Peg Gerrity.)

Anterior Cruciate Ligament Injuries

Michael D'Amato, MD, and Bernard R. Bach, Jr., MD

Background

As our understanding of the biology and biomechanics regarding the knee and graft reconstruction techniques has improved, rehabilitation after ACL injury has also changed. In the 1970s, ACL reconstructions were done through large arthrotomies, using extra-articular reconstructions, and patients were immobilized in casts for long periods after surgery. In the 1980s, arthroscopic techniques led to intra-articular reconstructions and eliminated the need for a large arthrotomy, which allowed the use of "accelerated" rehabilitation protocols that focused on early motion. In the 1990s, the concept of "accelerated" rehabilitation evolved in an effort to return athletes to the playing field quicker than ever. With this emphasis on quick return to sports, issues regarding open– and closed–kinetic chain exercises and graft strain have come to the forefront, as has the role of postoperative and functional bracing. In addition, the value of preoperative rehabilitation to prevent postoperative complications has been recognized.

Rehabilitation Rationale

Nonoperative treatment of the ACL-deficient knee may be indicated in older, sedentary people, but in active people, young or old, the ACL-deficient knee has a high incidence of instability, often leading to meniscal tears, articular injury, and subsequent degenerative changes in the knee. Adequate knee function may be maintained in the short term, particularly after hamstring strengthening programs, but this is unpredictable and function is usually below the preinjury level.

Surgical reconstruction of the ACL can now predictably restore the stability of the knee, and rehabilitation is focused on restoring motion and strength while maintaining knee stability by protecting the healing graft and donor site. Aggressive "accelerated" rehabilitation programs have been made possible through advances in graft materials and graft fixation methods and an improved understanding of graft biomechanics and the effects of various exercises and activities on graft strains. Whereas these protocols may ultimately prove to be safe and appropriate, they must be viewed cautiously until continued research into graft healing further delineates the limits to which rehabilitation after ACL reconstruction can be "accelerated."

Protocols for rehabilitation after ACL reconstruction follow *several basic guiding principles*.

- Achieving full ROM and reduction of inflammation and swelling before surgery to avoid arthrofibrosis.

- Early weight-bearing and ROM, with emphasis on obtaining early full extension.
- Early initiation of quadriceps and hamstring activity.
- Efforts to control swelling and pain to limit muscular inhibition and atrophy.
- Appropriate use of open– and closed–kinetic chain exercises, avoiding early open-chain exercises that may shear or tear the weak immature ACL graft (see section on open- and closed-kinetic chain exercises, following).
- Comprehensive lower extremity muscle stretching and strengthening and conditioning.
- Neuromuscular and proprioception retraining.
- Functional training.
- Cardiovascular training.
- Stepped progression based on achievement of therapeutic goals.

Basic Science and Biomechanics

The ACL is the primary restraint to anterior translation of the tibia and a secondary restraint to tibial rotation and to varus and valgus stress. An intact ACL resists forces up to **2500 N** and strain of about 20% before failing. Older ACLs fail under lower loads than younger ACLs. The forces placed on an intact ACL range from about 100 N during passive knee extension to about 400 N with walking and 1700 N with cutting and acceleration-deceleration activities. Loads exceed the ACL's failure capacity only with unusual combinations of loading patterns on the knee.

Graft Material Properties

The central third bone–patellar tendon bone graft has an initial failure strength of up to **2977 N**, and the strength of a quadrupled semitendinosis–gracilis graft complex has been estimated as high as **4000 N**. However, these strengths are greatly reduced after surgical implantation. Current thought is that the initial graft strength must exceed that of the normal ACL to maintain sufficient strength, because strength is lost during the healing phase, and that a stronger graft will allow for a safer rehabilitation and return to activity.

Graft Healing

After implantation, ACL grafts undergo sequential phases of avascular necrosis, revascularization, and remodeling. The graft material properties change as the process of *ligamentization* proceeds. Ultimate load to failure in a patellar tendon autograft can drop as low as 11% of the normal ACL, and the graft stiffness can fall to as low as 13% of the normal ACL during graft maturation. **Data on human grafts indicate that implanted grafts begin to re-** semble a native ACL structure as early as 6 months after implantation, but that final maturation does not occur until after 1 year.

Graft Fixation

In the first 6 to 12 weeks of rehabilitation, the fixation of the graft rather than the graft itself is the limiting factor for strength in the graft complex. The exercises and activities used in rehabilitation during this time must be carefully chosen so as not to exceed the ability of the fixation to resist graft slippage.

For **central third–patellar tendon grafts,** interference screw fixation of the bone blocks in the femoral and tibial tunnels has been shown to exceed **500 N** for both metallic and bioabsorbable screws. Graft slippage has not been a problem with this construct.

With **hamstring grafts,** soft tissue fixation and graft slippage vary greatly depending on the fixation (Fig. 4–13). The strongest fixation, with the least amount of graft slippage, is with soft tissue washers, which can provide a construct strength above **768 N**. Interference screw fixation has not been as successful, with yield strengths less than 350 N and graft slippage or complete fixation failure with low-level loading.

Open– and Closed–Kinetic Chain Exercise

Considerable debate has occurred in recent years regarding the use of closed–kinetic chain activity versus open–kinetic chain activity after ACL reconstruction (see Glossary for definition of open- and closed-chain exercises). An example of an open–kinetic chain exercise is the use of a leg extension machine (Fig. 4–14). An example of closed–kinetic chain exercise is the use of a leg press machine (Fig. 4–15). **In theory, closed–kinetic chain exercises provide a more significant compression force across the knee while activating cocontraction of the quadriceps and hamstring muscles.** It has been suggested that these two factors help decrease the anterior shear forces in the knee that would otherwise be placed upon the maturing ACL graft. Because of this, closed–kinetic chain exercises have been favored over open– kinetic chain exercises during rehabilitation after ACL reconstruction. However, the literature supporting this theory is not definitive. Many common activities cannot be clearly classified as open– or closed–kinetic chain, which adds to the confusion. Walking, running, stair climbing, and jumping all involve a combination of open– and closed–kinetic chain components to them.

Jenkins and colleagues (1997) measured side-to-side difference in anterior displacement of the tibia in subjects with unilateral ACL-deficient knees during open–kinetic chain exercise (knee extension) and closed–kinetic chain exercises (leg press) at 30 and 60 degrees of knee flexion

Figure 4–13. *A–F,* Hamstring ACL graft fixation methods. Femoral Endo button fixation with a variety of tibial fixation methods. (*A–F,* From Steiner ME, Kowalk DL: Anterior cruciate ligament reconstruction using hamstrings for a two-incision technique. In Drez D Jr, DeLee JC [eds]: Oper Tech Sports Med 7:172–178, 1999.)

and concluded that **open-chain exercises at low flexion angles may produce an increase in anterior shear forces, that may cause laxity in the ACL.**

Side-to-side Difference in Anterior Displacement

	30 degrees knee flexion (mm)	60 degrees knee flexion (mm)
Open–kinetic chain (knee extension)	4.7	1.2
Closed–kinetic chain (leg press)	1.3	20.1

(3–5 mm = abnormal; >5 mm = arthrometric failure)

Yack and colleagues (1993) also found increased anterior displacement during open–kinetic chain exercise (knee extension) compared with closed–kinetic chain exercise (parallel squat) through a flexion range of 0 to 64 degrees. Kvist and Gillquist (1999) demonstrated that displacement occurs with even low levels of muscular activity: generation of the first 10% of the peak quadriceps torque produced 80% of the total tibial translation seen with maximal quadriceps torque. Mathematical models also have predicted that shear forces on the ACL are greater with open-chain exercises. Jurist and Otis (1985), Zavetsky and coworkers (1994), and Wilk and Andrews (1993) all noted that changing the position of the resistance pad on isokinetic open–kinetic chain devices could modify anterior shear force and anterior tibial displacement. Wilk and Andrews also found greater anterior tibial displacements at slower isokinetic speeds.

Beynnon and associates (1997) used implanted transducers to measure the strain in the intact ACL during various exercises and found no consistent distinction between closed–kinetic chain and open–kinetic chain activities.

Rank Comparison of Peak Anterior Cruciate Ligament Strain Values during Commonly Prescribed Rehabilitation Activities

Rehabilitation Activity	Peak Strain (%)	Number of Subjects
Isometric quads contraction at 15 degrees (30 Nm of extension torque)	4.4	8
Squatting with Sport Cord	4.0	8
Active flexion-extension of the knee with 45 N weight boot	3.8	9
Lachman test (150 N of anterior shear load)	3.7	10
Squatting	3.6	8
Active flexion-extension (no weight boot) of the knee	2.8	18
Simultaneous quads and hams contraction at 15 degrees	2.8	8
Isometric quads contraction at 30 degrees (30 Nm of extension torque)	2.7	18
Anterior drawer (150 N of anterior shear load)	1.8	10
Stationary bicycling	1.7	8
Isometric hamstring contraction at 15 degrees (to −10 Nm of flexion torque)	0.6	8
Simultaneous quadriceps and hamstring contraction at 30 degrees	0.4	8
Passive flexion-extension of the knee	0.1	10
Isometric quadriceps contraction at 60 degrees (30 Nm of extension torque)	0.0	8
Isometric quadriceps contraction at 90 degrees (30 Nm of extension torque)	0.0	18
Simultaneous quadriceps and hamstring contraction at 60 degrees	0.0	8
Simultaneous quadriceps and hamstring contraction at 90 degrees	0.0	8
Isometric hamstring contraction at 30, 60, and 90 degrees (to −10 Nm of flexion torque)	0.0	8

From Beynnon BD, Fleming BC; Anterior cruciate ligament strain in-vivo: A review of previous work. J Biomech 31:519-525, 1998.

This finding contradicts the previous studies, and indicates that certain closed-chain activities, such as squatting, may not be as safe as the mathematical force models would predict, particularly at low flexion angles.

A *protective effect of the hamstrings has been suggested based on the findings of minimal or absent strain in the ACL with isolated hamstring contraction or when the hamstrings were simultaneously contracted along with the quadriceps.* Cocontraction of the quadriceps and hamstrings occurs in closed–kinetic chain exercises, with a progressive decrease in hamstring activity as the flexion angle of the knee increases. Cocontraction does not occur to any significant degree during open–kinetic chain exercise.

Other differences between open– and closed–kinetic chain exercise have been demonstrated. Closed–kinetic chain exercises generate greater activity in the vasti musculature, and open–kinetic chain exercises generate more rectus femoris activity. Open-chain activities generate more isolated muscle activity and thus allow for more specific muscle strengthening. However, with fatigue, any stabilizing effect of these isolated muscles may be lost and can put the ACL at greater risk. Closed-chain exercises, by allowing agonist muscle activity, may not provide

Figure 4–14. Example of an open-kinetic chain exercise (leg extension).

Figure 4–15. Example of a closed-kinetic chain exercise (leg press).

focused muscle strengthening, but may provide a safer environment for the ACL in the setting of fatigue.

In summary, closed-chain exercises can be used safely during rehabilitation of the ACL because they appear to generate low anterior shear force and tibial displacement through most of the flexion range, although some evidence now exists that low flexion angles during certain closed–kinetic chain activities may strain the graft as much as open-chain activities and may not be as safe as previously thought. At what level strain becomes detrimental and whether some degree of strain is beneficial during the graft healing phase are currently unknown. Until these answers are realized, current trends have been to recommend activities that minimize graft strain, so as to put the ACL at the lowest risk for developing laxity. Open-chain flexion that is dominated by hamstring activity appears to pose little risk to the ACL throughout the entire flexion arc, **but open-chain extension places significant strain on the ACL, as well as the patellofemoral joint, and should be avoided.**

Rehabilitation Considerations after ACL Reconstruction

Pain and Effusion

Pain and swelling are common after any surgical procedure. Because they cause reflex inhibition of muscle activity and thus postoperative muscle atrophy, it is important to control these problems quickly to facilitate early ROM and strengthening activities. Standard therapeutic modalities to reduce pain and swelling include cryotherapy, compression, and elevation.

Cryotherapy is commonly used to reduce pain, inflammation, and effusion after ACL reconstruction. Cryotherapy acts through local effects, causing vasoconstriction, which reduces fluid extravasation; inhibiting afferent nerve conduction, which decreases pain and muscle spasm; and preventing cell death, which limits the release of chemical mediators of pain, inflammation, and edema. Complications such as superficial frostbite and neuropraxia can be prevented by avoiding prolonged placement of the cold source directly on the skin. *Contraindications* to the use of cryotherapy include hypersensitivity to cold, such as Raynaud's phenomenon, lupus erythematosus, periarteritis nodosa, and rheumatoid arthritis.

Motion Loss

Loss of motion is perhaps the most common complication after ACL reconstruction. Loss of extension is more common than loss of flexion **and is poorly tolerated.** Loss of motion can result in anterior knee pain, quadriceps weakness, gait abnormalities, and early articular degenerative changes. **A number of factors can cause loss of motion after ACL reconstruction** (Schelbourne et al., 1996a):

- Arthrofibrosis, infrapatellar contracture syndrome, patella infera.
- Inappropriate ACL graft placement or tensioning.
- "Cyclops" syndrome.
- Acute surgery on a swollen inflamed knee.
- Concomitant MCL repair.
- Poorly supervised or poorly designed rehabilitation program.
- Prolonged immobilization.
- RSD.

Prevention is the first and most effective method of treatment for loss of motion after surgery. Many of the factors leading to loss of knee motion can be prevented with proper surgical timing and technique.

Anterior placement of the tibial tunnel and inadequate notchplasty both can lead to impingement of the graft on the roof of the intercondylar notch with a subsequent loss of extension (Fig. 4–16). Anterior femoral tunnel placement may lead to increased graft tension in flexion with subsequent limitation of flexion. Inappropriate tensioning of the graft may overconstrain the knee and also lead to difficulty regaining terminal motion. Inadequate notch preparation and ACL stump débridement may predispose the patient to formation of a fibroproliferative scar nodule, called a **"cyclops" lesion,** which may impinge anteriorly in the knee causing pain and limiting extension (Fig. 4–17). Symptoms suggestive of a cyclops lesion include loss of extension and a large, painful clunk on attempted terminal extension of the knee.

ACL reconstruction should be delayed until the acute posttraumatic inflammation and swelling have subsided, full ROM

Figure 4–16. ACL graft impingement as a result of an anterior tibial tunnel placement.

Figure 4–17. "Cyclops" lesion. A fibroproliferative scar nodule (Cyclops) causing a popping or clunking noted on extension of the knee. Cyclops lesions typically occur after inadequate débridement of soft tissue at the tibial plateau interface with the tibial tunnel.

has returned, and the patient has regained strong quadriceps activation.

To meet these goals, preoperative rehabilitation should be started shortly after injury. Modalities to control pain and swelling, such as cryotherapy, elevation, compression, and anti-inflammatory medication, are helpful in eliminating reflex muscular inhibition of the quadriceps. Quadriceps setting, SLR, and closed-chain exercises, accompanied by electrical muscle stimulation and biofeedback, are useful to reactivate the lower extremity musculature, prevent atrophy, and promote strength gain. Proprioception activities can also be started to improve neuromuscular retraining. Activities to increase motion, aided by modalities such as prone hangs, wall slides, and the use of extension boards, are also used in the preoperative period.

There is no single time frame (such as 3 weeks) for surgical delay to avoid postoperative arthrofibrosis. The condition of the patient's knee rather than any predeter-

mined waiting period determines the appropriate timing for surgery. Less motion loss and faster return of quadriceps strength have been reported when surgery was delayed until motion was restored. **Early ACL reconstruction, before return of motion and "cooling" of the knee, increases the risk of postoperative arthrofibrosis.**

Early passive and active ROM are begun immediately after surgery and may be augmented with the use of a continuous passive motion (CPM) machine. Postoperative immobilization increases the risk that later manipulation will be required to regain motion. Control of pain and swelling, early reactivation of the quadriceps musculature, and an early return to weight-bearing all improve the return of motion. Patellar mobilization techniques should be started to prevent patellar tendon shortening or retinacular contracture, both of which can lead to motion loss.

The most important immediate goal is to obtain and maintain full knee extension almost immediately after surgery.

Knee flexion to 90 degrees should be achieved by 7 to 10 days after surgery. Failure to do so should prompt the early initiation of countermeasures to prevent a chronic problem from occurring. These are discussed in detail in the complications/troubleshooting section.

Continuous Passive Motion

The efficacy of CPM after ACL reconstruction is controversial (Fig. 4–18). Historically, its use was advocated to improve cartilage nutrition and limit motion loss during a time when immobilization was common after surgery. With the growing popularity of accelerated rehabilitation emphasizing early motion and weight-bearing, the benefits of CPM have waned. Few recent studies have demonstrated a significant long-term benefit of CPM. We currently do not believe the added cost is justified by any short-term benefit and, since 1993, have not routinely recommended the use of CPM. However, there is a role for CPM after manipulation and arthroscopic surgery in patients who have developed arthrofibrosis.

Figure 4–18. Continuous passive motion (CPM) machine.

Weight-bearing Status

Theoretical advantages of weight-bearing include improved cartilage nutrition, decreased disuse osteopenia, reduced peripatellar fibrosis, and quicker quadriceps recovery. Tyler and colleagues (1998) showed that immediate weight-bearing reduced muscle inhibition at the knee joint in the early postoperative period, as demonstrated by an increased return of electromyographic (EMG) activity in the vastus medialis oblique (VMO) muscle within the first 2 weeks after surgery. They also demonstrated a reduction in the development of anterior knee pain in patients who began immediate weight-bearing. No differences in knee laxity, ROM, or functional scores were noted between weight-bearing and non–weight-bearing groups.

One theoretical concern about weight-bearing in the first 4 to 6 weeks after surgery is donor site morbidity in patients in whom a bone–patellar tendon–bone autograft is used. The frequency of proximal tibial fracture, patellar fracture, and patellar tendon rupture in association with weight-bearing is unknown at this time, but certainly is less than 1%. Although rare, these complications can be difficult to treat and can lead to poor results.

We currently recommend maintaining the knee in a brace locked in full extension during ambulation for the first 4 to 6 weeks after surgery to limit the forces transmitted through the extensor mechanism and to protect the extensor mechanism if the patient slips or falls.

Note: The editors maintain the knee locked in full extension during ambulation for only 2 to 3 weeks.

Muscle Training

The early initiation of muscle training is crucial to prevent muscle atrophy and weakness. *Electrical muscle stimulation* may be helpful to initiate muscle activation in patients who are unable to voluntarily overcome reflex inhibition. *Biofeedback* (such as VMO biofeedback) can be used to enhance the force of muscular contraction. Weight-bearing has also been shown to be beneficial in promoting muscle reactivation. *Muscle balance*, achieving the appropriate hamstring-to-quadriceps ratio, improves dynamic protection of the ACL. Barratta and colleagues (1988) reported an increased risk of injury with reduced hamstring antagonist activity and demonstrated improved coactivation ratios in response to exercise. *Fatigue* has been shown to significantly affect not only the strength of muscular contraction but also the electromechanical response time and rate of muscular force generation. Because deficits in these critical elements of dynamic knee stabilization reduce the ability to protect the knee during activity, endurance training should be included in the rehabilitation program.

Electrical Muscle Stimulation and Biofeedback

Electrical muscle stimulation (Fig. 4–19) and biofeedback (Fig. 4–20) may be useful as adjuncts to conven-

Figure 4–19. Electrical stimulation of the quadriceps.

tional muscle training techniques. Although there is no convincing evidence that *electrical muscle stimulation* alone is superior to voluntary muscle contraction alone in promoting muscle strength after surgery, it may be of benefit in the early postoperative period when reflex inhibition of the quadriceps owing to pain and swelling prevents the initiation of voluntary muscle activity. Anderson and Lip-

Figure 4–20. Electromyographic biofeedback of the vastus medialis oblique muscle.

scomb (1989) noted a positive effect of electrical muscle stimulation in limiting quadriceps strength loss and patellofemoral crepitus after ACL reconstruction. **The most appropriate use of electrical muscle stimulation seems to be in combination with volitional muscle activity in the early postoperative period.**

Biofeedback may be useful for reeducation of the muscles. Using EMG monitoring, a visual or auditory signal is provided to the patient when a preset threshold of muscle activity is achieved. The threshold limits can be modified as the patient progresses. Through the use of positive "rewards," biofeedback encourages increased muscular contraction, which is beneficial during strength training. It can also promote the improved timing of muscle activation, which in turn benefits dynamic stabilization of the knee.

Proprioception

The role of the ACL in proprioception of the knee is still under investigation. Altered proprioception has been reported to reduce the effectiveness of the individual to protect the knee and perhaps predispose the ACL to repetitive microtrauma and ultimately failure. Patients with ACL-deficient knees have been shown to have decreased proprioceptive abilities, which in turn has a detrimental effect on the dynamic hamstring stabilization reflex. Differences in proprioception have been demonstrated in asymptomatic and symptomatic patients after ACL injury, and a relationship between proprioception and outcome after ACL reconstruction has been noted. The mechanism by which rehabilitation after ACL reconstruction has a beneficial effect on improving proprioception is not clear. However, improvement has been shown in both ACL-reconstructed and ACL-deficient patients after proprioceptive training programs.

Lephart and coworkers (1992 and 1998) recommended a program designed to affect all three levels of neuromuscular control. *Higher brain center control* is developed through conscious, repetitive positioning activities, which maximize sensory input to reinforce proper joint stabilization activity. *Unconscious control* is developed by incorporating *distraction techniques* into the exercises, such as the addition of ball throwing or catching while performing the required task (Fig. 4–21).

To improve *brain stem control*, balance and postural maintenance activities are implemented, beginning with visual activities with the eyes open and progressing to exercises with the eyes closed to remove the visual input. The rehabilitation program also includes a progression of activities from stable to unstable surfaces and from bilateral to unilateral stance.

To enhance proprioceptive control at the *spinal level*, activities involving sudden changes in joint position are used. Plyometric activities and rapid movement exercises on changing surfaces improve the reflex dynamic stabilization arc.

Figure 4–21. Distraction technique to develop unconscious control. Mini-tramp, single-leg balance during ball toss.

ACL Bracing

The effectiveness of and need for bracing after ACL reconstruction are controversial. Two forms of braces are currently in use, *rehabilitation* (transitional) braces (Fig. 4–22A) and *functional* braces (Fig. 4–22B). Rehabilitation braces are used in the early postoperative period to protect the donor site while ROM, weight-bearing, and muscle activity are initiated. Functional braces are used when the patient returns to strenuous activity or athletics to provide increased stability to the knee and to protect

Figure 4–22. *A*, Transitional ACL rehabilitation brace. *B*, Functional knee brace (ACL).

the reconstructed ligament while it matures. **The efficacy of prophylactic functional bracing preventing reinjury after graft maturation has not been supported in the literature and is not recommended.** Beynnon and associates (1997) demonstrated a protective effect from bracing under low-level loading conditions, but this effect was diminished with progressively increasing loads. Bracing has been shown to increase quadriceps atrophy and inhibit the return of quadriceps strength after surgery. These effects appear to resolve once brace use is discontinued.

No long-term benefits of bracing on knee laxity, ROM, or function have been demonstrated.

We currently recommend use of a drop-lock rehabilitation brace for the first 4 to 6 weeks after surgery. The brace is locked in extension during sleep to prevent potential loss of extension, and for patients with bone–patellar tendon–bone autografts, it is locked in extension during weight-bearing to protect the extensor mechanism. The brace is removed or unlocked several times a day during ROM and non–weight-bearing exercises. We believe that the risk of postoperative patellar fracture or patellar tendon rupture, although rare, outweighs the cost and inconvenience of transitional brace use.

Gender Issues

In recent years, a tremendous increase in women's participation in athletics has made it apparent that **women are at an increased risk for ACL injury.** A number of differences between women and men have been hypothesized as possible causes for this increased susceptibility.

Specific rehabilitation modifications may help to compensate for these anatomic, neuromuscular, and flexibility differences and should be incorporated into the standard protocol being used.

The *anatomic differences* (a wider pelvis, increased genu valgum, increased external tibial torsion, and under-developed musculature) place a woman's ACL at an inherent mechanical disadvantage, especially during jumping activities when increased rotational forces at landing may overload the ligament.

Among the differences in *neuromuscular characteristics* of men and women is a decreased ability in women to generate muscular force, even when corrections are made for size differences. This limits the ability to resist displacing loads through dynamic stabilization of the knee. Other differences in dynamic knee stabilization that place women at greater risk for ACL injury include slower muscle activation and force generation, and the recruitment of the quadriceps muscles rather than the hamstrings or gastrocnemius muscles. An inherently lower hamstring-to-quadriceps muscle ratio may further strain the ACL.

Women have greater *laxity* than men. There may be a hormonal basis for this difference because changes in laxity have been documented during the menstrual cycle. As a result, women have increased hyperextension at the knee, placing the knee in a less favorable position for the hamstrings to generate a protective force. Women also generate less dynamic knee stability than men in response to muscle contraction. These factors lead to greater anterior tibial displacement in women and may place the ACL at greater risk for injury.

Hewett and colleagues (1996) developed a *prophylactic training program* designed specifically for women to try to reduce the risk of knee injury. They demonstrated a reduction in landing forces, increased muscle power, and improved hamstring-to-quadriceps ratio with a 6-week training program. They also found that the program, when done before a sport season, significantly reduced the number of knee injuries in women athletes.

Wilk and colleagues (1999) proposed *eight key factors that should be considered during rehabilitation after reconstruction of the ACL in women* and designed a set of specific exercises to counteract problem areas. Another key to avoiding ACL injuries in female athletes is to train the athlete to land from a jump with both knees slightly flexed. This will help avoid a hyperextension mechanism and reduce the risk of ACL injury.

Gender Issues That May Contribute to Increased Risk of ACL Injuries in Females

Anatomic Differences	Muscular and Neuromuscular Differences	Laxity and Range of Motion
Wider pelvis	Diminished muscular force	Greater ROM
Increased flexibility	Dependence on quadriceps muscle for stability	Genu recurvatum
Less well-developed thigh musculature	Longer time to develop force	Increased knee laxity
Narrower femoral notch	Longer electromechanical response time	Increased hip rotation
Smaller ACL		
Increased genu valgum		
Increased external tibial torsion		

From Wilk KE, Arrigo C, Andrews JR, Clancy WG: Rehabilitation after anterior cruciate ligament reconstruction in the female athlete. J Athletic Train 34:177–193, 1999.

Rehabilitation Protocol
Jump-training Program for Prevention of Anterior Cruciate Ligament Injuries in Female Athletes
Hewett

Exercise	Duration or Repetitions by Week	
Phase 1: Technique	**Week 1**	**Week 2**
1. Wall jumps	20 sec	25 sec
2. Tuck jumps*	20 sec	25 sec
3. Broad jump stick (hold) landing	5 reps	10 reps
4. Squat jumps*	10 sec	15 sec
5. Double-legged cone jumps*	30 sec/30 sec	30 sec/30 sec (side-to-side and back-to-front)
6. 180-degree jumps	20 sec	25 sec
7. Bounding in place	20 sec	25 sec
Phase 2: Fundamentals	**Week 3**	**Week 4**
1. Wall jumps	30 sec	30 sec
2. Tuck jumps*	30 sec	30 sec
3. Jump, jump, jump, vertical jump	5 reps	8 reps
4. Squat jumps*	20 sec	20 sec
5. Bounding for distance	1 run	2 runs
6. Double-legged cone jumps*	30 sec/30 sec	30 sec/30 sec (side-to-side and back-to-front)
7. Scissors jump	30 sec	30 sec
8. Hop, hop, stick landing*	5 reps/leg	5 reps/leg
Phase 3: Performance	**Week 5**	**Week 6**
1. Wall jumps	30 sec	30 sec
2. Step, jump up, down, vertical	5 reps	20 reps
3. Mattress jumps	30 sec/30 sec	30 sec/30 sec (side-to-side and back-to-front)
4. Single-legged jumps, distance*	5 reps/leg	5 reps/leg
5. Squat jumps*	25 sec	25 sec
6. Jump into bounding*	3 runs	4 runs
7. Hop, hop, stick landing	5 reps/leg	5 reps/leg

Glossary of Jump-training Exercises

- 180-degree jump: two-footed jump. Rotate 180 degrees midair, hold landing for 2 sec, repeat in reverse direction.
- Bounding for distance: start bounding in place, slowly increase distance with each step, keeping knees high.
- Bounding in place: jump from one leg to the other, straight up and down, progressively increasing rhythm and height.
- Broad jump stick (hold) landing: two-footed jump as far as possible, hold landing for 5 sec.
- Cone jump: double-legged jump with feet together, quickly jump side-to-side over cones, repeat forward and backward.
- Hop, hop, stick landing: single-legged hop, stick second landing for 5 sec, increase distance of hop as technique improves.
- Jump into bounding: two-footed broad jump, land on single leg, then progress into bounding for distance.
- Jump, jump, jump, vertical jump: three broad jumps with vertical jump immediately after landing the third broad jump.
- Mattress jump: two-footed jump on mattress, trampoline, or other easily compressed device, perform side-to-side and back-to-front.
- Scissors jump: start in stride position with one foot well in front of other.
- Single-legged jump, distance: single-legged hop for distance, hold landing (knees bent) for 5 sec.
- Squat jump: standing jump raising both arms overhead, land in squatting position, touching both hands to floor.
- Step, jump up, down, vertical: two-footed jump onto 6- to 8-inch step, jump off step with two feet, then vertical jump.
- Tuck jump: from standing position, jump and bring both knees up to chest as high as possible, repeat quickly
- Wall jump (ankle bounces): with knees slightly bent and arms raised overhead, bounce up and down off toes.

continued

Rehabilitation Protocol
Jump-training Program for Prevention of Anterior Cruciate Ligament Injuries in Female Athletes *(Continued)*

Stretching and Weight-training Program

Stretches[†]	Weight-training Exercises[‡]	Stretches[†]	Weight-training Exercises[‡]
1. Calf stretch with bent knee	1. Abdominal curl	6. Iliotibial band/lower back	6. Bench press
2. Calf stretch with straight knee	2. Back hyperextension	7. Posterior deltoids	7. Latissimus dorsi pull-down
3. Quadriceps	3. Leg press	8. Latissimus dorsi	8. Forearm curl
4. Hamstring	4. Calf raise	9. Pectorals/biceps	9. Warm-down short stretch
5. Hip flexors	5. Pullover		

Note: Before jumping exercises: stretching (15–20 min), skipping (2 laps), side shuffle (2 laps).
During training: Each jump exercise is followed by a 30-sec rest period.
Post-training: cool-down walk (2 min), stretching (5 min), weight training (after 15-min rest).
*These jumps performed on mats.
[†]Stretching consists of three sets of 30 sec each.
[‡]Weight training consists of one set of each exercise, generally 12 repetitions for upper body exercises and 15 repetitions for the trunk and lower body exercise.
From Hewett TE, Lindenfeld TN, Riccobene JV, Noyes FR: The effect of neuromuscular training on the incidence of knee injury in female athletes. Am J Sports Med 27:699–706, 1999.

Factors That Potentially Increase the Risk of ACL Injuries in Female Athletes, and Measures for Prevention

Factor	Measure for Prevention
Females exhibit a wider pelvis and increased genu valgum.	Establish dynamic control of valgus moment at the knee joint.
Female athletes recruit quadriceps muscle to stabilize the knee.	Retrain the neuromuscular pattern for the female athlete to use the hamstrings.
Females generate muscular force more slowly than males.	Train for fast speeds and reaction timing.
Jumping athletes lose hip control on landing.	Train hip and trunk control.
Less developed thigh musculature.	Train the hip musculature to assist in stabilization.
Genu recurvatum and increased knee laxity.	Train athlete to control knee extension (stability position).
Exhibit less effective dynamic stabilization.	Enhance neuromuscular control and protective pattern reflexes.
Poorer muscular endurance rates.	Train female athlete to enhance muscular endurance.

From Wilk KE, Arrigo C, Andrews JR, Clancy WG: Rehabilitation after anterior cruciate ligament reconstruction in the female athlete. J Athletic Train 34:177–193, 1999.

Rehabilitation Protocol
Eight Specific Exercise Drills Used after Anterior Cruciate Ligament Reconstruction in Women
Wilk, Arrigo, Andrews, and Clancy

Hip Musculature to Stabilize Knee

- Lateral step-overs (regular, fast, very slow)
- Step-overs with ball catches
- Step-overs with rotation
- Lateral step-ups on foam
- Dip walk
- Squats (foam) (Balance Master)
- Front diagonal lunges onto foam

Retrain Neuromuscular Pattern Hamstring Control

- Lateral lunges straight
- Lateral lunges
- Lateral lunges with rotation
- Lateral lunges onto foam
- Lateral lunges with ball catches
- Squats unstable pattern
- Lateral lunges jumping
- Lateral unstable pattern
- Coactivation balance through biofeedback
- Slide board
- Fitter (Fitter International, Calgary, Alberta, Canada)

Control Valgus Moment

- Front step-downs
- Lateral step-ups with Thera-Band (The Hygienic Corporation, Akron, Ohio)
- Tilt board balance throws

Control Hyperextension

- Plyometric leg press
- Plyometric leg press with four corners
- Plyometric jumps
  - 1 box
  - 2 boxes

- 4 boxes
- 2 boxes rotation
- 2 boxes with catches
- Bounding drills
- Forward and backward step-over drills

High-speed Training, Especially Hamstrings

- Isokinetics
- Backward lunging
- Shuttle
- Lateral lunges (fast jumps)
- Resistance tubing for hamstrings
- Backward running

Neuromuscular Reaction

- Squats on tilt board
- Balance beam with cords
- Dip walk with cords
- Balance throws
- Balance throws perturbations
- Lateral lunges with perturbations onto tilt board

Less Well-developed Thigh Musculature

- Knee extensor and flexor strengthening exercises
- Squats
- Leg press
- Wall squats
- Bicycling

Poorer Muscular Endurance

- Stair climbing
- Bicycling
- Weight training (low weights, high repetitions)
- Cardiovascular training
- Balance drills for longer durations

From Wilk KE, Arrigo C, Andrews JR, Clancy WG: Rehabilitation after anterior cruciate ligament reconstruction in the female athlete. J Athletic Train 34:177–193, 1999.

Older Patients with Anterior Cruciate Ligament Injuries

An awareness of the health benefits of improved physical fitness has led to an increase in the activity level of the older population and an increase in ACL injuries. Traditionally, ACL injures in older patients were treated nonoperatively, but much better outcomes have been demonstrated with surgical treatment.

Patients older than 35 years do benefit from ACL reconstruction and can expect results comparable with those of younger patients; however, the ACL deficiency must be treated early after injury, before chronic degenerative changes occur.

Results of ACL reconstruction in older patients with long-term, chronic ACL deficiency are not as predictable. Rehabilitation protocols developed specifically for the older population have not been studied, and it is unclear whether modifications in the standard programs are needed. *Patients older than 26 years have been shown to have decreased muscle strength after reconstructive surgery compared with younger patients.* An awareness of this fact and emphasis on quadriceps along with hamstring strengthening may help to improve outcomes in older patients. We routinely offer the option of nonirradiated patellar tendon allografts to patients older than 40 years to further reduce potential extensor mechanism complications.

Effect of Graft Selection on Postoperative Rehabilitation Protocol

We currently use a single rehabilitation protocol after all ACL reconstructions regardless of graft material, with only slight weight-bearing and bracing modification depending on the graft source (see p. 284). The current trend in rehabilitation after ACL reconstruction has been toward an increasingly aggressive restoration of motion and strength, with an accelerated return to sporting activities at 4 months after surgery. A number of prospective studies have demonstrated the efficacy and safety of these accelerated programs for patients with *patellar tendon autografts.*

The benefits of *hamstring grafts* have been cited as decreased donor site morbidity, improved cosmesis, and less residual anterior knee pain. However, questions have arisen regarding fixation strength, residual graft laxity, and the safety of accelerated rehabilitation protocols. Improved fixation methods for soft tissue grafts continue to be developed and currently approach the strength of patellar tendon–bone fixation. Studies comparing patellar tendon autografts with hamstring autografts show a trend toward greater laxity with the use of hamstring grafts, but this has not correlated consistently with a functional deficit. Howell and Taylor (1996) demonstrated the safety of an accelerated rehabilitation protocol with hamstring autografts. They allowed full return to sports at 4 months after brace-free rehabilitation, with clinical results similar to those with patellar tendon autografts. Results did not deteriorate between evaluations at 4 months and 2 years after surgery.

Allografts typically have been reserved for use in multiple ligament injuries or in revision surgery. Initially, fears of disease transmission and questions about weakened structural properties or delayed healing discouraged the use of allografts in primary reconstructions. Advances in screening techniques have virtually eliminated the risk of disease transmission, and the abandonment of ethylene oxide and irradiation for sterilization has resulted in stronger graft properties. The advantages of allografts are no donor site morbidity, larger graft constructs, and shorter surgical time. Although questions about the increased time for graft incorporation in the host remain, comparison studies of nonirradiated, fresh-frozen patellar tendon allografts and patellar tendon autografts have demonstrated few differences in outcomes using similar accelerated rehabilitation protocols.

Anterior Cruciate Ligament Reconstruction with Meniscal Repair

A lack of firm basic science and prospective outcome studies has resulted in a wide array of opinions regarding issues such as immobilization, ROM restrictions, and weight-bearing status after meniscal repair combined with ACL reconstruction. An accelerated return to activities, with immediate weight-bearing and no ROM limitations in the early postoperative period, has had results similar to those with more conservative rehabilitation programs. We have found little justification for modifying the standard rehabilitation protocol after meniscal repair done with ACL reconstruction. Rehabilitation after isolated meniscal repair is discussed separately later in this chapter (see pgs. 290 and 317).

Functional Training

Rehabilitation after ACL reconstruction is focused on the whole athlete to maintain cardiovascular conditioning, proprioception, and muscular coordination with appropriate exercises and activities that are gradually phased into the rehabilitation program. Functional training is also a useful way to maintain the patient's interest during therapy sessions because it takes some of the focus away from the knee and is often perceived as more fun than the standard rehabilitation exercises. The use of aids such as balance boards, mini-tramps, steps, balls, and the pool adds variety, breaks up the "routine" of therapy, and maintains patient motivation. Sport-specific drills can also speed the return of skills patients will need to relearn when they return to their sports after rehabilitation. The activities used in functional training must be appropriate and safe for each recovery phase.

In the early phase of recovery, protection of the healing graft prevents significant lower extremity activities, but upper extremity ergometry and well-leg bicycling can promote aerobic conditioning, and some early proprioception training can begin. As progression to unprotected walking begins, additional proprioception drills can be added, and stair-walking exercises can be started to aid in retraining the musculature for eccentric loading patterns. When running is safely allowed, more advanced proprioception drills and plyometric exercises can be added. Figure-of-eight pattern running may be started at this time, but should advance slowly, beginning first with large circles at a walking or jogging pace, and progressing to smaller circles at a faster pace as the return of muscular strength and graft healing allow. Cutting and agility drills are added during the late phases of recovery. Sport-specific drills, such as dribbling and shooting drills for basketball and throwing and fielding drills for baseball, are added slowly when safely allowed and become the main focus of the late rehabilitation phases.

Rehabilitation Protocol
Guidelines for Functional Training after Anterior Cruciate Ligament Reconstruction

Phase 1

Aerobic Conditioning
- Upper extremity ergometry.
- Well-leg bicycling.

Proprioception
- Active/passive joint positioning.
- Balancing activities.
- Stable platform, eyes open.
- Stable platform, eyes closed.
- Seated ball throwing and catching.

Phase 2

Aerobic Conditioning
- Advance to two-leg bicycling.
- Continue upper extremity ergometry.

Plyometrics/Eccentric Muscle Training
- Stair walking
  - Up/down, forward/backward

Aquatherapy
- Pool walking.
- Pool jogging (deep-water running).

Proprioception
- Balancing activities.
- Unstable platform (Kinesthetic Ability Trainer [KAT] or Biomechanical Ankle Platform System [BAPS] board) with eyes open/closed.
- Mini-tramp standing.
- Standing ball throwing and catching.

Phase 3

Aerobic Conditioning
- Continue bicycling/upper extremity ergometry.
- Pool running/swimming.
- Stair stepper/elliptical stepper.
- Cross-country skiing machine.

Plyometrics
- Stair jogging.
- Box jumps
  - 6- to 12-inch heights.

Running
- Straight ahead jogging, progressing to running.
- Figure-of-eight pattern.
- Large circles, walking or slow jogging.

Proprioception
- Mini-tramp bouncing.
- Pogoball balancing.
- Lateral slide board.
- Ball throwing and catching on unstable surface.

Phase 4

Aerobic Conditioning
- Continue as above.

Agility
- Start at slow speed, advance slowly.
- Shuttle run.
- Lateral slides.
- Carioca cross-overs.

Proprioception
- Continue as above.
- Add sport-specific activities ($1/4$ to $1/2$ speed).

Running
- Figure-of-eight pattern.
- Small circles, running.

Plyometrics
- Stair running.
- Box jumps
  - 1- to 2-ft height.

Phase 5

Aerobic Conditioning
- Continue as above.

Agility
- Continue as above.
- Cutting drills.

Proprioception
- Reaction drills.
- Advanced sport-specific drills (full speed).

Running
- Continue as above.

Plyometrics
- Advance heights.

Functional Testing after Anterior Cruciate Ligament Reconstruction

After ACL reconstruction and rehabilitation, clinical testing, including strength testing and laxity measurements, does not correlate well with functional ability in all patients. Functional testing was developed to help evaluate surgical and therapeutic outcomes and a patient's readiness to return to unrestricted activity. The most commonly used tests are the single hop for distance, the triple hop for distance, and the 6-m timed hop. Other proposed tests include the vertical jump, the cross-over hop for distance, and the figure-of-eight hop. The literature supporting the reliability and reproducibility of many of the functional tests is limited. No single test has been shown to be adequate for evaluating the dynamic function of the knee, and many surgeons recommend the use of a series of functional tests for testing dynamic function.

Noyes and coworkers (1991a) developed a battery of functional tests consisting of the single hop for distance, the triple hop for distance, the cross-over hop for distance, and the 6-m timed hop (Table 4–2). Independent testing has shown good reliability and reproducibility for

---

Table 4–2

Functional Testing after Anterior Cruciate Ligament Rupture

Rationale: Ruptures of the ACL result in varying amounts of functional limitations of the lower extremity. In order to assess these limitations quantitatively, objective testing under simulated conditions is required. Four one-legged hop function tests were devised. Their effectiveness and sensitivity in detecting limitations was assessed in two studies. These tests should be used with other clinical measuring tools (isokinetic testing, questionnaires) to verify functional limitations.

Methods

One-Legged Single Hop for Distance	One-Legged Timed Hop	One-Legged Triple Hop for Distance	One-Legged Crossover Hop for Distance
The patient stands on one limb, hops as far as possible, and lands on the same limb. The total distance is measured. Each limb is tested twice; the means of each are calculated and used to determine limb symmetry.	The patient hops on one limb a distance of 6 m as fast as possible. The total time to cover the distance is recorded. Each limb is tested twice; the times are calculated to the nearest 0.01 sec with a stopwatch. The means of each limb are calculated and used to determine limb symmetry.	The patient stands on one limb, performs three consecutive hops as far as possible, and lands on the same limb. The total distance hopped is measured; each limb is tested twice. The means of each limb are calculated and used to determine limb symmetry.	A distance of 6 m long with a 15-cm-long strip marked in the center of the floor is designated. The patient hops three consecutive times on one limb, crossing over the center strip on each hop. The total distance hopped is measured; each limb is tested twice. The means of each limb are calculated and used to determine limb symmetry.

Calculation

Limb symmetry = mean score of the involved limb divided by mean score of the noninvolved limb, result is multiplied by 100 involved/noninvolved × 100	Limb symmetry = mean time of the involved limb divided by the mean time of the noninvolved limb, result is multiplied by 100 involved/noninvolved × 100	Limb symmetry = involved/noninvolved × 100	Limb symmetry = involved/noninvolved × 100

Study Results

Normal limb symmetry was determined to be 85%. Approximately one half of the ACL-deficient knees demonstrated abnormal test scores. Results of normals and ACL-deficient knees showed low false-positive and high specificity rates. The indicated test is of value in confirming lower limb limitations. The low sensitivity rates found exclude the use of this test as a screening tool.	Normal limb symmetry was determined to be 85%. Approximately 42–49% of ACL-deficient knees had abnormal scores. Low false-positive and high specificity rates allow the test to be used to confirm lower limb limitations. Low sensitivity rates exclude its effectiveness in screening for limitations.	Data available for 26 ACL-deficient knees only. One half of the patients had abnormal symmetry scores. The low sensitivity rate excludes the test as a screening tool.	Data available for 26 ACL-deficient knees only. Fifty-eight percent of the patients had abnormal symmetry scores. Test showed highest percentage of abnormal symmetry scores compared with the other three; however, the low sensitivity rate does not allow it to be used as a screening test.

Conclusion/summary: The tests designed and the statistical analyses performed in these two studies attempted to correct deficiencies found in previous reports. The data collected on 93 normal knees showed no effect of gender, sports activity level, or dominance on limb symmetry. This allowed an overall normal symmetry limb score to be determined from the population as a whole, which was 85%, and simplified analysis of test scores of ACL-deficient knees. The percentage of ACL-deficient knees that had abnormal symmetry scores increased when the results of the two tests were analyzed versus just one test. Any two tests can be used: An analysis of the six possible two-test combinations failed to reveal that any one combination had a higher sensitivity rate. These tests should be used with other clinical measuring tools (isokinetic testing, questionnaires) to confirm abnormal lower limb symmetry. "Patients with normal symmetry scores should still be considered at risk for giving-way during sports activities."

From Andrews JR, Zarin B, Wilk KE: Injuries in Baseball. Philadelphia, Lippincott-Raven, 1997, p. 44.

this combination of testing. **More recently, it has been suggested that force absorption may be a more important factor in knee function than force production.** Alternative functional tests are being developed and tested, but at this time, the support for these tests is limited. We currently use a battery consisting of the single-leg hop, the timed single-leg hop for 20 feet, and the vertical jump (see p. 280).

Criteria for Return to Sports after Anterior Cruciate Ligament Reconstruction

Correlation between functional testing, clinical testing, and subjective testing methods is poor when evaluating a patient after ACL reconstruction, perhaps because each method evaluates a different aspect of the recovery process. For this reason, we advocate the use of multiple criteria, drawn from each area of evaluation, in determining when a patient can return to full activity.

Criteria for Return to Sports after Anterior Cruciate Ligament Reconstruction

Full ROM

KT-1000 side-to-side difference < 3 mm

Quadriceps strength 85% or more of contralateral side

Hamstring strength 100% of contralateral side

Hamstring-to-quadriceps strength ratio 70% or greater

Functional testing battery 85% or greater compared with contralateral side

- Single-leg hop
- Timed leg hop for 20 ft
- Vertical jump

No effusion

No pain or other symptoms

Complications and Troubleshooting after Anterior Cruciate Ligament Reconstruction

Loss of Motion

Loss of motion is often cited as the most common complication after ACL reconstruction and can result for a number of causes as shown in the next paragraph. The definition of loss of motion varies in the literature. Harner and colleagues (1992) use a loss of knee extension of 10 degrees or knee flexion of less than 125 degrees to define loss of motion, and Shelbourne and coworkers (1996b) define loss of motion as any symptomatic deficit of extension or flexion compared with that of the opposite knee. The term "arthrofibrosis" has been

used when the limitation of motion is symptomatic and resistant to rehabilitative measures. Often, it is used synonymously with loss of motion in the literature.

Shelbourne and coworkers also developed a *classification system for* **arthrofibrosis** *or loss of motion:*

Type 1   ≤10 degrees flexible extension loss and normal flexion; no capsular contracture; anterior knee pain common.

Type 2   >10 degrees fixed extension loss and normal flexion; possibly mechanical block to motion and posterior capsular tightness.

Type 3   >10 degrees extension loss and >25 degrees flexion loss with decreased medial and lateral movement of the patella (patellar tightness).

Type 4   >10 degrees extension loss and ≥30 degrees of flexion loss and patella infera with marked patellar tightness.

Patella infera, or "infrapatellar contracture syndrome" as Paulos and associates (1987) first called it, results from a hypertrophic healing response in the anterior soft tissues of the knee. The exuberant fibrosclerotic tissue entraps and tethers the patella, limiting knee motion. The term "patella infera" refers to the lower position of the affected patella on a lateral radiograph when compared with the uninvolved side (Fig. 4–23). A painful, restricted ROM, inflammation and induration of the peripatellar soft tissues, an extensor lag, and a "shelf sign," which is a step-off between the swollen patellar tendon and the tibial tubercle,

Figure 4–23. Patella infera. Note the lower position of the affected patella on the lateral radiograph.

all should raise the suspicion of a developing patella infera. The most effective prevention or treatment is early quadriceps activity and knee flexion. The quadriceps maintains tension in the patellar tendon, which limits shortening or contracture of the tendon. Knee flexion stretches the tendon and surrounding soft tissues, which also prevents any shortening or contracture from developing.

Prevention of arthrofibrosis is the most effective treatment.

- Full knee extension should be obtained and maintained immediately after surgery.
- Prone heel height side-to-side difference should be less than 5 cm by 7 to 10 days after surgery.

- Knee flexion to 90 degrees should be achieved by 7 to 10 days after surgery.
- Patellar mobility should show steady progression after surgery with proper mobilization techniques.

If any of the criteria are not met, aggressive countermeasures should be implemented to prevent fixed motion loss. To improve extension, prone hangs, an extension board, manual pressure extension against a theraband, and backward walking can be used (Fig. 4–24). To improve flexion, wall and heel slides, supine, prone, or sitting leg hangs, and manual pressure are used (Fig. 4–25). CPM and extension bracing, modalities to control pain and inflammation and to increase quadriceps and ham-

A   B

C   D

Figure 4–24. *A,* Prone extension hangs for gravity-assisted knee extension. Ankle weights may be added to increase the extension movement. *B,* A hyperextension device is used when a patient has difficulty regaining or maintaining extension. The patient lies supine to allow the hamstrings to relax. The patient's heel rests on the elevated cushion, and resistive straps are applied to the front of the knee. As the patient's leg becomes more extended and relaxed, the straps can be adjusted to apply more pressure. The device, which can be used in phases 1, 2, and 3 of rehabilitation, is used for 5–10 min several times a day. *C,* Knee extension against a padded Theraband (starting position). *D,* Knee extension against a Theraband (ending position). (*B,* From Shelbourne D: ACL rehabilitation. Physician Sports Med 28:[1]:31–44, 2000.)

A

B

Figure 4–25. *A,* Wall slides. Place the socked foot or the bare foot on a towel against the wall and slowly lower with gravity to a flexed knee position. *B,* Supine leg hang.

string activity, and the judicious use of cryotherapy, non-steroidal anti-inflammatory drugs (NSAIDs), electrical stimulation, ionophoresis, and phonophoresis are all helpful. If inflammation is prolonged after surgery, we occasionally use a Medrol Dose-Pak.

Surgical intervention is required when the motion loss becomes fixed and progress through nonoperative therapy has reached a plateau. When surgical intervention is necessary, aggressive rehabilitation to gain motion should be slowed to allow reduction of the inflammation in the knee, although strengthening should continue as tolerated. Surgery for arthrofibrosis is contraindicated in an acutely inflamed knee according to some surgeons who believe a better outcome is gained by waiting for the inflammation to resolve.

The first step in *surgical management of arthrofibrosis* is examination of the knee with the patient under anes-

thesia to delineate the extent of motion loss with the patient fully relaxed. Arthroscopy in conjunction with manipulation under anesthesia allows the direct examination of the knee joint to confirm the presence of a cyclops lesion, areas of exuberant scar formation, or other lesions that may be blocking motion. Any abnormal scar tissue or hypertrophic fat pad is débrided. For more severe motion loss, medial and lateral patellar releases may be performed, and an open posterior capsular release may be necessary. Depending on the severity of the arthrofibrosis, multiple manipulations may be required during the arthroscopic procedure to evaluate the progress of the débridement. (Recommended reading for indications and surgical techniques for treatment of arthrofibrosis includes Shelbourne and associates [1996b].)

Rehabilitation must start immediately after surgical resection for arthrofibrosis, with emphasis on maintaining and improving ROM. Particular attention should be given to maintaining extension, before directing efforts toward flexion. An extension brace may be beneficial, particularly in patients with severe arthrofibrosis.

Anterior Knee Pain

Anterior knee pain is another common problem after ACL reconstruction. Symptoms can occur anywhere along the extensor mechanism. It has been suggested that anterior knee pain after ACL reconstruction may be related to the choice of graft material. Whereas the literature remains mixed on this subject, most studies show a significant tendency for a decrease in anterior knee pain with the use of hamstring autografts when compared with patellar tendon autografts. Interestingly, no difference has been noted between patellar tendon autografts and allo-

grafts, suggesting that the relationship between donor site morbidity and anterior knee pain may not be as clear as previously thought.

Early rehabilitation to regain ROM and promote quadriceps control is important in the prevention of patellofemoral symptoms. Patellar mobilization techniques should be included to prevent contracture of the retinacular structures surrounding the patella, which may irritate the patellofemoral joint. For a patient who begins to show signs of anterior knee pain, the rehabilitation program should be modified to eliminate exercises that may place undue stress on the patellofemoral joint. Activities that increase the patellofemoral joint reaction forces (PFJRFs) should be avoided; these include deep squats, Stairmaster use, jogging, and excessive weight during leg presses. Terminal knee extension exercises also often elicit anterior knee pain.

Rehabilitation Protocol
After Anterior Cruciate Ligament Reconstruction
D'Amato and Bach

Phase 1: Weeks 0–2

Goals
- Protect graft fixation.
- Minimize effects of immobilization.
- Control inflammation.
- No CPM.
- Achieve full extension, 90 degrees of knee flexion.
- Educate patient about rehabilitation progress.

Brace
- Locked in extension for ambulation and sleeping (drop-lock brace).

Weight-bearing
- Weight-bearing as tolerated with two crutches.
- Discontinue crutches as tolerated after 7 days (with demonstrated good quadriceps control).

Therapeutic Exercises
- Heel slides/wall slides.
- Quadriceps sets, hamstring sets (electrical stimulation as needed).
- Patellar mobilization.
- Non–weight-bearing gastrocsoleus, hamstring stretches.
- Sitting assisted flexion hangs.
- Prone leg hangs for extension.
- Straight leg raises (SLR) all planes with brace in full extension until quadriceps strength is sufficient to prevent extension lag.
- Phase 1 functional training (see p. 279).

Phase 2: Weeks 2–4

Criteria for Progression to Phase 2
- Good quad set, SLR without extension lag (Fig. 4–26).
- Approximately 90 degrees knee flexion.

Figure 4–26. Straight leg raises. Ankle weights may be added to the ankle or thigh (1–5 pounds) for progressive resistance exercises (PREs).

- Full extension.
- No signs of inflammation.

Goals
- Restore normal gait.
- Restore full ROM.
- Protect graft fixation.
- Improve strength, endurance, and proprioception to prepare for functional activities.

Weight-bearing
- Patellar tendon graft—continue ambulation with brace locked in extension, may unlock brace for sitting and sleeping, may remove brace for ROM exercises.

Rehabilitation Protocol
After Anterior Cruciate Ligament Reconstruction *(Continued)*
D'Amato and Bach

- Hamstring graft and allograft—may discontinue brace use when normal gait pattern and quadriceps control are achieved.

Therapeutic Exercises
- Mini-squats 0–30 degrees.
- Stationary bike (begin with high seat, low tension).
- Closed-chain extension (leg press 0–30 degrees).
- Toe raises.
- Continue hamstring stretches, progress to weight-bearing gastrocsoleus stretches.
- Continue prone leg hangs with progressively heavier ankle weights until full extension is achieved.
- Phase 2 functional training (see p. 279).

Phase 3: Week 6–Month 4

Criteria for Progression to Phase 3
- Normal gait.
- Full ROM.
- Sufficient strength and proprioception to initiate functional activities.
- Stable graft on Lachman and KT1000 testing.

Goals
- Improve confidence in the knee.
- Avoid overstressing graft fixation.
- Protect the patellofemoral joint.
- Progress strength, power, and proprioception to prepare for functional activities.

Therapeutic Exercises
- Continue flexibility exercises as appropriate for patient.
- Advance closed–kinetic chain strengthening (one-leg squats, leg press 0–60 degrees).
- Elliptical stepper, stair stepper.
- Cross-country skiing machine.
- Phase 3 functional training (6–12 wk) (see p. 279).
- Phase 4 functional training (12+ wk).

Phase 4: Month 4

Criteria for Progression to Phase 4
- Full, painless ROM.
- No evidence of patellofemoral joint irritation.
- Sufficient strength and proprioception to progress functional activities (see p. 279).
- Physician clearance to initiate advanced closed–kinetic chain exercises and functional progression.
- Stable graft on Lachman and KT1000 testing.

Goal
- Return to unrestricted activities.

Therapeutic Exercises
- Continue and progress flexibility and strengthening programs.
- Phase 5 functional training (see p. 279).

Phase 5: Return to Sports

Criteria for Progression to Phase 5
- No patellofemoral joint or soft tissue complaints.
- All criteria met for return to sports.
- Physician clearance to resume full activity.

Goals
- Safe return to athletics.
- Maintenance of strength, endurance, and proprioception.
- Patient education concerning any possible limitations.

Brace
- Functional brace may be recommended by physician for use during sports for the first 1–2 yr after surgery for psychological confidence.

Therapeutic Exercises
- Gradual return to sports participation.
- Maintenance program for strength and endurance.
- Agility and sport-specific drills progressed.

Rehabilitation Protocol
After Anterior Cruciate Ligament Reconstruction
Wilk

General Rehabilitation Approach
- Full passive extension immediately after surgery.
- Immediate motion.
- Closed-chain exercises.
- Emphasis on proprioception return and neuromuscular control drills.

- Drop-lock brace locked in extension during ambulation
  - 2 wk for athletes.
  - 3 wk for general orthopaedic patients.
- More gradual progression of flexion
  - Week 1—90 degrees.
  - Week 2—105–115 degrees.

continued

Rehabilitation Protocol
After Anterior Cruciate Ligament Reconstruction *(Continued)*
Wilk

- Week 3—115–125 degrees.
- Week 4—beyond 125 degrees.

If restoration of flexion is too aggressive, swelling often occurs and the regimen is slowed.

- Not all closed-chain exercises produce cocontraction; closed-chain exercises that have been shown to produce actual cocontraction are used early
  - Vertical squats (0–45 degrees).
  - Lateral lunges.
  - Balance drills.
  - Slide board.
  - Fitter.
- Neuromuscular training and proprioception must be incorporated into every phase of the rehabilitation program.
- Progression of proprioception and neuromuscular drills
  - Level 1 drills (immediate after surgery)
    - Joint reproduction, closed–kinetic chain drills, knee sleeve, proprioception drills, weight shifts, and weight distribution.
- Level 2 drills (2–5 wk after surgery)
  - Weight-bearing drills, squats, postural balance drills, single-leg stance, lateral lunges, pool.
- Level 3 drills (5–10 wk after surgery)
  - Plyometrics, agility drills, neuromuscular control drills, perturbations.
- Level 4 drills (10 weeks or more after surgery)
  - Sport-specific training drills and gradual return to play.
- Emphasis is placed on obtaining muscular endurance
  - Fatigued muscles result in increased translation (possible strain or tear of graft).
  - Fatigued muscles also result in diminished proprioception.
- Progression is criteria-based, not time-based.

Rehabilitation Protocol
Accelerated Rehabilitation after Anterior Cruciate Ligament Reconstruction with Central–Third Patellar Tendon
Wilk

Preoperative Phase

Goals
- Diminish inflammation, swelling, and pain.
- Restore normal ROM (especially knee extension).
- Restore voluntary muscle activation.
- Provide patient education to prepare patient for surgery.

Brace
- Elastic wrap or knee sleeve to reduce swelling.

Weight-bearing
- As tolerated with or without crutches.

Exercises
- Ankle pumps.
- Passive knee extension to 0 degrees (Fig. 4–27).
- Passive knee flexion to tolerance.
- SLR: three-way, flexion, abduction, adduction.
- Closed–kinetic chain exercises: 30-degree mini-squats, lunges, step-ups.

Muscle Stimulation
- Electrical muscle stimulation to quadriceps during voluntary quadriceps exercises (4–6 hr/day)

Cryotherapy/Elevation
- Apply ice 20 min of every hour, elevate leg with knee in full extension (knee must be above heart).

Figure 4–27. Passive knee extension to 0 degrees.

Patient Education
- Review postoperative rehabilitation program.

Rehabilitation Protocol
Accelerated Rehabilitation after Anterior Cruciate Ligament Reconstruction with Central–Third Patellar Tendon (Continued)
Wilk

- Review instructional video (optional).
- Select appropriate surgical date.

Phase 1: Immediate Postoperative—Days 1–7
Goals
- Restore full passive knee extension.
- Diminish joint swelling and pain.
- Restore patellar mobility.
- Gradually improve knee flexion.
- Reestablish quadriceps control.
- Restore independent ambulation.

Day 1
Brace
- Transitional hinged brace locked in full extension during ambulation (Protonics Rehab System as directed by physician).

Weight-bearing
- Weight-bearing as tolerated with two crutches.

Exercises
- Ankle pumps.
- Overpressure into full passive knee extension.
- Active and passive knee flexion (90 degrees by day 5).
- SLR (flexion, abduction, adduction).
- Quadriceps isometric setting.
- Hamstring stretches.
- Closed–kinetic chain exercises, 30-degree mini-squats, weight shifts.

Muscle Stimulation
- Used during active muscle exercises (4–6 hr/day).

Continuous Passive Motion
- As needed, 0–45/50 degrees (as tolerated by patient and directed by physician).

Ice and Elevation
- Ice 20 min out of every hour and elevate with knee in full extension (elevated above the heart with pillows below the ankle, not the knee).

Days 2–3
Brace
- EZ Wrap brace/immobilizer, locked at 0-degrees extension for ambulation and unlocked for sitting (or Protonics Rehab System as directed by physician).

Weight-bearing
- As tolerated with two crutches.

Range of Motion
- Brace removed during ROM exercises four to six times a day.

Exercises
- Multiangle isometrics and 90 degrees and 60 degrees (knee extension).

- Knee extension 90–40 degrees.
- Overpressure into extension.
- Ankle pumps.
- SLR (three-way).
- Mini-squats and weight shifts.
- Standing hamstring curls.
- Quadriceps isometric setting.
- Proprioception and balance activities.

Muscle Stimulation
- Continue electrical muscle stimulation 6 hr/day.

Continuous Passive Motion
- 0–90 degrees as needed.

Ice and Elevation
- Ice 20 min of every hour and elevate leg with full knee extension.

Phase 2: Early Rehabilitation—Weeks 2–4
Criteria for Progression to Phase 2
- Quadriceps control (ability to perform good quad set and SLR).
- Full passive knee extension.
- Passive ROM 0–90 degrees.
- Good patellar mobility.
- Minimal joint effusion.
- Independent ambulation.

Goals
- Maintain full passive knee extension.
- Gradually increase knee flexion.
- Decrease swelling and pain.
- Muscle training.
- Restore proprioception.
- Patellar mobility.

Week 2
Brace
- Discontinue at 2–3 wk.

Weight-bearing
- As tolerated (goal is to discontinue crutches 10 days after surgery).

Range of Motion
- Self-ROM stretching exercises four to five times daily, emphasis on maintaining full passive ROM.

KT 2000 Testing
- 15-pound anterior-posterior test only.

Exercises
- Muscle stimulation to quadriceps exercises.
- Isometric quadriceps sets.
- SLR (four planes).
- Leg press (Fig. 4–28).
- Knee extension 90–40 degrees.

continued

Rehabilitation Protocol
Accelerated Rehabilitation after Anterior Cruciate Ligament Reconstruction with Central–Third Patellar Tendon *(Continued)*
Wilk

Figure 4–28. Leg press. Closed-chain exercise.

- Half squats (0–40 degrees).
- Weight shifts.
- Front and side lunges.
- Hamstring curls (Fig. 4–29).
- Bicycling.
- Proprioception training.
- Overpressure into extension.
- Passive ROM 0–50 degrees.
- Patellar mobilization.
- Well-leg exercises.
- Progressive resistance program: start with 1 pound and progress 1 pound per week.

Swelling Control
- Ice, compression, elevation.

Figure 4–29. Prone hamstring curls with a 1- to 5-pound weight.

Week 3
Brace
- Discontinue.

Range of Motion
- Continue ROM stretching and overpressure into extension.

Exercises
- Continue all exercises as in week 2.
- Passive ROM 0–115 degrees.
- Bicycling for ROM stimulus and endurance.
- Pool walking program (if incision is closed).
- Eccentric quadriceps program 40–100 degrees (isotonic only).
- Lateral lunges.
- Lateral step-ups.
- Front step-ups.
- Lateral step-overs (cones).
- Stair-stepper machine or elliptical trainer.
- Progress proprioception drills, neuromuscular control drills.

Phase 3: Controlled Ambulation—Weeks 4–10

Criteria for Progression to Phase 3
- Active ROM 0–115 degrees.
- Quadriceps strength 60% of contralateral side (isometric test at 60 degrees knee flexion).
- Unchanged KT test bilateral values (+1 or less).
- Minimal or no full joint effusion.
- No joint line or patellofemoral pain.

Goals
- Restore full knee ROM (0–125 degrees).
- Improve lower extremity strength.
- Enhance proprioception, balance, and neuromuscular control.
- Restore limb confidence and function.

Brace
- No immobilizer or brace, may use knee sleeve.

Range of Motion
- Self-ROM (four to five times daily using the other leg to provide ROM), emphasis on maintaining 0 degrees passive extension.

KT 2000 Testing
- Week 4, 20-pound anterior and posterior tests.

Week 4
Exercises
- Progress isometric strengthening program.
- Leg press.
- Knee extension 90–40 degrees.
- Hamstring curls.
- Hip abduction and adduction.

Rehabilitation Protocol
Accelerated Rehabilitation after Anterior Cruciate Ligament Reconstruction with Central–Third Patellar Tendon *(Continued)*
Wilk

- Hip flexion and extension.
- Lateral step-overs.
- Lateral lunges.
- Lateral step-ups.
- Front step-downs.
- Wall squats (Fig. 4–30).
- Vertical squats.
- Toe calf raises.
- Biodex Stability System (e.g., balance, squats).
- Proprioception drills.
- Bicycling.
- Stair-stepper machine.
- Pool program (backward running, hip and leg exercises).

Week 6
KT 2000 Testing
- 20- and 30-pound anterior and posterior tests.

Exercises
- Continue all exercises.
- Poor running (forward), agility drills.
- Balance on tilt boards.
- Progress to balance and board throws.

Week 8
KT 2000 Testing
- 20- and 30-pound anterior and posterior tests.

Exercises
- Continue all exercises.
- Plyometric leg press.

Figure 4–30. Thirty-degree wall squats performed with the back against the wall.

- Perturbation training.
- Isokinetic exercises (90–40 degrees) (120–240 degrees/sec.
- Walking program.
- Bicycling for endurance.
- Stair-stepper machine for endurance.

Week 10
KT 2000 Testing
- 20- and 30-pound and manual maximum tests.

Isokinetic Test
- Concentric knee extension-flexion at 180 and 300 degrees/sec.

Exercises
- Continue all exercises.
- Plyometric training drills.
- Continue stretching drills.

Phase 4: Advanced Activity—Weeks 10–16
Criteria for Progression to Phase 4
- Active ROM 0–125 degrees or greater.
- Quadriceps strength 79% of contralateral side.
- Knee extension flexor:extensor ratio 70–75%.
- No change in KT values (comparable with contralateral side, within 2 mm).
- No pain or effusion.
- Satisfactory clinical examination.
- Satisfactory isokinetic test (values at 180 degrees)
  - Quadriceps bilateral comparison 75%.
  - Hamstrings equal bilateral.
  - Quadriceps peak torque–to–body weight ratio.
  - Hamstrings:quadriceps ratio 66–75%.
- Hop test 80% of contralateral leg.
- Subjective knee scoring (modified Noyes system) 80 points or better.

Goals
- Normalize lower extremity strength.
- Enhance muscular power and endurance.
- Improve neuromuscular control.
- Perform selected sport-specific drills.

Exercises
- Continue all exercises.

Phase 5: Return to Activity—Months 16–22
Criteria for Progression to Phase 5
- Full ROM.
- Unchanged KT 2000 test (within 2.5 mm of opposite side).
- Isokinetic test that fulfills criteria.
- Quadriceps bilateral comparison ≥ 80%.
- Hamstring bilateral comparison ≥ 110%.

continued

Rehabilitation Protocol
Accelerated Rehabilitation after Anterior Cruciate Ligament Reconstruction with Central–Third Patellar Tendon (Continued)
Wilk

- Quadriceps torque:body weight ratio ≥ 70%.
- Proprioceptive test 100% of contralateral leg.
- Functional test ≥ 85% of contralateral side.
- Satisfactory clinical examination.
- Subjective knee scoring (modified Noyes system) ≥ 90 points.

Goals
- Gradual return to full unrestricted sports.
- Achieve maximal strength and endurance.
- Normalize neuromuscular control.
- Progress skill training.

Tests
- KT 2000 test.
- Isokinetic.
- Functional.

Exercises
- Continue strengthening exercises.
- Continue neuromuscular control drills.
- Continue plyometrics drills.
- Progress running and agility program.
- Progress sport-specific training.

6- and 12-Month Follow-up
- Isokinetic test.
- KT 2000 test.
- Functional test.

Note: We utilize the **orthovid.com** patient ACL instructional videotape and handout series for these patients. This videotape was produced by the senior author of this book.

Rehabilitation Protocol
Additional Guidelines for Rehabilitation after Anterior Cruciate Ligament Reconstruction
Wilk

After Reconstruction with Concomitant Meniscal Repair
- Immediate motion.
- Immediate weight-bearing.
- Restrictions/limitations
  - No isolated hamstring contraction for 8–10 wk.
  - No squatting past 60 degrees knee flexion for 8 wk.
  - No squatting with rotation or twisting for 10–12 wk.
  - No lunges past 75 degrees knee flexion for 8 wk.
- Return to sports at 5–7 mo.

After Reconstruction Using Contralateral Patellar Graft

Donor Leg
- Cryotherapy, ROM, and gradual strengthening exercises.
- Emphasis on quadriceps strengthening.
- Full ROM usually within 3 wk.

Anterior Cruciate Ligament Reconstructed Knee
- Less painful, faster ROM.
- Quadriceps weakness still present despite contralateral leg graft harvest.

- Rehabilitation same as after use of ipsilateral graft.
- Able to return to sports faster.
- Risk of contralateral knee complications (e.g., RSD).

After Reconstruction and Concomitant Articular Chondral Injury
- Weight-bearing modifications
  - Microfracture technique—toe-touch weight-bearing.
  - Mosaicplasty—non–weight-bearing for 6–8 wk.
- Pool program once wounds are healed (see Aqua-aerobics section).
- Immediate motion—stimulus for articular cartilage healing.
- No excess loading for 3–4 mo.
- Return to sports in 6–9 mo.

Rehabilitation Protocol
After Anterior Cruciate Ligament Reconstruction Using Ipsilateral Autogenous Patellar Tendon Graft
Shelbourne

Time Frame	Goals	Exercises	Comments
Preoperative	Obtain full ROM.	Prone hangs. Hyperextension device (see Fig. 4–24B). Heel slides.	This preoperative rehabilitation approach has decreased the incidence of postoperative ROM problems to <1%.
	Reduce swelling. Achieve good leg control. Maintain good mental attitude. Understand postoperative rehabilitation program.	Cold/compression device. Quad sets, step-ups, bike. Explanation of program.	
Surgery	Intravenous ketoroloc pain prevention program. Both knees moved through full ROM from full hyperextension to flexion with heel touching buttocks. Cold/compression device applied over light sterile dressing.		
Day 1–Week 1	Get the knee into a "quiet state" (decrease inflammation). Minimize hemarthrosis.	Bedrest except for bathroom privileges. Cold/compression; elevation in CPM machine.	
	Full passive hyperextension. Increase flexion to 110 degrees.	Heel prop exercise. Heel slide exercise with use of measuring stick: place stick so that zero is at heel when leg is extended; do heel slide exercise and observe number of centimeters at level of heel.	This measurement gives the patient a point of reference to evaluate improvement.
	Obtain good leg control.	Quadriceps contraction exercises. SLR.	
Weeks 1–2	Maintain hyperextension.	Heel props. Prone hang. Hyperextension device if needed.	
	Increase flexion to 125 degrees.	Heel slide (using measuring stick for reference).	Although physical therapist measures ROM with a goniometer, patient is given a flexion goal that relates to the number of centimeters of bend in the opposite, normal knee.
	Achieve normal gait.	Gait training in front of a mirror.	
	Increase leg strength.	Step-ups. Step-down exercise at low level. Proper gait with stairs.	
	Keep effusion to minimum.	Cold/compression continually as able.	

continued

Rehabilitation Protocol
After Anterior Cruciate Ligament Reconstruction Using Ipsilateral Autogenous Patellar Tendon Graft (Continued)
Shelbourne

Time Frame	Goals	Exercises	Comments
	Resume normal daily activities (school, sedentary work).	If activities cause increased swelling or soreness, reduce activities, elevate the leg, and use the cold/compression cuff more.	
Weeks 2–4	Maintain hyperextension.	Heel props. Prone hangs as needed.	
	Increase flexion to 135 degrees.	Heel slides.	
	Increase leg strength.	Step-down exercise at higher levels (Fig. 4–31). Stationary bike. Stair-climbing machine. Leg extension exercise. Single-leg press. Squats.	Program is designed according to type of equipment available to the patient.
	Maintain minimal effusion.	Adjust activities as needed. Cold/compression several times a day. Elevation as needed.	
Months 1–2	Maintain full ROM.	Check for ROM each morning and perform ROM exercises as needed; should be able to sit on heels.	We have observed that during this time when patients begin to increase activities, terminal flexion may decrease. Patients should monitor this daily.
	Increase leg strength.	Stair-climbing exercise. Stationary bike.	

Figure 4–31. Step-down exercise using a small step.

Rehabilitation Protocol
After Anterior Cruciate Ligament Reconstruction Using Ipsilateral Autogenous Patellar Tendon Graft (Continued)
Shelbourne

Time Frame	Goals	Exercises	Comments
		Single-leg strengthening as needed. Leg press. Squats.	
	Increase proprioception.	Progression of • Functional agility program. • Sport-specific drills (solo). • Sport-specific drills (controlled). • Part-time competition.	The progression of these activities varies according to the patient's individual goals and the sports involved; monitor for swelling and loss of motion.
Months 2 and Beyond	Maintain full ROM.	Monitor daily and perform exercises as needed.	
	Increase leg strength.	Continue strengthening exercises.	Patients sometimes need to be reminded to continue leg strengthening exercises owing to their level of excitement for returning to sports. Time should be devoted to single-leg strengthening to ensure that the patient does not favor the leg with sports activities.
	Increase proprioception.	Sport-specific drills and practice as needed, gradually returning to full participation and contact.	Monitor for swelling or loss of motion.

Posterior Cruciate Ligament Injuries

Michael D'Amato, MD, and Bernard R. Bach, Jr., MD

Information concerning PCL injuries has expanded greatly in the past few years. Despite these advances, significant controversy still exists concerning many aspects of the evaluation and treatment of PCL injuries, especially the natural history of the PCL-injured knee. Our improved understanding of the anatomy and biomechanics of the PCL has led to a more rational and sound basis for the design of rehabilitation programs for treatment both in the nonoperative setting and after surgery.

Rehabilitation Rationale

Normal Posterior Cruciate Ligament

The normal PCL is a complex ligamentous structure with insertions on the posterior aspect of the proximal tibia and the lateral aspect of the medial femoral condyle.

The ligament is composed of two functional bundles, a larger anterolateral bundle, which develops tension as the knee flexes, and the smaller posteromedial bundle, which develops tension in knee extension. **The PCL functions as the primary restraint to posterior translation of the tibia and a secondary restrain to external rotation.**

Mechanism of Injury

Rupture of the PCL is usually caused by a direct blow to the proximal tibia, a fall on the knee with the foot in a plantar-flexed position, or with hyperflexion of the knee (Fig. 4–32). Less common causes include hyperextension or combined rotational forces. Typically, the ligament fails in its midsubstance, but avulsions of the tibial or femoral attachments have been described. The injury may be isolated to the PCL or associated with multiple ligament injuries or knee dislocation. Isolated injuries tend to occur during athletics, and combined injuries are usually the result of high-energy trauma.

Figure 4–32. PCL injury mechanisms. *A,* Direct posterior blow to the anterior aspect of the proximal tibia. *B,* Hyperflexion of the knee with an anterior-directed force on the femur. *C,* Hyperextension of the knee. (*A–C,* From Miller MD, Harner CD, Koshiwaguchi S: Acute posterior cruciate ligament injuries. In Fu FH, Harner CD, Vince KG [eds]: Knee Surgery. Baltimore, Williams & Wilkins, 1994, pp. 749–767.)

Evaluation

A number of tests are available to clinically assess the integrity of the PCL. The *posterior drawer test* at 90 degrees of knee flexion has been shown to be the most sensitive (see Fig. 4–7). Other tests include the *posterior sag test* (see Fig. 4–8), the *quadriceps active test*, and the *reverse pivot shift test* (Fig. 4–33). The rotational stability of the knee must also be evaluated to rule out any associated injury to the posterolateral ligament complex. **One must also be wary when performing a Lachman test in the setting of a PCL injury. It is easy to assume that the anterior translation represents an injury to the ACL, when in fact it may be the tibia returning to a normal position from a previously abnormal posteriorly subluxated position.** The collateral ligaments and menisci should also be appropriately evaluated.

Biomechanical studies have produced several key points that should be considered in the evaluation of PCL injury.

- The PCL is the primary restraint to posterior translation at all positions of knee flexion.
- PCL tear is best detected at 70 to 90 degrees of knee flexion with posterior drawer testing.
- *Isolated* PCL tear does not cause varus-valgus laxity or increased rotation.

- *Isolated* PCL tear and isolated posterolateral corner injury will produce about the same degree of posterior translation at 30 degrees of knee flexion.
- If there is varus or valgus laxity in full extension, by definition there is combined injury to the PCL and collateral complex.
- If the knee hyperextends asymmetrically, there is a combined cruciate and posterolateral corner injury.
- Posterolateral corner injury may produce mild degrees of varus laxity, but more severe degrees of varus laxity indicate PCL injury.
- Combination of PCL tear and posterolateral corner tear produces much more severe posterior translation and external rotation than either injury in isolation.
- It is difficult to have *severe* posterolateral corner instability without injury to the PCL, fibular collateral ligament, *and* popliteus.

Classification

Classification of PCL injuries is based on the relationship of the medial tibial plateau to the medial femoral condyle during a posterior drawer test (Fig. 4–34). *Grade 1* injuries have 0 to 5 mm of posterior translation and maintain the position of the medial tibial plateau anterior to the medial femoral condyle. *Grade 2*

Figure 4–33. Reverse pivot shift test. *A,* With the patient in the supine position, the knee is flexed 90 degrees. External rotation, varus, and axial loads are applied as the leg is extended. With a PCL injury, the lateral tibial plateau will translate from a posterior subluxed position to a reduced position as the leg is extended. *B,* In the reverse pivot shift test, used to identify injury to posterolateral structures, the examiner lifts the patient's leg and stabilizes it with one hand on the heel against the pelvis. The other hand supports the lateral calf with the palm on the proximal fibula. *Left,* In the first step of the test, the patient's knee is flexed to 70 to 80 degrees and the foot is externally rotated, causing the tibia on the injured side to sublux posteriorly. *Right,* In the second step, the examiner extends the patient's leg while applying valgus stress to the knee. The test is positive if the subluxation reduces. A positive test indicates that the PCL, arcuate complex, and fibular collateral ligament are torn. (*A,* From Miller MD, Harner CD, Koshiwaguchi S: Acute posterior cruciate ligament injuries. In Fu FH, Harner CD, Vince KG [eds]: Knee Surgery. Baltimore, Williams & Wilkins, 1994, pp. 749-767; *B,* from Morgan EA, Wroble RR: Diagnosing PCL injuries. Physician Sports Med 25[11]:29–37, 1997.)

A

B

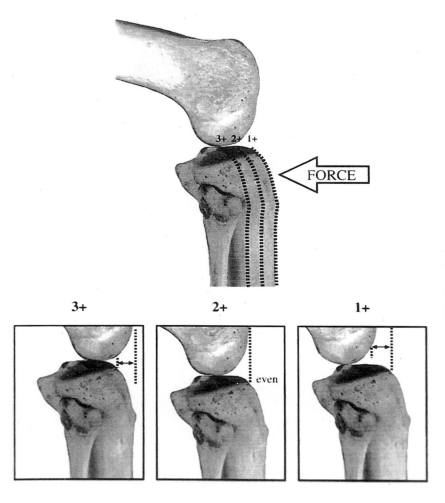

Figure 4–34. PCL injury grading. Grading is based on the relationship of the anterior aspect of the medial tibial plateau to the anterior aspect of the medial femoral condyle. In grade 1, the tibia remains anterior to the femur. In grade 2, the tibia is even with the femur. In grade 3, the tibia moves posterior to the femur. (From Miller MD, Bergfield JA, Fowler PJ, et al: The posterior cruciate ligament injured knee: principles of evaluation and treatment. In Zuckerman JD [ed]: Instr Course Lect 48:199–207, 1999.)

injuries have 5 to 10 mm of posterior translation and the medial tibial plateau rests flush to the medial femoral condyle. *Grade 3* injuries have more than 10 mm of posterior translation and the medial tibial plateau falls posterior to the medial femoral condyle.

Radiographic Evaluation

Radiographs are usually negative; however, they may identify the presence of a bony avulsion that can be reattached (Fig. 4–35). Stress radiographs have been shown to compare favorably with clinical examination techniques in the diagnosis of PCL injury. MRI is helpful to confirm the diagnosis of a PCL rupture as well as to evaluate the remaining structures of the knee (Fig. 4–36). Bone scans can be used to demonstrate increased subchondral stress resulting from changes in knee kinematics after PCL injury. The increased stresses may predispose the knee to early degeneration, and some surgeons use the abnormal bone scan as an indication of the need for operative PCL stabilization (Fig. 4–37).

Figure 4–35. PCL avulsion injury noted on x-ray. The tibial insertion of the PCL is avulsed with its bony attachment from the posterior aspect of the tibia.

Figure 4–36. MRI of the PCL injury. Note the interruption of the black posterior vertical structure (PCL).

DR BACH

Figure 4–37. Bone scan of the knee demonstrating degenerative changes. In chronic PCL injury, degenerative changes tend to occur in the medial and patellofemoral compartments.

Biomechanics of the Posterior Cruciate Ligament–Deficient Knee

Injury to the PCL results in changes in the kinematics of the knee. **Changes in contact pressure have been demonstrated in both the patellofemoral and the medial tibiofemoral compartments after sectioning of the PCL, with significant increases in joint forces.** This alteration in the normal kinematics may explain the tendency for the development of degenerative changes in these two compartments after PCL injury.

Biomechanics of Exercise

Markolf and colleagues (1997) demonstrated that passive ROM of the knee results in the generation of minimal force in the intact PCL throughout the entire motion arc. After reconstruction, no significant change in force production was noted except for a small increase at flexion angles greater than 60 degrees.

The *shear forces* generated in the knee during open– and closed–kinetic chain exercises have been closely examined. A posterior shear force occurs during closed–kinetic chain exercise throughout the entire ROM of the knee, with greater forces generated as knee flexion increases. **With open–kinetic chain activities, there appears to be a tremendous force exerted on the PCL during flexion exercises. However, with open–kinetic chain extension, minimal or no force appears to be generated in the PCL from 0 to 60 degrees, but from 60 to 90 degrees, significant stress is produced in the PCL.** It has been demonstrated that altering the position of the resistance pad can modify the forces generated with open–kinetic chain exercises.

The magnitude of force generated in the PCL during exercise is much greater than that in the ACL, which may be a factor in the tendency for PCL grafts to stretch out after surgical reconstruction. The trend has been to avoid reconstruction of the PCL when possible, but it may be that proper rehabilitation can avoid the development of progressive laxity and improve the results of reconstruction.

O'Connor (1993) calculated that it is possible to unload the cruciate ligaments dynamically using cocontraction of the quadriceps, hamstrings, and gastrocnemius muscles. The role of the gastrocnemius in dynamically stabilizing the PCL is supported indirectly by the findings of Inoue and coworkers (1998), who demonstrated an earlier activation of the gastrocnemius before the generation of flexion torque in the knee in PCL-deficient knees compared with uninjured knees.

The goal should be to minimize the potentially deleterious generation of force during rehabilitation. It appears that passive motion can be safely performed through the entire range of flexion and extension. **Active closed–kinetic chain activities of any kind, in any ROM, should be used cautiously when rehabilitating the PCL, either as** nonoperative therapy or after reconstruction. **If these exercises are used, they should be carried out in a ROM that limits flexion of the knee to about 45 degrees or less to avoid generating higher forces in the PCL.** Open–kinetic chain flexion exercises generate extremely high forces in the PCL and should be avoided altogether, whereas open–kinetic chain extension appears to be safe when performed at lower flexion angles (from 60 to 0 degrees). However, in this range, the patellofemoral stresses are at their greatest and the risk for development of patellofemoral symptoms is significant. Therefore, **we do not routinely recommend the use of open-chain exercises during rehabilitation after PCL injury or reconstruction.**

Natural History

The natural history of isolated PCL injuries remains controversial. In a number of studies, isolated PCL injuries have been shown to do well with nonoperative treatment, whereas others have shown poor outcomes after conservative measures.

Attempts have been made to determine what variables may predict the outcome of conservatively treated PCL injuries. Increased quadriceps strength has been correlated with improved outcome in some studies, whereas others have not found a significant relationship. Shelbourne, Davis, and Patel (1999) demonstrated that subjective and objective functional outcomes were independent of knee laxity. However, all of their patients demonstrated grade 2 laxity or less. It is unclear what effect more severe laxity has on the results of conservative treatment.

The development of degenerative changes, particularly in the medial tibiofemoral and patellofemoral compartments, is also an area of controversy. Some studies have demonstrated increased degeneration with time after conservative treatment of PCL injuries, whereas others have not.

Unlike a torn ACL and more like a torn MCL, the PCL may regain continuity with time. Shelbourne and colleagues (1999) found that, at follow-up, 63 of 68 patients with PCL injuries had the same or less clinical laxity than at their initial evaluations. Athletes with isolated PCL injuries may be told that the amount of posterior laxity is likely to improve with time, but this does not mean a better knee subjectively.

Clearly, isolated PCL injuries may not be as benign as was once believed. **The problem is not one of instability, but rather one of progressive disability.** Most studies demonstrate reasonably good functional outcomes after conservative treatment of isolated PCL injuries, yet a significant number of patients develop pain and early degenerative change in the knee despite a good functional recovery. Unfortunately, **surgical management has not been shown to consistently alter the natural history of these injuries.**

Rehabilitation Considerations

In general, rehabilitation after PCL injury tends to be more conservative than after ACL injury. The severity of the PCL injury should also guide the aggressiveness of nonoperative therapy. Rehabilitation progression can be more rapid with grades 1 and 2 injuries, whereas rehabilitation after grade 3 injuries is advanced more slowly. After reconstruction, a different protocol is used, and again, a more conservative approach is used than after ACL reconstruction.

Motion

Because passive motion places negligible stress on the intact PCL and only a small stress on PCL grafts with knee flexion past 60 degrees, the use of CPM may be beneficial for grade 3 injuries treated nonoperatively and after reconstruction. Early active motion may expose the ligament to excessive force and lead to elongation and subsequent laxity. For grades 1 and 2 injuries treated nonoperatively, nonresisted active motion as tolerated is probably safe, but resisted motion, including weight-bearing, should be limited to a 0- to 60-degree flexion arc during the early treatment phase.

Weight-bearing

Weight-bearing is encouraged. For mild injuries treated nonoperatively, weight-bearing should be in a brace limited to 0 to 60 degrees of motion. For more severe injuries treated nonoperatively and after PCL reconstruction, weight-bearing should be in a brace locked in extension during the early treatment phases and progressed gradually.

External Support

After reconstruction or during nonoperative treatment of grade 3 isolated PCL injuries, **it is crucial to prevent posterior displacement of the tibia from the effects of gravity and the weight of the leg, as well as from the pull of the hamstrings.** Proper bracing is helpful to resist these forces, but the therapist must be aware of the potential for posterior sag to occur. If CPM devices are used, resistance straps must be included to support the proximal tibia posteriorly. Exercises must be carried out with manual support of the tibia as well. **Alternatively, flexion exercises can be done prone (Fig. 4–38) so that the posterior translational force of gravity on the tibia is eliminated.**

Limited information is available concerning the efficacy of *functional bracing* after PCL injury. At this time, use of a functional brace is commonly recommended, even though little scientific data supporting this recommendation can be found.

Muscle Training

Quadriceps strengthening is the foundation of rehabilitation after PCL injury. As noted earlier, the quadri-

Figure 4–38. *A,* Prone flexion exercises for knee flexion. *B,* Prone knee flexion with a rubber band or towel.

ceps functions to dynamically stabilize the tibia and counteract the posterior pull of the hamstrings. Open–kinetic chain extension activities place the lowest strains on the PCL, but result in elevated patellofemoral joint forces. **We recommend the use of closed–kinetic chain activities from 0 to 45 degrees as a compromise to protect both the PCL and the patellofemoral joint. Open–kinetic chain flexion activities, which produce high posterior shear forces, should be avoided.**

Patellofemoral Joint

The patellofemoral joint is at particular risk for the development of symptoms during rehabilitation after PCL injury. The altered kinematics of the knee place an increased force across the joint, resulting in early degeneration of the articular surfaces. Also, open–kinetic chain extension exercises at low levels of knee flexion (0 to 60 degrees) create an extremely high joint reaction force across the patellofemoral joint.

Treatment

There is still a great deal of debate regarding the treatment of PCL injuries. Currently, most agree that combined ligamentous injuries of the knee require surgical repair or reconstruction; however, there is no clear consensus as to when reconstruction is indicated for isolated PCL injuries. **For acute isolated grade 1 or 2 PCL injuries, the common recommendation is nonoperative rehabilitation. For acute isolated grade 3 injuries, the clear indication for surgery is an avulsion or "pull-off" injury of the ligament at the bony insertion site.** Less clear are the indications for surgical treatment of midsubstance rupture of the ligament. Some advocate nonoperative treatment for all acute isolated grade 3 PCL injuries, whereas others recommend reconstruction in younger, high-demand patients. For *chronic* injuries, grade 1 and most grades 2 and 3 injuries are treated with rehabilitation and activity modification. Surgery is indicated for symptomatic chronic grades 2 and 3 injuries. The symptoms are typically pain or instability. A positive bone scan, indicating kinematic changes leading to early joint degeneration, may prompt surgical reconstruction in an attempt to forestall the progression of joint arthrosis.

Nonoperative Treatment

For grades 1 and 2 injuries, progression can proceed rapidly, with minimal immobilization, early strengthening, and a return to full activity as soon as 3 to 4 weeks in some patients. Outcomes after grade 3 injuries are less predictable, and the likelihood of an undetected posterolateral corner injury is significant. Therefore, with grade 3 injuries, a more conservative approach is recommended. These injuries are generally treated with a short course of immobilization, with passive rather than active motion in the early healing phase, and a less aggressive strengthening program.

Rehabilitation Protocol
Nonoperative Treatment of Posterior Cruciate Ligament Injuries
D'Amato and Bach

Phase 1

Days 1–7
- ROM 0–60 degrees.
- Weight-bearing with two crutches.
- Electrical muscle stimulation to quadriceps.
- Exercises
  - Quadriceps sets.
  - SLR.
  - Hip adduction and abduction.
  - Mini-squats/leg press (0–45 degrees).

Weeks 2–3
- ROM 0–60 degrees.
- Weight-bearing without crutches.
- Progress exercises using weights.
- Bike (week 3) for ROM.
- Pool program (see section on aquatic therapy in Chapter 7).
- Leg press (0–60 degrees).

Phase 2

Week 3
- ROM to tolerance.
- Discontinue brace.

- Bike, Stairmaster, rowing.
- Progress exercises with weights.
- Mini-squat (0–60 degrees).
- Leg press (0–60 degrees).
- Step-ups.
- Hip abduction and adduction.
- Toe-calf raises.

Weeks 5–6
- Continue all exercises.
- Fit functional brace.
- Pool running.

Phase 3

Weeks 8–12
- Begin running program.
- Continue all strengthening exercises.
- Gradual return to sports activities.
- Criteria to return to sports
  - No change in laxity.
  - No pain, tenderness, or swelling.
  - Satisfactory clinical examination.
  - Functional testing 85% of contralateral knee.
  - Quadriceps strength 85% of contralateral knee.

Operative Treatment

The rehabilitation protocol after reconstruction of the PCL is quite conservative when compared with that after ACL reconstruction, primarily because of the greater posterior shear forces generated during activity and motion of the knee. **Prevention of posterior sag and hamstring activity is paramount in avoiding residual laxity.** Despite this conservative approach, motion problems are rare after PCL reconstruction. As the biology of graft healing becomes better understood and surgical techniques improve, accelerated rehabilitation protocols may be shown to be safe, but at present, the information regarding aggressive rehabilitation is limited and protection of the graft from potentially deleterious forces must be enforced.

Rehabilitation Protocol
After Surgical Reconstruction of the Posterior Cruciate Ligament
D'Amato and Bach

General Guidelines
- No open-chain exercises.
- Caution against posterior tibial translation (gravity, muscle action).
- No CPM.
- Resistance for hip PREs is placed above the knee for hip abduction and adduction; resistance may be distal for hip flexion.

Phase 1: Weeks 0–4

Goals
- Protect healing bony and soft tissue structures.
- Minimize the effects of immobilization
  - Early protected ROM (protection against posterior tibial sagging).
  - PREs for quadriceps, hip, and calf, with emphasis on limiting patellofemoral joint compression and posterior tibial translation.

Rehabilitation Protocol
After Surgical Reconstruction of the Posterior Cruciate Ligament (Continued)
D'Amato and Bach

- Patient education for a clear understanding of limitations and expectations of the rehabilitation process and need for supporting proximal tibia and avoiding sag.

Bracing
- Brace locked at 0 degrees for 1 wk.
- At 1 wk after surgery, brace is unlocked for passive ROM done by physical therapist or athletic trainer.
- Patient is instructed in self-administered passive ROM with the brace on, with emphasis on supporting the proximal tibia.

Weight-bearing
- As tolerated with crutches, brace locked in extension.

Special Considerations
- Pillow under proximal posterior tibia at rest to prevent posterior sag.

Therapeutic Exercises
- Patellar mobilization.
- Prone passive flexion and extension.
- Quadriceps sets.
- SLR.
- Hip abduction and adduction.
- Ankle pumps.
- Hamstring and calf stretching.
- Calf exercise with Theraband, progressing to standing calf raise with full knee extension.
- Standing hip extension from neutral.
- Functional electrical stimulation (may be used for trace to poor quadriceps contraction).

Phase 2: Weeks 4–12

Criteria for Progression to Phase 2
- Good quadriceps control (good quadriceps set, no sag with SLR).
- Approximately 60 degrees knee flexion.
- Full knee extension.
- No signs of active inflammation.

Goals
- Increase ROM (flexion).
- Restore normal gait.
- Continue quadriceps strengthening and hamstring flexibility.

Bracing
- 4–6 wk: brace is unlocked for controlled gait training only (patient may walk with brace unlocked while attending physical therapy or when at home).
- 6–8 wk: brace is unlocked for all activities.
- 8 wk: brace is discontinued (as allowed by physician).

Weight-bearing
- 4–8 wk: weight-bearing as tolerated with crutches.
- 8 wk: may discontinue crutches if patient exhibits
  - No quadriceps lag with SLR.
  - Full knee extension.
  - Knee flexion 90–100 degrees.
  - Normal gait pattern (patient can use one crutch or cane until normal gait is achieved).

Therapeutic Exercises
Weeks 4–8
- Wall slides (0–45 degrees).
- Mini-squats (0–45 degrees).
- Leg press (0–60 degrees).
- Four-way hip exercises for flexion, abduction, adduction, extension from neutral with knee fully extended.
- Ambulation in pool (work on restoration of normal heel-toe gait pattern in chest-deep water).

Weeks 8–12
- Stationary bike (foot placed forward on pedal without use of toe clips to minimize hamstring activity, seat set slightly higher than normal).
- Stairmaster, elliptical stepper, Nordic-Trac.
- Balance and proprioception activities.
- Seated calf raises.
- Leg press (0–90 degrees).

Phase 3: Months 3–6

Criteria for Progression to Phase 3
- Full, pain-free ROM (*Note:* it is not unusual for flexion to be lacking 10–15 degrees for up to 5 mo after surgery).
- Normal gait.
- Good to normal quadriceps strength.
- No patellofemoral complaints.
- Clearance by physician to begin more concentrated closed–kinetic chain progression.

Goals
- Restore any residual loss of motion that may prevent functional progression.
- Progress functionally and prevent patellofemoral irritation.
- Improve functional strength and proprioception using closed–kinetic chain exercises.
- Continue to maintain quadriceps strength and hamstring flexibility.

Therapeutic Exercises
- Continue closed–kinetic chain exercise progression.
- Treadmill walking.
- Jogging in pool with wet vest or belt.
- Swimming (no frog kick).

continued

Rehabilitation Protocol
After Surgical Reconstruction of the Posterior Cruciate Ligament *(Continued)*
D'Amato and Bach

Phase 4: Month 6—Full Activity

Criteria for Progression to Phase 4
- No significant patellofemoral or soft tissue irritation.
- Presence of necessary joint ROM, muscle strength, endurance, and proprioception to safely return to athletic participation.

Goals
- Safe and gradual return to athletic participation.
- Maintenance of strength, endurance, and function.

Therapeutic Exercises
- Continue closed–kinetic chain exercise progression.

- Sport-specific functional progression, which may include but is not limited to
  - Slide board.
  - Jog/run progression.
  - Figure-of-eight, carioca, backward running, cutting.
  - Jumping (plyometrics).

Criteria for Return to Sports
- Full, pain-free ROM.
- Satisfactory clinical examination.
- Quadriceps strength 85% of contralateral leg.
- Functional testing 85% of contralateral leg.
- No change in laxity testing.

Rehabilitation Protocol
After Posterior Cruciate Ligament Reconstruction with a Two-Tunnel Graft Technique
Wilk

Important Rehabilitation Points
- Emphasize quadriceps strengthening.
- Monitor closely patellofemoral and medial joint line degeneration.
- Monitor capsular laxity, especially posterolateral corner.
- Gradual return to sports.

Phase 1: Immediate Postoperative—Weeks 1–2

Goals
- Control swelling and inflammation.
- Obtain full passive knee extension.
- Gradually increase flexion to 90 degrees.
- Voluntary quadriceps control.
- Patellar mobility.

Days 1–3
Brace
- EZ Wrap locked at 0 degrees extension, patient sleeps in brace.

Weight-bearing
- As tolerated with two crutches (50%).

Range of Motion
- Self ROM (0–90 degrees) out of brace, four or five times daily.

Exercises
- Patellar mobilization.
- Stretching of hamstrings and calf.
- Ankle pumps.

- Quadriceps sets.
- SLR (three-way) for hip flexion, abduction, and adduction.
- Knee extensions 0–60 degrees.

Muscle Stimulation
- Muscle stimulation to quadriceps (4 hr/day) during quadriceps sets.

Continuous Passive Motion
- 0–60 degrees as tolerated.

Ice and Elevation
- Ice 20 min out of every hour and elevate with knee in extension; do not allow proximal tibia to sag posteriorly.

Days 4–7
Brace
- EZ Wrap locked at 0 degrees extension for ambulation and sleep only.

Weight-bearing
- Two crutches (50%).

Range of Motion
- Self ROM (0–90 degrees) out of brace, four or five times daily for 10 min.
- Patellar mobilization.
- Stretching of hamstrings and calf.

Exercises
- Ankle pumps.
- Quadriceps sets.

Rehabilitation Protocol
After Posterior Cruciate Ligament Reconstruction with a Two-Tunnel Graft Technique *(Continued)*
Wilk

- SLR (three-way) for hip flexion, abduction, and adduction.
- Knee extensions 0–60 degrees.

Muscle Stimulation
- Muscle stimulation to quadriceps (4 hr/day) during quadriceps sets.

Continuous Passive Motion
- 0–60 degrees as tolerated.

Ice and Elevation
- Ice 20 min out of every hour and elevate with knee in extension; do not allow proximal tibia to sag posteriorly.

Phase 2: Maximum Protection—Weeks 2–6

Goals
- Control external forces to protect graft.
- Restore motion.
- Nourish articular cartilage.
- Decrease swelling.
- Decrease fibrosis.
- Prevent quadriceps atrophy.

Week 2
Brace
- EZ Wrap locked at 0 degrees extension.

Weight-bearing
- As tolerated (50% or more, approximately 75% of body weight), with one crutch.

Range of Motion
- Self ROM (0–90 degrees) out of brace, four or five times daily.
- Patellar mobilization.
- Stretching of hamstrings and calf.

Exercises
- Multiangle isometrics, 60, 40, and 20 degrees.
- Quadriceps sets.
- Knee extensions 0–60 degrees.
- Intermittent ROM 0–60 degrees (four or five times daily).
- Well-leg bicycling.
- Proprioception training squats (0–45 degrees) (Biodex Stability System).
- Leg press (0–60 degrees).
- Continue electrical stimulation to quadriceps.
- Continue ice and elevation.

Weeks 3–4
Brace
- EZ Wrap locked at 0 degrees extension.

Weight-bearing
- Full weight-bearing, no crutches.

Range of Motion
- 0–100 degrees by week 3, 0–110 degrees by week 4.
- Patellar mobilization.
- Hamstring and calf stretching.

Exercises
- Weight shifts.
- Mini-squats 0–45 degrees.
- Wall squats 0–50 degrees.
- Intermittent ROM 0–100/110 degrees.
- Knee extension 60–0 degrees.
- Proprioception drills (cup walking).
- Biodex Stability System.
- Pool walking.
- Bike for ROM and endurance.

Phase 3: Controlled Ambulation—Weeks 5–10

Goals
- Restore full motion.
- Improve quadriceps muscle strength.
- Restore proprioception and dynamic stabilization.
- Discontinue use of knee immobilizer.

Criteria for Full Weight-bearing with Knee Motion
- Passive ROM 0–120 degrees.
- Quadriceps strength 70% of contralateral side (isometric test).
- Decreased joint effusion.

Week 5
Range of Motion
- Passive ROM 0–120 degrees.

Exercises
- Knee extension 0–60 degrees.
- Multihip machine.
- Leg press 0–60/75 degrees.
- Vertical squats 0–45 degrees.
- Wall squats 0–60 degrees.
- Lateral step-ups.
- Front lunges.
- Side or lateral lunges.
- Proprioception drills.
- Single-leg balance.
- Cup walking.
- Heel-toe raises.
- Continue stretching hamstrings and calf.
- Progress pool exercises.

Week 6
Range of Motion
- Passive ROM 0–125/130 degrees.

continued

Rehabilitation Protocol
After Posterior Cruciate Ligament Reconstruction with a Two-Tunnel Graft Technique *(Continued)*
Wilk

KT 2000 Test
- 15- and 20-pound anterior-posterior force at 20–35 degrees and 15- and 20-pound anterior-posterior at Quad Neutral Angle (QNA) approximately 70 degrees of flexion as tolerated.

Exercises
- Continue all exercises.
- Initiate swimming.
- Increase closed–kinetic chain rehabilitation.
- Functional exercise program.

Weeks 8–10
Exercises
- Begin isokinetic 60–0 degrees ROM.
- Continue all exercises.
- Initial pool running (forward only).
- Initiate hamstring curls (0–60 degrees), low weight.
- Bicycle for endurance (30 min).
- Begin walking program.
- Stair-climbing machine, ski machine.

Phase 4: Light Activity—Months 3–4

Goals
- Develop strength, power, and endurance.
- Begin to prepare for return to functional activities.

Month 3
Exercises
- Begin light running program.
- Continue isokinetic exercises (light speed, full ROM).
- Continue eccentrics.
- Continue mini-squats, lateral step-ups, wall squats, front step-down, knee extension.
- Continue closed–kinetic chain rehabilitation.
- Continue endurance exercises.
- Begin light agility drills (side shuffle, cariocas).

Month 4
Tests
- Isokinetic test (week 15).
- KT 2000 test (week 16).
- Functional test (before running program).

Criteria for Beginning Running Program
- KT 2000 test unchanged.
- Functional test 70% of contralateral leg.
- Isokinetic test interpretation satisfactory.

Exercises
- Progress all strengthening exercises, with emphasis on quadriceps strength.
- Initiate plyometrics (box jumps [Fig. 4–39], double-leg jumps).

Phase 5: Return to Activity—Months 5–6

Goals
- Advance rehabilitation to competitive sports, usually at 6–7 mo.

A

B

Figure 4–39. Plyometric box jumps. *A*, Patient starts on top of the box. *B*, Patient hops off the box, landing on the floor in a controlled fashion. The box height is gradually increased as strength progresses. The exercise may be performed in a single-leg mode as well.

- Achieve maximal strength and further enhance neuromuscular coordination and endurance.

Exercises
- Closed-kinetic rehabilitation.
- High-speed isokinetics.

Rehabilitation Protocol
After Posterior Cruciate Ligament Reconstruction with a Two-Tunnel Graft Technique *(Continued)*
Wilk

- Running program.
- Agility drills.
- Balance and proprioception training.
- Plyometrics training.

Criteria for Return to Sports
- Full, nonpainful ROM.
- Satisfactory isokinetic test (85% or better).

- Satisfactory KT 2000 test.
- Functional hop test 85% of contralateral leg.
- Satisfactory clinical examination by physician.

6-Month and 12-Month Follow-up
- KT 2000 test.
- Isokinetic test.
- Functional test.

Rehabilitation Protocol
After Combined Reconstruction of the Posterior Cruciate Ligament and Posterolateral Structures (Biceps Tenodesis)
Wilk

Preoperative Instructions
- Gait training, weight-bearing as tolerated with crutches.
- Instruction in immediate postoperative activities and hospital course.
- Brace stays on for all exercises; can open brace to put on muscle stimulator and to do patellar mobilizations.

Phase 1: Immediate Postoperative—Days 1–4

Brace
- EZ Wrap locked at 0 degrees or full extension.

Weight-bearing
- Two crutches, progress to full weight-bearing as tolerated.

Ice and Elevation
- Ice 20 min out of every hour, elevate with knee in extension.

Exercises
- Ankle pumps.
- Patella mobilization and passive extension to 0 degrees.
- Quadriceps sets, adductor sets with Quadriceps Setting (QS), glut sets.

Phase 2: Maximal Protection—Day 5–Week 8

Day 5–Week 2
Brace
- Locked in full extension.

Weight-bearing
- Progress to full weight-bearing without crutches.

Exercises
- Continue all exercises.
- Begin PREs with leg raises.

Week 6
Brace
- Discontinue brace.

Exercises
- Work toward regaining full active flexion seated, not against gravity.
- Start exercise bike and swimming, emphasizing ROM.
- Starts for PREs for quadriceps only.

Week 10
Exercises
- Begin hamstring work against gravity, and then start PREs.
- Continue all strengthening exercises.

Week 12
- KT 2000 test.

Exercises
- Continue mini-squats.
- Initiate lateral step-ups.
- Initiate pool running (forward only).
- Hamstrings curls (0–60 degrees), low weight.
- Bicycle for endurance (30 min).
- Begin walking program.

Phase 4: Light Activity—Months 3–4

Goals
- Develop strength, power, and endurance.
- Begin to prepare for return to functional activities.

Exercises
- Begin light running program.
- Initiate isokinetics (light speed, full ROM).
- Continue eccentrics.

continued

Rehabilitation Protocol
After Combined Reconstruction of the Posterior Cruciate Ligament and Posterolateral Structures (Biceps Tenodesis) *(Continued)*
Wilk

- Continue mini-squats and lateral step-ups.
- Continue closed-kinetic rehabilitation.
- Continue endurance exercises.

Tests
- Isokinetic test (week 15)
- KT 2000 test (before running program).
- Functional test (before running program).

Criteria for Running
- Isokinetic test interpretation satisfactory.
- KT 2000 test unchanged.
- Functional test 70% of contralateral leg.

Phase 5: Return to Activity—Months 5–6

Goals
- Advance rehabilitation to competitive sports.
- Achieve maximal strength and further enhance neuro-muscular coordination and endurance.

Exercises
- Closed-kinetic rehabilitation.
- High-speed isokinetics.

- Running program.
- Agility drills.
- Balance drills.
- Plyometrics initiated.
- Gradual return to sport activities.

Criteria for Return to Sport Activities
- Isokinetic quadriceps torque to body weight ratio.
- Isokinetic test 85% of contralateral side.
- No change in laxity.
- No pain, tenderness, or swelling.
- Satisfactory clinical examination.

6-Month and 12-Month Follow-up
- KT 2000 test.
- Isokinetic test.
- Functional test.

Rehabilitation Protocol
After Combined Reconstruction of the Posterior and Anterior Cruciate Ligaments
Wilk

Phase 1: Immediate Postoperative—Days 1–14

Brace
- EZ Wrap brace locked at 0 degrees extension.

Weight-bearing
- As tolerated with two crutches (50%).

Muscle Stimulation
- Muscle stimulation to quadriceps (4 hr/day) during quadriceps set.

Ice and Elevation
- Ice 20 min out of every hour and elevate with knee in extension.

Continuous Passive Motion
- 0–60 degrees as tolerated.

Exercises
- Ankle pumps.
- Quadriceps sets.

- SLR (three-way) for hip flexion, abduction, and adduction.
- Knee extension 0–60 degrees.

Phase 2: Maximal Protection—Weeks 2–6

Goals
- Absolute control of external forces to protect graft.
- Nourish articular cartilage.
- Decrease swelling.
- Decrease fibrosis.
- Prevent quadriceps atrophy.

Week 2

Brace
- Brace locked at 0 degrees, continue intermittent ROM exercises.

Weight-bearing
- As tolerated, 50% or more.

Rehabilitation Protocol
After Combined Reconstruction of the Posterior and Anterior Cruciate Ligaments *(Continued)*
Wilk

KT Testing
- 15-pound maximal force at 70 degrees of flexion.

Exercises
- Multiangle isometrics, 60, 40, and 20 degrees.
- Quadriceps sets.
- Knee extension 60–0 degrees.
- Intermittent ROM 0–60 degrees (four or five times a day).
- Patellar mobilization.
- Well-leg bicycling.
- Proprioception training squats (0–45 degrees).
- Continue electrical stimulation to quadriceps.
- Leg press 0–60 degrees.
- Continue ice and elevation.

Week 4
Brace
- Brace locked at 0 degrees, continue intermittent ROM exercises.

Weight-bearing
- Full weight-bearing, no crutches; one crutch if necessary.

KT Testing
- 15-pound maximal force at 70 degrees of flexion.

Exercises
- Weight shifts.
- Mini-squats 0–45 degrees.
- Intermittent ROM 0–90 degrees.
- Knee extension 80–40 degrees (therapist discretion).
- Pool walking.
- Bike for ROM and endurance.

Week 5
Brace
- Fit for functional PCL brace.

Exercises
- Initiate pool exercises.

Phase 3: Controlled Ambulation—Weeks 6–9

Criteria for Progression to Phase 3
- Active ROM 0–115 degrees.
- Quadriceps strength 60% of contralateral side (isometric test, 60-degree knee flexion angle).
- Unchanged KT test (+1 or less).

Goal
- Control forces during ambulation.

Brace
- Discontinued locked brace, brace open 0–125 degrees.

KT Testing
- Testing at weeks 6 and 8, 20-pound and 30-pound test.

Exercises
- Continue all exercises.
- Passive ROM 0–130 degrees.

- Initiate swimming.
- Initiate step-ups (start with 2 ft and gradually increase).
- Increase closed–kinetic chain rehabilitation.
- Increase proprioception training.

Phase 4: Moderate Protection—Weeks 9–14

Criteria for Progression to Phase 4
- Active ROM 0–125 degrees.
- Quadriceps strength 60% of contralateral leg (isokinetic test).
- No change in KT scores (+2 or less).
- Minimal effusion.
- No patellofemoral complaints.
- Satisfactory clinical examination.

Goals
- Protect patellofemoral joint articular cartilage.
- Maximal strengthening of quadriceps, lower extremity.

Testing
- KT 2000 test, week 12.
- Isokinetic test, weeks 10–12.

Exercises
- Emphasis on eccentric quadriceps work.
- Continue closed-chain exercises, step-ups, mini-squats, leg press.
- Continue knee extension 90–40 degrees.
- Hip abduction and adduction.
- Hamstring curls and stretches.
- Calf raises.
- Bicycle for endurance.
- Pool running (forward and backward).
- Walking program.
- Stair-master.
- Initiate isokinetic work 100–40 degrees.

Phase 5: Light Activity—Months 3–4

Criteria for Progression to Phase 5
- Active ROM 0–125 degrees or more.
- Quadriceps strength 70% of contralateral side, knee flexor-extensor rated 70–79%.
- No change in KT scores (+2 or less).
- Minimal or no effusion.
- Satisfactory clinical examination.

Goals
- Develop strength, power, and endurance.
- Begin to prepare for return to functional activities.

Tests
- Isokinetic test, weeks 10–12 and 16–18.

Exercises
- Continue strengthening exercises.
- Initiate plyometric program.
- Initiate running program.

continued

Rehabilitation Protocol
After Combined Reconstruction of the Posterior and Anterior
Cruciate Ligaments (Continued)
Wilk

- Initiate agility drills.
- Sport-specific training and drills.

Criteria for Beginning Running Program
- Satisfactory isokinetic test.
- Unchanged KT 2000 results.
- Functional test 70% of contralateral leg.
- Satisfactory clinical examination.

Phase 6: Return to Activity—Months 5–6

Criteria for Returning to Activities
- Isokinetic test that fulfills criteria.
- KT 2000 test unchanged.
- Functional test 80% of contralateral leg.
- Satisfactory clinical examination.

Goals
- Achieve maximal strength and further enhance neuro-muscular coordination and endurance.

Tests
- Isokinetic test before return to activity.
- KT 2000 test.
- Functional test.

Exercises
- Continue strengthening programs.
- Continue closed-chain strengthening program.
- Continue plyometric program.
- Continue running and agility program.
- Accelerate sport-specific training and drills.

6-Month and 12-Month Follow-up
- KT 2000 test.
- Isokinetic test.
- Functional test.

Medial Collateral Ligament Injuries

Bruce Reider, MD, and Kenneth J. Mroczek, MD

Clinical Background

The anatomy of the medial knee has been divided into three layers, consisting of the deep investing fascia of the thigh, the superficial MCL and the deep MCL, or knee joint capsule. The superficial MCL is the primary restraint to valgus loading, and the deep MCL and postero-medial capsule are secondary valgus restraints at full extension.

Most isolated MCL injuries result from direct trauma to the lateral aspect of the knee creating a valgus force (Fig. 4–40). An indirect or noncontact mechanism, especially involving rotation, typically produces associated injuries, usually involving the cruciate ligaments.

The patient may report a popping or tearing sensation on the medial aspect of the knee. Most injuries occur at the femoral origin or in the midsubstance over the joint line, although tibial avulsions do occur. MCL sprains may be isolated or combined with other knee injuries. Associated injuries may be diagnosed by an alert clinician who looks for clues that appear in the history and examination or while monitoring the clinical progress of the patient.

Classification of Medial Collateral Ligament

Grade	Damage to Ligament	Clinical Examination	Laxity on Examination (mm)
1	Microtrauma with no elongation	Tender ligament Normal valgus laxity	0–5
2	Elongated but intact	Increased valgus laxity with firm endpoint on valgus stress at 20 degrees of knee flexion	5–10
3	Complete disruption	Increased valgus laxity with soft endpoint on valgus stress at 30 degrees of knee flexion	>10

Figure 4–40. MCL injury mechanism. A direct blow to the lateral aspect of the knee creates a valgus stress, disrupting the MCL. (From Baker CL Jr, Liu SH: Collateral ligament injuries of the knee: operative and nonoperative approaches. In Fu FH, Harner CD, Vince KG [eds]: Knee Surgery. Baltimore, Williams & Wilkins, 1994, pp. 787–808.)

Physical Examination

The physical examination begins with the patient seated. Inspection of the knee may reveal localized edema over the MCL. A visible enlargement of the normal prominence of the medial epicondyle characterizes injuries to the femoral origin. The presence of a large effusion should alert the clinician to a possible intra-articular injury, such as a fracture, meniscal tear, or cruciate ligament injury. **Because the MCL is extra-articular, isolated MCL injuries seldom produce large intra-articular swelling.** Careful palpation along the course of the MCL from the origin on the femoral epicondyle to the insertion on the proximal medial tibia will reveal maximal tenderness over the injured portion of the ligament.

Valgus laxity should be evaluated with the patient supine and relaxed (see Fig. 4–5). The examiner supports the leg with one hand under the heel and, with the other hand, applies a gentle valgus force to the fully extended knee. In a normal knee, the examiner will feel firm resistance with virtually no separation of the femur and tibia. In an abnormal knee, the femur and tibia will be felt to separate in response to the valgus force and to "clunk" back together when the force is relaxed.

Increased laxity on valgus stress testing of the MCL in full extension (0 degrees) indicates severe injury to the MCL, the posteromedial capsule, and usually one or both cruciate ligaments.

If the valgus stress test is normal with the knee in full extension, the examiner flexes the knee about 30 degrees and repeats the test. This flexion relaxes the posterior capsule and permits more isolated testing of the MCL. With the knee flexed, the examiner again evaluates the firmness of the resistance (the "endpoint") and the amount of joint separation. The opposite knee should be examined to determine normal laxity; generalized ligamentous laxity may be incorrectly identified as abnormal opening to valgus stress.

The physical examination findings progress with higher grades of injuries. In a *grade 1* sprain, the ligament is tender, but the knee is stable to valgus stress testing in 30 degrees of knee flexion. A *grade 2* sprain demonstrates abnormal valgus laxity compared with the contralateral knee, but with a firm endpoint. The firm endpoint may be difficult to appreciate owing to involuntary guarding. Because a *grade 3* sprain represents a complete rupture, valgus laxity is abnormal with a soft or indefinite endpoint.

Differential Diagnosis

The differential diagnosis of an isolated MCL injury includes medial knee contusion, medial meniscal tear, patellar subluxation or dislocation, and physeal fracture (in a skeletally immature patient).

A careful physical examination will help to differentiate an MCL sprain from the other diagnostic possibilities. A *bone contusion* also produces tenderness, but does not result in abnormal valgus laxity. Tenderness near the adductor tubercle or medial retinaculum adjacent to the patella can be caused by a *patellar dislocation* or subluxation with VMO avulsion or medial retinaculum tear. A positive patellar apprehension sign aids in distinguishing an episode of patellar instability from MCL injury. Physeal fractures in skeletally immature patients are tender over the growth plate, and the growth plate opens up on gentle stress-testing radiographs.

Joint line tenderness may be present in either a *medial meniscal tear* or an MCL sprain. Opening of the joint line on valgus laxity examination should differentiate between a meniscal tear and a grade 2 or 3 MCL sprain. The differentiation between a grade 1 MCL sprain and a medial meniscal tear is more difficult. An MRI can be obtained, or the patient can be observed for a few weeks. Tenderness usually resolves with a MCL sprain, but persists with a meniscal injury.

Radiographic Examination

Routine plain radiographs of the knee, including AP, lateral sunrise, and tunnel views, should be obtained to exclude a fracture or osteochondral injury.

Figure 4–41. MRI of an MCL injury.

Bony avulsions of the cruciates or a tibial flake avulsion of the lateral capsule (Segond sign—associated with an ACL injury) may indicate associated injuries. **The Pelligrini-Steida sign does not indicate an avulsion fracture, but rather an ectopic calcification that may develop near the medial epicondyle after a proximal MCL sprain.** Its presence on radiographs suggests a previous MCL injury. An MRI is not indicated for evaluation of an isolated MCL injury but may be helpful if the examination is equivocal (Fig. 4–41). Isolated MCL sprains are rarely associated with meniscal tears.

Treatment of Isolated and Combined Medial Collateral Ligament Injuries

The treatment of all grades of isolated MCL sprains is an aggressive, nonoperative rehabilitation program. Numerous studies have shown that a functional rehabilitation treatment program allows more rapid recovery with results equal or superior to those obtained with surgery or prolonged immobilization. When abnormal MCL laxity is present, a functional hinged brace is used to support and protect the MCL while allowing full knee ROM during rehabilitation.

When an **associated cruciate ligament injury** is present, treatment of the cruciate injury assumes paramount importance, and surgery is usually recommended. For MCL sprains associated with ACL tears, surgical reconstruction of the ACL **without** direct surgical repair of the MCL is recommended by most authors. It has been shown that injuries to both ligaments (ACL and MCL) adversely affect the healing of the MCL. Reconstruction of the ACL improved the healing response of the MCL.

Some surgeons advocate primary repair of the MCL in association with ACL reconstruction in a knee that opens widely to valgus stress in full extension. Documentation to support this practice is scarce because these cases are relatively infrequent and difficult to compare in a controlled fashion.

For *combined PCL and MCL injuries,* primary repair of the injured medial structures and PCL reconstruction are usually recommended.

For *isolated MCL sprains,* we stress the functional rehabilitation treatment outlined later. The healing MCL is protected with a lightweight hinged brace at all times, and the patient is encouraged to return to full weight-bearing and to begin an endurance activity such as cycling or stair climbing as soon as possible. This minimizes secondary muscle atrophy so that the factor limiting the patient's return to sports is the rate of healing of the MCL and not weakness or stiffness owing to imposed restrictions. The paramount feature of this program is that progression of rehabilitation activities and return to sports are based on the attainment of functional goals rather than arbitrary time periods.

When MCL injury occurs with ACL rupture, the athlete is treated with the same brace and rehabilitation program until full weight-bearing and nearly full motion are attained and swelling is minimized. ACL reconstruction usually is then carried out **without** direct repair of the MCL. Rarely, in a knee with gross increased valgus laxity at full extension, primary repair of injured medial structures is done at the time of ACL reconstruction. In this case, surgery should be done within 7 to 10 days of injury to facilitate primary repair of the medial structures. When the superficial MCL is too compromised to permit a strong repair, it is reinforced with the semitendinosus tendon, which is left attached to the tibia and fixed at the most isometric point on the medial epicondyle. This same technique is also useful for reconstruction of the MCL in the rare case in which it does not heal primarily. Finally, for combined injuries of the PCL and MCL or of the ACL, PCL, and MCL, the medial structures usually are repaired primarily during the cruciate ligament surgery.

Rehabilitation after MCL Injury

The rehabilitation program is divided into three phases. Successful completion of each phase and progression into the next phase are based on attaining specific goals. The time in each phase varies. The average time to return to sport varies with both grade and sport.

On the average, grade 1 injuries require about 10 days, and grades 2 and 3 need about 3 to 6 weeks.

Sports that place more stress on the MCL, such as soccer, may require a longer period of healing before return to play.

Rehabilitation Protocol
Isolated Medial Collateral Ligament Injury
Reider and Mroczek

Phase 1

Goals
- Normal gait.
- Minimal swelling.
- Full ROM.
- Baseline quadriceps control.

Cryotherapy
- Therapeutic cold via ice packs or other means is applied to the medial aspect of the knee for 20 min every 3–4 hr for the first 48 hr.
- Early cryotherapy provides anesthesia and local vasoconstriction to minimize initial hemorrhage and reduce secondary edema. Leg elevation also helps limit swelling.

Weight-bearing
- Weight-bearing is allowed as tolerated.
- Crutches are used until the patient ambulates without a limp, which takes approximately 1 wk.
- For grades 2 and 3 sprains, a lightweight hinged brace is worn. The brace should protect against valgus stresses of daily living, but not restrict motion or inhibit muscle function. The brace is worn at all times except for bathing during the initial 3–4 wk.
- **Knee immobilizers and full-leg braces are discouraged because they tend to inhibit motion and prolong the period of disability.**

Exercises
- ROM exercises are begun immediately. A cold whirlpool may make these exercises easier.
- Exercises such as towel extension exercises and prone hangs are used to obtain extension or hyperextension equal to the contralateral side. A heavy shoe or light ankle weight can be used with prone hangs to aid extension.
- To promote flexion, the patient sits at the end of a table, allowing gravity to aid in flexion. The uninjured limb assists by gently pushing the injured leg into further flexion.
- A similar technique of the uninjured limb assisting can be used during supine wall slides.
- To achieve greater than 90 degrees of flexion, heel slides are done with the patient sitting and grabbing the ankle to flex the knee farther.
- A stationary bicycle also aids in the restoration of motion. The bicycle seat is initially set as high as possible and gradually lowered to increase flexion.
- Isometric quadriceps sets and SLR are begun immediately to minimize muscle atrophy.
- Electrical stimulation may be helpful by limiting reflex muscle inhibition.

Phase 2

Goal
- Restoration of the strength of the injured leg to approximately 80–90% of the uninjured leg.

Bracing
- Continued use of the lightweight hinged brace.

Exercises
- Strengthening exercise begins with 4-inch step-ups and 30-degree squats without weights.
- Light resistance exercises of knee extensions, leg presses, and curls on a standard isotonic weight bench or dedicated resistance machine. Sets with lighter weights but a higher number of repetitions are usually used.
- Recurrent pain and swelling are signs of too rapid progression. If they occur, the strengthening program should be slowed.
- Upper body, aerobic, and further lower extremity conditioning are achieved with swimming, stationary cycling, and/or a stair climber.

Phase 3

Goals
- Completion of a running program.
- Completion of series of sport-specific activities.

Bracing
- Continued use of the brace is recommended during this phase and for the rest of the athletic season. This may protect against further injury and at least provides psychologic support.

Exercises
- A progressive running program commences with fast-speed walking and advances to light jogging, straight-line running, and then sprinting. Next, agility is achieved with cutting and pivoting activities such as figure-of-eight drills and cariocas.
- If pain or swelling occurs, the program is amended appropriately.
- Continued input from a trainer or physical therapist will be helpful in providing progress reports and guidance in appropriate performance of the activities.

Return to Sport
- Permitted when the athlete can complete a functional testing program including a long run, progressively more rapid sprints, cutting and pivoting drills, and appropriate sport-specific tests.

Rehabilitation Protocol
Progression of Rehabilitation after Medial Collateral Ligament Injury
Reider and Mroczek

	Phase 1	Phase 2	Phase 3
Bracing			
• Lightweight brace	X	X	X
Weight-bearing			
• Full	X	X	X
• Crutches until normal gait	X		
Range of Motion			
• Cold whirlpool	X		
• Extension exercises			
• Towel extensions	X		
• Prone hangs	X		
• Flexion exercises			
• Sitting off table	X		
• Wall slides	X		
• Heel slides	X		
Strengthening			
• Isometric quadriceps sets	X	X	
• SLR	X	X	
• Step-ups		X	X
• Squats		X	X
• Knee extensions		X	X
• Leg presses		X	X
• Leg curls		X	X
Conditioning			
• Stationary bike	X	X	X
• Swimming		X	X
• Stair climber		X	X
Agility/Sport-specific Training			
• Running program			
• Fast-speed walking			X
• Light jogging			X
• Straight-line running			X
• Sprinting			X
• Figure-of-eight drills			X
• Cariocas			X
• Sport-specific drills			X

Rehabilitation Protocol
Progression of Rehabilitation after Medial Collateral Ligament Injury
(Continued)
Reider and Mroczek

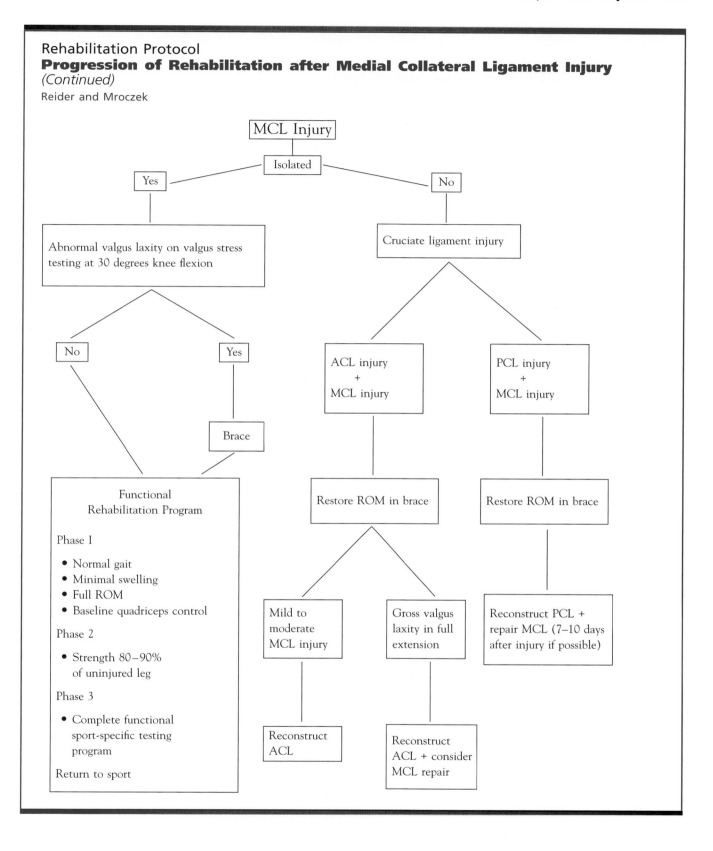

Rehabilitation Protocol
Isolated Medial Collateral Ligament Sprains
Wilk

Phase 1: Maximal Protection

Goals
- Early protected ROM.
- Prevent quadriceps atrophy.
- Decrease effusion and pain.

Day 1
- Ice, compression, and elevation.
- Knee hinge brace, nonpainful ROM, if needed.
- Crutches, weight-bearing as tolerated.
- Passive ROM, active-assisted ROM.
- Electrical muscle stimulation to quadriceps (8 hr/day).
- Quadriceps isometrics: quad sets, SLR (flexion).
- Emphasize hamstring stretches, active-assisted ROM knee flexion stretching to tolerance.

Day 2
- Continue above exercises.
- Quadriceps sets.
- SLR (flexion, abduction).
- Hamstring isometric sets.
- Well-leg exercises.
- Whirlpool for ROM (cold for first 3–4 days, then warm).
- High-voltage galvanic stimulation to control swelling.

Days 3–7
- Continue above exercises.
- Crutches, weight-bearing as tolerated.
- ROM as tolerated.
- Eccentric quadriceps work.
- Bicycle for ROM stimulus.
- Resisted knee extension with electrical muscle stimulation.
- Initiate hip adduction and extension.
- Initiate mini-squats.
- Initiate leg press isotonics.
- Brace worn at night, brace during day as needed.
- Continue ROM and stretching exercises.

Phase 2: Moderate Protection

Criteria for Progression to Phase 2
- No increase in instability.
- No increase in swelling.
- Minimal tenderness.
- Passive ROM 10–100 degrees.

Goals
- Full painless ROM.
- Restore strength.
- Ambulation without crutches.

Week 2
- Continue strengthening program with PREs.
- Continue electrical muscle stimulation to quadriceps during isotonic strengthening.
- Continue ROM exercises and stretching.

- Emphasize closed–kinetic chain exercises (lunges, squats, lateral lunges, wall squats, lateral step-ups).
- Bicycle for endurance and ROM stimulus.
- Water exercises, running in water forward and backward.
- Full ROM exercises.
- Flexibility exercises: hamstrings, quadriceps, iliotibial band, etc.
- Proprioception training (balance drills).
- Stairmaster endurance work.

Days 11–14
- Continue all exercises in week 2.
- PREs with emphasis on quadriceps, hamstrings, and hip abduction.
- Initiate isokinetics, progress from submaximal to maximal fast contractile velocities.
- Begin running program if full painless extension and flexion are present.

Phase 3: Minimal Protection

Criteria for Progression to Phase 3
- No instability.
- No swelling or tenderness.
- Full painless ROM.

Goal
- Increase power and strength.

Week 3
- Continue strengthening program
  - Wall squats.
  - Lateral lunges.
  - Knee extension.
  - Vertical squats.
  - Step-ups.
  - Hip abduction-adduction.
  - Lunges.
  - Leg press.
  - Hamstring curls.
- Emphasize
  - Functional exercise drills.
  - Fast-speed isokinetics.
  - Eccentric quadriceps.
  - Isotonic hip adduction, medial hamstrings.
- Isokinetic testing.
- Proprioception testing.
- Endurance exercises.
- Stationary bike 30–40 min.
- Nordic-Trac, swimming, etc.
- Initiate agility program, sport-specific activities.

Phase 4: Maintenance

Criteria for Return to Competition
- Full ROM.
- No instability.

Rehabilitation Protocol
Isolated Medial Collateral Ligament Sprains (Continued)
Wilk

- Muscle strength 85% of contralateral side.
- Satisfactory proprioception ability.
- No tenderness over MCL.
- No effusion.
- Quadriceps strength, torque–to–body weight ratio that fulfills criteria.
- Lateral knee brace (if necessary).

Maintenance Program
- Continue isokinetic strengthening exercises.
- Continue flexibility exercises.
- Continue proprioceptive exercises.

Meniscal Injuries

Michael D'Amato, MD, and Bernard R. Bach, Jr., MD

Clinical Background

The importance of the menisci in preserving the health and function of the knee has been well established. Most of the functions performed by the menisci relate to protecting the underlying articular cartilage.

- By increasing the effective contact area between the femur and the tibia, the menisci lower the load–per–unit area borne by the articular surfaces. Total meniscectomy results in a 50% reduction in contact area.
- The menisci transmit central compressive loads out toward the periphery, further decreasing the contact pressures on the articular cartilage.
- Half of the compressive load in the knee passes through the menisci with the knee in full extension and 85% of the load passes through the knee with the knee in 90 degrees of flexion.

Meniscectomy has been shown to reduce the shock absorption capacity of the knee by 20%.

Meniscal Movement

The lateral meniscus has been shown to be more mobile than the medial meniscus. In each meniscus, the anterior horn has greater mobility than the posterior horn. The reduced mobility of the posterior medial meniscus may result in greater stresses in this area, leading to increased vulnerability to injury. This would explain the higher rate of meniscal tears that occur in the posterior medial meniscus.

Weight-bearing has been shown to effect few changes in the movement of the menisci, although it has been suggested that meniscal loading may lead to distraction of radial tears. ROM of the knee, especially increasing rotation and flexion of the knee past 60 degrees, results in significant changes in the AP position of the menisci. **Clinically, second-look arthroscopy has shown that extension of the knee maintains a posterior horn meniscal tear in a reduced position, and knee flexion results in displacement of the tear.**

Meniscal Healing

King, in 1936, first noted that communication with the peripheral blood supply was critical for meniscal healing. Arnoczky and Warren, in 1982, described the microvasculature of the menisci. In children, the peripheral blood vessels permeate the full thickness of the meniscus. With age, the penetration of the blood vessels decreases. In adults, the blood supply is limited to only the outer 6 mm or about a third of the width of the meniscus. It is in this vascular region that the healing potential of a meniscal tear is greatest (Fig. 4–42). This potential drops off dramatically as the tear progresses away from the periphery.

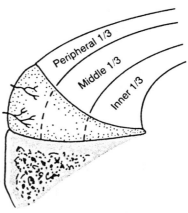

Figure 4–42. Meniscal tear zones. Peripheral meniscal tears at the red/white zone often have an intact perimeniscal capillary plexus and thus the potential for healing (blood supply present).

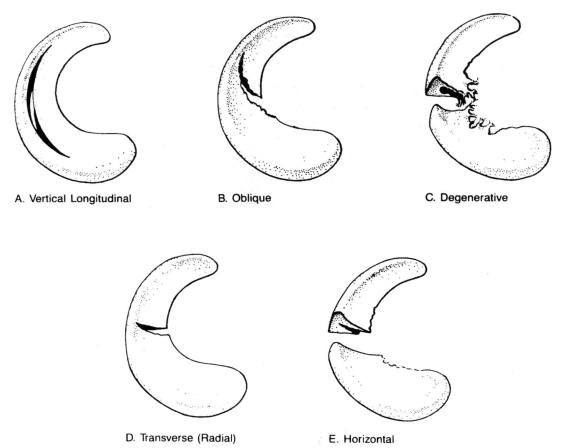

A. Vertical Longitudinal   B. Oblique   C. Degenerative

D. Transverse (Radial)   E. Horizontal

Figure 4–43. *A–E,* Variation in meniscal tear patterns. (*A–E,* From Ciccotti MG, Shields CL Jr, El Attrache NS: Meniscectomy. In Fu FH, Harner CD, Vince KG [eds]: Knee Surgery. Baltimore, Williams & Wilkins, 1994, pp. 749–767.)

Meniscal healing is also influenced by the pattern of the tear (Fig. 4–43). Longitudinal tears have a more favorable healing potential compared with radial tears. Simple tear patterns are more likely to heal than complex tears. Traumatic tears have higher healing rates than degenerative tears, and acute tears more so than chronic tears.

Rehabilitation Considerations

Weight-bearing and Motion

Although weight-bearing has little effect on displacement patterns of the meniscus and may be beneficial in approximating longitudinal tears, weight-bearing may place a displacing force across radial tears. Several studies have confirmed the benefits of early motion by demonstrating meniscal atrophy and decreased collagen content in menisci after immobilization. ROM of the knee before 60 degrees of flexion has little effect on meniscal displacement, but flexion angles greater than 60 degrees translate the menisci posteriorly. This increased translation may place detrimental stresses across a healing meniscus. As knee flexion increases, compressive loads across the meniscus also increase. The combination of weight-bearing and increasing knee flexion must be carefully balanced in the development of a rehabilitation protocol.

Axial Limb Alignment

Varus malalignment tends to overload the medial compartment of the knee, with increased stress placed on the meniscus, and **valgus malalignment** has the same effect on the lateral compartment and lateral meniscus. These increased stresses may interfere or disrupt meniscal healing after repair. Patients with limb malalignment tend to have more degenerative meniscal tears, which have been suggested to have an inherently poorer healing capacity. The use of an "unloader" brace has been recommended to help protect the healing meniscus, although no scientific data exist to support this approach.

Rehabilitation after Meniscectomy

Because there is no anatomic structure that must be protected during a healing phase, rehabilitation may progress aggressively. The goals are early control of pain and swelling, immediate weight-bearing, obtaining and maintaining a full ROM, and regaining quadriceps strength.

Rehabilitation after Meniscal Repair

Current studies support the use of unmodified accelerated ACL rehabilitation protocols after combined ACL reconstruction and meniscal repair. In tears with decreased healing potential (such as white-white tears, radial tears, or complex pattern tears), **limiting weight-bearing and limiting flexion to 60 degrees for the first 4 weeks have been suggested to better protect the repair and increase the healing potential of these difficult tears. However, we are unaware of any published studies that support these measures.**

Rehabilitation after isolated meniscal repair remains controversial. The healing environment clearly is inferior to that with concomitant ACL reconstruction, but good results have been obtained with accelerated rehabilitation protocols after isolated meniscal repairs.

Rehabilitation Protocol
After Arthroscopic Partial Medial or Lateral Meniscectomy
Wilk

Phase 1: Acute Phase

Goals
- Diminish inflammation and swelling.
- Restore ROM.
- Reestablish quadriceps muscle activity.

Days 1–3
- Cryotherapy.
- Electrical muscle stimulation to quadriceps.
- Quadriceps sets.
- SLR.
- Hip adduction and abduction.
- Knee extension.
- $^1/_2$ squats.
- Active-assisted ROM stretching, emphasizing full knee extension (flexion to tolerance).
- Weight-bearing as tolerated (two crutches).
- Light compression wrap.

Days 4–7
- Cryotherapy.
- Electrical muscle stimulation to quadriceps.
- Quadriceps sets.
- Knee extension 90–40 degrees.
- SLR.
- Hip adduction and abduction.
- $^1/_2$ squats.
- Balance/proprioceptive drills.
- Active-assisted and passive ROM exercises.
- ROM 0–115 degrees (minimal).
- Stretching (hamstrings, gastrocsoleus, quadriceps).
- Weight-bearing as tolerated (one crutch).
- Continued use of compression wrap or brace.
- High-voltage galvanic stimulation/cryotherapy.

Days 7–10
- Continue all exercises.
- Leg press (light weight).
- Toe raises.
- Hamstring curls.
- Bicycle (when ROM is 0–102 degrees with no swelling).

Phase 2: Internal Phase

Goals
- Restore and improve muscular strength and endurance.
- Reestablish full nonpainful ROM.
- Gradual return to functional activities.

Days 10–17
- Bicycle for motion and endurance.
- Lateral lunges.
- Front lunges.
- $^1/_2$ squats.
- Leg press.
- Lateral step-ups.
- Knee extension 90–40 degrees.
- Hamstring curls.
- Hip abduction and adduction.
- Hip flexion and extension.
- Toe raises.
- Proprioceptive and balance training.
- Stretching exercises.
- Active-assisted and passive ROM knee flexion (if necessary).
- Stairmaster or elliptical trainer.

Day 17–Week 4
- Continue all exercises.
- Pool program (deep-water running and leg exercises).
- Compression brace may be used during activities.

Phase 3: Advanced Activity Phase—Weeks 4–7*

Criteria for Progression to Phase III
- Full, nonpainful ROM.
- No pain or tenderness.
- Satisfactory isokinetic test.
- Satisfactory clinical examination (minimal effusion).

Goals
- Enhance muscular strength and endurance.
- Maintain full ROM.
- Return to sport/functional activities.

continued

Rehabilitation Protocol
After Arthroscopic Partial Medial or Lateral Meniscectomy *(Continued)*
Wilk

Exercises
- Continue to emphasize closed–kinetic chain exercises.
- May begin plyometrics.
- Begin running program and agility drills.

Note: We utilize the **Orthovid.com** meniscectomy instructional videotape with its concomitant handouts for all postoperative patients. This videotape was produced by the senior author of this book.

*Patients can begin phase III when criteria are met, which may be earlier than week 4.

Rehabilitation Protocol
Accelerated Rehabilitation after Meniscal Repair
D'Amato and Bach

Phase 1: Weeks 0–2

Goals
- Full motion.
- No effusion.
- Full weight-bearing.

Weight-bearing
- As tolerated.

Treatment
- ROM as tolerated (0–90 degrees).
- Cryotherapy.
- Electrical stimulation as needed.
- Isometric quadriceps sets.
- SLR.

Phase 2: Weeks 2–4

Criteria for Progression to Phase 2
- Full motion.
- No effusion.
- Full weight-bearing.

Goals
- Improved quadriceps strength.
- Normal gait.

Therapeutic Exercises
- Closed–kinetic chain resistance exercises 0–90 degrees.
- Bike and swim as tolerated.
- Early-phase functional training.

Phase 3: Weeks 4–8

Criteria for Progression to Phase 3
- Normal gait.
- Sufficient strength and proprioception for advanced functional training.

Goals
- Strength and functional testing at least 85% of contralateral side.
- Discharge from physical therapy to full activity.

Therapeutic Exercises
- Strength work as needed.
- Sport-specific functional progression.
- Advanced-phase functional training.

Rehabilitation Protocol
After Meniscal Repair
Wilk

Key factors in determining progression of rehabilitation after meniscal repair

- Anatomic site of tear.
- Suture fixation (too vigorous rehabilitation can lead to failure).
- Location of tear (anterior or posterior).
- Other pathology (PCL, MCL, or ACL injury).

Phase 1: Maximum Protection—Weeks 1–6

Stage 1: Immediate Postoperative Day 1–Week 3
- Ice, compression, elevation.
- Electrical muscle stimulation.
- Brace locked at 0 degrees.

Rehabilitation Protocol
After Meniscal Repair (Continued)
Wilk

- ROM 0–90 degrees.
  - Motion is limited for the first 7–21 days, depending on the development of scar tissue around the repair site. Gradual increase in flexion ROM is based on assessment of pain (0–30, 0–50, 0–70, 0–90 degrees).
- Patellar mobilization.
- Scar tissue mobilization.
- Passive ROM.
- Exercises
  - Quadriceps isometrics.
  - Hamstring isometrics (if posterior horn repair, no hamstring exercises for 6 wk).
  - Hip abduction and adduction.
- Weight-bearing as tolerated with crutches and brace locked at 0 degrees.
- Proprioception training.

Stage 2: Weeks 4–6
- Progressive resistance exercises (PREs)—1–5 pounds.
- Limited-range knee extension (in range less likely to impinge or pull on repair).
- Toe raises.
- Mini-squats.
- Cycling (no resistance).
- Surgical tubing exercises (diagonal patterns).
- Flexibility exercises.

Phase 2: Moderate Protection—Weeks 6–10

Criteria for Progression to Phase II
- ROM 0–90 degrees.
- No change in pain or effusion.
- Quadriceps control ("Good MMT").

Goals
- Increase strength, power, endurance.
- Normalize ROM of knee.
- Prepare patients for advanced exercises.

Exercises
- Strength—PRE progression.
- Flexibility exercises.

- Lateral step-ups (30 sec × 5 sets → 60 sec × 5 sets).
- Mini-squats.
- Isokinetic exercises.

Endurance Program
- Swimming (no frog kick).
- Cycling.
- Nordic-Trac.
- Stair machine.
- Pool running (see aquatic therapy section in Chapter 7).

Coordination Program
- Balance board.
- High-speed bands.
- Pool sprinting.
- Backward walking.

Plyometric Program

Phase 3: Advanced Phase—Weeks 11–15

Criteria for Progression to Phase 3
- Full, nonpainful ROM.
- No pain or tenderness.
- Satisfactory isokinetic test.
- Satisfactory clinical examination.

Goals
- Increase power and endurance.
- Emphasize return-to-skill activities.
- Prepare for return to full unrestricted activities.

Exercises
- Continue all exercises.
- Increase tubing program, plyometrics, pool program.
- Initiate running program.

Return to Activity: Criteria
- Full, nonpainful ROM.
- Satisfactory clinical examination.
- Satisfactory isokinetic test.

Patellofemoral Disorders

William R. Post, MD, John W. Brautigan, PT, ATC, and S. Brent Brotzman, MD

Clinical Background

Patellofemoral disorders (anterior knee pain) are one of the most commonly treated conditions in orthopaedic and primary care practices. The patellofemoral joint is a complex articulation that depends on both dynamic and static restraints for stability. Anterior knee pain encompasses numerous underlying disorders and **cannot be treated by a single treatment algorithm.**

Possible Etiologies of Patellofemoral Pain

Acute patellar dislocation

Patellar subluxation (chronic)

Recurrent patellar dislocation

Jumper's knee (patellar tendinitis)

continued

Possible Etiologies of Patellofemoral Pain
(Continued)

Osgood-Schlatter disease

Sinding-Larsen-Johanssen syndrome (inferior pole of patella)

Excessive lateral patellar compression syndrome (ELPS)

Global patellar pressure syndrome (GPPS)

Iliotibial band friction syndrome (lateral knee at Gerdy's tubercle)

Hoffa's disease (inflamed fat pad)

Bursitis

Medial patellofemoral ligament pain or tear

Trauma

Patellofemoral arthritis

Sickle cell disease

Anterior blow to patella

Osteochondritis dissecans (OCD)

RSD

Hypertrophic plica (runner)

Turf knee, wrestler's knee

Patellar fracture

Quadriceps rupture

Contusion

Tibial tubercle fracture

Prepatellar bursitis (housemaid's knee)

Patella baja

Patella alta

Medial retinaculitis

Referred hip pain

Gout

Pseudogout (chondrocalcinosis)

The key to successful treatment of patellofemoral pain is obtaining an accurate diagnosis by a thorough history and physical examination. For example, the treatment of RSD is very different than that for excessive lateral pressure syndrome (ELPS) and the correct diagnosis must be made to allow appropriate treatment.

"Chondromalacia" has been incorrectly used as an all-inclusive diagnosis for anterior knee pain. Chondromalacia actually is a pathologic diagnosis that describes articular cartilage changes seen on direct observation. This term should not be used as a synonym for patellofemoral or anterior knee pain. Often, the articular cartilage of the patella and femoral trochlea is normal, and the pain originates from the densely innervated peripatellar retinaculum or synovium. All peripatellar structures should be palpated and inspected. Other nociceptive input is possible from the subchondral bone, paratenon, tendon, and subcutaneous nerves in the patellofemoral joint.

Dye (1996) introduced the concept of loss of normal tissue homeostasis after overload of the extensor mecha-nism. The presence of excessive biomechanical load overwhelms the body's capacity to absorb energy and leads to microtrauma, tissue injury, and pain. Dye described the knee as a biologic transmission system that functions to accept, transfer, and dissipate loads. During normal ambulation, the muscles about the knee actually absorb more energy than they produce for propulsive forces.

Dye also described an "envelope of function" that considers both the applied loads at the knee and the frequency of loading. This model is useful in conceptualizing both direct trauma and overuse repetitive trauma as a cause of patellofemoral pathology. Either an excessive single loading event or multiple submaximal loading variables over time could exceed the limits of physiologic function and disrupt tissue homeostasis. For healing and homeostasis to occur, the patient must keep activities and rehabilitation efforts within the available envelope of function. **Therefore, submaximal, pain-free exercise and avoidance of "flaring" activities (increased PFJRFs) is a very important part of rehabilitation of patellofemoral injuries.**

Clinical Pearls for Patellofemoral Pain

- Approximately 70% of patellofemoral disorders will improve with conservative (nonoperative) treatment and time.
- When thinking about and evaluating patellofemoral knee pain, first try to decide if the problem stems from **instability or pain.** Once the diagnosis is correctly placed into one of these two categories, appropriate work-up and treatment decisions can be reached.
- **Arthroscopic release may be effective in patients with a positive lateral tilt (i.e., tight lateral structures) after failure of conservative measures. However, a lateral release should not be used to treat patellar instability.** A common complication of this procedure incorrectly used for instability is iatrogenic medial patellar subluxation or instability.
- Osteochondral fractures of the lateral femoral condyle or the medial facet of the patella have been documented by arthroscopy in 40 and 50% of patellar dislocations.
- Success rates of patellar operative procedures are related to the procedure selected and the number of previous surgeries.
- PFJRFs (Fig. 4–44) increase with flexion of the knee from 0.5 times body weight during level walking to 3 to 4 times body weight during stairclimbing to 7 to 8 times body weight with squatting.
- Females generally have a greater Q-angle than males. However, critical review of available studies found no evidence that Q-angle measures correlated with the presence or severity of anterior knee pain.
- Quadriceps flexibility deficits are common in these patients, especially in the chronic cases. Quadriceps

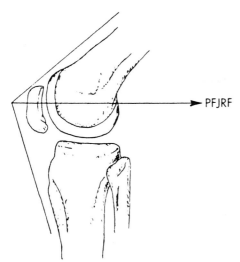

Figure 4–44. Increased patellofemoral joint reaction force (PFJRF) with knee flexion (e.g., squatting, kneeling, stair climbing).

stretching exercises produce dramatic improvement in symptoms in these patients.
- Restoration of flexibility (iliotibial band, quadriceps, hamstrings) is often overlooked but is extremely helpful in patients with flexibility deficits. ELPS with a tight lateral retinaculum and tight iliotibial band often responds dramatically to iliotibial band stretching and low-load, long-duration stretching of the lateral retinaculum.

Classification

Confusion over classification of patellofemoral disorders exists in the literature. Wilk and associates (1998) noted that a comprehensive patellofemoral classification scheme should (1) clearly define diagnostic categories, (2) aid in the selection of appropriate treatment, and (3) allow the comparison of treatment approaches for a specific diagnosis.

- Patellar instability
  - Acute patellar dislocation
  - Chronic patellar subluxation
  - Recurrent patellar dislocation
- Overuse syndromes
  - Patellar tendinitis (jumper's knee)
  - Quadriceps tendinitis
  - Osgood-Schlatter disease (tibial tubercle)
  - Sinding-Larsen-Johanssen syndrome (inferior aspect of the patella)
- Patellar compression syndrome
  - Excessive lateral pressure syndrome (ELPS)
  - Global patellar pressure syndrome (GPPS)
- Soft tissue lesions
  - Iliotibial band friction syndrome (lateral knee)
  - Symptomatic plica syndrome
  - Inflamed hypertrophic fat pad (Hoffa's disease)

- Bursitis
- Medial patellofemoral ligament pain
- Biomechanical linkage problems
  - Foot hyperpronation
  - Limb-length discrepancy
  - Loss of flexibility
- Direct trauma
  - Articular cartilage lesion (isolated)
  - Fracture
  - Fracture-dislocation
- Osteochondritis dissecans
- RSDS

Evaluation of the Patellofemoral Joint

Signs and Symptoms

- *Instability.* Often, patients complain of the knee "giving way" during straight-ahead activities or stairclimbing (versus instability owing to ACL or PCL injury, which typically is associated with giving way during pivoting or changing directions). Patellar subluxation typically lacks a history of trauma found with ACL-related instability. With frank episodes of patellar dislocation, the patella may spontaneously reduce or reduction may require pushing the patella medially and/or extending the knee. Dislocations typically are followed by a large bloody effusion (versus recurrent subluxation).
- *Overuse or training errors.* Training errors or overuse should be suspected in athletes, obese patients who climb stairs or squat all day, etc.
- *Localization of pain.* Pain may be diffuse or discretely localized to the patellar tendon (patellar tendinitis), medial or lateral retinaculum, quadriceps tendon, or inferior patella (Sinding-Larsen-Johanssen syndrome).
- *Crepitance.* Crepitance is often due to underlying articular cartilage damage in the patellofemoral joint, but may be due to soft tissue impingement. Many patients describe asymptomatic crepitance with stairclimbing.
- *Aggravating activities.* Painful popping with hill running only may indicate plica or iliotibial band syndrome. Aggravation of symptoms by stair climbing, squatting, kneeling, rising from sitting to standing (movie theater sign) suggests a patellofemoral articular cartilage or retinacular source (often GPPS or ELPS).
- *Swelling.* Perceived knee swelling with patellofemoral pain is infrequently due to an actual effusion, but is more commonly due to synovitis and fat pad inflammation. Large effusions are seen after patellar dislocations, but otherwise an effusion should imply other intra-articular pathology.
- *Weakness.* Although uncommon, weakness may represent quadriceps inhibition secondary to pain or may be indicative of extensive extensor mechanism damage (patellar tendon rupture, fractured patella, or patellar dislocation).

- *Night pain.* Pain at night or without relation to activity may imply tumor, advanced arthritis, infection, and the like. Unrelenting pain out of proportion to the injury, hyperesthesia, and so on implies RSD, neurogenic origin, postoperative neuroma, symptom magnification, etc.

Physical Examination

Both lower extremities should be examined with the patient in shorts only and without shoes. The patient should be examined and observed standing, walking, sitting, and lying supine. The ipsilateral knee, hip, foot, and ankle should be examined and compared with the opposite limb for symmetry, comparison of thigh muscular girths, Q-angles, and other factors.

Physical examination also should include evaluation of:

- Generalized ligamentous laxity (thumb to wrist, elbow or finger hyperextension, sulcus sign of shoulder) raises a red flag for possible patellar subluxation (Fig. 4–45).
- Gait pattern.
- Extensor mechanism alignment
  - Q-angle (standing and sitting) (see Fig. 4–1).
  - Genu valgum, varum, recurvatum (see Fig. 4–2).
  - Tibial torsion.
  - Femoral anteversion.
  - Patellar malposition (baja, alta, squinting).
  - Pes planus or foot pronation.
  - Hypoplastic lateral femoral condyle.
  - Patellar glide test: lateral glide, medial glide, apprehension (Fairbank sign).
  - Patellofemoral tracking.
  - J-sign (if present).

- Patellofemoral crepitance.
- VMO atrophy, hypertrophy.
- Effusion (large, small, intra-articular, extra-articular).
- Peripatellar soft tissue point tenderness
  - Medial retinaculum.
  - Lateral retinaculum.
  - Bursae (prepatellar, pes anserinus, iliotibial).
  - Quadriceps tendon.
  - Patellar tendon.
  - Palpable plica.
  - Iliotibial band/bursa.
  - Enlarged fat pad.
- Atrophy of thigh, VMO, calf.
- Flexibility.
  - Hamstrings.
  - Quadriceps.
  - Iliotibial band (Ober test).
- Leg-length discrepancy.
- Lateral pull test.
- Areas of possible referred pain (back, hip).
- RSD signs (temperature or color change, hypersensitivity).
- Hip ROM, flexion contracture.

Clinical Tests for Patellofemoral Disorders

Q-angle

The Q-angle is the angle formed by the intersection of lines drawn from the anterior superior iliac spine to the center of the patella and from the center of the patella to the tibial tubercle (see Fig. 4–1). In essence, these lines represent the lines of action of the quadriceps musculature and patellar tendons, respectively, on the patella. It should

A   B

Figure 4–45. Generalized ligamentous laxity. *A,* The patient is able to place the thumb to the wrist. *B,* The patient is able to hyperextend the finger joints (i.e., "double-jointed").

be measured with the knee slightly flexed, to center the patella in the trochlear groove. **Foot pronation (pes planus or flat feet) and limb internal rotation both increase the Q-angle.** The range of normal for the Q-angle varies in the literature, and there is controversy whether the wider pelvic anatomy in women contributes to a greater Q-angle. **The reported values of normal quoted are 10 degrees for men and 15 degrees for women.** It is well accepted that patellar alignment is somewhat affected by the degree of valgus at the knee; however, the degree of valgus present is not a dependable pathologic marker for severity of symptoms.

Soft Tissue Stabilizers of the Patella

In addition to the bony stabilizers, there are medial and lateral soft tissue restraints to the patella. The medial restraints consist of the medial retinaculum, the medial patellofemoral ligament, and the VMO. **The VMO is the most important dynamic stabilizer of the patella to resist lateral displacement.** Its fibers are oriented at about a 50- to 55 degree angle to the long axis of the femur (Fig. 4–46). It inserts normally into the superomedial aspect of

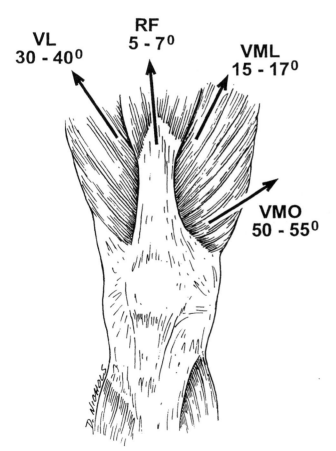

Figure 4–46. Fiber orientation of quadriceps muscle groups. RF, rectus femoris; VL, vastus lateralis; VML, vastus medialis lateral; VMO, vastus medialis oblique. (From Wilk KE, Davies GJ, Mangine RE, Malone TR: Patellofemoral disorders: a classification system and clinical guideline for nonoperative rehabilitation. J Orthop Sports Phys Ther 28:307–322, 1998.)

the patella along about one third to one half its length. However, in some cases of instability, the muscle may be absent or hypoplastic or may insert proximal to the patella.

The lateral restraints consist of the lateral retinaculum, the vastus lateralis, and the iliotibial band. Contracture in any of these structures may exert a tethering effect on the patella (e.g., ELPS), and they must be appropriately assessed during evaluation of the patellofemoral region.

Standing Alignment of the Extensor Mechanism

Inspection of the entire lower extremity should be performed not only to assess the alignment of the extensor mechanism but also to look for pes planus, tibial torsion, genu varum or valgum, genu recurvatum, femoral anteversion, or limb-length discrepancy, all of which can contribute to patellofemoral dysfunction. **It is important to evaluate the patient in a standing position.** The weight-bearing position may unmask otherwise hidden deformities such as excessive forefoot pronation (which increases the relative standing Q-angle) or limb-length discrepancies. Observation of the gait pattern may reveal abnormalities in mechanics, such as foot hyperpronation, or avoidance patterns during stair descent. Muscular atrophy can be visualized qualitatively or measured quantitatively (circumferentially from a fixed point) with a tape measure. The presence of erythema or ecchymosis in a particular area may offer an additional clue to the underlying pathology.

Local Palpation

Palpation also reveals any tenderness that may be present in the soft tissues around the knee. Tenderness along the medial retinacular structures may be the result of injury occurring with patellar dislocation. As the patella dislocates laterally, the medial retinaculum has to tear to allow the lateral displacement of the knee cap.

Lateral pain may be secondary to inflammation in lateral restraints, including the iliotibial band. Joint line tenderness typically indicates an underlying meniscal tear. Tenderness due to tendinitis or apophysitis in the quadriceps or patellar tendon will typically present with distinctly localized point tenderness at the area of involvement. Snapping or painful plicae may be felt, typically along the medial patellar border.

Range of Motion (Hip, Knee, Ankle)

ROM testing should include not only the knee but also the hip, ankle, and subtalar joints. Pathology in the hip may present as referred knee pain, and abnormal mechanics in the foot and ankle can lead to increased stresses in the soft tissue structures of the knee that may present as pain. While ranging the knee, the presence of crepitation and patellar tracking should be assessed. Palpable crepitus may or may not be painful and may or may not indicate significant underlying pathology, although it

Figure 4–47. Patellar grind or compression test. The examiner evaluates articular pain and crepitus by compressing the patella into the trochlea at various angles of knee flexion. Avoid compressing the peripatellar soft tissues by pressing the patella with the thenar eminence of the hand. The flexion angles that elicit pain during compression will indicate the likely location of the lesions.

Figure 4–48. Testing hamstring flexibility. In this test, the hip is flexed with the leg extended until the pelvis begins to move or the knee begins to flex. The angle formed between the leg and the table represents the flexibility of the hamstrings (popliteal angle).

should raise the suspicion of articular cartilage injury or soft tissue impingement. The *patella grind or compression test* (Fig. 4–47) will help to elucidate the etiology. To perform this test, one applies a compressive force to the patella as the knee is brought through a ROM. The reproduction of pain with or without accompanying crepitus is indicative of articular cartilage damage. More experienced examiners may be able to further localize the pain to specific regions of the patella or trochlea with subtle changes in the site of compression.

Flexibility of the Lower Extremity

Flexibility of the lower extremity must be evaluated. Quadriceps, hamstring, or iliotibial band tightness may all contribute to patellofemoral symptoms. Quadriceps flexibility may be tested with the patient in a prone or lateral position. The hip is extended and the knee progressively flexed. Limitation of knee flexion or compensatory hip flexion is indicative of quadriceps tightness. Hamstring flexibility can be tested (Fig. 4–48).

The **Ober test** (Fig. 4–49) is used to assess iliotibial band flexibility. The test is done with the patient in a side-lying position with the leg being measured up above the other. The lower hip is flexed to flatten lumbar lordosis and stabilize the pelvis. The examiner, positioned behind the patient, gently grasps the leg proximally just below the knee, flexes the knee to apply a mild stretch on the quadriceps, and flexes the hip to 90 degrees to flatten the lumbar lordosis. The hip is then extended to neutral, and any flexion contracture is noted. With the opposite hand at the iliac crest to stabilize the pelvis and prevent the patient from rolling backward, the examiner maximally abducts and extends the hip. The abducted and extended hip is then allowed to adduct by gravity while the knee is kept flexed, the pelvis stabilized, and the femur in

neutral rotation. Generally, the thigh should adduct to a position at least parallel to the examining table. Palpation proximal to the lateral femoral condyle with the iliotibial band on stretch is frequently painful to patients with iliotibial band and lateral retinacular tightness. When this is found, iliotibial band stretches become a valuable part of the treatment plan. Again, bilateral comparison is important. Ober's position is useful in the treatment (stretching) as well as in the diagnosis of iliotibial band tightness.

J-sign

Evaluation of patellar tracking begins with the knee in full extension. In this position, the patella typically rests just lateral to the midline. As the knee moves into flexion, at around 10 to 30 degrees, the patella centers into the trochlear groove and proceeds to track in a relatively straight path with progressive knee flexion. This normal path should progress smoothly. A sharp jump of the patella into the trochlear groove sometimes referred to as the *J-sign,* or late centering of the patella, should raise the suspicion of patellar instability.

Examination for knee instability should include a full evaluation of the cruciate and collateral ligaments to assess for any rotatory component, as well as to examine the patellar restraints. Patients with posterolateral corner knee instability may develop secondary patellar instability owing to a dynamic increase in the Q-angle. Similarly, patients with chronic MCL laxity may also develop secondary patellar instability. Apprehension on medial or lateral displacement testing of the patella should raise the

Figure 4–49. Ober test. With the patient in the lateral position and the involved leg up, the pelvis is stabilized and the hip is abducted and extended. The leg is then allowed to adduct toward the table. In a normal test, the upper knee will reach the table. In an abnormal test, the knee will remain tethered by a tight iliotibial band and will fail to reach the table.

suspicion of *underlying instability* in the patellar restraints. Superior and inferior patellar mobility should also be assessed; they may be decreased in situations of global contracture.

Patellar Glide Test

The patellar glide test is useful to assess the medial and lateral patellar restraints. In extension, the patella lies above the trochlear groove and should be freely mobile both medially and laterally. As the knee is flexed to 20 degrees, the patella should center in the trochlear groove, providing both bony and soft tissue stability.

Lateral Glide Test

The lateral glide test evaluates the integrity of the medial restraints. Lateral translation is measured as a percentage of patellar width (Fig. 4–50). Translations of 25% of patellar width are considered normal; translations greater than 50% indicate laxity within the medial restraints. The *medial patellofemoral ligament* has been noted to provide 53% of the stabilizing force to resist lateral subluxation, and normally presents with a solid endpoint when the lateral glide test is performed. Reproduction of the patient's symptoms with passive lateral translation of the patella pulling on the medial structures is referred to as a *positive lateral apprehension sign*. This signals lateral patellar instability.

Medial Glide Test

The medial glide test is performed with the knee in full extension. The patella is centered on the trochlear groove and medial translation from this "zero" point is measured in millimeters. Greater than 10 mm of translation is abnormal. The lateral retinacular laxity may be due to a hypermobile patella or, less commonly, medial

instability. *Medial patellar instability is rare and usually presents as an iatrogenic complication following patellar realignment surgery, typically from an overaggressive lateral release.* Six to 10 mm of translation is considered normal. Translation less than 6 mm medially indicates a tight lateral restraint and may be associated with ELPS.

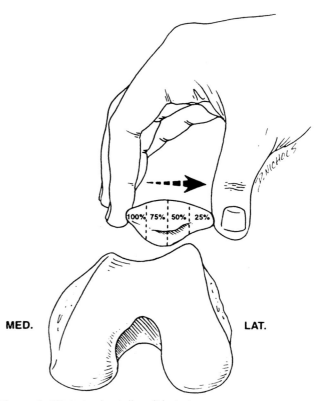

Figure 4–50. Lateral patellar glide test.

Patellar Tilt

A *tight lateral restraint* may contribute to patellar tilt. Patellar tilt is evaluated as the knee is brought to full extension and an attempt is made to elevate the lateral border of the patella (Fig. 4–51). Normally, the lateral border should be able to be elevated 0 to 20 degrees above the medial border. Less than 0 degrees indicates tethering by a tight lateral retinaculum, vastus lateralis, or iliotibial band. Presence of clinical and radiographic lateral patellar tilt is indicative of tight lateral structures. This may be responsible for ELPS. If extensive rehabilitation fails, the presence of a lateral patellar tilt correlates with a successful outcome after lateral release.

Bassett Sign

Tenderness over the medial epicondyle of the femur may represent an injury to the medial patellofemoral ligament in the patient with an acute or recurrent patellar dislocation.

Lateral Pull Test

This test is performed by contraction of the quadriceps with the knee in full extension. It is a positive (abnormal) test if lateral displacement of the patellar is observed. This test demonstrates excessive dynamic lateral forces.

Figure 4–51. *A,* Patellar tilt test. The patella is gripped manually with the patient in the supine position and the knee extended. Gently grasp the patella and push down on its *medial* edge and attempt to rotate the patella in the coronal plane to see whether lateral patellar tilt exists, and if so, can the tilt be corrected to "neutral." Neutral is defined as the patella's anterior surface being parallel to the examination table. Compare the contralateral knee. *B,* Passive patellar tilt test. An excessively tight lateral restraint (lateral retinaculum) is demonstrated by a neutral or negative angle to the horizontal. This test is performed with the knee extended and the quadriceps relaxed. *C,* With excessive lateral pressure syndrome, the lateral retinaculum is excessively tight and pulls the patella laterally, usually resulting in a lateral tilt and a gradual stretching out of the medial retinaculum. (*B,* Redrawn from Kolowich P: Lateral release of the patella: indications and contraindications. Am J Sport Med 14:359, 1990; *C,* from Wilk KE, Davies GJ, Mangine RE, Malone TR: Patellofemoral disorders: a classification system and clinical guidelines for nonoperative rehabilitation. J Orthop Sports Phys Ther 28:307-320, 1998.)

Radiographic Evaluation

Three views of the patella, an AP, a lateral in 30 degrees of knee flexion, and an axial image, should be obtained. The AP view can assess for the presence of any fractures, which should be distinguished from a bipartite patella, a normal variant. The overall size, shape, and gross alignment of the patella can also be ascertained. The lateral view is used to evaluate the patellofemoral joint space and to look for patella alta (see Fig. 4–1) or baja. In addition, the presence of fragmentation of the tibial tubercle or inferior patellar pole can be seen. Both the AP and the lateral views can also be used to confirm the presence and location of any loose bodies or osteochondral defects that may exist. **An axial image, typically a Merchant (knee flexed 45 degrees and x-ray beam angled 30 degrees to axis of the femur) or skyline view, may be the most important. It is used to assess patellar tilt and patellar subluxation.** The anatomy of the trochlear groove is also well visualized and the depth and presence of any condylar dysplasia can be determined. One important point deserves mention. The radiographs visualize only the subchondral bone of the patella and trochlea and do not show the articular cartilage. The articular surfaces are not necessarily of uniform thickness in these regions. Therefore, any measurements made from plain radiographs are only an indirect indication of the actual anatomic structure.

Assessment begins with the measurement of the **sulcus angle** (Fig. 4–52). A line is drawn along the medial and lateral walls of the trochlea. The angle formed between them is the sulcus angle. Greater than 150 degrees

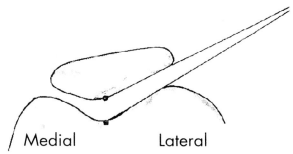

Figure 4–53. *Patellar tilt* is evaluated by the *patellofemoral angle*. Lines drawn along the lateral patellar facet (upper line) and the trochlear groove (lower line) should be parallel. Convergence of these two lines indicates lateral patellar tilt.

is abnormal and indicates a shallow or dysplastic groove that may have a predisposition for patellar instability.

Patellofemoral subluxation is evaluated by measurement of the **congruence angle** (see Fig. 4–52). The angle is formed by a line drawn from the apex of the trochlear groove bisecting the sulcus angle and a line drawn from the apex of the groove to the apex of the patella. A lateral position of the patella apex relative to the apex of the trochlea is considered positive. A normal congruence angle has been described as −6 degrees ±6 degrees.

Patellar tilt is evaluated by the patellofemoral angle (Fig. 4–53). This angle is formed by the lines drawn along the articular surfaces of the lateral patella facet and the lateral wall of the trochlear groove. The lines should be roughly parallel. Divergence is measured as a positive angle and is considered normal, whereas convergence of the lines is measured as a negative angle and indicates the presence of abnormal patellar tilt.

Important Points in Rehabilitation of Patellofemoral Disorders

Patellar Instability

- Patellar instability refers to symptoms secondary to episodic lateral (rarely medial) subluxation or dislocation of the patella. Lateral patellar subluxation is very common.
- Medial subluxation is typically rare, iatrogenic, and a result of excessive or ill-advised lateral release.
- **Predisposing risk factors** contributing to **patellar instability** include:
  - Femoral anteversion
  - Genu valgum
  - Patellar or femoral dysplasia
  - Patella alta
  - High Q-angle
  - Pes planus
  - Generalized laxity
  - Over-release of lateral retinaculum (medial instability)

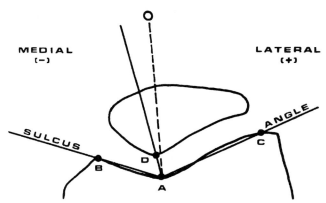

Figure 4–52. Sulcus angle and congruence angle. The *sulcus angle* is formed by lines BA and AC. The *congruence angle* is formed by a line bisecting the sulcus angle and a line drawn through the lowest point on the patella articular surface (represented by D in this diagram). A sulcus angle of greater than 150 degrees indicates a shallow trochlear groove, predisposing to patellar instability. Patellofemoral subluxation is evaluated by the congruence angle (see text). (From Merchant AC, Mercer RL, Jacobsen RH, Cool CR [eds]: Roentgenographic analysis of patellofemoral congruence. J Bone Joint Surg 56A:1391–1396, 1974.)

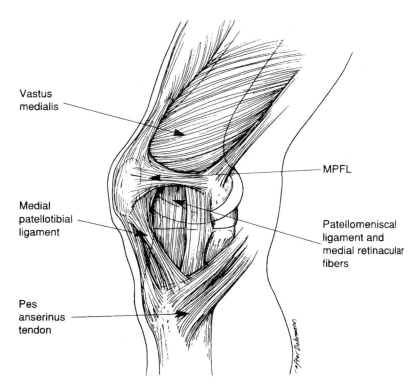

Vastus
medialis

MPFL

Medial
patellotibial
ligament

Patellomeniscal
ligament and
medial retinacular
fibers

Pes
anserinus
tendon

Figure 4–54. Anatomy of the medial aspect of the knee. The medial patellofemoral ligament (MPFL) provides 53% of the restraining force in preventing lateral displacement of the patella; the patellomeniscal ligament and medial retinacular fibers, on average, 22%. (From Boden BP, Pearsall AW, Garrett WE, Feagin JA [eds]: Patellofemoral instability: evaluation and management. J Am Acad Orthop Surg 5:47–57, 1997.)

- Previous patellar dislocation
- Atrophy of VMO
- Patellar subluxation generally describes the transient lateral movement of the patellar during early knee flexion. Often, this subluxation is reported as "something jumps or comes out of place" or is "hung up."
- Palpation often elicits medial retinacular tenderness.
- Patient apprehension (positive Fairbank sign) is common on displacing the patella laterally.
- Patellar mobility should be evaluated by displacing the patellar medially and laterally with the knee flexed 20 to 30 degrees. If more than 50% of the total patellar width can be displaced laterally over the

edge of the lateral femoral condyle, patellar instability should be suspected.
- Inspection of patellar tracking should be done with particular attention to the entrance and exit of the patella into the trochlea between 10 and 25 degrees of knee flexion. An abrupt lateral movement of the patella on terminal knee extension (extension subluxation) indicates patellar instability or subluxation.
- Conlan and coworkers (1993) in a biomechanical study of medial soft tissue restraints that prevent lateral patellar subluxation found that the medial patellofemoral ligament provides 53% of the total restraining force (Fig. 4–54).

Rehabilitation Protocol
General Guidelines for Nonoperative Treatment of Recurrent (Not Acute) Patellar Instability (Lateral)

Goals

- Decrease symptoms and instability.
- Increase quadriceps strength and endurance (VMO > lateral structures).
- Use of passive restraints (Palumbo-type bracing, McConnell taping) to augment stability during transition.
- Enhance patellar stability by dynamic stabilization or passive mechanisms.

Exercises

- Modify or avoid activities that aggravate or induce symptoms (running, squatting, stair-climbing, jumping, high-impact activities).
- Rest, ice, limb elevation.
- Use of cane or crutches if needed.
- NSAIDs (if not contraindicated) for anti-inflammatory effect; no steroid injection.
- Modalities to modify pain, reduce effusion and edema.

Rehabilitation Protocol
General Guidelines for Nonoperative Treatment of Recurrent (Not Acute) Patellar Instability (Lateral) *(Continued)*

- Electrical stimulation.
- VMO biofeedback for VMO strengthening.
- External Palumbo-type lateral buttress bracing (Fig. 4–55) or McConnell taping (Fig. 4–56) based on patient preference and skin tolerance to taping.
- Orthotics posted in subtalar neutral to control foot pronation, decrease Q-angle, or correct leg-length discrepancy.
- General conditioning and cross-training
  - Aqua exercises, deep pool running.
  - Swimming.
  - Avoid bicycling in the early phases.
- Pain-free quadriceps strengthening exercises with VMO efficiency enhancement.

Figure 4–56. McConnell taping (patellofemoral).

- No exercises isolate the VMO but several produce high EMG activity of the VMO
  - Leg press.
  - Lateral step-ups.
  - Isometric quadriceps setting.
  - Hip adduction exercises.
- Gradual restoration of flexibility (stretching) for noted deficits
  - Iliotibial band.
  - Quadriceps.
  - Hamstrings.
  - Gastrocnemius soleus.
  - Avoid mobilization of the medial retinaculum.
- Reestablish knee proprioception skills.

A   **B**

Figure 4–55. *A* and *B*, Patellar stabilizing braces.

Rehabilitation Protocol
McConnell Patellar Taping Techniques
D'Amato and Bach

- Figure 4–57 illustrates McConnell taping.
- The knee is cleaned, shaved, and prepared with an adhesive spray. If possible, try to avoid shaving immediately before taping to decrease the likelihood of skin irritation.

- Patellar taping is done with the knee in extension.
- Leukotape P is the taping material used.
- Correction is based on the individual malalignment, with each component corrected as described following.

continued

Rehabilitation Protocol
McConnell Patellar Taping Techniques *(Continued)*
D'Amato and Bach

Figure 4–57. *A,* Assessment of the glide component of the patella. *B,* Lateral glide is corrected with tape placed across the patella and pulled medially. *C,* Correction of the lateral glide component by applying a medial glide to the patella with Leukosport tape. *D,* Assessment of the tilt component of the patella.

Correcting Lateral Glide

- The tape is started at the midlateral border.
- It is brought across the face of the patella and secured to the medial border of the medial hamstring tendons while the patella is pulled in a medial direction.

- The medial soft tissues are brought over the medial femoral condyle toward the patella to obtain a more secure fixation.

Rehabilitation Protocol
McConnell Patellar Taping Techniques *(Continued)*
D'Amato and Bach

Figure 4–57 *continued.* *E,* Frequently, the lateral patellar border is pulled posteriorly (tight) by tightened lateral retinacular structures rather than the patellar borders being horizontal. *F,* Lateral tilt correction. *G,* External rotation correction.

Correcting Lateral Tilt

- The tape is started in the middle of the patella.
- It is brought across the face of the patella and secured to the medial border of the medial hamstring tendons, lifting the lateral border of the patella.
- The medial soft tissues are brought over the medial femoral condyle toward the patella to obtain a more secure fixation.

Correcting External Rotation

- The tape is applied to the middle of the inferior border of the patella.
- The inferior pole of the patella is manually rotated internally.

- The tape is secured to the medial soft tissues in superior and medial direction while the manual correction is maintained.

Alternatively, if there is also a component of **inferior tilt,** the tape can be started on the middle of the superior pole. After manual correction of the rotational deformity, the tape is secured in a superior and lateral direction. This not only corrects patellar rotation but also lifts the inferior pole away from the fat pad. Care must be taken not to create a lateral patellar glide when using this alternative method.

continued

Rehabilitation Protocol
McConnell Patellar Taping Techniques *(Continued)*
D'Amato and Bach

Correcting Inferior Patellar Tilt

- Correction of inferior tilt is always combined with correction of lateral tilt or glide component.
- To correct the inferior tilt component, the starting position of the tape is shifted from the midportion of the patella to the superior portion of the patella. Correction is then carried out as above for each individual component of glide or tilt. The superior starting position of the tape lifts the inferior pole of the patella away from the fat pad.

Technical Taping Considerations

- The tape is never left on for more than 24 hr at a time and should not be worn during nighttime sleep.
- The average duration of continuous taping treatment is 2 wk, followed by a weaning period during which the tape is worn only during strenuous activities. Taping may be continued as long as 6 wk, if tolerated.
- The tape must be removed slowly and carefully to prevent skin irritation, which will limit further taping. Commercial solvents are available to aid in tape removal.
- The application of rubbing alcohol to the skin after tape removal helps toughen the skin and prevent skin breakdown.
- Application of a skin moisturizer overnight will nourish the skin; the moisturizer is removed before tape is applied the next day.
- Allergic reaction to the tape may occur in a few first-time patients. The knee will develop an itchy rash, usually at 7–10 days after the start of taping. Topical cortisone creams may limit the rash. Only hypoallergenic tape should be used in patients who develop an allergic reaction.

Rehabilitation Protocol
Principles of McConnell Taping

- Taping is used as an adjunct to exercise and muscular balancing.
- The VMO–to–vastus lateralis ratio has been shown to improve during taping.
- The ability to truly change patellar position is debated.
- To tape correctly, the position of the patella relative to the femoral condyle must be evaluated.
- Four positional relationships are evaluated statically (sitting with the legs extended and quadriceps relaxed) then dynamically by doing a quadriceps set.

Glide component is the relationship of the medial and lateral poles of the patella to the femoral condyles. Statically, the patella should be centered in the condyles; dynamically this relationship should be maintained. With a quadriceps set, the patella should move superiorly without noticeable lateral movement. Most athletes require correction of the glide component for static or dynamic malalignment.

Tilt component is evaluated by comparing the anterior and posterior relationships of the medial and lateral borders of the patella. With the patient supine and the knee extended, the borders should be horizontal, both statically and dynamically. Frequently, the lateral border will be pulled posteriorly by the lateral retinaculum into the lateral condyle. This may also occur after the glide is corrected by taping.

Rotational component is the relationship between the long axis of the patella and the long axis of the femur. The ideal position is for the axes to be parallel. Frequently, the inferior pole of the patella is lateral to the axis of the femur, which would be described as lateral rotation.

Anteroposterior tilt is the anterior and posterior relationship of the superior and inferior poles of the patella. When the inferior pole of the patella is posterior, fat pad irritation is common.

After the patellar position is evaluated, an activity is identified that consistently provokes the patient's symptoms. Stepping off from an 8-inch-step is often effective. After taping, the test should be done again to ensure the effectiveness of taping in eliminating pain.

Taping Procedure

- Corrections are typically done in the order of evaluation, but the most significant alteration in position should be corrected first.
- Leukosport tape (Beiersdorf, Inc) is commonly used.
- Tape that is strong and tacky enough to be effective requires a protective cover next to the skin, such as "Cover Roll Stretch."
- To correct the **glide component,** the tape is anchored on the lateral pole of the patella, the patella is manually glided medially and taped in this position.
- The **tilt component** is corrected by starting the tape in the middle of the patella and pulling the medial pole of

Rehabilitation Protocol
Principles of McConnell Taping *(Continued)*

the patella posteriorly and anchoring over the tape used for the glide correction.

- A **rotational fault** is corrected by anchoring on the lateral aspect of the inferior pole of the patella and pulling toward the medial joint line.
- If an **anteroposterior tilt** is present, it is corrected by taping the glide or tilt on the superior aspect of the patella to pull the inferior aspect of the patella out of the fat pad.

- Not all components have to be corrected if the pain is eliminated with one or two corrections.
- **A provocation test should be done after each stage of taping to check its effectiveness.**
- Taping is worn during activities that produce pain: just with athletics or with all activities of daily living.
- Once muscular control of the patella is improved, the patient is weaned from the tape; it is not intended for long-term use.

Patellar Excess Pressure Syndromes (GPPS versus ELPS)

The most important clinical finding differentiating GPPS from ELPS is patella mobility. In GPPS, mobility is restricted in both the medial and the lateral directions. Often, superior mobility is also restricted. With ELPS, tightness is present **only** in the lateral retinacular structures.

The rehabilitation program for **ELPS** focuses on stretching the tight lateral retinacular structures and includes medial mobilization with medial glides and tilts, McConnell taping to "medialize" or normalize the patella (correct the tilt), and low-load long-duration stretching of the tight lateral structures. Musculotendinous stretching should include the hamstrings, quadriceps, and iliotibial band. Improving quadriceps strength, especially the VMO, is emphasized. Open-chain knee extension and bicycling are not used in early rehabilitation. NSAIDs can be used for synovitis and inflammation, as well as modalities such as high-voltage galvanic stimulation and cryotherapy. Daily home exercises are done, and the patient is educated about which activities to avoid (stairs,

squatting, kneeling, jumping, running) and counseled about changing sports.

GPPS is treated in a similar manner, with a few important changes. **Patellar mobility in all planes must be reestablished or improved before initiation of any aggressive rehabilitation to decrease inflammation and cartilage degeneration.** Modalities such as a warm whirlpool and ultrasound can be used before mobilization of the patella. The glide is held for at least 1 to 2 minutes, 10 to 12 minutes if possible, during mobilization. Mobilization of the quadriceps insertion is used. The patient performs unrestricted knee motion several times a day to maintain soft tissue mobility. Restoration of full passive knee extension is vital to preseve the integrity of patellofemoral articular cartilage. Initially, multiangle quadriceps isometric contraction, straight-leg raises, and 40-degree mini-squats are used until patellar mobilization improves. Then leg press, lunge, and wall squat can be added. Bicycling, deep knee bends, deep squats, and resisted knee extension **should be avoided** until patellar mobility is restored. Bracing or taping is **not** used in patients with GPPS because it restricts and compresses the patella.

Rehabilitation Protocol
Patellofemoral Compression Syndromes: Excessive Lateral Pressure Syndrome (ELPS) and Global Patellar Pressure Syndrome (GPPS)
D'Amato and Bach

Phase 1

Goals
- Reduce pain and inflammation.
- Increase patellar mobility, mobilize contracted peripatellar structures.

- Regain quadriceps control.
- Improve patellofemoral movements.

Taping/Bracing
- ELPS: McConnell taping to correct tilt.
- GPPS: no bracing or taping.

continued

Rehabilitation Protocol
Patellofemoral Compression Syndromes: Excessive Lateral Pressure Syndrome (ELPS) and Global Patellar Pressure Syndrome (GPPS) *(Continued)*
D'Amato and Bach

Therapeutic Exercises
- Ice, electrical stimulation, and NSAIDs to decrease inflammation and pain.
- Quadriceps sets and straight-leg raises, multiangle quadriceps isometrics.
- Hip adduction and abduction, flexion and extension exercises.
- Begin patellar mobilization techniques
  - ELPS: mobilize tight lateral patellar tissues.
  - GPPS: mobilize medial, lateral, superior peripatellar tissue.

Phase 2

Criteria for Progression to Phase 2
- Minimal pain.
- Minimal inflammation.

Goals
- Good quadriceps set with no extension lag.
- Improve ROM.
- Increase patellar mobility (*Note:* Avoid aggressive strengthening with GPPS until patellar mobility is significantly improved).

Therapeutic Exercises
- Continue patellar mobilization.
- Fit patella stabilizing brace or use McConnell taping (ELPS) to correct patellar tilt.
- Continue ice and electrical stimulation (especially after exercise) and NSAIDs.
- SLR, quadriceps sets.
- Flexibility exercises for quadriceps, hamstrings, iliotibial band, gastrocnemius, soleus.
- Closed-chain exercises: mini-lunges, wall slides, lateral step-ups, mini-squats.
- Avoid bicycling, deep knee bends, deep squats, resisted knee extension.
- Pool exercises, swimming.
- Advance exercises for hip flexors and extensors, abductors and adductors, and muscles of the lower leg and foot, increasing weight as tolerated, doing 3 to 10 sets and increasing weight by 2 pounds.

Phase 3

Criteria for Progression to Phase 3
- No increase in pain or inflammation.
- Good quadriceps strength.

Goals
- Full knee motion.
- Improved strength and flexibility.

Bracing
- Continue using brace or taping if helpful.

Therapeutic Exercises
- Advance hamstring strengthening exercises.
- Bicycling, swimming, stair-stepping, or walking for cardiovascular and muscle endurance; increase duration, then speed.
- Continue flexibility exercises.
- Progress closed-chain activities.

Phase 4

Criteria for Progression to Phase 4
- Full knee motion.
- Quadriceps strength 80% of normal.

Goal
- Return to full activity.

Brace
- Brace or tape is worn for sports participation if desired. Tape up to 6 wk, then discontinue. Continue brace as needed.

Therapeutic Exercises
- Add slow return to running if desired; increase distance, then speed.
- Warm up well.
- Use ice after workout.
- Continue aerobic cross-training.
- Start jumping, cutting, and other sport-specific exercises.

Return to Full Activity
- Full pain-free motion.
- Strength and functional tests 85% of normal.

Rehabilitation Protocol
After First-time Acute Lateral Patellar Dislocation
D'Amato and Bach

Phase 1
Goals
- Decrease pain and avoid recurrent dislocation.
- Return of muscle function.

- Decrease swelling.
- Limit ROM to protect healing tissues.
- Limit weight-bearing to protect healing tissues.

Rehabilitation Protocol
After First-time Acute Lateral Patellar Dislocation *(Continued)*
D'Amato and Bach

- Avoid leading patient into pain dysfunction syndrome with overaggressive therapy.

Bracing
- Limited-range brace set at 0 degrees with ambulation initially; lateral buttress doughnut pad in brace.
- Patella stabilizing brace or McConnell taping.
- Light compressive dressing.

Weight-bearing
- Partial weight-bearing with crutches.

Therapeutic Exercises
- Cryotherapy.
- Electrical stimulation to promote quadriceps activity, emphasising VMO (high-voltage galvanic stimulation).
- Supine SLR when pain level allows.
- Passive ROM in pain-free range.
- Ankle pumps if swelling is present.
- Isometric hamstrings.
- Aspiration of blood if effusion is inhibiting quadriceps.

Phase 2
Criteria for Progression to Phase 2
- No significant joint effusion.
- No quadriceps extension lag.
- **Avoid performing apprehension to patellar mobility test.**
- Little or no pain with activities of daily living.

Goals
- Improve quadriceps muscle function.
- Obtain full pain-free ROM.
- Begin low-level functional activities.
- Initiate conditioning program.
- Avoid patellofemoral symptoms or instability.

Bracing
- Continue patellar bracing or taping.

Weight-bearing
- As tolerated.
- Discard crutches when quadriceps control with no extension lag is achieved.

Therapeutic Exercises
- Continue electrical stimulation as needed.
- Continue supine SLR and add PREs, adduction and abduction SLR.
- Toe raises with equal weight-bearing bilaterally.
- Modalities as needed.
- Closed–kinetic chain exercises (wall sitting, toe raises).
- Low-level endurance training (well-leg cycling).
- Low-level pool activities.

Phase 3
Criteria for Progression to Phase 3
- Full active ROM.
- Good to normal quadriceps function.
- Full weight-bearing without gait deviations.

Goals
- Improve functional capabilities.
- Gradual return to sports activity or other high-level activity.

Bracing
- Wean from patellar brace or taping as quadriceps strength improves.

Therapeutic Exercises
- Four-way hip exercises (i.e., SLR with adduction, abduction, flexion, extension).
- Aqua therapy, walking progressing to running in water.
- Sport- and skill-specific training.
- Proprioceptive training.
- Patient education.

Criteria for Return to Full Activity (8–12 Weeks)
- ROM equal to opposite limb.
- No pain or effusion.
- Strength 85% of opposite limb.
- Satisfactory 1-min hop test, two-legged hop test.
- Patellar stability on clinical examination.

Rehabilitation Protocol
After Lateral Retinacular Release
D'Amato and Bach

Indications for Lateral Release
- Recalcitrant patellofemoral pain with a positive lateral tilt of the patella (see p. 326).
- Tight lateral retinaculum—positive ELPS.
- Lateral retinacular pain with positive lateral tilt.

Phase 1: Immediately after Surgery—2 Weeks
Goals
- Protect healing soft tissue structures.
- Improve knee flexion and extension.

continued

Rehabilitation Protocol
After Lateral Retinacular Release *(Continued)*
D'Amato and Bach

- Increase lower extremity strength, including quadriceps muscle re-education.
- Education of patient regarding limitations and rehabilitation process.

Weight-bearing
- As tolerated with two crutches.

Therapeutic Exercises
- Quadriceps sets and isometric adduction with biofeedback for VMO.
- Heel slides.
- Ankle pumps.
- Non–weight-bearing gastrocsoleus and hamstring exercises.
- SLR in flexion with turnout, adduction, and extension; begin hip abduction at approximately 3 wk.
- Functional electrical stimulation can be used for trace to poor quadriceps contraction.
- Begin aquatic therapy at 2 wk (when wound is healed), with emphasis on normalization of gait.
- Stationary bike for ROM when sufficient knee flexion is present.

Phase 2: Weeks 2–4

Criteria for Progression to Phase 2
- Good quadriceps set.
- Approximately 90 degrees active knee flexion.
- Full active knee extension.
- No signs of active inflammation.

Goals
- Increase flexion.
- Increase lower extremity strength and flexibility.
- Restore normal gait.
- Improve balance and proprioception.

Weight-bearing
- Ambulation as tolerated without crutches if following criteria are met
  - No extension lag with SLR.
  - Full active knee extension.
  - Knee flexion of 90–100 degrees.
  - Nonantalgic gait pattern.
- May use one crutch or cane to normalize gait before walking without assistive device.

Therapeutic Exercises
- Wall slides from 0–45 degrees knee flexion, progressing to mini-squats.
- Four-way hip exercises for flexion, extension, and adduction.
- Calf raises.
- Balance and proprioception activities (including single-leg stance, KAT, and BAPS board).

- Treadmill walking with emphasis on normalization of gait pattern.
- Iliotibial band and hip flexor stretching.

Phase 3: Weeks 4–8

Criteria for Progression to Phase 3
- Normal gait.
- Good to normal quadriceps strength.
- Good dynamic control with no evidence of patellar lateral tracking or instability.
- Clearance by physician to begin more concentrated closed–kinetic chain progression.

Goals
- Restore any residual loss of ROM.
- Continue improvement of quadriceps strength.
- Improve functional strength and proprioception.

Therapeutic Exercises
- Quadriceps stretching when full knee flexion has been achieved.
- Hamstring curl.
- Leg press from 0–45 degrees knee flexion
- Closed–kinetic chain progression.
- Abduction on four-way hip exercises.
- Stairmaster or elliptical trainer.
- Nordic-Trac.
- Jogging in pool with wet vest or belt.

Phase 4: Return to Full Activity—Week 8

Criteria for Progression to Phase 4
- Release by physician to resume full or partial activity.
- No patellofemoral or soft tissue complaints.
- No evidence of patellar instability.
- Necessary joint ROM, muscle strength and endurance, and proprioception to safely return to athletic participation.

Goals
- Continue improvements in quadriceps strength.
- Improve functional strength and proprioception.
- Return to appropriate activity level.

Therapeutic Exercises
- Functional progression, which may include but is not limited to
  - Slide board.
  - Walk/jog progression.
  - Forward and backward running, cutting, figure-of-eight, and carioca.
  - Plyometrics.
  - Sport-specific drills.

Rehabilitation Protocol
After Lateral Retinacular Release
Wilk

Phase 1: Immediate Postoperative Phase

Goals
- Diminish swelling and inflammation (control hemarthrosis).
- Initiate quadriceps muscle training.
- Medial mobilization of patella.
- Independent ambulation.

Weight-bearing
- As tolerated with two crutches.

Control Swelling and Inflammation
- Cryotherapy.
- Lateral "C" buttress pad (felt).
- Compression bandage.
- Elevation and ankle pumps.

Range of Motion
- ROM to tolerance.
- At least 75 degrees flexion by days 2–3.
- Patellar mobilization (especially medial).

Muscle Retraining
- Quadriceps isometrics.
- SLR (flexion).
- Hip adduction.
- Knee extension (pain-free arc).

Flexibility
- Hamstring stretches.
- Calf stretches.
- Active-assisted ROM knee flexion (to tolerance).

Phase 2: Acute Phase

Goals
- Control swelling and inflammation.
- Gradual improvement in ROM.
- Quadriceps strengthening, especially VMO.

Note: rate of progression is based on swelling and inflammation.

Weight-bearing
- Progress weight-bearing as tolerated with one crutch (progression based on pain, swelling, and quadriceps control).
- Discontinue crutch use when appropriate.

Control Swelling and Inflammation
- Continue use of lateral "C" buttress pad (felt).
- Compression bandage.
- Cryotherapy and elevation five or six times a day.

Range of Motion
- At least 90–100 degrees flexion (wk 1).
- At least 105–115 degrees flexion (wk 2).
- At least 115–125 degrees flexion (wk 3).

Note: rate of progression based on swelling and inflammation.

Muscle Retraining
- Electrical stimulation to quadriceps.
- Quadriceps setting isometrics.
- SLR (flexion).
- Hip adduction.
- Knee extension 60–0 degrees (pain-free arc).
- Mini-squats with adduction (squeeze ball).
- Leg press (squeeze ball).
- Stationary bicycle if ROM and swelling permit.
- Proprioception training.

Flexibility
- Continue hamstring and calf stretches.
- Initiate quadriceps muscle stretching.

Phase 3: Subacute, Moderate Protection Phase

Criteria for Progression to Phase 3
- Minimal inflammation.
- ROM 0–125 degrees.
- Voluntary quadriceps contraction.

Goals
- Eliminate any joint swelling.
- Improve muscular strength and control without exacerbation of symptoms.
- Functional exercise movements.

Exercises
- Continue muscle stimulation to quadriceps, if needed.
- Quadriceps setting isometrics.
- Four-way hip machine (adduction, abduction, flexion, extension).
- Lateral step-ups (if able to do pain-free).
- Front step-ups (if able to do pain-free).
- Half-squats against wall (0–60 degrees).
- Leg press.
- Knee extension (90–0 degrees) pain-free arc.
- Bicycle.
- Pool program (walking, strengthening, running).
- Proprioceptive training.

Flexibility
- Continue all stretching exercises.

Control Swelling and Inflammation
- Continue use of ice, compression, and elevation as needed.

Phase 4: Advanced, Minimal Protection Phase

Criteria for Progression to Phase 4
- Full, nonpainful ROM.
- Absence of swelling or inflammation.
- Knee extension strength 70% of contralateral knee.

continued

Rehabilitation Protocol
After Lateral Retinacular Release (Continued)
Wilk

Goals
- Achieve maximal strength and endurance.
- Functional activities and drills.

Exercises
- Wall squats (0–70 degrees) pain-free arc.
- Half vertical squats (0–60 degrees).
- Leg press.
- Forward lunges.
- Lateral lunges.
- Lateral step-ups.
- Front step-ups.
- Knee extension, pain-free arc.
- Hip strengthening (four-way).
- Bicycle.
- Stairmaster.
- Proprioception drills.
- Sport-specific functional drills (competitive athletes).

- Continue all stretching.
- Continue use of ice as needed.

Phase 5: Return to Activity Phase

Criteria for Progression to Phase 5
- Full, nonpainful ROM.
- Appropriate strength level (80% or more of contralateral leg).
- Satisfactory clinical examination.

Goal
- Functional return to work or sport.

Exercises
- Functional drills.
- Strengthening exercises (selected).
- Flexibility exercises.

Rehabilitation Protocol
After Distal and/or Proximal Patellar Realignment Procedures
D'Amato and Bach

General Guidelines
- No closed–kinetic chain exercises for 6 wk.
- Same rehabilitation protocol is followed for proximal and distal realignments, except for weight-bearing limitations as noted.
- After a combined proximal and distal realignment, the protocol for distal realignment is used.

Phase 1: Immediately Postoperative—Weeks 1–6

Goals
- Protect fixation and surrounding soft tissues.
- Control inflammatory process.
- Regain active quadriceps and VMO control.
- Minimize adverse effects of immobilization through CPM and heel slides in the allowed ROM.
- Full knee extension.
- Patient education regarding the rehabilitation process.

Range of Motion
- 0–2 wk: 0–30 degrees of flexion.
- 2–4 wk: 0–60 degrees of flexion.
- 4–6 wk: 0–90 degrees of flexion.

Brace
- 0–4 wk: locked in full extension for all activities except therapeutic exercises and CPM use; locked in full extension for sleeping.
- 4–6 wk: unlocked for sleeping, locked in full extension for ambulation.

Weight-bearing
- As tolerated with two crutches for proximal realignment procedure 50% with two crutches for distal realignment procedure.

Therapeutic Exercises
- Quadriceps sets and isometric adduction with biofeedback and electrical stimulation for VMO (no electrical stimulation for 6 wk with proximal realignment).
- Heel slides from 0–60 degrees of flexion for proximal realignment, 0–90 degrees for distal realignment.
- CPM for 2 hr, twice daily, from 0–60 degrees of flexion for proximal realignment, 0–90 degrees of flexion for distal realignment.
- Non–weight-bearing gastrocnemius soleus, hamstring stretches.
- SLR in four planes with brace locked in full extension (can be done standing).
- Resisted ankle ROM with Theraband.
- Patellar mobilization (begin when tolerated).
- Begin aquatic therapy at 3–4 wk with emphasis on gait.

Rehabilitation Protocol
After Distal and/or Proximal Patellar Realignment Procedures *(Continued)*
D'Amato and Bach

Phase 2: Weeks 6–8

Criteria for Progression to Phase 2
- Good quadriceps set.
- Approximately 90 degrees of flexion.
- No signs of active inflammation.

Goals
- Increase range of flexion.
- Avoid overstressing fixation.
- Increase quadriceps and VMO control for restoration of proper patellar tracking.

Brace
- Discontinue use for sleeping, unlock for ambulation as allowed by physician.

Weight-bearing
- As tolerated with two crutches.

Therapeutic Exercises
- Continue exercises, with progression toward full flexion with heel slides.
- Progress to weight-bearing gastrocnemius soleus stretching.
- Discontinue CPM if knee flexion is at least 90 degrees.
- Continue aquatic therapy.
- Balance exercises (single-leg standing, KAT, BAPS board).
- Stationary bike, low-resistance, high-seat.
- Wall slides progressing to mini-squats, 0–45 degrees flexion.

Phase 3: 8 Weeks–4 Months

Criteria for Progression to Phase 3
- Good quadriceps tone and no extension lag with SLR.
- Nonantalgic gait pattern.
- Good dynamic patellar control with no evidence of lateral tracking or instability.

Weight-bearing
- May discontinue use of crutches when following criteria are met

- No extension lag with SLR.
- Full extension.
- Nonantalgic gait pattern (may use one crutch or cane until gait is normalized).

Therapeutic Exercises
- Step-ups, begin at 2 inches and progress toward 8 inches.
- Stationary bike, add moderate resistance.
- Four-way hip for flexion, adduction, abduction, extension.
- Leg press for 0–45 degrees of flexion.
- Swimming, Stairmaster for endurance.
- Toe raises.
- Hamstring curls.
- Treadmill walking with emphasis on normalization of gait.
- Continue proprioception exercises.
- Continue flexibility exercises for gastrocnemius soleus and hamstrings, add iliotibial band and quadriceps as indicated.

Phase 4: 4–6 Months

Criteria for Progression to Phase 4
- Good to normal quadriceps strength.
- No evidence of patellar instability.
- No soft tissue complaints.
- Clearance from physician to begin more concentrated closed–kinetic chain exercises and resume full or partial activity.

Goals
- Continue improvements in quadriceps strength.
- Improve functional strength and proprioception.
- Return to appropriate activity level.

Therapeutic Exercises
- Progression of closed–kinetic chain activities.
- Jogging/running in pool with wet vest or belt.
- Functional progression, sport-specific activities.

Rehabilitation Protocol
After Patellofemoral Distal Realignment Procedure
Wilk

Phase 1: Immediate Postoperative Phase—Days 1–5

Goals
- Diminish swelling, inflammation (control hemarthrosis).
- Diminish postoperative pain.

- Initiate voluntary quadriceps control.
- Independent ambulation.

Brace
- Brace for ambulation only (days 1–4).

continued

Rehabilitation Protocol
After Patellofemoral Distal Realignment Procedure *(Continued)*
Wilk

Weight-bearing
- As tolerated with two crutches (approximately 50% weight-bearing).

Control Swelling and Inflammation
- Cryotherapy.
- Compression bandage.
- Elevation and ankle pumps.

Range of Motion
- Full passive knee extension.
- Flexion to 45 degrees (days 1–4).
- Flexion to 60 degrees (day 5).
- Passive ROM and gentle active-assisted ROM only.

Muscle Retraining
- Quadriceps setting isometrics.
- SLR (flexion).
- Hip adduction and abduction.
- No active knee extension.

Flexibility
- Hamstring and calf stretches.
- Passive and active-assisted ROM within ROM limitations.

Phase 2: Acute Phase—Weeks 2–4

Goals
- Control swelling and pain.
- Promote healing of realigned tibial tuberosity.
- Strengthen quadriceps.

Brace
- Continue brace for ambulation only.
- Discontinue brace at 4 wk.

Weight-bearing
- Progress weight-bearing as tolerated (two crutches for four wk).

Control Swelling and Inflammation
- Continue use of cryotherapy.
- Compression bandage.
- Elevation.

Range of Motion
- Passive and active-assisted ROM exercises.
- ROM 0–75 degrees (wk 1–3).
- Range of motion 0–90 degrees (wk 4).

Muscle Retraining
- Electrical muscle stimulation to quadriceps.
- Quadriceps setting isometrics.
- SLR (flexion).
- Hip adduction and abduction.
- Hip extension.
- **Gentle** submaximal isometric knee extension (multiangle).

Week 4
- Light leg press.
- Vertical squats (no weight).

Flexibility
- Continue hamstring and calf stretches.

Phase 4: Motion Phase—Weeks 5–8

Goals
- Gradual improvement in ROM.
- Improve muscular strength and endurance.
- Control forces on extension mechanism.

Weight-bearing
- One crutch (wk 4–6).
- Discontinue crutch at week 6.

Range of Motion
- Passive ROM 0–115 degrees (wk 5).
- Passive ROM 0–125 degrees (wk 6).
- Passive ROM 0–125/135 degrees (wk 8).

Therapeutic Exercises
- Continue electrical muscle stimulation to quadriceps.
- Quadriceps setting isometrics.
- Hip adduction, abduction, and extension.
- Vertical squats.
- Leg press.
- Knee extension, light (0–60 degrees).
- Bicycle (wk 6–8).
- Pool program, walking and strengthening (when able).

Flexibility
- Continue all stretching exercises for lower extremity.

Phase 4: Strengthening Phase—Weeks 9–16

Criteria for Progression to Phase 4
- ROM at least 0–115 degrees.
- Absence of swelling and inflammation.
- Voluntary control of quadriceps.

Goals
- Gradual improvement of muscular strength.
- Functional activities and drills.

Therapeutic Exercises
- Half vertical squats (0–60 degrees).
- Wall squats.
- Leg press.
- Forward lunges.
- Lateral lunges.
- Lateral step-ups.
- Knee extension (60–0 degrees).
- Hip adduction and abduction.
- Bicycle.
- Stairmaster.

Rehabilitation Protocol
After Patellofemoral Distal Realignment Procedure *(Continued)*
Wilk

Phase 5: Return to Activity Phase

Criteria for Progression to Phase 5
- Full, nonpainful ROM.
- Appropriate strength level (80% or more of contralateral leg).
- Satisfactory clinical examination.

Goal
- Functional return to specific drills.

Therapeutic Exercises
- Functional drills.
- Strengthening exercises.
- Flexibility exercises.

Overuse Syndromes of the Knee

Overuse syndromes involving the extensor mechanism are commonly grouped together under the term **"jumper's knee."** **Patellar tendinitis** is the most common, typically presenting with pain near the insertion of the tendon at the inferior pole of the patella (Fig. 4–58). Less commonly, the symptoms may be localized to the distal tendon insertion at the tibial tubercle or the quadriceps tendon insertion at the proximal pole of the patella. In adolescents, it typically presents as a form of apophysitis, occurring at the tibial tubercle **(Osgood-Schlatter)** or distal patellar pole **(Sinding-Larsen-Johanssen)** (Fig. 4–59).

History of Patellar Tendinitis (Jumper's Knee)

The typical history is that of an insidious onset of anterior knee pain, localized to the site of involvement, that develops during or soon after repetitive running or jumping activities. The pain usually resolves after a short period of rest, but recurs with renewed activity. It occurs most often in basketball, volleyball, and track-and-field athletes. One theory is that it results from the accumulation of damage after recurrent episodes of microtrauma to the tendon. It has been shown that, compared with asymptomatic athletes, athletes with jumper's knee have an ability to generate greater force during jumping activities, indicating an overload phenomena as a possible cause. The type of playing surface may also play a role, with activities on hard surfaces leading to an increased incidence of tendinitis symptoms.

Classification

The classification of tendinitis by Blazina and associates (1973) is the most commonly cited and is useful in organizing a treatment plan.

Figure 4–59. Sinding-Larsen-Johansson disease is an osteochondritis of the inferior pole of the patella in the skeletally immature. Conservative treatment leads to healing in 3–12 mos. (From Colosimo A [ed]: Lower extremity problems in the skeletally immature patient. Orthop Rev 19:139, 1990.)

25%

65%

10%

Figure 4–58. Typical locations of pain in the jumper's knee.

Rehabilitation Protocol
Patellar Tendinitis
D'Amato and Bach

Phase 1

Goals
- Patient education.
- Promote healing time.
- Resolve or control pain.

Therapeutic Exercises
- Rest.
- NSAIDs.
- Cryotherapy, electrical stimulation, iontophoresis, phonophoresis.
- Flexibility exercises, with specific focus on hamstrings.
- Lower extremity strengthening in pain-free range (closed-chain only).
- General conditioning, hip strengthening of flexors, abductors, and adductors.
- SLR with progressive resistance.

Phase 2

Criteria for Progression to Phase 2
- No pain at rest.
- Decreased tenderness to palpation.
- No pain with activities of daily living.
- Decreased swelling.

Goals
- Increase strength.
- Increase flexibility.

- Control inflammation.
- Promote healing.

Therapeutic Exercises
- Use of a chopat "counterforce" strap.
- Continue flexibility exercises.
- Closed–chain kinetic exercises.
- Four-position hip strengthening.
- Start endurance training (pool, bike, cross-country ski machine).
- Balance training.

Phase 3

Criteria for Progression to Phase 3
- No pain with activities of daily living.
- No pain with running.
- Quadriceps strength 70–80% of contralateral extremity.

Goals
- Pain-free return to activity.
- Patient education to prevent recurrent episodes and modify activities.
- Maintain strength and flexibility.

Therapeutic Exercises
- Continue flexibility exercises.
- Continue strengthening.
- Running program and skill-specific activities.
- Aerobic conditioning.
- Patient education.

Classification of Patellar Tendinitis

Phase 1	Pain only after participation.
Phase 2	Pain during participation that does not limit performance.
Phase 3	Pain during participation that limits performance.
Phase 4	Complete tendon disruption.

Patients in phases 1 and 2 typically respond to nonoperative therapy. Patients with phase 3 symptoms have a more variable response to conservative treatment. Surgery is indicated for patients in phase 1, 2, or 3 in whom at least 3 to 6 months of conservative therapy fails and for all patients with phase 4 involvement.

Iliotibial Band Friction Syndrome

Repetitive activity can also lead to irritation of the soft tissues, such as the iliotibial band friction syndrome, which is common in runners. The iliotibial band is a thick fibrous tissue band that runs along the **lateral** aspect of the thigh and inserts at Gerdy tubercle on the anterolateral aspect of the proximal tibia. It has small attachments to the lateral patellar retinaculum and to the biceps femoris. As the knee moves from full extension to flexion, the iliotibial band shifts from a position anterior to the lateral femoral epicondyle to a position posterior to the epicondyle (Fig. 4–60). The transition occurs at about 30 degrees of knee flexion. The repetitive flexion and extension of the knee in running can lead to irritation of the iliotibial band as it passes back and forth over the lateral femoral epicondyle. Subsequently, the surrounding tissues and bursa become inflamed and painful.

History and Examination

Patients typically complain of a gradual onset of pain, tightness, or burning at the lateral aspect of the knee that develops during the course of a run. Symptoms usually re-

Figure 4–60. *A,* Anatomy of the lateral aspect of the knee showing the location of the iliotibial band. *B,* With the knee in approximately 30 degrees of flexion, the iliotibial band lies over the lateral femoral epicondyle. *C,* With the knee between 30 degrees of flexion and full extension, the iliotibial band is anterior to the lateral femoral epicondyle and assists in extension. *D,* With knee flexion greater than 30 degrees, the iliotibial band is posterior to the lateral femoral epicondyle and assists in flexion. (*A,* From Lineger JM, Christensen CP: Is the iliotibial band syndrome often overlooked? Physician Sports Med 20:98–108, 1992; *B–D,* from Aronen JG, Chronister R, Regan K, Hensien MA: Practical conservative management of iliotibial band syndrome. Physician Sports Med 21:[9]: 59–69, 1993.)

solve with rest. Examination reveals tenderness and possibly localized swelling at the lateral femoral epicondyle or at Gerdy's tubercle, and when the knee is put through ROM, pain, snapping, popping, or crepitation may be felt as the iliotibial band crosses the epicondyle. Iliotibial band contracture is associated with the presence of symptoms and this can be evaluated by the Ober test (see p. 325).

Predisposing Factors

Factors that predispose runners to iliotibial band friction syndrome include inexperience, a recent increase in distance, and running on a track. Other potential etiologies include leg-length discrepancies, hyperpronation of the foot, and running repetitively in one direction on a pitched surface.

Treatment of Iliotibial Band Friction Syndrome

The basic progression of treatment is early reduction of the acute inflammation, followed by stretching of the iliotibial band and strengthening of the hip abductors to alleviate soft tissue contracture, and finally, education in proper running techniques and institution of an appropriate running program to prevent recurrence (see following rehabilitation protocol).

Rehabilitation Protocol
Iliotibial Band Friction Syndrome in Runners
Brotzman

- Rest from running until asymptomatic.
- Ice area before and after exercise.
- Oral NSAIDs.
- Relative rest from running and high–flexion-extension activities of the knee (cycling, running, stair descent, skiing).

- Avoid downhill running.
- Avoid running on pitched surfaces with a pitched drainage grade to the road.
- Use of soft, new running shoes rather than hard shoes.
- Use of iontophoresis if helpful.
- Steroid injection into bursa if required.

A

B

C

D

E

F

Figure 4–61. *A,* Two-person Ober stretch. *B,* Self-Ober stretch. *C,* Cross-over lateral fascial stretch (the involved leg crosses behind the uninvolved leg). *D,* Leaning lateral fascial stretch (the involved leg is closer to the wall). *E,* Posterior fascial stretch, including gluteus maximus and piriformis. *F,* Quadriceps self-stretch.

Rehabilitation Protocol
Iliotibial Band Friction Syndrome in Runners *(Continued)*
Brotzman

- Stretching exercises (Fig. 4–61).
  - Two-man Ober stretch.
  - Self-Ober stretch.
  - Lateral fascial stretch.
  - Posterior fascial stretch plus gluteus maximus and piriformis self-stretch.

- Standing wall lean for lateral fascial stretch.
- Rectus femoris self-stretch.
- Iliopsoas with rectus femoris self-stretch.
- Use of lateral heel wedge in shoe, especially for iliotibial band tightness.
- Built-in correction in shoe for leg-length discrepancy.

Patellar Tendon Ruptures

Matthew J. Matava, MD, and Sue Million, MHS, PT

Background

Rupture of the patellar tendon is a relatively uncommon injury, occurring primarily during athletic pursuits in patients younger than 40 years. Most of these injuries are unilateral, although bilateral ruptures have been described in patients with systemic illnesses known to weaken collagen structures. Technically, the term "patellar tendon" is a misnomer because the tendon is actually a ligament connecting the patella and the tibial tubercle. However, this term is widely accepted because the patella is technically a sesamoid bone merely encompassed by the thickened condensation of the quadriceps tendon.

Anatomy and Biomechanics

The patellar tendon comprises the thickened fibers of the rectus femoris tendon that traverse the anterior surface of the patella. It converges medially and laterally, with the extensor retinaculum proximal to its insertion into the tibial tubercle. This relationship is important because rupture of the tendon usually involves the retinaculum as well.

The greatest force in the tendon is generated during active knee extension with the joint at approximately 60 degrees of flexion. **It has been shown that the tensile strain in the tendon is much higher at the bony insertion sites than in the tendon's midsubstance.** Collagen fiber stiffness is also decreased at these peripheral regions. These differences in force transmission may explain why rupture occurs most commonly near the proximal insertion rather than in the midsubstance.

Etiology

Rupture is invariably caused by a forceful quadriceps contraction against a fixed structure or by a sudden load of the patient's body weight against an actively contracting quadriceps. **The common denominator in both of these modes of injury is an eccentric quadriceps contraction with muscle lengthening during the contraction.**

Acute patellar tendon rupture usually occurs when there is long-standing tendon degeneration. Pathologic findings include hypoxic and calcifying tendonopathy, mucoid degeneration, and tendolipomatosis. Patients with preexisting systemic disorders such as diabetes mellitus, chronic renal failure, and various autoimmune conditions are susceptible to tendon rupture during nonstrenuous activity. These ruptures are occasionally bilateral because of the overall weakened state of the collagenous tissues.

Rupture may also occur after the injection of a corticosteroid medication in or around the tendon. We recommend against corticosteroid injection in or around the patellar tendon. These medications are known to cause necrosis and disorganization of the collagen fibrils, resulting in a weakened structure.

Patellar tendon rupture can also occur after surgical procedures that disturb the extensor mechanism of the knee, such as total knee arthroplasty or ACL reconstruction with harvest of the central third of the patellar tendon. In these situations, the rupture tends not to disrupt the reconstructive procedure, but the long-term outcome varies because of the alteration in the anatomy and the necessity of reconstructive grafts to reestablish knee extension when local tissues are deficient.

Clinical Evaluation

Physical Examination

After an acute injury, the patient usually has a tense hemarthrosis of the knee and cannot bear weight on the involved extremity. Active knee extension is usually impossible, especially if the rupture extends into the medial and lateral retinaculi. Active knee flexion, although possible, is limited because of pain. A gap may be palpable at the rupture site, and the patella may feel proximally displaced because the unopposed pull of the quadriceps muscle. Associated intra-articular injuries (such as an ACL tear) may occur and must also be ruled out.

Radiographic Evaluation

Plain radiographs usually are the only imaging modality required to confirm the diagnosis of an acute rupture.

The most common finding is a high-riding patella (patella alta), which is noted best on the lateral view.

Occasionally, one or more bony fragments are attached to the tendon if the injury resulted from an avulsion.

High-resolution ultrasonography has also been used effectively to confirm both acute and chronic ruptures. Sagittal images obtained with a linear array transducer allow identification of a confluent area of hypoechogenicity, signifying a complete rupture. With chronic tears, thickening of the tendon along with disruption of the normal tendon echo pattern is seen. Ultrasonography, although inexpensive and easy to perform, is operator dependent, which results in accuracy rates occasionally differing between institutions.

MRI has emerged as an excellent, although expensive, means of evaluating the extensor mechanism. With rupture, tendon discontinuity is seen along with waviness of the tendon ends and hemorrhage in the intervening space. This imaging modality is also helpful in evaluating the knee for concomitant intra-articular injuries.

Classification

Patellar tendon ruptures have been classified based on the location, configuration, and chronicity of the tear, but no universally accepted classification system currently exists. The most widely used system is that of Siwek and Rao (1981), who grouped ruptures into two categories based on the interval between injury and repair: *immediate* versus *delayed* (repair more than 2 weeks after injury). This system is the only one that has successfully correlated the type of rupture with the method of treatment (primary repair versus tendon reconstruction) and final outcome. The difference in rehabilitation between the two types of rupture is affected most by the method of treatment rather than by the type of rupture.

Treatment

Surgical repair of the ruptured patellar tendon is required for optimal function of the extensor mechanism of the knee. *There is no place for nonoperative treatment of this injury.* Surgical repair should be done as soon after the injury as possible. Multiple methods for repair have been described, although simple end-to-end repair, with or without a reinforcing cerclage suture, has been the method most commonly used.

With a chronic rupture (more than 6 weeks), simple reapproximation of the tendon ends is often impossible because of contraction of the quadriceps muscle and resulting proximal patellar migration. In this situation, preoperative patellar traction and passive ROM exercises are necessary.

A number of reconstructive procedures have been used after the reestablishment of knee motion: primary repair combined with autogenous graft augmentation with the hamstring tendons or fascia lata, inert carbon fiber or nonabsorbable tape suture repair, and allograft tissues in the form of the Achilles tendon or an intact patellar tendon.

Rehabilitation after Repair of Patellar Tendon Rupture

General Principles

Successful rehabilitation after patellar tendon repair requires an integration of the concepts of tissue healing and biomechanics with muscle strengthening and conditioning techniques. Essential to optimal recovery is early joint mobilization, gradual introduction of forces across the patellar tendon, normalization of movement, and progressive quadriceps strengthening. The ideal program uses a multiphase approach that includes functional rehabilitation strategies to allow the full resumption of activities of daily living and return to sport. The following protocol is designed for the rehabilitation of an acute, unilateral tendon repair.

Rehabilitation Protocol
Outline after Repair of Acute Unilateral Patellar Tendon Tear
Matava and Millions

Weeks 0–2

- Hinged knee immobilizer locked at 15 degrees flexion, braced in extension.
- Touch-down weight-bearing.
- Quadriceps isometric exercises.
- Upper body ergometer.

Weeks 3–6

- Hinged knee immobilizer locked at 0 degrees flexion.
- Weight-bearing as tolerated.
- 0–45 degrees active flexion with passive extension (in brace).
- Active flexion ROM increased by 15 degrees each week.

Rehabilitation Protocol
Outline after Repair of Acute Unilateral Patellar Tendon Tear *(Continued)*
Matava and Millions

- Full ROM achieved by 6 wk.
- Quadriceps isometrics.
- Upper body ergometer.
- Stationary bike, no resistance.

Weeks 7–8

- Hinged knee immobilizer discontinued.
- Full weight-bearing.
- Quadriceps isometrics.
- Open-chain exercises
  - Short arc quadriceps.
  - SLR.
- Closed-chain exercises
  - Double-leg mini-squats.
  - Leg press.
- Stationary bike, progressive resistance.

Weeks 9–12

- Open-chain exercises.
- Closed-chain exercises.

- Isokinetics.
- Stationary bike, progressive resistance.
- Treadmill walking.

Months 4–6

- Open-chain exercises.
- Closed-chain exercises.
- Isokinetics.
- Stationary bike, progressive resistance.
- Treadmill walking.
- Jogging/running.
- Sport-specific conditioning
  - Plyometrics.
  - Slide board.
  - Running, sprinting, figures-of-eight.
  - Advanced isokinetics.

Rehabilitation Protocol
After Repair of Acute Unilateral Patellar Rupture
Matava and Millions

Phase 1: Immobilization—0–2 Weeks

Bracing
- Hinged knee brace fixed at 15 degrees of knee flexion.
- All activities, including exercise, are done in the brace through postoperative week 6. The brace can be removed for bathing or showering once the surgical incision has healed.

Edema Control
- The patient is instructed on aggressive edema management including the use of cold, compression, and elevation throughout the initial postoperative period.

Weight-bearing
- Touchdown weight-bearing with axillary crutches and hinged knee brace.

Placement of a heel lift in the *opposite* shoe will facilitate swing-through of the involved leg during gait.

Therapeutic Exercises
- Quadriceps isometrics (postoperative day 1).
- Ankle pumps and gluteal and hamstring isometric exercises.

- Isometric exercises are done for four sets of six repetitions twice daily. Each repetition is held for 5 sec followed by a 2-sec rest.

Active ankle dorsiflexion has been shown to be effective in facilitating quadriceps muscle contraction force and may help decrease discomfort.

- Use of electrical stimulation is recommended, especially if the patient is unable to generate a strong quadriceps muscle contraction. Electrical stimulation should be provided for 15 min per session, three to five times per week.

A burst modulated medium frequency current has been found to be most effective in producing muscle force.

- Gentle patellar mobilizations using both inferior-superior and medial-lateral glides to maintain normal patellofemoral joint mobility.
- Maintenance of aerobic fitness through the use of an upper body ergometer.

continued

Rehabilitation Protocol
After Repair of Acute Unilateral Patellar Rupture *(Continued)*
Matava and Millions

Phase 2: Range of Motion—3–6 Weeks

Weight-bearing

- Crutch ambulation is progressed to weight-bearing as tolerated with the brace locked in full extension.
- Progression to full weight-bearing should be achieved by week 6.

Range of Motion

- Active knee flexion, 0–45 degrees in the hinged knee brace. *Knee extension should be passive.* Active flexion range is increased 15 degrees per week. Full knee flexion range should be achieved by week 6. ROM exercises should be done for 3 min, three times per day.
- A stationary bike for passive knee ROM once 95–105 degrees of knee flexion has been achieved (approximately week 5). *No pedal resistance should be used.*

Therapeutic Exercises

- Resistive exercise routine for hip abduction and adduction and prone hip extension applying resistance at the knee.
- Resistive ankle plantar flexion exercise with a band or sport cord.
- Edema management and patellar mobilization are continued.
- Modalities such as hot packs or TENS can be used to decrease pain and facilitate movement.
- Closed-chain exercises (in the brace) may be considered once full weight-bearing has been achieved.
- Appropriate exercises include weight shifting, standing bilateral heel raises, and standing balance and proprioception exercises.

A

B

C

D

Figure 4–62. Closed-chain exercises. *A,* Heel raises—starting position. *B,* Heel raises—ending position. *C* and *D,* Leg press (*C* on an inverted hack squat machine, *D* on total gym).

Rehabilitation Protocol
After Repair of Acute Unilateral Patellar Rupture *(Continued)*
Matava and Millions

Phase 3: Strengthening—7–12 Weeks

Weight-bearing

- Crutch ambulation, full weight-bearing with hinged knee brace allowing 0–60 degrees of active knee flexion.
- Use of axillary crutches is gradually discontinued as the patient is able to demonstrate a normal, symmetrical gait pattern.
- Bracing is discontinued once the patient is able to perform an SLR without an extensor lag.

Therapeutic Exercises

- Closed-chain exercises, including double-leg mini-squats, heel raises, and leg press (0–60 degrees of knee flexion) (Fig. 4–62). In addition to strengthening critical muscles, these exercises are designed to introduce coordinated movement patterns and normal joint forces. Therefore, the patient should be encouraged to perform these exercises in a slow, controlled fashion while maintaining proper trunk and limb alignment.
- Multiangle, *submaximal* quadriceps isometrics as tolerated. Exercises are done at 0, 30, 60, and 90 degrees of knee flexion.
- Open-chain quadriceps exercise program, such as short arc quadriceps (from 0–30 degrees), and SLR. Resistance is gradually added, using a PRE protocol as the patient is able to tolerate.
- Quadriceps sets and SLR are discontinued when patient is able to lift 10 pounds with PREs.

- Double-leg balance and proprioception tasks on firm, level surfaces, gradually progressing to single-leg standing on firm and flexible surfaces (e.g., pillow, balance board).
- Progressive addition of resistance to stationary bike program for lower extremity conditioning.
- Lower extremity stretching program for quadriceps, hamstring, calf, and iliotibial band flexibility as appropriate.

Weeks 9–12

- Ambulation on a treadmill at comfortable walking speeds. Continue to emphasize a normal, symmetrical gait pattern. **To encourage a normal gait pattern, use a mirror to provide visual feedback.**
- Progression of closed–kinetic chain exercises from double leg to single leg as tolerated.
- Two-inch lateral step-ups (Fig. 4–63), side steps with band resistance, lunges, and wall sitting as pain allows.
- Gradual multiangle *maximum* quadriceps isometrics.
- Progression of open–kinetic chain quadriceps PRE program. Exercise should be done two to three times per week, three sets of 8 to 12 repetitions. Load is increased when 12 repetitions per set are attained, with 1- to 2-min rest periods between sets. Exercise range is increased to 0–60 degrees.
- Isokinetic strengthening program of the quadriceps and hamstrings (concentric only) at 180 degrees/sec through a full knee ROM once the patient is able to ambulate with good quadriceps control.

A   B

Figure 4–63. Two-inch lateral step-ups. *A,* Starting position. *B,* Ending position.

continued

Rehabilitation Protocol
After Repair of Acute Unilateral Patellar Rupture (Continued)
Matava and Millions

- Edema management to control postexercise pain and swelling.

Phase 4: Sport-specific Functional Rehabilitation—4–6 Months

Therapeutic Exercises

- Closed-chain and open-chain exercises two to three times per week, progressing resistance as tolerated.
- Multispeed isokinetic exercise program (90, 180, and 300 degrees/sec) for quadriceps and hamstring musculature.
- Plyometric exercises, beginning with double-leg activities such as jumping jacks and double-leg landing off of 4-, 6-, and 8-inch steps. Gradual progression to advanced plyometric exercises including single-leg jumping tasks, hopping, and bounding as patient tolerates.
- Plyometric exercises are initiated after the patient demonstrates normal balance and controlled limb movements with all single-leg closed-chain exercises.
- *Running program* once the following criteria are met

- Quadriceps strength 65% of uninvolved extremity (determined by isokinetic testing).
- Normal leg and trunk alignment maintained during all closed-chain exercises.
- Symmetrical gait pattern.

Initially, the running program should be limited to 5 min on a firm, level surface three to five days per week. Jogging time should be progressed 5 min per week until the patient is able to tolerate continuous jogging for 15 min (or 1 mile). The patient should not advance running time or distance if significant pain, effusion, or movement asymmetry is experienced.

- If strengthening and running programs are done on the same day, running should precede strengthening.
- Speed and agility training should include sprints, rapid starts and stops, and figures-of-eight. Speed and agility drills should be tailored to meet sport-specific demands.

Termination of Rehabilitation

Rehabilitation is terminated when the patient demonstrates full joint ROM and 85 to 90% of contralateral lower extremity strength on isokinetic testing. **Resumption of strenuous athletic activity is prohibited for 4 to 6 months.**

In addition to isokinetic testing, a functional assessment of lower extremity performance is recommended before return to sport. The one-legged hop test for distance should be included as a way to compare lower extremity functional capacity and assess readiness to return to previous activity.

An athlete should display symmetrical movement patterns and normal static alignment before release to sport. ∎

Articular Cartilage Procedures of the Knee

G. Kelley Fitzgerald, PhD, PT, and James J. Irrgang, PhD, PT, ATC

Clinical Background

Designing successful rehabilitation programs after articular cartilage surgical procedures requires careful consideration of the healing process and a thorough understanding of the potential stresses applied to articular surfaces during therapeutic exercise. Although it is important to begin early rehabilitation to promote tissue healing and to restore joint motion, muscular strength, and functional ca-

pacity, rehabilitation procedures must be applied in a manner that does not interfere with or disrupt the healing articular lesion.

Types of Motion

Evidence from animal studies suggests that early active and passive motion exercises after articular cartilage lesions can enhance the quality of tissue healing, limit the adverse effects of joint immobilization on the remaining healthy articular cartilage, and reduce the risk of adhesions. **Complete immobilization is not recommended after surgical procedures that involve the articular cartilage.**

However, the application of shear stress while the healing articular lesion is under compression may have adverse effects on the healing process. ROM exercises should be done in a controlled manner to avoid excessive shear loads while the joint is under compression. This can be accomplished by emphasizing passive, active-assisted, and unloaded-active ROM exercises in the early postoperative period (0–6 weeks).

Muscle Strengthening

Muscle performance training is an essential component of postoperative rehabilitation after articular cartilage surgical procedures. Muscles need to be strong enough to assist in absorbing shock and dissipating loads across the joint. The resistance exercise program should be tailored to minimize shear loading across the lesion during the healing period. In general, exercises that have the potential for producing high shear stress coupled with compression, such as closed-chain exercises, should be avoided in the early phases of rehabilitation.

We believe isometric exercises are the safest option for restoring muscle strength during early rehabilitation.

Isometric quadriceps exercises in full knee extension may be effective in preventing or resolving a knee extensor lag, and most articular lesions will not be engaged with the knee in full extension. Isometric exercise at 90 degrees of flexion may also be a safe option because it is unlikely to result in excessive compression or shear loads across most articular cartilage lesions. In addition, it has been shown that isometric quadriceps training at 90 degrees of flexion can result in increased muscle force production at other joint angles. Isometric exercises at angles between 20 and 75 degrees should be used with caution because most articular lesions would be engaged in this arc of motion. If open-chain leg extension exercises are to be used, it is essential that the arc of motion is limited to ranges that do not engage the lesion. This requires effective communication between the surgeon and the therapist regarding ROM limitations for resistive exercises.

Weight-bearing Progression

Progression of weight-bearing and functional activities is a gradual process that begins in the intermediate phase of postoperative rehabilitation. The weight-bearing status after surgery is dependent on the size, nature, and location of the lesion, as well as the surgical procedure that has been used to treat it. Progression of weight-bearing is also dependent on the resolution of joint motion and muscular strength impairments in the early rehabilitation period.

After **arthroscopic débridement,** patients are usually permitted to bear weight as tolerated with crutches. Weight-bearing can be progressed as long as increased loading does not result in increased pain or effusion. Crutches can be discontinued when the patient has full passive knee extension and at least 100 degrees of knee flexion, can perform an SLR without an extensor lag, and can walk without pain or limp.

When patients have undergone **abrasion arthroplasty, microfracture procedure, fixation of an articular cartilage defect, or osteochondral graft,** weight-bearing is usually delayed for 6 weeks to allow adequate initial healing of the lesion. Non–weight-bearing or touch-down weight-bearing with crutches is allowed in the immediate postoperative period. In some cases, depending on the location of the lesion or stability of fixation, partial weight-bearing or weight-bearing as tolerated with crutches may be permitted in conjunction with use of a rehabilitation brace locked in full knee extension. Progressive weight-bearing is usually begun 6 weeks after surgery. At this time, fibrocartilage should have begun to fill in the articular defect and an osteochondral graft or articular cartilage fragment should have united with adjacent subchondral bone. Crutches can be discontinued when the patient has full passive knee extension and at least 100 degrees of knee flexion, can perform an SLR without an extensor lag, and can walk without pain or limp. Therapists should monitor patients for increases in pain or effusion during progressive weight-bearing and reduce the progression if these iatrogenic effects arise.

The progression from protected weight-bearing to full weight-bearing can be facilitated by using techniques that gradually increase the load on the knee. Deweighting devices can be used for treadmill ambulation and running. Unloading of body weight by the deweighting device is increased to the point that allows performance of the activity without pain or gait abnormalities. The unloading is then gradually reduced over time until the patient can perform the activity in full weight-bearing without pain. A pool can also be used to unload body weight for ambulation and running activities. These activities can be initiated in shoulder-deep water and then gradually progressed by decreasing the depth of the water.

Once the patient has progressed to pain-free full weight-bearing, a variety of low-impact aerobic activities, such as walking, cycling, and use of step or cross-country ski machines, can be employed to improve local muscular and cardiovascular endurance. Returning to sports activities may not be possible for some patients, depending on the severity of joint damage. These patients should be counseled with respect to appropriate activity modifications. For patients who wish to return to recreational or sports activities, a functional retraining program, involving agility training and sport-specific skill training, should be incorporated into the program. These activities should be delayed until the patient can perform low-impact aerobic activities without recurrent pain or effusion. Agility and sport-specific skill training should be progressed gradually from 50% effort to full effort. The therapist should continue to monitor the patient for changes in pain and effusion as these activities are progressed.

Important Rehabilitation Considerations

- The surgeon should include on the physical therapy referral form the type of surgical procedure, the location of the lesion, and restrictions in ROM during exercise. A diagram of the lesion site is also helpful. Therapists must adhere to the surgeon's ROM limitations so that the lesion is not engaged during exercise.
- Unloaded passive or active-assisted ROM exercises should begin as soon as possible after surgery. Closed-chain exercises should be avoided in the first 6 weeks after surgery.
- Isometric exercises with the knee in full extension or 90 degrees of flexion should be emphasized for early strength training. Open-chain exercises can be used in arcs of motion that do not engage the lesion.

- Protected weight-bearing with the use of crutches, and in some cases, a rehabilitation brace, should be incorporated in the first 6 weeks after surgery. Assistive devices can be discontinued when the patient has full knee extension and 100 degrees of knee flexion, can perform an SLR without an extensor lag, and can walk without pain or limp.
- Progression of weight-bearing activities can be made easier by gradually increasing the load on the knee. This can be accomplished with the use of deweighting devices or pool activities. A gradual progression of agility and sport-specific skill training should be completed before the patient is allowed to return to full sports activity.

Rehabilitation Protocol

Our rehabilitation protocol is divided into three phases: early postoperative phase (0–6 weeks), intermediate phase (6–12 weeks), and return to activity phase (12 weeks and beyond). The time frames for these phases are only estimated guidelines. Progression to each phase depends on meeting criteria based on the type of surgical procedure, estimated periods of healing, restoration of joint mobility and strength, and potential recurrence of pain and joint effusion. Individual patients are able to progress at different intervals, and the surgeon and therapist are required to use their clinical judgments in determining when progression should be delayed or can be accelerated.

Rehabilitation Protocol
After Articular Cartilage Procedures
Fitzgerald and Irrgang

Early Postoperative Phase (0–6 Weeks)

	Joint Mobility	Muscle Performance	Weight-bearing
Arthroscopic Débridement	Passive and active-assisted ROM with no restrictions on ROM. Full knee extension should be obtained in 1 wk, and full flexion in 3 wk.	Initiate training with isometric exercises. May progress to open-chain resisted exercises* when tolerated. Closed-chain resisted exercises† initiated when patient meets criteria for full weight-bearing.	Weight-bearing as tolerated with crutches until patient has full extension, 100 degrees of flexion, no knee extensor lag, and ambulates without pain or effusion. Initiate low-impact aerobic activities (walking program, stationary cycling, swimming) at 3–6 wk, when patient meets full weight-bearing status.
Abrasion Arthroplasty, Subchondral Drilling, Microfracture Procedures	Passive and active-assisted ROM in pain-free range for 6 wk. Full extension should be achieved in 1 wk, full flexion in 3 wk.	Isometric exercises in ROM that does not engage the lesion site. Open-chain exercises with light resistance may be initiated at 4–6 wk in ROM that does not engage lesion site. Avoid closed-chain exercises.	Non–weight-bearing or toe-touch weight-bearing with crutches.
Osteochondral Grafts	Passive and active-assisted ROM in range restrictions that do not engage lesion site. Full knee extension should be obtained in 1 wk, full flexion in 6 wk.	Isometric exercises in ROM that does not engage the lesion site. Open-chain exercises with light resistance may be initiated at 4–6 wk in ROM that does not engage lesion site. Avoid closed-chain exercises.	Non–weight-bearing or toe-touch weight-bearing with crutches.
Osteotomy	Passive and active ROM exercises in pain-free ROM. Full knee extension should be achieved in 1 wk, full flexion in 8 wk.	Isometric exercises for 4–6 wk. No open- or closed-chain resisted exercises for 4–6 wk, to avoid loading across the osteotomy site.	Touch-down weight-bearing for first 2 wk, partial weight-bearing 2–4 wk, weight-bearing as tolerated with crutches 4–8 wk. Rehabilitation brace locked in full extension.

Rehabilitation Protocol
After Articular Cartilage Procedures *(Continued)*
Fitzgerald and Irrgang

Intermediate Phase (6–12 Weeks)

	Joint Mobility and Muscle Performance	Weight-bearing and Functional Retraining
Arthroscopic Débridement	Full motion should be achieved at this time. Continue with maintenance active ROM. Progress open- and closed-chain resistance exercises[‡§] as tolerated.	Agility[‖] and sport-specific skill training initiated at 50% effort and progressed to full effort as tolerated. Initiate return to full activity when these activities to do not induce recurrent pain or effusion.
Abrasion Arthroplasty, Subchondral Drilling, Microfracture Procedures	Progress to full-range active ROM. Progress loading of resistive exercises. May initiate closed-chain exercise when full weight-bearing is achieved. Restrict to ranges that do not engage lesion site.	Discontinue use of crutches at 6–8 wk when patient has achieved full knee extension, 100 degrees of flexion, no extensor lag, and can ambulate without pain or effusion. May use deweighting device[¶] or pool activities in making transition to full weight-bearing.
Osteochondral Grafts	Progress to full-range active ROM. Progress loading of resistive exercises. May initiate closed-chain exercise when full weight-bearing is achieved. Restrict to ranges that do not engage lesion site.	Discontinue use of crutches at 6–8 wk when patient has achieved full knee extension, 100 degrees of flexion, no extensor lag, and can ambulate without pain or effusion. May use deweighting device or pool activities in making transition to full weight-bearing. Low-impact aerobic activities may be initiated when patient achieves full weight-bearing status.
Osteotomy	Progress to full-range active ROM. Progress loading of resistive exercises. May initiate closed-chain exercise when full weight-bearing is achieved. Restrict to ranges that do not engage lesion site.	Discontinue rehabilitation brace. Progress to full weight-bearing without crutches when patient has achieved full knee extension, 100 degrees of flexion, no extensor lag, and can ambulate without pain or effusion. May use deweighting device or pool activities in making transition to full weight-bearing. Low-impact aerobic activities may be initiated when patient achieves full weight-bearing status.

Return to Activity Phase (12 Weeks and Beyond)

	Joint Mobility and Muscle Performance	Functional Retraining and Return to Activity
Arthroscopic Débridement		Patients should have returned to full activity by this time period.
Abrasion Arthroplasty, Subchondral Drilling, Microfracture Procedures	Continue with maintenance full active ROM exercise. Continue with progression of resistance for open- and closed-chain exercises as tolerated in ranges that do not engage lesion site.	Initiate agility and sport-specific skill training when tolerating low-impact aerobic activities without recurrent pain or effusion. Agility and sport-specific skill training should be initiated at 50% effort and progressed to full effort as tolerated. Running should be delayed until 6 mo postsurgery. May initiate return to activity when tolerating running and agility and sport-specific skill training without recurrent pain or effusion.
Osteochondral Grafts	Continue with maintenance full active ROM exercise. Continue with progression of resistance for open- and	Initiate agility and sport-specific skill training when tolerating low-impact aerobic activities without recurrent pain or effusion. Agility and sport-specific skill training should be initiated at 50% effort and progressed to full effort as

continued

Rehabilitation Protocol
After Articular Cartilage Procedures *(Continued)*
Fitzgerald and Irrgang

Return to Activity Phase (12 Weeks and Beyond)

	Joint Mobility and Muscle Performance	Functional Retraining and Return to Activity
	closed-chain exercises as tolerated in ranges that do not engage lesion site.	tolerated. Running should be delayed until 6 mo post-surgery. May initiate return to activity when tolerating running and agility and sport-specific skill training without recurrent pain or effusion.
Osteotomy	Continue with maintenance full active ROM exercise. Continue with progression of resistance for open- and closed-chain exercises as tolerated in ranges that do not engage lesion site.	Initiate agility and sport-specific skill training when tolerating low-impact aerobic activities without recurrent pain or effusion. Agility and sport-specific skill training should be initiated at 50% effort and progressed to full effort as tolerated. Running should be delayed until 6 mo postsurgery. May initiate return to activity when tolerating running and agility and sport-specific skill training without recurrent pain or effusion.

*Resisted open-chain exercises refers to non–weight-bearing leg extensions for quadriceps strengthening and leg curls for hamstring strengthening.
†Resisted closed-chain exercises include leg press, partial range squats, wall slides, and step-ups.
‡Resisted open-chain exercises refers to non–weight-bearing leg extensions for quadriceps strengthening and leg curls for hamstring strengthening.
§Resisted closed-chain exercises include leg press, partial range squats, wall slides, and step-ups.
‖ Agility training includes activities such as side slides, cariocas, shuttle runs, cutting and pivoting drills, figure-of-eight running.
¶A deweighting device is a pelvic harness that is suspended above the treadmill from a frame. Cables attached to the harness are connected to an electric motor that can be programmed to apply an upward-lifting load on the pelvis through the harness, which, in turn, will reduce the loading effect of the patient's body weight on the lower extremities while the patient is ambulating on the treadmill. The upward-lifting load is set high enough to allow performance of walking on the treadmill without reproducing the patient's pain. Treatment is progressed over several sessions by gradually reducing the upward-lifting load as tolerated by the patient, until the patient is able to ambulate in full weight-bearing on the treadmill without pain.

Trouble-shooting Techniques after Articular Cartilage Procedures

Pain and Effusion with Exercise or Activity Progression

Monitoring of pain and effusion in response to exercise or activity progression is important to maintain a safe and effective rehabilitation process. Pain and effusion in response to exercise may indicate that the articular lesion is being harmed or the intensity of exercise is too rigorous. Therapists should reconsider the ROM restrictions that are being used and perhaps modify them to reestablish pain-free ranges. The frequency and duration of joint mobility exercise or the magnitude of loading during resistance exercises may also have to be reduced.

Recurrent pain and effusion that occur during progression of weight-bearing or functional retraining activities indicate that the joint is not ready to progress to higher levels of activity. Progression of activity may need to be delayed in these circumstances.

Footwear and activity surface–types should also be considered. Patients may need to obtain footwear that provides better cushioning or biomechanical foot or-

thotics to compensate for faulty foot mechanics. Activities may need to be begun on softer surfaces to acclimate to more rigorous ground reaction forces as higher activity levels are introduced.

Persistent effusion in the early postoperative period may result in quadriceps inhibition (reduced ability to voluntarily activate the quadriceps muscles). This can significantly retard progress with the rehabilitation program. Use of cold treatments, compression bandaging, limb elevation, and intermittent isometric contractions of the thigh and leg muscles may help resolve problems with effusion. If significant effusion persists more than 1 or 2 weeks after surgery, the therapist should notify the surgeon.

Quadriceps Inhibition or Persistent Knee Extensor Lag

Some patients may have difficulty with voluntary activation of the quadriceps muscles after surgery. This problem may be indicated by the inability to perform a full, sustained, isometric quadriceps contraction or the presence of a knee extensor lag on SLR. If patients exhibit this problem, they may not respond well to voluntary exercises alone. In addition, prolonged inability to actively achieve full knee extension may result in a knee flexion contracture that could, in turn, result in gait abnormalities and excessive loading of the knee during weight-bearing activities. Other treatment adjuncts to enhance quadriceps muscle activation such as *neuromuscular electrical stimulation or EMG biofeedback* may need to be incorporated into the program. If these treatment adjuncts are administered, the intensity of the treatment stimulus should be great enough to produce a full, sustained contraction of the quadriceps as evidenced by superior glide of the patella during the quadriceps contraction. Superior glide of the patella is important to prevent patellar entrapment in the intercondylar groove, which may sometimes be a causative factor in knee extensor lags. ■

Baker's Cyst (Popliteal Cyst)

S. Brent Brotzman, MD

Clinical Background

Popliteal cysts are often referred to by the eponym "Baker's cyst." In 1877, Baker described an enlarged popliteal cyst formed by trapping of fluid in a bursa related to the semimembranosus tendon. He noted *communication of the cyst with the joint* synovium with fluid that leaks into the bursa but cannot flow back in the reverse direction (see Fig. 4–3).

Wilson, in 1938, noted that the bursa under the medial head of the gastrocnemius and the bursa under the semimembranosus often had connections and concluded that the popliteal cyst arose from distention of the gastrocnemius semimembranosus bursa. In a dissection study, Taylor and Rana (1973) found that a large number of popliteal cysts had a valvular communication between the medial gastrocnemius bursa and the knee joint. Lindgren (1977) demonstrated that, with increased age, the frequency of communication of the bursa with the joint increased, which he believed to be secondary to the thinning of the posterior joint capsule.

The term "Baker's cyst" describes cysts that occur on the posteromedial aspect of the knee between the medial head of the gastrocnemius and the semimembranosus tendon.

Popliteal cysts are frequently associated with intra-articular pathology. Meniscal tears, rheumatoid arthritis, osteoarthritis, conditions causing synovitis, Charcot's joints, and tuberculosis have all been reported to be associated with formation of popliteal cysts. Fielding and coworkers (1991) found that 82% of popliteal cysts were associated with a meniscal tear, commonly a tear of the posterior portion of the medial meniscus. Only 38% of

tears involve the lateral meniscus. ACL tears were present in 13% of subjects. They also found that the overall prevalence of popliteal cysts was 5% and this increased with increased age.

Clinical Presentation

Popliteal cysts typically present as a mass in the posteromedial aspect of the knee. In the rare pediatric patient with a popliteal cyst, the mass is typically asymptomatic and is noticed by the patient who is concerned about the prominence of the posterior popliteal fossa. In adults, the complaint is typically an achy sensation and fullness in the back of the knee that is exacerbated with exercise or activities that involve significant flexion and extension. These symptoms are often accompanied by symptoms from the underlying pathologic condition, such as meniscal tear, torn ACL, or degenerative arthritis.

Rupture of a popliteal cyst may occur suddenly, causing severe pain and swelling in the calf region. This combination has been called **"pseudothrombophlebitis syndrome,"** because the signs and symptoms of a ruptured popliteal cyst are identical to those of thrombophlebitis, with a positive Homans sign and tenderness in the posterior aspect of the calf.

Venous Doppler sonography or venography should be used to rule out thrombophlebitis. On clinical examination, a hard cord corresponding to the thrombosed vein may be palpable in thrombophlebitis, but is *not* present in a ruptured popliteal cyst; however, this is not easily palpated in some patients.

Differential diagnoses of popliteal cysts include fibrosarcoma, synovial sarcoma, malignant fibrohistiocytoma, and degenerative meniscal cysts.

Because of the associated high incidence of intra-articular pathology with Baker's cyst, MRI is recommended in the evaluation of popliteal cysts.

On MRI, *degenerative meniscal cysts* typically have a communicating peripheral tear and are more medial or lateral than a true popliteal cyst. MRI can also distinguish popliteal cysts from solid lesions or tumors in the popliteal area. Because of the cyst's high content of free water, MRI typically shows features of a low signal intensity on T1-weighted images and a high signal intensity on T2-weighted images. Septa are often present within popliteal cysts, as well as hemorrhage, loose bodies, and debris.

Treatment

In *children*, popliteal cysts generally are benign, asymptomatic, self-limited, and rarely associated with intra-articular pathology. MRI is typically recommended to confirm the diagnosis and rule out a soft tissue tumor. Most popliteal cysts in children resolve spontaneously and surgery is not indicated.

In *adults,* injection of steroids into the cyst has been recommended. This is usually just a temporizing measure, and the cyst recurs unless the associated intra-articular disorder is corrected.

If MRI is negative for intra-articular pathology, the cyst is treated symptomatically and followed conservatively. *Arthroscopic evaluation* is indicated if MRI reveals an intra-articular lesion causing mechanical symptoms that do not respond to nonsurgical management (anti-inflammatories, compression sleeves, and physical therapy). If pain or persistent swelling interferes with activities of daily living despite conservative measures, surgical treatment is indicated. If arthroscopic intervention does not relieve symptoms, open excision may be necessary. The stalk leading from the joint to the cyst is located and sutured or cauterized, and the cyst is removed. The reported recurrence rate of open popliteal cyst excision varies widely, with some studies reporting frequent recurrences.

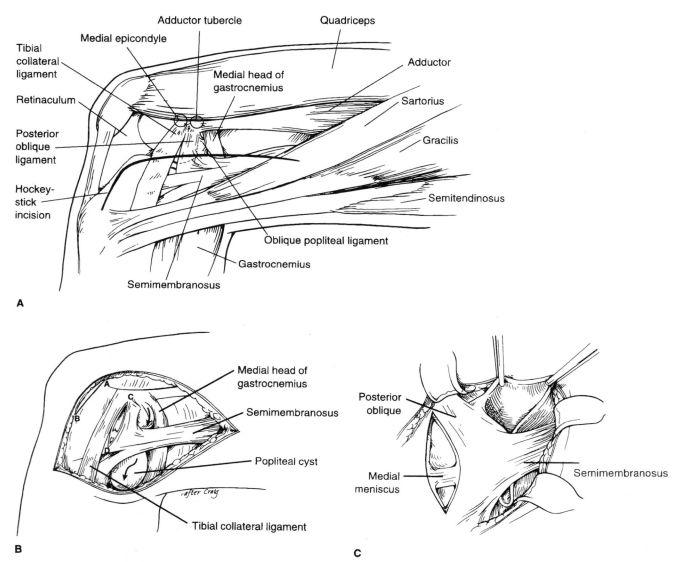

Figure 4–64. Hughston and colleagues' posteromedial surgical approach for popliteal cyst incision. *A,* Medial hockey-stick incision and the underlying anatomic structures in the right knee. *B,* Area exposed by the incision. The skin and subcutaneous tissues have been removed to demonstrate the relationship of the popliteal cyst to the anterior medial retinacular incision (*A–B*) and the posterior capsular incision (*C–D*). The posterior oblique ligament can be retracted posteriorly for inspection of the medial meniscus and the intra-articular aspect of the posterior capsule. *C,* Opening and retraction of the cyst demonstrates adherence to the surrounding tissues. The cyst can then be isolated and excised in its entirety. (*A–C,* From Curl WW: Popliteal cysts: historical background and current knowledge. © 1996 American Academy of Orthopaedic Surgeons. Reprinted from the Journal of the American Academy of Orthopaedic Surgeons, vol. 4[3], pp. 129–133 with permission.)

Treatment of the intra-articular disorder often leads to resolution of the popliteal cyst. Jayson (1972) reported good results with anterior synovectomy in patients with rheumatoid arthritis and popliteal cysts.

Open Surgical Technique

Hughston and colleagues (1991) described a surgical procedure in a series of 30 patients with only 2 recurrences. In this procedure, a posteromedial approach is made through a medial hockey-stick incision with the knee flexed at 90 degrees (Fig. 4–64). The capsular incision begins between the medial epicondyle and the adductor tubercle and is extended distally along the posterior edge of the tibial collateral ligament (anterior to the popliteal oblique ligament). The popliteal oblique ligament is retracted posteriorly. The cyst is found between the semimembranosus tendon and the medial head of the gastrocnemius. The cyst is dissected free of its surrounding adhesions and excised with the capsular origin of the cyst identified. The rent in the capsule is repaired with nonabsorbable sutures, and this can be reinforced with a pedicle flap from the medial head of the gastrocnemius as described by Rauschning (1980).

Postoperative Rehabilitation

After the wound is closed, the knee is immobilized in a large hinged cast, which is worn for 2 to 3 days with crutch-assisted weight-bearing as tolerated. For the first few days after surgery, SLR and gentle ankle pumps are done and icing is used for edema and pain control. Gentle active ROM of the knee is begun between postoperative days 3 and 7 with care to *avoid excess tension* on the medial hockey-stick incision. ■

Patella Fractures

S. Brent Brotzman, MD

Anatomy and Background

- The patella is the largest human sesamoid bone and a very important *functional* component of the extensor mechanism.
- The patella serves to increase the magnitude of the quadriceps moment arm. The contribution to an increase of extension "strength" made by the patella increases with progressive extension of the knee, being almost 30% at full extension.

For this reason, **total** patellectomy should be avoided in the treatment of patellar fractures if possible.

- The patella is subject to complex loading. In knee *extension*, the patella is loaded primarily in tension.

However, in knee *flexion*, the articular surface contacts the distal femur and is subject to compressive force, termed *patellofemoral joint reactive forces* (PFJRFs) (see Fig. 4–44).

Evaluation of Patellar Fractures

- A history of a direct blow, a severe muscle contraction, or an unexpected, rapid knee flexion while the quadriceps was contracted is often elicited.
- The examiner should look for a possible palpable defect of the patella, localized contusion or tenderness over the patella, weak extension of the knee, or inability to actively extend the knee (i.e. perform an SLR).

The inability to perform active extension of the knee with radiographic evidence of a displaced patella fracture is an absolute indication for surgical open reduction and internal fixation or surgical repair of a patella fracture in an operative candidate. Operative intervention may include open reduction and internal fixation, and partial patellectomy.

Bipartate Patella

- Secondary ossification centers that never fused to the body of the patella may sometimes be confused with the rare marginal or peripheral fracture. **Obtaining radiographs of the opposite patella** are often helpful in this differentiation **because bipartate patellas almost never occur unilaterally.** Bipartate patellas typically are *not tender on palpation* of the suspicious area, in contrast to a marginal or peripheral fracture.

Classification of Patella Fractures

Patellar fractures are classified according to their *mechanism of injury* (direct and indirect) and *fracture morphology*.

Direct blows (e.g., dashboard) usually cause significant comminution but often little displacement. The important articular cartilage of the contact area is typically significantly injured by this type of mechanism.

Indirect blows (e.g., jumping) are typically less comminuted than those from direct blows, but are often displaced and transverse. The articular cartilage is less damaged than with direct blows.

To help with treatment planning, patellar fractures are classified morphologically (Fig. 4–65).

- *Transverse* fractures occur in the medial-lateral direction. They usually occur in the central or distal third of the patella. Displaced transverse patella fractures typically require open reduction and internal fixation; nondisplaced transverse fractures are usually treated nonoperatively.
- *Vertical* fractures are rare and occur in the superior-inferior direction. Usually, the extensor mechanism remains intact (nonoperative treatment).

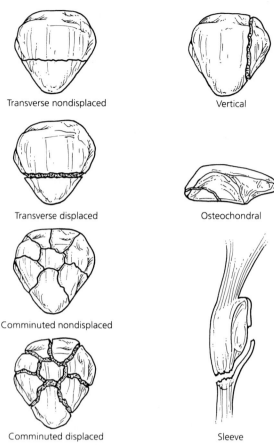

Transverse nondisplaced

Vertical

Transverse displaced

Osteochondral

Comminuted nondisplaced

Comminuted displaced

Sleeve

Figure 4–65. Patellar fractures are classified according to radiographic pattern. Displaced fractures are treated surgically. Nondisplaced fractures with the patient having the ability to perform a straight-leg raise are generally treated nonoperatively. (From Carpenter JE, Matthews LS: When the kneecap and kneecap extensors are injured. J Musculoskel Med 14[2]: 83–90, 1997. Artist: Charles H. Boyter.)

- *Marginal* fractures occur at the edge of the patella and do not disrupt the function of the extensor mechanism (nonoperative).
- *Sleeve* fractures typically occur in children. The inferior (or occasionally superior) pole of the patella is pulled off (avulsion) with a large amount of important articular cartilage that is very hard to identify radiographically. The diagnosis of a sleeve fracture is typically made on clinical findings of local pain and tenderness, inability to fully actively extend the knee, and radiographs showing a high-riding patella (alta) in comparison with the uninjured side. We follow Houghton and Ackroyd's (1979) recommendation of operative treatment of these fractures.
- *Osteochondral* fractures include sleeve fractures (see above) and osteochondral fragments as a result of a patellar dislocation or direct blow. The latter types may result in a displaced fragment that becomes a troublesome loose body (surgical excision or trans-

osseous fixation for large fragments) or result in a fracture fragment that never displaces (nonoperative treatment).

Radiographs

AP, lateral, and "sunrise" views of the knee should be taken. On the lateral view, Insall's method (see Fig. 4–1B) of assessing patellar height should be used to rule out associated patellar tendon rupture, with its resultant "patella alta" as the unopposed quadricep pulls the patella superiorly.

The length of the patellar tendon (from distal pole of the patella to the tibial tubercle) is measured and compared with the height of the patella. If the ratio of patella–to–patellar tendon height is less than 0.8 then the patella is too high (i.e., patella alta) and a patellar tendon rupture with proximal retraction is suspected.

The sunrise view most commonly used is Merchant's (45 degrees of knee flexion).

Treatment

Restoration of articular congruity of the articular portion of the patella is very important to avoid post-traumatic arthritis.

- **The most important factors in treatment of patella fractures are restoration of articular congruity and retaining the ability to actively extend the knee.**

Patella fractures with **articular incongruity** (step-off) of **more than 2 mm** or **separation** (displacement) of the two fragments (inferior and superior pole) of **more than 3 mm** require surgical treatment. Lack of the ability to actively extend the knee (disruption of the extensor mechanism) is also a surgical indication.

Nonoperative Treatment

- Nonoperative treatment is indicated for most vertical fractures, nondisplaced fractures, and fractures with less than 2 mm articular incongruity of the articular surface (step-off) and an intact extensor mechanism on SLR testing. For example, a patient with a nondisplaced, transverse fracture who can perform an SLR is treated nonoperatively.
- Frequently, a few degrees of extreme flexion are lost with nonoperative treatment, but patient satisfaction is high (>95%). Bostrom (1972) had slight or no pain in 89% of these patients and normal or slightly impaired function in 91%. Ninety percent of nonoperative patients had 0 to 120 degrees of ROM.
- Four to 6 weeks of immobilization in extension in a cast or large hinged brace followed by gentle, progressive ROM exercises and, later, quadriceps strengthening exercises.

Rehabilitation Protocol
Nonoperative Patella Fracture

Weeks 0–6

- Continue icing until effusion resolves.
- Wear a straight-leg cylinder cast for 2–3 wk or controlled motion brace locked at 0 degrees in a very compliant patient.
- Allow weight-bearing to tolerance with crutches.
- Employ a 1/4-inch heel lift (shoe insert) on the *contralateral* extremity to help with ground clearance of the involved "stiff" leg.
- Begin quadriceps sets, gluteal sets, hamstring sets, and SLR in all planes (supine and standing) before discharge from the hospital (quadriceps sets help decrease adhesion formation during the healing process).
- May begin open- and closed-chain exercises with the cast on, especially for hip strengthening.
- Replace cast with controlled motion brace at 2–3 wk.
- Begin electrical muscle stimulation for quadriceps re-education.
- Progress weight-bearing to tolerance with crutches to weight-bearing with the use of a cane.
- In general, begin strengthening and ROM exercises at week 3 or 4 (open- and closed-chain exercises).
- Begin gentle patellar mobilization; the patient should be independent with this exercise.
- At approximately 6 wk, begin stationary bicycling with the seat elevated and no resistance for ROM and strengthening.
- Begin isokinetic exercises at speeds of 60–120 degrees/sec to strengthen the quadriceps musculature and decrease the forces on the patellofemoral joint that occur at lower speeds.
- Use stool scoots for hamstring strengthening.

Weeks 6–12

- Begin and progress closed-chain exercises, such as 40-degree mini-squats and step-ups.
- May use a Theraband for resistance in hip exercises and mini-squats.
- Start BAPS board exercises.
- Begin lunges (usually 8–10 wk).
- Can use stationary bicycling with affected leg only with added resistance to aid strengthening.
- Because most patients with patellar fractures eventually develop some degree of chondromalacia, emphasize that restoration of quadriceps strength is essential to assist in the absorption of body weight load that is transmitted up the kinetic chain.
- The exercise program should emphasize restoration of lower extremity strength and flexibility. After this is achieved, implement a maintenance program with emphasis on closed-chain exercises. All exercises should be in a pain-free ROM.
- Evaluate the entire lower extremity, especially for excessive pronation of the feet, which add stresses to the knee and exacerbate patellofemoral-type symptoms. Use orthotics if excessive pronation is noted.

Operative Treatment

Most patella fractures will be treated operatively.

Treatment is aimed at **preservation** of patellar **function** whenever possible, preferably through open reduction and internal fixation if bone quality allows. **Restoring articular congruity** is key to avoid posttraumatic arthritis.

- It is important to obtain secure, stable fixation for anticipated knee motion during rehabilitation. If significant or poor bone quality exists, a major (usually superior) fragment with a large amount of articular cartilage is retained and partial patellectomy is performed (Fig. 4–66).

Patellar Operative Technique (General Principles)

- Minimize further soft tissue trauma caused by excess knee flexion, direct contact with ice, or splints with excessive compression.
- If a tense hematoma is stretching the anterior skin, consider hematoma aspiration.
- Use of a *longitudinal* incision (not transverse). Although transverse incisions are better from a cosmetic standpoint, this incision can seldom be used in future procedures (slough possible later).
- Avoid excess retractor tension or prolonged retraction during surgery.
- Often, comminution (especially inferior pole) is underestimated on x-rays and intraoperative reassessment is vital.
- **Partial patellectomy and patellar tendon repair is preferable to tenuous open reduction and internal fixation of comminuted soft bone.**
- Fractures with some comminution may often be converted to a simple transverse fracture by lag-screw fixation of the comminuted fragments.

The most important goal is restoration of articular congruity under direct visualization and palpation.

- Extension of the exposure with a small medial parapatellar capsular incision to allow *direct* visual-

Figure 4–66. Modified AO tension band technique for patella fracture fixation (see text). *A,* Retrograde drilling of the proximal fragment. K-wires mark the proximal ends of the holes during reduction. *B,* Reduction, clamping, and antegrade partial drilling of the distal fragment. K-wires with prebent proximal ends are then hammered through the remaining bone of the distal pole. *C,* With a large-bore needle, the 1.2-mm tension band wire is placed deep to the proximal and distal ends of the K-wires immediately adjacent to the patella through the stout soft tissue attachments of the quadriceps tendon and patellar ligament. Medially and laterally, the tension band wire lies anterior to the patella and is not usually crossed. It is tightened and twisted securely, and the "pigtail" end is bent flush with the bone surface. A twist or a square knot is reliable. The AO bent wire fastening technique is not secure enough for definitive fixation. *D,* The prebent proximal ends of the K-wires are driven into the proximal pole, and the distal ends are trimmed if necessary. (*A–D,* From Sanders R, Gregory PR: Patellar fractures and extensor mechanism injuries. In Browner BD, Jupiter JB, Levine AM, Trafton PG [eds]: Skeletal Trauma, 2nd ed. Philadelphia, WB Saunders, 1998.)

ization and palpation of articular congruity is recommended.

- A modified tension band technique is currently the most widely accepted operative technique.
- The anterior tension band (18-gauge wire looped over Kirshner wires and over the anterior patella) acts to neutralize the large distraction force across the patella with quad contraction and knee flexion.
- Avoid making the most common error in the tension band technique, which involves failure to bring the tension board *directly* into contact with the distal and proximal poles of the patella, leaving intervening soft tissue.
- Irrigate and remove all comminuted fragments and debris that may later act as loose bodies intraarticularly.
- Place knee through a gentle ROM intraoperatively after operative fixation to observe the stability of the surgical construct. Document the degree of flexion the repair is stable to (e.g., 90 degrees) and give to the therapist.

Partial Patellectomy

- Number 2 braided polyester sutures are used to reattach the patellar tendon to the patella through multiple drill holes.
- Preserve as much of the length of the patellar tendon as possible.
- The holes drilled through the patella should enter as near to the articular surface as possible so that there is minimal step-off between the tendon and the remaining patellar articular cartilage.
- Postoperative complications can be minimized by careful attention to wound care, accurate fracture reduction, secure fixation, and early ROM.

Postoperative Management (General Principles)

- Monitor the wound closely postoperative.
- It is essentially impossible to completely unload the patella postoperatively. The fracture is loaded with each quadriceps contraction.
- **Weight-bearing itself does not increase quadriceps force; therefore, weight-bearing with the use of a brace locked in extension is permitted.**

Rehabilitation Protocol
Postoperative Patellar Fracture after Open Reduction and Internal Fixation
S. Brent Brotzman, MD

Note: Rehabilitation protocols vary depending on the type of fracture, the surgical technique, and the rehabilitation philosophy of the surgeon. Gentle ROM intraoperatively

after tension band wiring (or partial patellectomy) is often performed to observe the stability of the fracture and construct. This information (e.g., stable to 90 degrees of flex-

Rehabilitation Protocol
Postoperative Patellar Fracture after Open Reduction and Internal Fixation
(Continued)

S. Brent Brotzman, MD

ion) is helpful for timing of postoperative ROM progression. Document the degrees of flexion reached intraoperatively with good stability of construct and give to the therapist.

Postoperative Days 1–7

- Weight-bearing as tolerated with crutches or walker with long-leg straight-leg cylinder cast or commercial full-length knee brace locked in extension (0 degrees.) Brace may be unlocked during ambulation at approximately 3 wk if good quadriceps control.
- Maximal elevation + ice for 3–5 days.
- Gentle quad sets, SLR if surgeon feels construct is *very* stable.
- Use heel elevation for *contralateral* shoe to help ground clearance of involved straight-leg cast during ambulation.

Weeks 2–6

- Begin gentle patellar mobilization exercises, the patient should become independent in this exercise.

- Electrical muscle stimulation for quadriceps reeducation.
- Stationary bicycling with seat elevated and no resistance. Begin at 5–6 wk.

Week 6

- Ensure radiographic evidence of healed fracture.
- Progress isometric exercises with 1- to 2-pound weights on thigh for SLR.
- Stool scoots.
- Increase bicycling distance, speed, and endurance.
- Begin gentle closed-chain exercises
  - 30-degree mini-squats.
  - Wall sits.
  - Stool scoots.
  - Lateral step-ups (4-inch platform).
- Hamstring curls with 2–5 pounds at ankle.
- We employ a hinged brace until the patient reaches 90 degrees of flexion and has excellent quadriceps control.

Typical Findings in Common Knee Conditions

Acute Patellar Dislocation

Patient often reports "the knee shifted"

Tender over medial retinaculum (torn)

Usually a tense effusion (hemarthrosis)

Positive patellar apprehension test and increased lateral excursion on lateral glide test

May have an osteochondral fracture of patella or subluxed position of patella on sunrise view

Anterior Cruciate Ligament Tear

Acute injury

Rapid effusion (<2 hr)

Inability to continue play

Subjective instability

Positive Lachman test, pivot shift test

Positive anterior drawer sign (usual)

Baker's Cyst

Posterior mass in back of knee

May transilluminate

High incidence of associated intraarticular pathology (e.g., meniscal tear)

Iliotibial Band Syndrome

Lateral knee pain and tenderness over the iliotibial band

Runner

Training errors such as hill climbing, rapid progression (variable)

Pain on hill climbing, Stairmaster, or deep flexion exercises

Jumper's Knee

Pain at the patellar tendon

Tender on the palpation of the patellar tendon

History of repetitive jumping, running, or overuse syndrome

Medial Collateral Ligament Injury

Forced valgus mechanism (acute)

Medial pain and tenderness over medial collateral ligament

Minimal localized effusion (variable) over MCL

Pain or opening on valgus stress testing at 30 degrees of knee flexion with type 2 or 3 MCL injury

Meniscal Tears

True locking is almost pathognomic (also seen with a loose body)

Medial or lateral joint line pain and tenderness

Pain with twisting or deep knee flexion at joint line

Positive McMurray test

Locked knee or lack of extension if a large (bucket-handle) tear

Apley compression test positive (variable)

continued

Typical Findings in Common Knee Conditions *(Continued)*

Osgood-Schlatter Disease

Active, skeletally immature athlete

Tender tibial tubercle

Prominent tibial tubercle

Osteoarthritis

Insidious or gradual onset

Angular deformity (variable)

Effusion (variable)

Joint line narrowing on standing AP films

Tenderness and pain over affected joint lines

Osteophytes (variable)

Osteochondritis Dissecans

Vague, insidious onset of clicking, popping, locking, mild swelling

Radiographs (tunnel view) often reveal an OCD lesion

MRI useful to some degree for diagnosis and staging

Patellofemoral Syndrome (Anterior Knee Pain)

Anterior knee pain

Often bilateral

Exacerbated by activities that increase patellofemoral joint reaction forces (squatting, jumping, running, stair climbing)

Often underlying biomechanical changes (see patellofemoral section) such as increased Q-angle, patellar tilt, pes planus, patella alta

No mechanical symptoms or findings

Tender on patellar facet palpation, may have crepitance

Posterior Cruciate Ligament Tear

Abnormal posterior drawer test

Posterior cruciate ligament mechanism of injury (see section)

Effusion (variable)

Drop-back sign

Posterolateral Capsuloligamentous Injury

Dropback sign

Posterior Drawer sign positive

External rotation (Loomer) test positive

Often other ligament injuries associated

Prepatellar Bursitis (Housemaid's Knee)

Swollen, large bursa noted over anterior aspect of knee

Often a history of repetitive shearing force to anterior aspect of knee (repetitive kneeling on knee [e.g., carpet layer], etc.)

Aspiration of knee joint is negative—NO intraarticular effusion

Sinding-Larsen-Johanssen Syndrome

Tender at inferior pole of patella

Radiographic changes noted at inferior pole of patella (traction apophysitis)

May have bump palpable at inferior pole of patella

Bibliography

Knee Ligaments/Meniscal/Anterior Knee Pain

Aglietti P, Insall JN, Cerulli G: Patellar pain and incongruence. I: Measurements of incongruence. Clin Orthop 176:217–224, 1983.

Ahmed AM: The load-bearing role of the knee menisci. In Mow VC, Arnoczky SP, Jackson DW (eds): Knee Meniscus: Basic and Clinical Foundations. New York, Raven, 1992, pp. 59–73.

Ahmed AM: Burke DL, Hyder A: Force analysis of the patellar mechanism. J Orthop Res 5:69–85, 1987.

Anderson AF, Lipscomb AB: Analysis of rehabilitation techniques after anterior cruciate reconstruction. Am J Sports Med 17:154–160, 1989.

Anderson DR, Weiss JA, Takai S, et al: Healing of the MCL following a triad injury: a biomechanical and histological study of the knee in rabbits. J Orthop Res 10:485–495, 1992.

Arms S, Boyle J, Johnson R, Pope M: Strain measurement in the medial collateral ligament of the human knee: an autopsy study. J Biomech 16:491–496, 1983.

Arnoczky SP: Meniscus. In Fu FH, Harner CD, Vince KG (eds). Knee Surgery. Baltimore, Williams & Wilkins, 1994, pp. 131–140.

Arnoczky SP, Tarvin GB, Marshall JL: Anterior cruciate ligament replacement using patellar tendon: an evaluation of graft revascularization in the dog. J Bone Joint Surg 64A:217–224, 1982.

Arnoczky SP, Warren RF: Microvasculature of the human meniscus. Am J Sports Med 10:90–95, 1982.

Bach BR Jr, Levy ME, Bojchuk J, et al: Single-incision endoscopic anterior cruciate ligament reconstruction using patellar tendon autograft—minimum two year follow-up evaluation. Am J Sports Med 26:30–40, 1998.

Bach BR Jr, Tradonsky S, Bojchuk J, et al: Arthroscopically assisted anterior cruciate ligament reconstruction using patellar tendon autograft. Am J Sports Med 26:20–29, 1998.

Ballock RT, Woo SL-Y, Lyon RM, et al: Use of patellar tendon autograft for anterior cruciate ligament reconstruction in the rabbit: a long term histological and biomechanical study. J Orthop Res 7:474–485, 1989.

Barber FA: Accelerated rehabilitation for meniscus repairs. Arthroscopy 10:206–210, 1994.

Barber FA, Click SD: Meniscus repair rehabilitation with concurrent anterior cruciate reconstruction. Arthroscopy 13:433–437, 1997.

Barber FA, Elrod BF, McGuire DA, Paulos LE: Is an anterior cruciate ligament reconstruction outcome age dependent? Arthroscopy 12:720–725, 1996.

Barber-Westin SD, Noyes FR, Heckmann TP, Shaffer BL: The effect of exercise and rehabilitation on anterior-posterior knee displacements after anterior cruciate ligament autograft reconstruction. Am J Sports Med 27:84–93, 1999.

Barrack RL, Skinner HB, Buckley SL: Proprioception in the anterior cruciate deficient knee. Am J Sports Med 17:1–6, 1989.

Barratta R, Solomonow M, Zhou BH, et al: Muscular coactivation: the role of the antagonist musculature in maintaining knee stability. Am J Sports Med 16:113–122, 1988.

Barrett DS: Proprioception and function after anterior cruciate ligament reconstruction. J Bone Joint Surg 73B:833–837, 1991.

Beard DJ, Kyberd PJ, Ferguson CM, Dodd CAF: Proprioception enhancement for ACL deficiency: a prospective randomized trial of two physiotherapy regimens. J Bone Joint Surg 76B:654–659, 1994.

Bell DG, Jacobs I: Electro-mechanical response times and rate of force development in males and females. Med Sci Sports Exerc 18:31–36, 1986.

Bellemans J, Cauwenberghs F, Brys P, et al: Fracture of the proximal tibia after fulkerson anteromedial tibial tubercle transfer. Am J Sports Med 26:300–302, 1998.

Beynnon BD, Fleming BC: Anterior cruciate ligament strain in-vivo: a review of previous work. J Biomech 31:519–525, 1998.

Beynnon BD, Johnson RJ: Anterior cruciate ligament injury rehabilitation in athletes: biomechanical considerations. Sports Med 22:54–64, 1996.

Beynnon BD, Johnson RJ, Fleming BC, et al: The effect of functional knee bracing on the anterior cruciate ligament in the weightbearing and nonweightbearing knee. Am J Sports Med 25:353–359, 1997.

Blazina ME, Kerlan RK, Jobe FW, et al: Jumper's knee. Orthop Clin North Am 4:665–673, 1973.

Bockrath K, Wooden C, Worrell T, et al: Effects of patella taping on patella position and perceived pain. Med Sci Sports Exerc 25:989–992, 1993.

Bolgla LA, Keskula DR: Reliability of lower extremity functional performance tests. J Orthop Sports Phys Ther 26:138–142, 1997.

Bose K, Kanagasuntheram R, Osman MBH: Vastus medialis obliquis: an anatomic and physiologic study. Orthopedics 3:880–883, 1980.

Boynton MD, Tietjens BR: Long-term followup of the untreated isolated posterior cruciate ligament–deficient knee. Am J Sports Med 24:306–310, 1996.

Brody LT, Thein JM: Nonoperative treatment for patellofemoral pain. J Orthop Sports Phys Ther 28:336–344, 1998.

Bush-Joseph CA, Bach BR Jr: Arthroscopic assisted posterior cruciate ligament reconstruction using patellar tendon autograft. In Fu FH (ed): Sports Med Arthrosc Rev 2: 106–119, 1994.

Butler DL, Grood ES, Noyes FR, Sodd AN: On the interpretation of our ACL data. Clin Orthop 196:26–34, 1985.

Butler DL, Guan Y, Kay MD, et al: Location-dependent variations in the material properties of the anterior cruciate ligament. J Biomech 25:511–518, 1992.

Butler DL, Noyes FR, Grood ES: Ligamentous restraints to anterior-posterior drawer in the human knee. J Bone Joint Surg 62A:259–270, 1980.

Bylski-Austrow DI, Ciarelli MJ, Kayner DC, et al: Displacements of the menisci under joint load: an in vitro study in human knees. J Biomech 27:421–431, 1994.

Caborn DNM, Coen M, Neef R, et al: Quadrupled semitendinosis-gracilis autograft fixation in the femoral tunnel: a comparison between a metal and a bioabsorbable interference screw. Arthroscopy 14:241–245, 1998.

Caborn DNM, Urban WP Jr, Johnson DL, et al: Biomechanical comparison between BioScrew and titanium alloy interference screws for bone–patellar tendon–bone graft fixation in anterior cruciate ligament reconstruction. Athroscopy 13:229–232, 1997.

Caylor D, Fites R, Worrell TW: The relationship between the quadriceps angle and anterior knee pain syndrome. J Orthop Sports Phys Ther 17:11–16, 1993.

Cerny K: Vastus medialis oblique/vastus lateralis muscle activity ratios for selected exercises in persons with and without patellofemoral pain syndrome. Phys Ther 75: 672–683, 1995.

Chang PCC, Lee LKH, Tay BK: Anterior knee pain in the military population. Ann Acad Med Singapore 26:60–63, 1997.

Clancy WG Jr, Shelbourne KD, Zoellner GB, et al: Treatment of knee joint instability secondary to rupture of the posterior cruciate ligament: report of a new procedure. J Bone Joint Surg 65A:310–322, 1983.

Cohn BT, Draeger RI, Jackson DW: The effects of cold therapy in the postoperative management of pain in patients undergoing anterior cruciate ligament reconstruction. Am J Sports Med 17:344–349, 1989.

Colby SM, Hintermeister RA, Torry MR, Steadman JR: Lower limb stability with ACL impairment. J Orthop Sports Phys Ther 29:444–451, 1999.

Conlan T, Garth WP Jr, Lemons JE: Evaluation of the medial soft-tissue restraints of the extensor mechanism of the knee. J Bone Joint Surg 75A:682–693, 1993.

Cooper DE, Xianghua HD, Burstein AL, Warren RF: The strength of the central third patellar tendon graft. Am J Sports Med 21:818–824, 1993.

Corry IS, Webb JM, Clingeleffer AJ, Pinczewski LA: Arthroscopic reconstruction of the anterior cruciate ligament: a comparison of patellar tendon autograft and four-strand hamstring tendon autograft. Am J Sports Med 27:444–454, 1999.

Cosgarea AJ, Sebastianelli WJ, DeHaven KE: Prevention of arthrofibrosis after anterior cruciate ligament reconstruction using the central third patellar tendon autograft. Am J Sports Med 23:87–92, 1995.

Cross MJ, Powell JF: Long-term followup of posterior cruciate ligament rupture. Am J Sports Med 12:292–297, 1984.

Denham RA, Bishop RED: Mechanics of the knee and problems in reconstructive surgery. J Bone Joint Surg 60B:345–351, 1978.

Doucette SA, Child DP: The effect of open and closed chain exercise and knee joint position on patellar tracking in lateral patellar compression syndrome. J Orthop Sports Phys Ther 23:104–110, 1996.

Doucette SA, Goble EM: The effect of exercise on patellar tracking in lateral patellar compression syndrome. Am J Sports Med 20:434–440, 1992.

Dowdy PA, Miniaci A, Arnoczky SP, et al: The effect of cast immobilization on meniscal healing: an experimental study in the dog. Am J Sports Med 23:721–728, 1995.

Dye SF: The knee as a biologic transmission with an envelope of function: a theory. Clin Orthop 325:10–8, 1996.

Eng JJ, Pierrynowski MR: Evaluation of soft foot orthotics in the treatment of patellofemoral pain syndrome. Phys Ther 73:62–70, 1993.

Engle CP, Noguchi M, Ohland KJ, et al: Healing of the rabbit medial collateral ligament following an O'Donoghue triad injury: the effects of anterior cruciate ligament reconstruction. J Orthop Res 12:357–364, 1994.

Escamilla RF, Fleisig GS, Zheng N, et al: Biomechanics of the knee during closed kinetic chain and open kinetic chain exercises. Med Sci Sports Exerc 30:556–569, 1998.

Falconiero RP, DiStefano VJ, Cook TM: Revascularization and ligamentization of autogenous anterior cruciate ligament grafts in humans. Arthroscopy 14:197–205, 1998.

Feretti A: Epidemiology of jumper's knee. Sports Med 3:289–295, 1986.

Fetto JF, Marshall JL: Medial collateral ligament injuries of the knee: a rationale for treatment. Clin Orthop 132:206–218, 1978.

Frank CB, Jackson DW: The science of reconstruction of the anterior cruciate ligament. J Bone Joint Surg 79A:1556–1576, 1997.

Fukibayashi T, Torzilli PA, Sherman MF, Warren RF: An in-vitro biomechanical evaluation of anterior-posterior motion of the knee. J Bone Joint Surg 64A:258–264, 1982.

Fulkerson JP, Kalenak A, Rosenberg TD, Cox JS: Patellofemoral pain. In Eilert RE (ed): Instr Course Lect 41: pp. 57–70, 1992.

Gerrard B: The patellofemoral pain syndrome in young, active patients: a prospective study. Clin Orthop 179:129–133, 1989.

Gilleard W, McConnell J, Parsons D: The effect of patellar taping on the onset of vastus medialis obliquus and vastus lateralis muscle activity in persons with patellofemoral pain. Phys Ther 78:25–31, 1998.

Giove TP, Miller SJ III, Kent BE, et al: Non-operative treatment of the torn anterior cruciate ligament. J Bone Joint Surg 65A:184–192, 1983.

Giurea M, Zorilla P, Amis AA, Aichroth P: Comparative pull-out and cyclic-loading strength tests of anchorage of hamstring tendon grafts in anterior cruciate ligament reconstruction. Am J Sports Med 27:621–625, 1999.

Goldfuss AJ, Morehouse CA, LeVeau BF: Effect of muscular tension on knee stability. Med Sci Sports Exerc 5:267–271, 1973.

Gollehon DL, Torzilli PA, Warren RF: The role of the posterolateral and cruciate ligaments in the stability of the human knee: a biomechanical study. J Bone Joint Surg 69A:233–242, 1987.

Gomez MA, Woo SL-Y, Amiel D, et al: The effects of increased tension on healing medial collateral ligaments. Am J Sports Med 19:347–354, 1991.

Goodfellow J, Hungerford DS, Zindel M: Patello-femoral mechanics and pathology. I: Functional anatomy of the patello-femoral joint. J Bone Joint Surg 58B:287–290, 1976.

Grabiner MD, Koh TJ, Draganich LF: Neuromechanics of the patellofemoral joint. Med Sci Sports Exerc 26:10–21, 1994.

Greenwald AE, Bagley AM, France EP, et al: A biomechanical and clinical evaluation of a patellofemoral knee brace. Clin Orthop 324:187–195, 1996.

Grelsamer RP, Klein JR: The biomechanics of the patellofemoral joint. J Orthop Sports Phys Ther 28:286–298, 1998.

Grood ES, Noyes FR, Butler DL, et al: Ligamentous and capsular restraints preventing straight medial and lateral laxity in intact human cadaver knees. J Bone Joint Surg 63A:1257–1269, 1981.

Grood ES, Stowers SF, Noyes FR: Limits of movement in the human knee: effect of sectioning the posterior cruciate ligament and posterolateral structures. J Bone Joint Surg 70A:88–97, 1988.

Grood ES, Suntay WJ, Noyes FR, Butler DL: Biomechanics of the knee-extension exercise. J Bone Joint Surg 66A:725–734, 1984.

Habata T, Ishimura M, Ohgushi H, et al: Axial alignment of the lower limb in patients with isolated meniscal tear. J Orthop Sci 3:85–89, 1998.

Hakkinen K: Force production characteristics of leg extensor, trunk flexor, and extensor muscles in male and female basketball players. J Sports Med Phys Fitness 31:325–331, 1991.

Hardin GT, Bach BR Jr: Distal rupture of the infrapatellar tendon after use of its central third for anterior cruciate ligament reconstruction. Am J Knee Surg 5:140–143, 1992.

Hardin GT, Bach BR Jr, Bush-Joseph CA: Extension loss following arthroscopic ACL reconstruction. Orthop Int 1:405–410, 1993.

Harner CD, Hoher J: Evaluation and treatment of posterior cruciate ligament injuries. Am J Sports Med 26:471–482, 1998.

Harner CD, Irrgang JJ, Paul J, et al: Loss of motion after anterior cruciate ligament reconstruction. Am J Sports Med 20:499–506, 1992.

Harner CD, Olson E, Irrgang JJ, et al: Allograft versus autograft anterior cruciate ligament reconstruction. Clin Orthop 325:134–144, 1996.

Hewett TE, Lindenfeld TN, Riccobene JV, Noyes FR: The effect of neuromuscular training on the incidence of knee injury in female athletes. Am J Sports Med 27:699–706, 1999.

Hewett TE, Noyes FR, Lee MD: Diagnosis of complete and partial posterior cruciate ligament ruptures: stress radiography compared with KT-1000 Arthrometer and posterior drawer testing. Am J Sports Med 5:648–655, 1997.

Hewett TE, Stroupe AL, Nance TA, Noyes FR: Plyometric training in female athletes: decreased impact forces and increased hamstring torques. Am J Sports Med 24:765–773, 1996.

Holmes SW, Clancy WG: Clinical classification of patellofemoral pain and dysfunction. J Orthop Sports Phys Ther 28:299–306, 1998.

Howell SM, Taylor MA: Brace-free rehabilitation, with early return to activity, for knees reconstructed with a double-looped semitendinosis and gracilis graft. J Bone Joint Surg 78A:814–825, 1996.

Huberti HH, Hayes WC: Contact pressures in chondromalacia patellae and the effects of capsular reconstructive procedures. J Orthop Res 6:499–508, 1988.

Huberti HH, Hayes WC, Stone JL, Shybut GT: Force ratios in the quadriceps tendon and ligamentum patellae. J Orthop Res 2:49–54, 1984.

Hull ML, Berns GS, Varma H, Patterson HA: Strain in the medial collateral ligament of the human knee under single and combined loads. J Biomech 29:199–206, 1996.

Huston LJ, Wojtys EM: Neuromuscular performance characteristics in elite female athletes. Am J Sports Med 24:427–436, 1996.

Indelicato PA: Non-operative treatment of complete tears of the medial collateral ligament of the knee. J Bone Joint Surg 65A:323–329, 1983.

Ingersoll C, Knight K: Patellar location changes following EMG biofeedback or progressive resistive exercises. Med Sci Sports Exerc 23:1122–1127, 1991.

Inoue M, Yasuda K, Ohkoshi Y, et al: Factors that affect prognosis of conservatively treated patients with isolated posterior cruciate ligament injury. In Programs and Abstracts of the 64th Annual Meeting of the American Academy of Orthopaedic Surgeons, San Francisco, 1997, p. 78.

Inoue M, Yasuda K, Yamanaka M, et al: Compensatory muscle activity in the posterior cruciate ligament–deficient knee during isokinetic knee motion. Am J Sports Med 26:710–714, 1998.

Insall J, Falvo KA, Wise DW: Chondromalacia patellae. A prospective study. J Bone Joint Surg 58A:1–8, 1976.

Itoh H, Kurosaka M, Yoshiya S, et al: Evaluation of functional deficits determined by four different hop tests in patients with anterior cruciate ligament deficiency. Knee surg Sports Traumatol Arthrosc 6:241–245, 1998.

Jenkins WL, Munns SW, Jayaraman G, et al: A measurement of anterior tibial displacement in the closed and open kinetic chain. J Orthop Sports Phys Ther 25:49–56, 1997.

Juris PM, Phillips EM, Dalpe C, et al: A dynamic test of lower extremity function following anterior cruciate ligament reconstruction and rehabilitation. J Orthop Sports Phys Ther 26:184–191, 1997.

Jurist KA, Otis JC:. Anteroposterior tibiofemoral displacements during isometric extension efforts. Am J Sports Med 13:254–258, 1985.

Karst GM, Willett GM: Onset timing of electromyographic activity in the vastus medialis oblique and vastus lateralis muscles in subjects with and without patellofemoral pain syndrome. Phys Ther 75:813–837, 1995.

Kartus J, Magnusson L, Stener S, et al: Complications following arthroscopic anterior cruciate ligament reconstruction. Knee Surg Sports Traumatol Arthrosc 7:2–8, 1999.

Keller PM, Shelbourne KD, McCarroll JR, Rettig AC: Non-operatively treated isolated posterior cruciate ligament injuries. Am J Sports Med 21:132–136, 1993.

King D: The healing of semilunar cartilages. J Bone Joint Surg 18:333–342, 1936.

Klein L, Heiple KG, Torzilli PA, et al: Prevention of ligament and meniscus atrophy by active joint motion in a non–weight-bearing model. J Orthop Res 7:80–85, 1989.

Kleipool AEB, Zijl JAC, Willems WJ: Arthroscopic anterior cruciate ligament reconstruction with bone–patellar tendon–bone allograft or autograft. Knee Surg Sports Traumatol Arthrosc 6: 224–230, 1998.

Klingman RE, Liaos SM, Hardin KM. The effect of subtalar joint posting on patellar glide position in subjects with excessive rearfoot pronation. J Orthop Sports Phys Ther 25:185–191, 1997.

Kolowich PA, Paulos LE, Rosenberg TD, Farnsworth S: Lateral release of the patella: indications and contraindications. Am J Sports Med 18:359–365, 1990.

Komi PV, Karlsson J: Physical performance, skeletal muscle enzyme activities, and fibre types in monozygous and dizygous twins of both sexes. Acta Physiol Scand 462(Suppl):1–28, 1979.

Kowall MG, Kolk G, Nuber GW, et al: Patellofemoral taping in the treatment of patellofemoral pain. Am J Sports Med 24:61–66, 1996.

Kvist J, Gillquist J: Anterior tibial translation during eccentric, isokinetic quadriceps work in healthy subjects. Scand J Med Sci Sports 9:189–194, 1999.

Kwak SD, Colman WW, Ateshian GA, et al: Anatomy of the human patellofemoral joint articular cartilage: a surface curvature analysis. J Orthop Res 15:468–472, 1997.

Laprade J, Culham E, Brouwer B: Comparison of five isometric exercises in the recruitment of the vastus medialis oblique in persons with and without patellofemoral pain. J Orthop Sports Phys Ther 27:197–204, 1998.

Larsen B, Andreasen E, Urfer A, et al: Patellar taping: a radiographic examination of the medial glide technique. Am J Sports Med 23:465–471, 1995.

Larsen NP, Forwood MR, Parker AW: Immobilization and re-training of cruciate ligaments in the rat. Acta Orthop Scand 58:260–264, 1987.

Laurin CA, Levesque HP, Dussault R, et al: The abnormal lateral patellofemoral angle. A diagnostic roentgenographic sign of recurrent patellar subluxation. J Bone Joint Surg 60A:55–60, 1978.

Lephart SM, Kocher MS, Fu FH, et al: Proprioception following anterior cruciate ligament reconstruction. J Sports Rehabil 1:188–196, 1992.

Lephart SM, Pincivero DM, Rozzi SL: Proprioception of the ankle and knee. Sports Med 3:149–155, 1998.

Lian O, Engebretsen L, Ovrebo RV, Bahr R: Characteristics of the leg extensors in male volleyball players with jumper's knee. Am J Sports Med 24:380–385, 1996.

Lieb FJ, Perry J: Quadriceps function: an anatomical and mechanical study using amputated limbs. J Bone Joint Surg 53A:749–758, 1971.

Lieber RL, Silva PD, Daniel DM: Equal effectiveness of electrical and volitional strength training for quadriceps femoris muscles after anterior cruciate ligament surgery. J Orthop Res 14:131–138, 1996.

Lipscomb AB Jr, Anderson AF, Norwig ED, et al: Isolated posterior cruciate ligament reconstruction: long-term results. Am J Sports Med 21:490–496, 1993.

Lundberg M, Messner K: Long-term prognosis of isolated partial medial collateral ligament ruptures. Am J Sports Med 24:160–163, 1996.

Lutz GE, Palmitier RA, An KN, Chao EYS: Comparison of tibiofemoral joint forces during open-kinetic-chain and closed-kinetic-chain exercises. J Bone Joint Surg 75A:732–739, 1993.

MacDonald P, Miniaci A, Fowler P, et al: A biomechanical analysis of joint contact forces in the posterior cruciate deficient knee. Knee Surg Sports Traumatol Arthrosc 3:252–255, 1996.

Magen HE, Howell SM, Hull ML: Structural properties of six tibial fixation methods for anterior cruciate ligament soft tissue grafts. Am J Sports Med 27:35–43, 1999.

Mangine RE, Eifert-Mangine M, Burch D, et al: Postoperative management of the patellofemoral patient. J Orthop Sports Phys Ther 28:323–335, 1998.

Marder RA, Raskind JR, Carroll M: Prospective evaluation of arthroscopically assisted anterior cruciate ligament reconstruction: patellar tendon versus semitendinosis and gracilis tendons. Am J Sports Med 19:478–484, 1991.

Mariani PP, Santori N, Adriani E, Mastantuono M: Accelerated rehabilitation after arthroscopic meniscal repair: a clinical and magnetic resonance imaging evaluation. Arthroscopy 12:680–686, 1996.

Markolf KL, Burchfield DM, Shapiro MM, et al. Biomechanical consequences of replacement of the anterior cruciate ligament with a patellar ligament allograft. Part II: Forces in the graft compared with forces in the intact ligament. J Bone Joint Surg 78A:1728–1734, 1996.

Markolf KL, Mensch JS, Amstutz HC: Stiffness and laxity of the knee: the contributions of the supporting structures. J Bone Joint Surg 58A:583–593, 1976.

Markolf KL, Slauterbeck JR, Armstrong KL, et al: A biomechanical study of replacement of the posterior cruciate lig-

ament with a graft. Part II: Forces in the graft compared with forces in the intact ligament. J Bone Joint Surg 79A:381–386, 1997.

McConnell J: The management of chondromalacia patellae: a long term solution. Aust J Physiother 32:215–223, 1986.

McDaniel WJ, Dameron TB: Untreated ruptures of the anterior cruciate ligament. J Bone Joint Surg 62A:696–705, 1980.

McDaniel WJ, Dameron TB: The untreated anterior cruciate ligament rupture. Clin Orthop 172:158–163, 1983.

McKernan DJ, Paulos LE: Graft Selection. In Fu FH, Harner CD, Vince KG (eds): Knee Surgery. Baltimore, Williams & Wilkins, 1994.

McLaughlin J, DeMaio M, Noyes FR, Mangine RE: Rehabilitation after meniscus repair. Orthopedics 17:463–471, 1994.

Merchant AC: Classification of patellofemoral disorders. Arthroscopy 4:235–240, 1988.

Merchant AC, Mercer RL, Jacobsen RH, Cool CR: Roentgenographic analysis of patellofemoral congruence. J Bone Joint Surg 56A:1391–1396, 1974.

Mirzabeigi E, Jordan C, Gronley JK, et al: Isolation of the vastus medialis oblique muscle during exercise. Am J Sports Med 27:50–53, 1999.

Mok DWH, Good C: Non-operative management of acute grade III medial collateral ligament injury of the knee. Injury 20:277–280, 1989.

Moller BN, Krebs B: Dynamic knee brace in the treatment of patellofemoral disorders. Arch Orthop Trauma Surg 104:377–379, 1986.

Morgan CD, Wojtys EM, Casscells CD, Cassells SW: Arthroscopic meniscal repair evaluated by second-look arthroscopy. Am J Sports Med 19:632–637, 1991.

Muhle C, Brinkmann G, Skaf A, et al: Effect of a patellar realignment brace on patients with patellar subluxation and dislocation. Am J Sports Med 27:350–353, 1999.

Muneta T, Sekiya I, Ogiuchi T, et al: Effects of aggressive early rehabilitation on the outcome of anterior cruciate ligament reconstruction with multi-strand semitendinosis tendon. Int Orthop 22:352–356, 1998.

Neeb TB, Aufdemkampe G, Wagener JH, Mastenbroek L: Assessing anterior cruciate ligament injuries: the association and differential value of questionnaires, clinical tests, and functional tests. J Orthop Sports Phys Ther 26:324–331, 1997.

Nissen CW, Cullen MC, Hewett TE, Noyes FR: Physical and arthroscopic examination techniques of the patellofemoral joint. J Orthop Sports Phys Ther 28:277–285, 1998.

Nogalski MP, Bach BR Jr: Acute anterior cruciate ligament injuries. In Fu FH, Harner CD, Vince KG (eds): Knee Surgery. Baltimore, Williams & Wilkins, 1994.

Novak PJ, Bach BR Jr, Hager CA: Clinical and functional outcome of anterior cruciate ligament reconstruction in the recreational athlete over the age of 35. Am Journal Knee Surg 9:111–116, 1996.

Noyes FR: Functional properties of knee ligaments and alterations induced by immobilization: a correlative biomechanical and histological study in primates. Clin Orthop 123:210–242, 1977.

Noyes FR, Barber SD, Mangine RE: Abnormal lower limb symmetry determined by function hop tests after anterior cruciate ligament rupture. Am J Sports Med 19:513–518, 1991a.

Noyes FR, Butler DL, Grood ES, et al: Biomechanical analysis of human ligament grafts used in knee-ligament repairs and replacements. J Bone Joint Surg 66A:344–352, 1984.

Noyes FR, DeMaio M, Mangine RE: Evaluation-based protocol: a new approach to rehabilitation. J Orthop Res 14:1383–1385, 1991b.

Noyes FR, Wojyts EM, Marshall MT: The early diagnosis and treatment of developmental patella infera syndrome. Clin Orthop 265:241–252, 1991c.

Nyland J: Rehabilitation complications following knee surgery. Clin Sports Med 18:905–925, 1999.

O'Connor JJ: Can muscle co-contraction protect knee ligaments after injury or repair. J Bone Joint Surg 75B:41–48, 1993.

Odensten M, Hamberg P, Nordin M, et al: Surgical or conservative treatment of the acutely torn anterior cruciate ligament. Clin Orthop 198:87–93, 1985.

O'Donoghue DH: Surgical treatment of fresh injuries to the major ligaments of the knee. J Bone Joint Surg 32A:721–738, 1950.

Ohno K, Pomaybo AS, Schmidt CC, et al: Healing of the MCL after a combined MCL and ACL injury and reconstruction of the ACL: comparison of repair and nonrepair of MCL tears in rabbits. J Orthop Res 13:442–449, 1995.

Ostenberg A, Roos E, Ekdahl C, Roos H: Isokinetic knee extensor strength and functional performance in healthy female soccer players. Scand J Med Sci Sports 8:257–264, 1998.

Osteras H, Augestad LB, Tondel S: Isokinetic muscle strength after anterior cruciate ligament reconstruction. Scand J Med Sci Sports 8:279–282, 1998.

Otero AL, Hutcheson L: A comparison of the doubled semitendinosis/gracilis and central third of the patellar tendon autografts in arthroscopic anterior cruciate ligament reconstruction. Arthroscopy 9:143–148, 1993.

Palumbo PM: Dynamic patellar brace: a new orthosis in the management of patellofemoral pain. Am J Sports Med 9:45–49, 1981.

Papagelopoulos PJ, Sim FH: Patellofemoral pain syndrome: diagnosis and management. Orthopedics 20:148–157, 1997.

Parolie JM, Bergfeld JA: Long-term results of nonoperative treatment of isolated posterior cruciate ligament injuries in the athlete. Am J Sports Med 14:35–38, 1986.

Paulos LE, Rosenberg TD, Drawbert J, et al: Infrapatellar contracture syndrome: an unrecognized cause of knee stiffness with patella entrapment and patella infera. Am J Sports Med 15:331–341, 1987.

Pincivero DM, Lephart SM, Henry TJ: The effects of kinesthetic training on balance and proprioception in anterior cruciate ligament injured knee. J Athletic Train 31(Suppl 2):S52, 1996.

Pope MH, Johnson RJ, Brown DW, Tighe C: The role of the musculature in injuries to the medial collateral ligament. J Bone Joint Surg 61A:398–402, 1979.

Popp JE, Yu JS, Kaeding CC: Recalcitrant patellar tendinitis: magnetic resonance imaging, histologic evaluation, and surgical treatment. Am J Sports Med 25:218–222, 1997.

Powers CM: Rehabilitation of patellofemoral joint disorders: a critical review. J Orthop Sports Phys Ther 28:345–354, 1998.

Powers CM, Landel R, Perry J: Timing and intensity of vastus muscle activity during functional activities in subjects with and without patellofemoral pain. Phys Ther 76:946–966, 1996.

Race A, Amis AA: The mechanical properties of the two bundles of the human posterior cruciate ligament. J Biomech 27:13–24, 1994.

Radin EL, Rose RM: Role of subchondral bone in the initiation and progression of cartilage damage. Clin Orthop 213:34–40, 1986.

Reider B: Medial collateral ligament injuries in athletes. Sports Med 21:147–156, 1996.

Reider B, Sathy MR, Talkington J, et al: Treatment of isolated medial collateral ligament injuries in athletes with early functional rehabilitation. Am J Sports Med 22:470–477, 1993.

Reinold MM, Fleisig GS, Wilk KE: Research supports both OKC and CKC activities. Biomechanics 2(2, Suppl):27–32, 1999.

Risberg MA, Holm I, Steen H, et al: The effect of knee bracing after anterior cruciate ligament reconstruction. Am J Sports Med 27:76–83, 1999.

Roberts D, Friden T, Zatterstrom R, et al: Proprioception in people with anterior cruciate ligament–deficient knees: comparison of symptomatic and asymptomatic patients. J Orthop Sports Phys Ther 29:587–594, 1999.

Rodeo SA: Arthroscopic meniscal repair with use of the outside-in technique. J Bone Joint Surg 82A:127–141, 2000.

Sachs RA, Daniel DM, Stone ML, Garfein RF: Patellofemoral problems after anterior cruciate ligament reconstruction. Am J Sports Med 17:760–765, 1989.

Schutzer SF, Ramsby GR, Fulkerson JP: Computed tomographic classification of patellofemoral pain patients. Orthop Clin North Am 144:16–26, 1986.

Schutzer SF, Ramsby GR, Fulkerson JP: The evaluation of patellofemoral pain using computerized tomography: a preliminary study. Clin Orthop 204:286–293, 1986.

Seitz H, Schlenz I, Muller E, Vecsei V: Anterior instability of the knee despite an intensive rehabilitation program. Clin Orthop 328:159–164, 1996.

Sernert N, Kartus J, Kohler K, et al. Analysis of subjective, objective, and functional examination tests after anterior cruciate ligament reconstruction. Knee Surg Sports Traumatol Arthrosc 7:160–165, 1999.

Shelbourne KD, Davis TJ: Evaluation of knee stability before and after participation in a functional sports agility program during rehabilitation after anterior cruciate ligament reconstruction. Am J Sports Med 27:156–161, 1999.

Shelbourne KD, Davis TJ, Patel DV: The natural history of acute, isolated, nonoperatively treated posterior cruciate ligament injuries. Am J Sports Med 27:276–283, 1999.

Shelbourne KD, Foulk AD: Timing of surgery in anterior cruciate ligament tears on the return of quadriceps muscle strength after reconstruction using an autogenous patellar tendon graft. Am J Sports Med 23:686–689, 1995.

Shelbourne KD, Nitz P: Accelerated rehabilitation after anterior cruciate ligament reconstruction. Am J Sports Med 18:292–299, 1990.

Shelbourne KD, Patel DV: Treatment of limited motion after anterior cruciate ligament reconstruction. Knee Surg Sports Traumatol Arthrosc 7:85–92, 1999.

Shelbourne KD, Patel DV, Adsit WS, Porter DA: Rehabilitation after meniscal repair. Clin Sports Med 15:595–612, 1996a.

Shelbourne KD, Patel DV, Martini DJ: Classification and management of arthrofibrosis of the knee after anterior cruciate ligament reconstruction. Am J Sports Med 24:857–862, 1996b.

Shelbourne KD, Wilckens JH, Mollabaashy A, DeCarlo MS: Arthrofibrosis in acute anterior cruciate ligament reconstruction: the effect of timing of reconstruction and rehabilitation. Am J Sports Med 9:332–336, 1991.

Shellock FG, Mink JH, Deutsch AL, Foo TK: Kinematic MR imaging of the patellofemoral joint: comparison of passive positioning and active movement techniques. Radiology 184:574–577, 1992.

Shelton WR, Papendick L, Dukes AD: Autograft versus allograft anterior cruciate ligament reconstruction. Arthroscopy 13:446–449, 1997.

Skyhar MJ, Warren RF, Oritz GJ, et al: The effects of sectioning of the posterior cruciate ligament and the posterolateral complex on the articular contact pressures within the knee. J Bone Joint Surg 75A:694–699, 1993.

Snyder-Mackler L, Ladin Z, Schepsis AA, Young JC: Electrical stimulation of thigh muscles after reconstruction of anterior cruciate ligament. J Bone Joint Surg 73A:1025–1036, 1991.

Steinkamp LA, Dillingham MF, Markel MD, et al: Biomechanical considerations in patellofemoral joint rehabilitation. Am J Sports Med 21:438–444, 1993.

Stetson WB, Friedman MJ, Fulkerson JP, et al: Fracture of the proximal tibia with immediate weightbearing after a Fulkerson osteotomy. Am J Sports Med 25:570–574, 1997.

Thompson WO, Thaete FL, Fu FH, Dye SF: Tibial meniscal dynamics using three-dimensional reconstruction of magnetic resonance images. Am J Sports Med 19:210–216, 1991.

Torg JS, Barton TM, Pavlov H, Stine R: Natural history of the posterior cruciate ligament–deficient knee. Clin Orthop 246:208–216, 1989.

Tyler TF, McHugh MP, Gleim GW, Nicholas SJ: The effect of immediate weightbearing after anterior cruciate ligament reconstruction. Clin Orthop 357:141–148, 1998.

Vedi V, Williams A, Tennant SJ, et al: Meniscal movement: an in-vivo study using dynamic MRI. J Bone Joint Surg 81B:37–41, 1999.

Voloshin AS, Wosk J: Shock absorption of the meniscectomized and painful knees: a comparative in vivo study. J Biomed Eng 5:157–161, 1983.

Vos EJ, Harlaar J, van Ingen-Schenau GJ: Electromechanical delay during knee extensor contractions. Med Science Sports Exerc 23:1187–1193, 1991.

Weiss JA, Woo SL-Y, Ohland KJ, Horibe S: Evaluation of a new injury model to study medial collateral ligament healing: primary repair versus non-operative treatment. J Orthop Res 9:516–528, 1991.

Wilk KE: Rehabilitation of isolated and combined posterior cruciate ligament injuries. Clin Sports Med 13(3):649–677, 1994.

Wilk KE, Andrews JR: The effects of pad placement and angular velocity on tibial displacement during isokinetic exercise. J Orthop Sports Phys Ther 17:24–30, 1993.

Wilk KE, Arrigo C, Andrews JR, Clancy WG: Rehabilitation after anterior cruciate ligament reconstruction in the female athlete. J Athletic Train 34:177–193, 1999.

Wilk KE, Davies GJ, Mangine RE, Malone TR: Patellofemoral disorders: a classification system and clinical guideline for nonoperative rehabilitation. J Orthop Sports Phys Ther 28:307–322, 1998.

Williams JS Jr, Bach BR Jr: Rehabilitation of the ACL deficient and reconstructed knee. In Grana W (ed): Sports Med Arthrosc Rev 3:69–82, 1996.

Woo SL-Y, Chan SS, Yamaji T: Biomechanics of knee ligament healing, repair, and reconstruction. J Biomech 30:431–439, 1997.

Woo SL-Y, Gomez MA, Sites TJ, et al: The biomechanical and morphological changes of the MCL following immobilization and remobilization. J Bone Joint Surg 69A:1200–1211, 1987.

Woo SL-Y, Hollis JM, Adams DJ, et al: Tensile properties of the human femur–anterior cruciate ligament complex. Am J Sports Med 19:217–225, 1991.

Woo SL-Y, Inoue M, McGurck-Burleson E, Gomez M: Treatment of the medial collateral ligament injury II. Structure and function of canine knees in response to differing treatment regimens. Am J Sports Med 15:22–29, 1987.

Woodland LH, Francis RS: Parameters and comparisons of the quadriceps angle of college-aged men and women in the supine and standing positions. Am J Sports Med 20:208–211, 1992.

Yack HJ, Collins CE, Whieldon TJ: Comparison of closed and open kinetic chain exercises in the anterior cruciate ligament–deficient knee. Am J Sports Med 21:49–54, 1993.

Yamaji T, Levine RE, Woo SL-Y, et al: MCL healing one year after a concurrent MCL and ACL injury: an interdisciplinary study in rabbits. J Orthop Res 14:223–227, 1996.

Yasuda K, Erickson AR, Beynnon BD, et al: Dynamic elongation behavior in the medial collateral and anterior cruciate ligaments during lateral impact loading. J Orthop Res 11:190–198, 1993.

Zavetsky AB, Beard DJ, O'Connor JJ: Cruciate ligament loading during isometric muscle contractions. Am J Sports Med 22:418–423, 1994.

Zheng N, Fleisig GS, Escamilla RF, Barrentine SW: An analytical model of the knee for estimation of the internal forces during exercise. J Biomech 31:963–967, 1998.

Patellar Tendon Ruptures

Antich T, Brewster C: Modification of quadriceps femoris muscle exercises during knee rehabilitation. Phys Ther 66:1246–1251, 1986.

Aoki M, Ogiwara N, Ohata T, Nabeta Y: Early active motion and weightbearing after cross-stitch Achilles tendon repair. Am J Sports Med 26:794–800, 1998.

Bonomo JJ, Krinick RM, Sporn AA: Rupture of the patellar ligament after use of its central third for anterior cruciate reconstruction: a report of two cases. J Bone Joint Surg 196A:253–255, 1985.

Burks RT, Delson RH: Allograft reconstruction of the patellar ligament: a case report. J Bone Joint Surg 76A:1077–1079, 1994.

Carroll TJ, Abernethy PJ, Logan PA, et al: Resistance training frequency: strength and myosin heavy chain responses to two and three bouts per week. Eur J Appl Physiol 78:270–275, 1998.

Davies SG, Baudouin CJ, King JD, et al: Ultrasound, computed tomography and magnetic resonance imaging in patellar tendinitis. Clin Radiol 43:52–56, 1991.

Dervin GF, Taylor DE, Keene G: Effects of cold and compression dressings on early postoperative outcomes for the arthroscopic anterior cruciate ligament reconstruction patient. J Orthop Sports Phys Ther 27:403–406, 1998.

Ecker ML, Lotke PA, Glazer RM: Late reconstruction of the patellar tendon. J Bone Joint Surg 61A:884–886, 1979.

Emerson RH Jr, Head WC, Malinin TI: Reconstruction of patellar tendon rupture after total knee arthroplasty with an extensor mechanism allograft. Clin Orthop 260:154–161, 1990.

Evans PD, Pritchard GA, Jenkins DHR: Carbon fibre used in the late reconstruction of rupture of the extensor mechanism of the knee. Injury 18:57–60, 1987.

Gould III JA, Davies GJ (eds): Orthopaedic and Sports Physical Therapy. St. Louis, Mosby, 1985.

Greenberger HB, Paterno MV: Relationship of knee extensor strength and hopping test performance in the assessment of lower extremity function. J Orthop Sports Phys Ther 22:202–206, 1995.

Hsu KY, Wang KC, Ho WP, et al: Traumatic patellar tendon ruptures: a follow-up study of primary repair and a neutralization wire. J Trauma 36:658–660, 1994.

Ismail AM, Balakrishnan R, Rajakumar MK: Rupture of patellar ligament after steroid infiltration: report of a case. J Bone Joint Surg 51B:503–505, 1969.

Jones D, Rutherford O: Human muscle strength training: the effects of three different regimes and the nature of the resultant changes. J Physiol 391:1–11, 1987.

Kannus P, Jozsa L: Histopathological changes preceding spontaneous rupture of a tendon: a controlled study of 891 patients. J Bone Joint Surg 73A:1507–1525, 1991.

Kennedy JC, Willis RB: The effects of local steroid injections on tendons: a biomechanical and microscopic correlative study. Am J Sports Med 4:11–21, 1976.

McNair PJ, Marshall RN, Maguire K: Swelling of the knee joint: effects of exercise on quadriceps muscle strength. Arch Phys Med Rehabil 77:896–899, 1996.

Mortensen NH, Skov O, Jensen PE: Early motion of the ankle after operative treatment of a rupture of the Achilles tendon. J Bone Joint Surg 81A:983–990, 1999.

Palmitier R, An K-N, Scott S, Chao E: Kinetic chain exercise in knee rehabilitation. Sports Med 11:402–413, 1991.

Rutherford O: Muscular coordination and strength training: implications for injury rehabilitation. Sports Med 5:196–202, 1998.

Siwek CW, Rao JP: Ruptures of the extensor mechanism of the knee joint. J Bone Joint Surg 63A:932–937, 1981.

Takai S, Woo S, Horibe S, et al: The effects of frequency and duration of controlled passive mobilization on tendon healing. J Orthop Res 9:705–713, 1991.

Tepperman PS, Mazliah J, Naumann S, Delmore T: Effect of ankle position on isometric quadriceps strengthening. Am J Phys Med 65:69–74, 1986.

Vergso J, Genuario S, Torg J: Maintenance of hamstring strength following knee surgery. Med Sci Sports Exerc 17:376–379, 1985.

Webb LX, Toby EB: Bilateral rupture of the patella tendon in an otherwise healthy male patient following minor trauma. J Trauma 26:1045–1048, 1986.

Wigerstad-Lossing I, Grimby G, Jonsson T, et al: Effects of electrical stimulation combined with voluntary contractions after knee ligament surgery. Med Sci Sports Exerc 20:93–98, 1988.

Woo S, Maynard J, Butler D, et al: Ligament, tendon, and joint capsule insertions to bone. In Woo SL-Y, Buckwalter JA (eds): injury and repair of the musculoskeletal soft tissues. Park Ridge, Ill: American Academy of Orthopaedic Surgeons, 1988, pp. 133–166.

Yu JS, Petersilge C, Sartoris DJ, et al: MR imaging of injuries of the extensor mechanism of the knee. Radiographics 14:541–551, 1994.

Articular Cartilage Repair

Bandy WD, Hanten WP: Changes in torque and electromyographic activity of the quadriceps femoris muscles following isometric training. Phys Ther 73:455–465, 1993.

Buckwalter J: Effects of early motion on healing musculoskeletal tissues. Hand Clin 12:13–24, 1996.

Rosenberg TD, Paulos LE, Parker RD, et al: The forty five degree posteroanterior flexion weight bearing radiograph of the knee. J Bone Joint Surg 70A:1479–1483, 1988.

Salter RB, Minster R, Bell R, et al: Continuous passive motion and the repair of full-thickness articular cartilage defects: a 1-year follow-up [abstract]. Trans Orthop Res Soc 7:167, 1982.

Salter RB, Simmonds DF, Malcolm BW, et al: The biological effect of continous passive motion on healing of full-thickness defects in articular cartilage: an experimental study in the rabbit. J Bone Joint Surg 62A:1232–1251, 1980.

Suh J, Aroen A, Muzzonigro T, et al: Injury and repair of articular cartilage: related scientific issues. Oper Tech Orthop 7:270–278, 1997.

Baker's Cyst (Popliteal Cyst)

Burleson RJ, Bickel WH, Dahlin DC: Popliteal cyst: a clinicopathological survey. J Bone Joint Surg 38A:1265–1274, 1956.

Bogumill GP, Bruno PD, Barrick EF: Malignant lesions masquerading as popliteal cysts: a report of three cases. J Bone Joint Surg 63A:474–477, 1981.

Curl WW. Popliteal cysts: historical background and current knowledge. J Am Acad Orthop Surg 4:129–133, 1996.

Dinham JM: Popliteal cysts in children: the case against surgery. J Bone Joint Surg 57B:69–71, 1975.

Fielding JR, Franklin PD, Kustan J: Popliteal cysts: a reassessment using magnetic resonance imaging. Skeletal Radiol 20(6):433–435, 1991.

Hermann G, Yeh HC, Lehr-Janus C, et al: Diagnosis of popliteal cyst: double-contrast arthrography and sonography. AJR Am J Roentgenol 137:369–372, 1981.

Hughston JC, Baker CL, Mello W: Popliteal cyst: a surgical approach. Orthopedics 14:147–150, 1991.

Janzen DL, Peterfy CG, Forbes JR, et al: Cystic lesions around the knee joint: MR imaging findings. AJR Am J Roentgenol 163:155–161, 1994.

Jayson MI, Dixon AS, Kates A, Pinder I, Coomes EH: Popliteal and calf cysts in rheumatoid arthritis. Treatment by anterior synovectomy. Ann Rheum Dis 31(1):9–15, 1972.

Katz RS, Zizic TM, Arnold WP, et al: The pseudothrombophlebitis syndrome. Medicine 56:151–164, 1977.

Lantz B, Singer KM: Meniscal cysts. Clin Sports Med 9:707–725, 1990.

Lindgren PG, Willen R: Gastrocnemio-semembranosus bursa and its relation to the knee joint. I. Anatomy and histology. Acta Radiol Diagn (Stockh) 18(5):497–512, 1977.

Rauschning W: Popliteal cysts (Baker's cysts) in adults II. Acta Orthop Scand 51(3):547–55, 1980.

Taylor AR, Rana NA: A valve. An explanation of the formation of popliteal cysts. Ann Rheum Dis 32(5):419–21, 1973.

Patella Fractures

Bostrom A: Fracture of the patella. A study of 422 patella fractures. Acta Orthop Scand Suppl. 143:1–80, 1972.

Houghton GR, Ackroyd CE: Sleeve fractures of the patella in children: a report of three cases. J Bone Joint Surg Br 61B(2):165–8, 1979.

Chapter 5

Foot and Ankle Injuries

Ken Stephenson, MD, Charles L. Saltzman, MD,
and S. Brent Brotzman, MD

Ankle Sprains

Ken Stephenson, MD

Ankle sprains make up about 15% of all athletic injuries, with a reported 23,000 ankle ligament injuries occurring each day in the United States. They are particularly common in basketball, volleyball, soccer, modern dance, and ballet. Most patients fully recover, but an estimated 20 to 40% develop chronic symptoms of pain and instability.

Relevant Anatomy

The stability of any joint depends on the inherent constraints provided by the bony configuration and the active and passive soft tissue restraints. The ankle joint is quite stable in the neutral position because the wider anterior portion of the talus fits snugly into the ankle mortise. Plantar flexion of the ankle rotates the narrower posterior talus into the mortise, resulting in a much looser fit, with a particular tendency toward inversion. Active soft tissue restraint depends on the muscle-tendon units involved in movement and support of the joint. The talus, however, has no tendinous insertions and must rely in an indirect way on the muscular actions on other bones adjacent to the ankle joint. Passive support of the ankle is provided by the medial, lateral, and posterior ligaments and the syndesmosis. The lateral ankle ligament complex is the structure most commonly involved in ankle sprains.

The three main components of the lateral ligament complex are the anterior talofibular ligament (ATFL), the calcaneofibular ligament (CFL), and the posterior talofibular ligament (PTFL) (Fig. 5–1). The ATFL is relaxed in neutral and taut in plantar flexion. It is the primary restraint against inversion while the foot is plantar flexed. The CFL is also relaxed in neutral, but it is taut in dorsiflexion.

The **most common ankle injury** involves an isolated tear of the ATFL, followed by a combined tear of the

Figure 5–1. A, Ankle stability is provided by the peroneus longus and brevis tendons on the posterolateral side and by the tibialis posterior, flexor digitorum longus, and flexor hallucis longus on the medial side. When the foot is plantar flexed, the anterior talofibular ligament (ATFL) tightens and is more likely to become injured that the calcaneofibular (CFL) and posterior talofibular (PTFL) ligaments. The growth plate in children is particularly vulnerable to fracture because it is weaker than the surrounding ligaments, bone, and periosteum. B, Structures crossing the medial ankle anteriorly include the tibialis anterior tendon and the saphenous vein and nerve. Behind the medial malleolus lie the important tibialis posterior, flexor digitorum longus, posterior tibial artery and veins, tibial nerve, and the posteriorly located flexor hallucis longus.

C

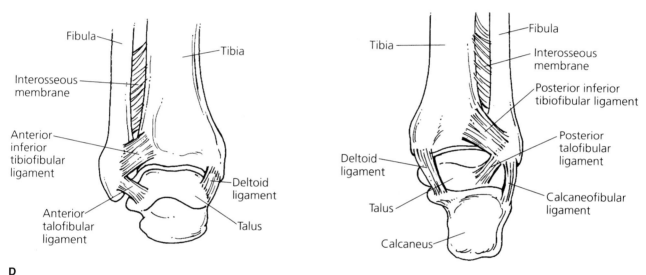

D

Figure 5–1 *Continued. C,* Lateral view of the ankle shows its chief musculotendinous and ligamentous stabilizers. *D,* Anterior *(left)* and posterior *(right)* views of the syndesmotic ligaments. The interosseous ligament is deep to the anterior inferior and posterior inferior tibiofibular ligament. Syndesmotic sprains are usually produced by high-impact external or internal rotational forces. Low-grade syndesmotic injury can occur alone or in conjunction with other ligamentous injury of the ankle or foot. Severe syndesmotic sprain can cause ankle mortise destabilization that is usually accompanied by fracture. (*A,* From Ganley TJ, Flynn JM, Pill SG, Hanlon PA: Ankle injury in the young athlete: fracture or sprain? J Musculoskel Med 17:311–325, 2000. Artist: C. Jones; *C,* from Trojian TH, McKeag DB: Ankle sprains: expedient assessment and management. Physician Sports Med 26[10]:29–40, 1998; *D,* from Veenema KR: Ankle sprain: primary care evaluation and rehabilitation. J Musculoskel Med 17:563–576, 2000. Artist: Robert Marguiles.)

ATFL and the CFL. The mechanism of injury is usually inversion of the plantar flexed foot (Fig. 5–2).

Classification of Lateral Collateral Ligament Sprains

A **grade 1,** or mild ankle sprain, is a stretch of the ligament with no macroscopic tear, little swelling or tender-

ness, minimal or no functional impairment, and no joint instability. A **grade 2,** or moderate ankle sprain, involves a partial tear of the ligament with moderate swelling and tenderness, some loss of joint function, and mild joint instability. A **grade 3,** or severe sprain, involves a complete tear of the ligaments (ATFL and CFL) with severe swelling, ecchymosis and tenderness, inability to bear weight on the extremity, and mechanical joint instability (Fig. 5–3).

Figure 5–2. The most typical injury mechanism in ankle sprain: plantar flexion, inversion, and adduction. The ATFL is most commonly torn in a plantar flexion inversion mechanism. (From Lane SE: Severe ankle sprains. Physician Sports Med 19[11]:43–51, 1990.)

Diagnosis

An inversion injury is commonly associated with a tearing sensation or a pop felt by the patient over the lateral ankle. Swelling can be immediate in grades 2 and 3 sprains, and the initial intense pain subsides after a few hours, only to return more intensely as the hemorrhage continues 6 to 12 hours after the injury.

Figure 5–3. Grade 3 ankle sprain. Note the significant ecchymosis and swelling associated with a grade 3 injury. (From Lane SE: Severe ankle sprains. Physician Sports Med 18[11]:43–51, 1990.)

Physical Examination

Physical examination reveals mild swelling in grade 1 sprains and moderate to severe swelling in a diffuse pattern in grades 2 and 3 sprains. Tenderness is usually elicited at the anterior edge of the fibula with ATFL injuries and at the tip of the fibula with CFL injuries. The region of the syndesmosis and the base of the fifth metatarsal should also be palpated to rule out injuries to these structures.

The **anterior drawer test** and the **talar tilt test** are commonly used to identify signs of joint instability (Fig. 5–4A and B). The anterior drawer test is performed by stabilizing the distal tibia anteriorly with one hand and pulling the slightly plantar flexed foot forward with the other hand from behind the heel. A positive finding of more than 5 mm of anterior translation indicates a tear of the ATFL. The talar tilt test is performed by stabilizing the distal tibia with one hand and inverting the talus and calcaneus as a unit with the other hand. A positive finding of more than 5 mm with a soft endpoint indicates a combined injury to the ATFL and CFL (see Fig. 5–4C). It is important to always compare the affected ankle with the contralateral side because some patients are naturally very flexible (generalized ligamentous laxity), and this could result in a false-positive test.

Examination of the Ankle after an Inversion Injury

Palpation of the lateral collaterals (ATFL and CFL)

Medial palpation of the deltoid ligament

Palpation of the proximal fibula close to the knee to rule out a Maisonneuve fracture (tearing of the interosseous membrane and proximal fibula fracture)

Squeeze test to rule out ankle syndesmosis tearing with resultant ankle mortise instability (Fig. 5–5A)

External rotation (Cotton) test (see Fig. 5–5B and C) to test for syndesmosis injury

Palpation of the proximal (base) fifth metatarsal to rule out avulsion fracture from peroneus brevis pull

Anterior drawer and inversion (talar tilt) stress testing

Motor testing of posterior tibial (inversion) and peroneal (eversion) tendons

---

Syndesmosis Injury

Disruption of the syndesmosis ligament complex (tibiofibular ligaments and interosseous membrane) may occur in as many as 10% of all ankle ligament injuries (Fig. 5–6). The examiner should always test for this injury (see squeeze test and external rotation test, p. 377). Rupture of the syndesmosis is often associated with deltoid (medial) ligament rupture, and concomitant fracture of the fibula is common (see ankle fracture section). The

Figure 5–4. *A, Left,* Test for ligamentous instability with the **anterior drawer test.** Grasp the patient's foot at the heel and pull forward while maintaining the tibia in a fixed position with the other hand at the anterior distal tibia. Translation greater than 3 mm or difference in anterior translation from the asymptomatic ankle suggests a tear of the ATFL. *Right,* Excessive anteroposterior (AP) translation of the tibia on the talus during the anterior drawer test indicates that the patient has injury to the ATFL.

mechanism may be pronation and eversion of the foot combined with internal rotation of the tibia on a fixed foot, such as occurs in football players who have an external rotation force applied to the foot (stepped on) while lying prone on the field.

Point tenderness and pain are located primarily on the anterior aspect of the syndesmosis (not over the lateral collaterals as with an ankle sprain), and the patient is usually unable to bear weight. These injuries are typically more severe than ankle sprains, with more pain, swelling, and difficulty in weight-bearing. Stress radiographs taken with the ankle in external rotation (in both dorsiflexion and plantar flexion) often display the diastasis (gap) between the tibia and the fibula. Bone scanning is useful if the diagnosis is suspected but hard to confirm.

Partial isolated syndesmosis tears are typically treated nonoperatively in a removable cast for 6 to 8 weeks (partial weight-bearing with crutches). With complete syndesmosis rupture, the fibula may shorten and externally rotate. A complete tear is treated by suture of the ligament

and temporary fixation of the tibia and fibula with a syndesmosis screw. The syndesmosis screw must be placed with the ankle dorsiflexed to neutral (the widest portion of the talus) to avoid postoperative limited dorsiflexion. A walking boot is used (touch-down weight-bearing) for 6 to 8 weeks postoperative. Early active and passive motion out of the boot is encouraged from day 7, and full weight-bearing is allowed at 6 weeks. An aggressive rehabilitation program stressing vigorous range of motion (ROM), strengthening, and proprioception exercises is undertaken (see ankle sprain rehabilitation protocol, p. 381). The patient should be informed about the longer recovery compared with ankle sprains and the potential for pain and late sequelae, such as heterotopic ossification.

Factors crucial for a good outcome after syndesmosis injuries are recognition of the injury and obtaining and maintaining an anatomic reduction of the ankle mortise and the distal lower extremity syndesmosis. Syndesmosis fixation is usually indicated to avoid the more catastrophic complications of mortise widening and joint incongruity (e.g., early post-traumatic arthritis).

B

C

Figure 5–4 *Continued. B,* **Talar tilt test (inversion stress test).** This tests the integrity of the CFL. This test may be performed with a commercial jig or leaded hands under radiographs. Invert the foot while stabilizing the tibia with one hand and the subtalar joint with the other. *C, Left,* AP view of the ankle prestress. *Right,* AP view of the ankle with inversion stress reveals marked lateral ligament injury. (*A, Left,* From Ganley TJ, Flynn JM, Pill SG, Hanlon PA: Ankle injury in the young athlete: fracture or sprain? J Musculoskel Med 17:311–325, 2000. Artist: Teri J. McDermott; *Right,* from Baker CL, Todd JL: Intervening in acute ankle sprain and chronic instability. J Musculoskel Med 12[7]:51–68, 1995; *B,* from Meisterling RC: Recurrent lateral ankle sprains. Physician Sports Med 21[3]:123–135, 1993; *C,* from Lassiter TE, Malone TR, Garrett WE: Injuries to the lateral ligaments of the ankle. Orthop Clin North Am 20:632, 1989.)

A   B   C

Figure 5–5. *A,* **Squeeze test** is used to evaluate the syndesmotic ligaments of the ankle. It is performed by grasping the anterior of the leg proximally and squeezing the fibula and tibia, thus compressing the interosseous ligaments. If syndesmotic injury exists, the player complains of distal ankle pain at the joint. *B,* **External rotation stress test** is performed with the patient's in neutral position and the knee flexed 90 degrees. Stabilizing the tibia and fibula with one hand, the physician externally rotates the ankle with the other hand. Pain in the syndesmotic area indicates injury to the syndesmosis. *C,* In the **tibiotalar shuck test (Cotton test),** the examiner holds the patient's lower leg with one hand while alternately applying medial and lateral force to the talus with the other. Pain in the syndesmosis or a feeling of looseness (comparison with the normal side may help) indicates syndesmotic ligament injury. (*A,* From Crosby LA, Davick JP: Managing common football injuries on the field. J Musculoskel Med 17:651–669, 2000. Artist: Robin Lazurus Clark; *B* and *C,* from Bassewitz HL, Shapiro MS: Persistent pain after ankle sprain. Physician Sports Med 25[12]:58–67, 1997.)

Radiographic Evaluation

Radiographs are taken to rule out fractures of the medial and lateral malleoli, the talus, and the fifth metatarsal base. Radiographs should include three views of the ankle on long cassettes that include the entire length of the fibula: anteroposterior [AP], lateral, and mortise views (Fig. 5–7A) and three views of the foot (AP, lateral, and oblique) (see Fig. 5–7B–D).

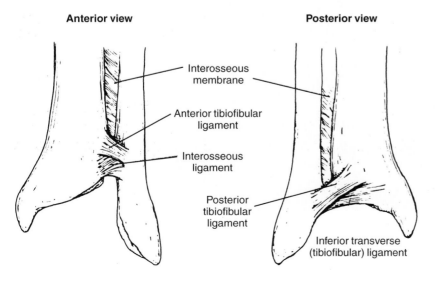

Anterior view   Posterior view

Interosseous membrane

Anterior tibiofibular ligament

Interosseous ligament

Posterior tibiofibular ligament

Inferior transverse (tibiofibular) ligament

Figure 5–6. Components of the distal lower extremity syndesmosis (DLES). The syndesmosis comprises four ligaments and the interosseous membrane. The ligaments are the anterior tibiofibular, posterior tibiofibular, transverse tibiofibular, and interosseous. (From Wuest TK: Injuries to the distal lower extremity syndemosis. © 1997 American Academy of Orthopaedic Surgeons. Reprinted from the Journal of the American Academy of Orthopaedic Surgeons, vol. 5[3]: pp. 172–181 with permission.)

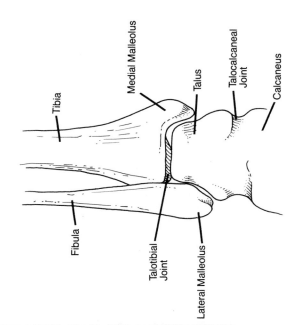

Tibia

Medial Malleolus

Talus

Talocalcaneal Joint

Calcaneus

Fibula

Talotibial Joint

Lateral Malleolus

A

Phalanges

Sesamoids

Metatarsals

Bases of Metatarsals

Lateral Cuneiform
Middle Cuneiform
Medial Cuneiform
Navicular
Talonavicular Joint

Talus

Metatarsal Heads

Base of Fifth Metatarsal

Cuboid

Calcaneocuboid Joint

Calcaneus

Figure 5–7. *A,* AP views of the ankle. *Left,* Radiograph illustrates the relationships of the ankle joint including the medial mortise. *Right,* Anatomic drawing for correlation. Typically, three views of the ankle are taken (AP, lateral, and mortise). *B,* AP projections of the foot. *Left,* Perpendicular x-ray beam demonstrates the forefoot anatomy, particularly the phalanges and MTP joints. Note the distal third and fourth metatarsal fractures. *Center,* Angled x-ray beam provides improved detail of the midfoot anatomy, particularly illustrating the normal alignment of the lateral border of the first MTP joint and the medial border of the second MTP joint. *Right,* Anatomic drawing for correlation.

B

Figure 5–7 *Continued. C,* Lateral projection of the foot. *Top,* Radiograph illustrates the anatomic relationships of the midfoot and hindfoot. *Bottom,* Anatomic drawing for correlation. *D,* Medial oblique projection of the foot. *Top,* Radiograph demonstrates the normal medial border alignment of the third and fourth MTP joints. It also allows evaluation of the talonavicular and calcaneocuboid relationships. *Bottom,* Anatomic drawing for correlation. (*A–D,* From Mann R, Coughlin M: Surgery of the Foot and Ankle. Philadelphia, Mosby, 1997).

Stress radiographs can be used to quantify instability during the anterior drawer and talar tilt stress tests. Anterior taluar subluxation of more than 10 mm or more than 5 mm difference from the contralateral ankle indicates a positive anterior drawer stress test. Talar tilt of 15 degrees or 10 degrees difference from the contralateral ankle indicates a positive talar tilt test.

Treatment for Lateral Collateral Sprains

The current literature supports functional rehabilitation as the preferred method of treatment for ankle sprains, allowing an earlier return to work and physical activity without a higher rate of late symptoms (ankle instability, pain, stiffness, or muscle weakness) when compared with cast immobilization.

Immediately after injury in the **acute phase,** the PRICE (protection, rest, ice, compression, and elevation) principle is followed (see rehabilitation protocol). The goal is to reduce hemorrhage, swelling, inflammation, and pain. A period of immobilization is initiated, depending on the severity of the injury. Some authors stress the importance of immobilizing the ankle in neutral rather than in plantar flexion because the ATFL is stretched out during plantar flexion. For grades 1 and 2 sprains, an ankle brace (Fig. 5–8) is used for immobilization. For grade 3 sprains, a removable cast boot offers more stability and protection and allows earlier weight-bearing with less pain. Immobilization is continued for several days in mild sprains and up to 3 weeks in severe grade 3 sprains. As grade 3 sprains improve, the cast boot is replaced with an ankle brace.

In the **subacute phase,** goals include continued reduction of swelling, inflammation, and pain, while some

Standard
ankle brace

Figure 5–8. Aircast ankle brace (1-800-526-8785). (From DeLee JC, Drez D Jr: Orthopaedic Sports Medicine: Principles and Practice. Philadelphia, WB Saunders, 1994.)

motion, strengthening, and appropriate controlled weight-bearing are started. This is the period of collagen fiber proliferation, and too much stress on the ligaments at this point could result in weaker tissue.

The **rehabilitative phase** focuses on improving strength, endurance, balance, and weight-bearing proprioception. During this maturation phase of the healing ligament, about 3 weeks after the injury, controlled stretching of the muscles and movement of the joint promote a more normal orientation of the collagen fibers parallel with the stress lines. Repeated exercise during this phase has been shown to increase the mechanical and structural strength of the ligaments.

Rehabilitation Protocol
After Ankle Sprains (Lateral Collateral Ligaments)
Stephenson

Phase 1: Acute Phase

Timing
- Grade 1 sprain: 1–3 days.
- Grade 2 sprain: 2–4 days.
- Grade 3 sprain: 3–7 days.

Goals
- Decrease swelling.
- Decrease pain.
- Protect from reinjury.
- Maintain appropriate weight-bearing status.

Protection Options
- Taping.
- Functional bracing.
- Removable cast boot (some grade 2 and most grade 3 sprains).
- Rest (crutches to promote ambulation without gait deviation).

continued

Rehabilitation Protocol
After Ankle Sprains (Lateral Collateral Ligaments) *(Continued)*
Stephenson

Ice
- Cryocuff ice machine.
- Ice bags.
- Ice with other modalities (interferential [Fig. 5–9A], high-voltage galvanic stimulation, ultrasound).

Light Compression
- Elastic (Ace) wrap.
- TED hose.
- Vasopneumatic pump.

Elevation
- Above the heart (combined with ankle pumps).

Phase 2: Subacute Phase
Timing
- Grade 1 sprain: 2–4 days.
- Grade 2 sprain: 3–5 days.
- Grade 3 sprain: 4–8 days.

Goals
- Decrease swelling.
- Decrease pain.
- Increase pain-free ROM.
- Begin strengthening.
- Begin non–weight-bearing proprioceptive training.
- Provide protective support as needed.

A

B

C

Figure 5–9. *A,* Interferential electrical stimulation. *B,* Aqua ankle. Ankle resistance training is performed with this device in a cold whirlpool, then eventually warm water (1-877-272-2376 or www.kineticinnovations.com). *C,* Isometric strengthening. Eversion against a fixed object (wall) with a pillow as a cushion.

Rehabilitation Protocol
After Ankle Sprains (Lateral Collateral Ligaments) *(Continued)*
Stephenson

Modalities to Decrease Pain and Swelling
- Ice or contrast baths.
- Electrical stimulation (high-voltage galvanic or interferential).
- Ultrasound.
- Cross-friction massage (gently).
- Soft orthotics with $1/8$- to $3/16$-inch lateral wedge if needed.

Weight-bearing
- Progress weight-bearing as symptoms permit.
- Partial weight-bearing to full weight-bearing if no signs of antalgic gait are present.

Therapeutic Exercises
- Active ROM exercises
  - Dorsiflexion
  - Inversion
  - Foot circles
  - Plantar flexion
  - Eversion
  - Alphabet
  - Use of Aqua Ankle in cold water for gentle strengthening and ROM (see Fig. 5–9B).
- Strength exercises
  - Isometric in pain-free range (see Fig. 5–9C).
  - Toe curls with towel (place weight on towel to increase resistance).
  - Pick up objects with toes (tissue, marbles).
- Proprioceptive training
  - Seated Biomechanical Ankle Platform System (BAPS board) (Fig. 5–10).
  - Wobble board.
  - Ankle disc.
- Stretching
  - Passive ROM—only dorsiflexion and plantar flexion in pain-free range, *not* eversion or inversion.
  - Achilles stretch (gentle).
  - Joint mobilizations (grades 1–2 for dorsiflexion/plantar flexion).

Phase 3: Rehabilitative Phase

Timing
- Grade 1 sprain: 1 wk.
- Grade 2 sprain: 2 wk.
- Grade 3 sprain: 3 wk.

Goals
- Increase pain-free ROM.
- Progress strengthening.
- Progress proprioceptive training.
- Increase pain-free activities of daily living.
- Pain-free full weight-bearing and uncompensated gait.

Figure 5–10. Patients can perform balancing exercises on a circular tilt board to improve proprioception, sitting or standing. (From Meisterling RC: Recurrent lateral ankle sprains. Physician Sports Med 21[5]:123–132, 1993.)

Therapeutic Exercises
- Stretching
  - Gastrocnemius and soleus with increased intensity.
  - Joint mobilization (grades 1, 2, and 3 for dorsiflexion, plantar flexion, and eversion; hold inversion).
- Strengthening
  - Weight-bearing exercises
    - Heel raises (see Fig. 5–11A).
    - Toe raises (see Fig. 5–11B).
    - Stair steps.
    - Quarter squats.
  - Eccentric/concentric and isotonics (Theraband and cuff weights)
    - Inversion (Fig. 5–12A).
    - Eversion (see Fig. 5–12B).
    - Plantar flexion (see Fig. 5–12C).
    - Dorsiflexion (see Fig. 5–12D).
    - Peroneal strengthening.
  - Isokinetics.

continued

Rehabilitation Protocol
After Ankle Sprains (Lateral Collateral Ligaments) *(Continued)*
Stephenson

A

B

Figure 5–11. *A,* Standing heel raises. The raises are done with the foot in neutral position *(i),* inversion *(ii),* and eversion *(iii). B,* Toe raise. (*A,* From Kovan JR, McKeag DB: Lower extremity overuse injuries in aerobic dancers. J Musculoskel Med 9[4]:33–46, 1992. Artist: Gwenn Alton-Bird.)

A

B

C

D

Figure 5–12. *A,* Inversion against Thera-band. *B,* Eversion against Thera-band. This is probably the most important of the Thera-band exercises. *C,* Plantar flexion against Thera-band. *D,* Dorsiflexion against Thera-band.

continued

Rehabilitation Protocol
After Ankle Sprains (Lateral Collateral Ligaments) *(Continued)*
Stephenson

A   B   C

Figure 5–13. *A,* Single-leg balance. *B,* Single-leg balance on trampoline. *C,* Single-leg balance with distraction.

- Proprioceptive training (progress from non–weight-bearing/controlled weight-bearing stage to full weight-bearing
  - Standing BAPS board.
  - Standing wobble board.
  - KAT system.
  - Single-leg balance activities (stable to unstable surfaces, without to with distractions) (Fig. 5–13).
- Continue modalities as needed, specifically after exercises to preven recurrence of pain and swelling.
- Supportive taping, bracing, and orthotics used as needed. Typically, we finish the athletic season with supportive bracing in an effort to avoid reinjury.

Phase 4: Return to Activity or Functional Phase
Timing
- Grade 1 sprain: 1–2 wk.
- Grade 2 sprain: 2–3 wk.
- Grade 3 sprain: 3–6 wk.

Goals
- Regain full strength.
- Normal biomechanics.

- Return to participation.
- Protection and strengthening of any mild residual joint instability.

Therapeutic Exercises
- Continue progression of ROM and strengthening exercises.
- Sport-specific strengthening and training are imperative.

Running progression
- Unloaded jogging on ZUNI (Fig. 5–14).
- Unloaded running on ZUNI.
- Alternate jog-walk-jog on smooth, straight surfaces.
- Alternate sprint-jog-sprint on smooth, straight surfaces.
- Figure-of-eights.
- Zig-zag cutting.
- Agility drills
  - Back pedaling.
  - Side stepping.
  - Carioca.
- Plyometrics specific to each sport.

Rehabilitation Protocol
After Ankle Sprains (Lateral Collateral Ligaments) *(Continued)*
Stephenson

Figure 5–14. Unloaded jogging.

- Progress weight-bearing multidirectional balance exercises and movement activities (Fig. 5–15).

Return to Competition
- When above skills are accomplished at full speed, athlete may return to practice.
- When full practice is tolerated, competition can be resumed.

- Some type of ankle support is recommended for the first several months. We typically use a low-profile Aircast or the Bledsoe Ultimate Ankle Brace.

Phase 5: Prophylactic Phase

Goal
- Prevent injury.

Therapeutic Exercises
- Functional drills.
- Multidirectional balance board activities.
- Prophylactic strengthening (emphasis on peroneal eversion).
- Prophylactive protective support as needed.

Figure 5–15. Use of a slide board.

Prevention of Ankle Sprains

Proper strengthening and rehabilitation are critical to help prevent inversion ankle injuries; however, some patients require additional biomechanical support. We routinely use ankle braces in athletes prone to ankle injuries in high-risk sports like basketball and volleyball. We prefer a lace-up brace with figure-of-eight straps or a functional stirrup brace that is placed beneath the insole of the shoe. The Ultimate Ankle Brace (Bledsoe Brace Company) effectively limits inversion injuries, but still allows the ankle to dorsiflex and plantar flex. However, some athletes, such as ballet dancers, may not be able to perform in a brace, which limits its usefulness in some sports. Another effective means of preventing inversion injuries is to apply a slight lateral flare to the sole of the tennis shoe or a lateral wedge to an insole. This, again, is effective only in certain sports in which a tennis shoe is worn.

Ankle taping may be of some benefit, but much of the strength is lost with loosening of the tape within the first 10 minutes. We use a closed basketweave technique (Fig. 5–16).

1. Have the seated athlete position the ankle at 90 degrees *(A)*.
2. Spray a tape adherent (e.g., Tuf-Skin, QDA) over the area to be taped.
3. Apply a heel and lace pad with skin lubricant on the anterior and posterior aspects of the ankle *(B)*.

A

B

4. Apply pre-wrap, starting at the midfoot and continuing up the leg, overlapping by half until approximately 5–6 inches above the medial malleolus *(C)*.
5. Apply an anchor strip at the proximal (#1) and distal (#2) ends of the pre-wrap with half of the tape covering the pre-wrap and the other half adhering to the skin *(D)*.

C

D

6. Starting posteromedially on the proximal anchor, apply a stirrup covering the posterior third of the medial malleolus and then under the foot and up the lateral side to the proximal anchor (#3) *(Ei and ii)*.

Ei

Eii

7. Starting at the distal anchor (#4), apply a horseshoe around the heel (approximately 2 inches from the plantar surface) to the other side of the distal anchor *(F)*.
8. Repeat steps 6 and 7 twice. Each time, overlap the previous strip by half the width of the tape *(G)*.

F

G

Figure 5–16. Ankle taping for ankle sprains. (Mark Bohling, AT-C.)

9. To apply a figure-of-8, start medially (*Hi*) at the position of the first stirrup (#5), pull the tape at an angle toward the medial longitudinal arch (approximately where the third stirrup goes under the foot), under the foot, across the anterior aspect of the ankle, and around the ankle (just above the third horseshoe strip) (*Hii*).

Hi

Hii

10. Close up the tape by applying single strips of tape around the leg, overlapping by half until the area from the ankle to the proximal anchor is covered (#6) (*I*).

I

11. To apply a heel lock, start at the anterior aspect of the proximal anchor laterally. Pull the tape at an angle (arrows) toward the posterior aspect of the lateral malleolus, around the posterior aspect of the ankle, under the heel, up the lateral side of the foot, and across the anterior aspect of the ankle (*Ji–iii*). To continue and apply a continuous double-heel lock, make one complete loop around the ankle (#7), continue around the ankle, then down around the posterior aspect of the ankle, under the heel, and up the medial side of the foot (*K*), across the anterior aspect of the ankle, and complete with another full loop around the ankle.

Ji

Jii

Jiii

K

Li   Lii

Liii   Liv

Lv

12. Apply one or two closure strips (dark tape) around the foot (#8) to hold the horseshoes down to the foot and the anchor strip *(Li–v)*.

Chronic Lateral Ankle Instability: Rehabilitation after Lateral Ankle Ligament Reconstruction

Mark Colville MD, and Ken Stephenson, MD

It is estimated that 20 to 40% of patients with ankle sprains develop long-term sequelae such as pain, swelling, or instability. Interestingly, the severity of the ankle sprain does not seem to correlate with the development of chronic symptoms. If a patient has received appropriate treatment for an ankle sprain and has completed a rehabilitation program but continues to have significant symptoms, another etiology of the symptoms must be sought. Etiologies to be considered in patients with chronic ankle pain include occult bony injuries such as fractures, osteochondral defects, or bone contusions; cartilage damage; ankle, subtalar, or syndesmosis instability secondary to ligament rupture; tendon pathology such as a peroneal tendon or posterior tibial tendon longitudinal tear; a neuropraxia of the superficial peroneal or sural nerves; or soft tissue problems such as anterolateral ankle soft tissue impingement.

Possible Etiologies of Chronic Ankle Pain

Chronic ankle ligament instability (instability with minor provocation, such as stepping off a curb)

Reflex sympathetic dystrophy (RSD) (see Chapter 8)

Undetected syndesmotic sprain or diastasis (see p. 374)

Undetected tear of the deltoid ligament (medially)

Stress fracture

Posterior tibial tendon (PTT) injury

Osteochondral fracture or osteochondritis dissecans (OCD) of the talus or tibial plafond

Os trigonum fracture (posterior pain, clicking, positive x-ray)

Subtalar joint sprain or instability

Tibiotalar synostosis (ossification of the syndesmosis impairing normal tibiofibular motion with restricted dorsiflexion on examination)

Midfoot sprain of the transverse tarsal (midtarsal), intertarsal, or tarsometatarsal joints

Bony impingement from osteophytes off the anterior tibia, with soft tissues trapped between the spur and the talus during dorsiflexion

Ankle arthrosis

Undetected fractures

- Lateral, medial, or posterior malleolus
- Posterior or lateral process of the talus
- Anterior process of the calcaneus
- Fifth metatarsal
- Navicular or other midtarsal bone

Nerve injuries

- Superficial peroneal nerve stretch after ankle sprain
- Common peroneal nerve entrapment
- Tarsal tunnel syndrome (entrapment of the posterior tibial nerve)

Tumor

Radiographic Examination

If the patient has a history or examination consistent with instability, stress radiographs (talar tilt and anterior drawer) are indicated. Although there is some controversy in the literature regarding normal values for stress radiographs, in general, a *positive talar tilt* is more than 15 degrees or more than 10 degrees difference from the contralateral side. A *positive anterior drawer* is 5 to 10 mm anterior subluxation of the talus or more than 5 mm difference from the contralateral side. MRI is useful for delineating bone contusions, avascular necrosis, osteochondral defects, and tendon or ligament injuries. The diagnosis of chronic lateral ankle ligament instability is based on a history of multiple inversion ankle sprains, often with fairly minor provocation (such as stepping off a curb). Instability, not pain alone, should be the primary criterion for ligament reconstruction.

Ankle Ligament Reconstruction

Numerous surgical procedures have been described for lateral ankle instability, but the most commonly used is the modified Brostrom procedure. This involves an anatomic repair of the ATFL and CFL augmented by suture of the superior edge of the inferior peroneal retinaculum to the anterior edge of the fibula. This procedure is particularly indicated in ballet dancers or patients whose livelihood depends on a full ROM and in most patients undergoing reconstruction for the first time. It is not the procedure of choice for revision surgery or patients with generalized ligamentous laxity or a connective tissue disorder. The use of the peroneus brevis tendon to augment the repair is indicated for revision surgery. The Watson-Jones, Chrisman-Snook, and Evans procedures have good success rates (80 to 85%) but each limits subtalar and ankle motion.

The goal of ankle ligament reconstruction in an unstable ankle is to restore stability while preserving normal ankle and subtalar motion whenever possible. Most patients with chronic instability have laxity of the ATFL and CFL and increased subtalar joint motion.

General Principles of Rehabilitation after Ankle Ligament Reconstruction

Postoperatively, a short-leg, well-padded splint is applied with the ankle in slight eversion, and the patient remains non–weight-bearing. One to 2 weeks after surgery, the patient is placed into a removable cast boot or short-leg walking cast with the foot in neutral position and is allowed to begin partial weight-bearing, progressing to full weight-bearing as tolerated. Four weeks postoperative, the patient is placed into a functional brace or removable cast boot, and active rehabilitation is started with gentle ROM exercises and isometric strengthening exercises. Usually at 6 weeks, proprioception and balancing exercises are started. In athletes, sport-specific exercises are started at about 8 weeks postoperative. Return to sports or dancing is allowed when peroneal strength is normal and the patient is able to perform multiple single-leg hops on the injured side without pain. A lace-up brace (such as the Rocket Sock) or functional stirrup brace should be worn for at least the first season, and most athletes prefer bracing or taping for sports indefinitely.

Rehabilitation Protocol
After Modified Brostrom Ankle Ligament Reconstruction
Modified Hamilton Protocol

Days 0–4

- Place ankle in anterior-posterior plaster splints in neutral dorsiflexion and discharge patient as non–weight-bearing.

Days 4–7

- When swelling has subsided, apply a short-leg walking cast with the ankle in neutral.
- Allow weight-bearing as tolerated in cast.

Week 4

- Remove cast.
- Apply air splint for protection, to be worn for 6–8 wk after surgery.
- Begin gentle ROM exercises of the ankle.
- Begin isometric peroneal strengthening exercises.
- Avoid adduction and inversion until 6 wk postoperative.
- Begin swimming.

Week 6

- Begin proprioception/balancing activities
  - Unilateral balancing for timed intervals.
  - Unilateral balancing with visual cues.

- Balancing on one leg and catching #2 plyoball.
- Slide board, increasing distance.
- Fitter activity, catching ball.
- Side-to-side bilateral hopping (progress to unilateral).
- Front-to-back bilateral hopping (progress to unilateral).
- Diagonal patterns, hopping.
- Mini-tramp jogging.
- Shuttle leg press and rebounding, bilateral and unilateral.
- Positive deceleration, ankle everters, Kin-Com.
- Complete rehabilitation of the peroneals is essential.
- Dancers should perform peroneal exercises in full plantar flexion, the position of function in these athletes (Fig. 5–17A).
- Early in rehabilitation, pool exercises may be beneficial (see Fig. 5–17B).
- Dancers should perform plantar flexion/eversion exercises with a weighted belt (2–20 pounds).

Weeks 8–12

- Patient can return to dancing or sport if peroneal strength is normal.

Figure 5–17. *A,* In plantar flexion, the ATFL is vertically oriented and is particularly vulnerable to inversion forces. Plantar flexion is the position of function for ballet dancers. *B,* During rehabilitation, barré exercises may also be performed in a pool, taking advantage of the buoyancy of the water. (*A* and *B,* From Malone T: Rehabilitation of the foot and ankle injuries in ballet dancers. J Orthop Sports Phys Ther 11:8, 1990.)

Inferior Heel Pain (Plantar Fasciitis)

S. Brent Brotzman, MD

Clinical Background

Heel pain is best classified by anatomic location (see box following). This section discusses *plantar fasciitis* (inferior heel pain). Posterior heel pain is discussed in the section on Achilles tendinitis.

Differential Diagnosis of Heel Pain

Plantar (Inferior) Signs and Symptoms

Plantar fasciitis/plantar fascia rupture/partial plantar fascia rupture

Calcaneal spur or heel spur (misnomer)

Fat pad syndrome

Calcaneal periostitis

Compression of the nerve to the abductor digiti quinti (rare)

Calcaneal apophysitis (skeletally immature patients), called Sever's disease

Medial

PTT disorders (insuffiency, tenosynovitis, or rupture)

Tarsal tunnel syndrome

Jogger's foot (medial plantar neuropraxia)

Medial calcaneal neuritis (very rare)

Lateral

Peroneal tendon disorders (tendinitis, rupture)

Lateral calcaneal nerve neuritis

Posterior

Retrocalcaneal bursitis

Haglund's deformity (pump bump)

Calcaneal exostosis

Tendinoachilles tendinitis/tendinosis/partial rupture/complete rupture

Diffuse

Calcaneal stress fracture

Calcaneal fracture

Other

Systemic disorders (often bilateral heel pain present)

Reiter's syndrome

Ankylosing spondylitis

Lupus

Gouty arthropathy

Pseudogout (chondrocalcinosis)

Rheumatoid arthritis

Systemic lupus erythematosus

Modified from Doxey GE: Calcaneal pain: a review of various disorders. J Orthop Sports Phys Ther 9:925, 1987.

Anatomy and Pathomechanics

The plantar fascia is a dense, fibrous connective tissue structure originating from the medial tuberosity of the calcaneus (Fig. 5–18). Of its three portions—**medial, lateral,** and **central** bands—the largest is the central portion. The central portion of the fascia originates from the medial process of the calcaneal tuberosity superficial to the origin of the flexor digitorum brevis, quadratus plantae, and abductor hallicus muscle. The fascia extends through the medial longitudinal arch into individual bundles and inserts into each proximal phalanx.

The medial calcaneal nerve supplies sensation to the medial heel. The nerve to the abductor digiti minimi may **rarely** be compressed by the intrinsic muscles of the foot. Some studies, such as those by Baxter and Thigpen (1984), suggest that nerve entrapment (abductor digiti quinti) does on rare occasions play a role in inferior heel pain (Fig. 5–19).

The plantar fascia is an important static support for the longitudinal arch of the foot. Strain on the longitudinal arch exerts its maximal pull on the plantar fascia, especially its origin on the medial process of the calcaneal tuberosity. The plantar fascia elongates with increased loads to act as a shock absorber, but its ability to elongate

Plantar view

Medial plantar fascia

Plantar aponeurosis

Lateral plantar fascia

Plantar aponeurosis

Medial view

Figure 5–18. From its origin at the calcaneal tubercle, the plantar fascia extends distally and attaches to the MTP joints and base of the toes. It is functionally divided into contiguous medial, central, and lateral bands. The fascia covers the intrinsic musculature and neurovascular anatomy of the plantar foot. (From McGarvey WC: Heel pain: front line management of a bottom line problem. J Musculoskel Med 15[4]:14–23, 1998. Artist: Robert Marguiles.)

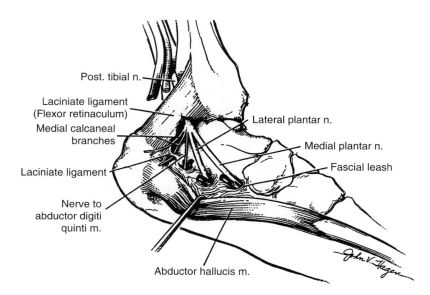

Figure 5-19. Site of entrapment of the posterior tibial nerve and its branches. Note the nerve to the abductor digiti minimi, which on rare occasions may be entrapped with resultant inferior heel burning, neurogenic pain. (From Baxter DE, Thigpen CM: Heel pain: operative results. Foot Ankle Int 5[1]:16.)

is limited (especially with decreasing elasticity common with age). Passive extension of the metatarsophalangeal (MTP) joints pulls the plantar fascia distally and also increases the height of the arch of the foot (Fig. 5-20).

Myth of the Heel Spur

The bony spur at the bottom of the heel does not cause the pain of plantar fasciitis. Rather, this is caused by the inflammation and microtears of the plantar fascia. *The spur is actually the origin of the short flexors of the toes.* Despite this, the misnomer persists in the lay public and the literature.

Heel spurs have been found in approximately 50% of patients with plantar fasciitis. This exceeds the 15% prevalence of radiographically visualized spurs in normal asymptomatic patients noted by Tanz (1963). However, spur formation is related to progression of age. The symptomatic loss of elasticity of the plantar fascia with the onset of middle age suggests that this subset of patients would be expected to show an increased incidence of spurs noted on radiographs.

Figure 5-20. The windlass effect: Dorsiflexion of the MTP joints results in increased arch height. (From Mann RA, Coughlin MJ: Survey of the Foot and Ankle, 6th ed. St. Louis, Mosby, 1993.)

Etiology

Inferior (subcalcaneal) pain may well represent a spectrum of pathologic entities including plantar fasciitis, nerve entrapment of the abductor digiti quinti nerve, periostitis, and subcalcaneal bursitis.

Plantar fasciitis is more common in sports that involve running and long-distance walking and is also frequent in dancers, tennis players, basketball players, and nonathletes whose occupations require prolonged weight-bearing. Direct repetitive microtrauma with heel strike to the ligamentous and nerve structures has been implicated, especially in middle-aged, overweight, nonathletic individuals who stand on hard, unyielding surfaces, as well as in long-distance runners.

Some anatomic features seem to make plantar fasciitis more likely. Campbell and Inman (1974) noted that in patients with *pes planus, heel pronation* increased the tension on the plantar fascia, predisposing the patient to heel pain. Pronation of the subtalar joint everts the calcaneus and lengthens the plantar fascia. A *tight gastrocnemius* (with increased compensatory pronation) also predisposes patients to plantar fasciitis. *Cavus feet* with relative rigidity have been noted to place more stress on the loaded plantar fascia. Several studies have shown an association with plantar fasciitis and *obesity.* However, other researchers have not obtained similar findings.

Bone spurs may be associated with plantar fasciitis, but are not believed to be the cause of it. Many studies show no clear association between spurs and plantar fasciitis. Studies of patients with plantar fasciitis report that 10 to 70% have an associated ipsilateral calcaneal spur; however, most also have a spur on the contralateral asymptomatic foot. Anatomic studies have shown the spur is located at the short flexor origin rather than at the plantar fascia origin, casting further doubt on its role in contributing to heel pain.

Natural History

Although plantar fasciitis can seem quite debilitating during the acute phase, it rarely causes lifelong problems. It is estimated that 90 to 95% of patients who have true plantar fasciitis recover with conservative treatment. However, it may take 6 months to 1 year, and patients often require much encouragement to continue stretching, wearing appropriate and supportive shoes, and avoiding high-impact activities or prolonged standing on hard surfaces. Operative treatment can be very helpful in selected "failed" patients, but the success rate of surgery is only 50 to 85%.

Bilateral Heel Involvement

Bilateral plantar fasciitis symptoms require ruling out systemic disorders such as Reiter's syndrome, ankylosing spondylitis, gouty arthropathy, and systemic lupus erythematosus. A high index of suspicion for a systemic disorder should accompany bilateral heel pain in a young male aged 15 to 35 years.

Causes of Inflammation of the Heel

Inflammation	Secondary Inflammation
Idiopathic	Local inflammatory conditions
	Sprain of the foot
Local factors	Nerve entrapment
Abnormal foot alignment	Medial branch of posterior
Cavus foot (high arch)	tibial nerve (rare)
Planovalgus foot	Nerve to the abductor
Pronated foot (flat foot)	digiti quinti (rare)
Leg-length discrepancy	Bony disorders
Externally rotated	Accessory coalition
lower limb	Tarsal coalition
Increased loading of	Subtalar instability
plantar fascia	Calcaneal periostitis
Tight Achilles tendon	Fracture
Fat pad atrophy	Haglund's deformity
Osteopenia of calcaneus	Subcalcaneal bursitis
Systemic factors	Retrocalcaneal bursitis
Overweight	Systemic inflammatory
Systematic disease	conditions
Inflammatory arthritis	Inflammatory
Gout	arthritis
Sarcoidosis	Gout
Hyperlipoproteinemia	Infection
Training errors	Gonorrhea
Overuse	Tuberculosis
Incorrect training	
Incorrect footware	
Hard surface	
Middle age	

Modified from Noyes FE, Demaio M, Mangine RE: Heel pain. Orthopedics 16:1154, 1993.

Signs and Symptoms

The **classic presentation** of plantar fasciitis includes a gradual, insidious onset of inferomedial heel pain at the insertion of the plantar fascia (Fig. 5–21). Pain and stiffness are **worse with rising in the morning** or after prolonged ambulation and may be exacerbated by climbing stairs or doing toe raises. It is rare for patients with plantar fasciitis not to have pain or stiffness with the first few steps in the morning or after a prolonged rest.

Evaluation of Patients with Inferior Heel Pain

- History and examination
- Biomechanical assessment of foot
  - Pronated or pes planus foot
  - Cavus-type foot (high arch)
  - Assessment of fat pad (signs of atrophy)
  - Presence of tight Achilles tendon
- Squeeze test of calcaneal tuberosity (medial and lateral sides of calcaneus) to evaluate for possible calcaneal stress fracture.
- Evaluation for possible training errors in runners (e.g., rapid mileage increase, running on steep hills, poor running shoes, improper techniques).
- Radiographic assessment with 45-degree oblique view and standard three views of foot.
- Bone scan if recalcitrant pain (>6 wk after treatment initiated) or suspected stress fracture from history.
- Rheumatologic work-up (Table 5–1) for patients with suspected underlying systemic process (patients with bilateral heel pain, recalcitrant symptoms, or associated sacroiliac joint or multiple joint pain).
- Electromyographic (EMG) studies if clinical suspicion of nerve entrapment.
- Establish correct diagnosis and rule out other possible etiologies (Tables 5–2 and 5–3).

Text continues on p. 403

Figure 5–21. Plantar fasciitis pain is inferior, located at the origin of the plantar fascia.

Table 5-1

Rheumatologic Findings for Patients with Suspected Underlying Systemic Process Associated with Heel Pain

	Rheumatoid Arthritis	Reiter's Syndrome	Ankylosing Spondylitis	Hyperlipoproteinemia Type II	Gout
Signs	Retrocalcaneal bursitis, most common Cocking-up of toes Subluxation of metatarsal heads Fibular deviation of toes two to five Swelling of tibiotalar joint Loss of subtalar motion	Plantar fasciitis Acute diffuse swelling of digits Pain at medial calcaneal tuberosity or swelling over Achilles insertion Low back pain	Plantar fasciitis May follow Reiter's syndrome Limited chest expansion Low back pain Painful sacroiliac joints	Plantar nodules and fasciitis Xanthomatous nodules in plantar fascia	Plantar fasciitis Tophi Swelling of ankle Pain Metatarsal pain and swelling
Radiographic signs	Changes at metatarsal and interphalangeal joints of great toe	Enthesopathy Periostitis	Enthesopathy Periostitis Spine x-rays characteristic	Asymmetrical arthritis of small and large joints	Bony erosion Calcific tophi

From Noyes FE, DeMaio M, Mangine RE: Heel pain. Orthopedics 16(10):115, 1993.

Table 5-2

Helpful Findings in Evaluating Etiologies of Heel Pain

Etiology	Findings
Plantar fasciitis	Pain and tenderness located **inferiorly** at the plantar fascia origin (not posteriorly). Almost all patients complain of inferior heel pain in the mornings with the first few steps and may complain of pain after prolonged walking or standing.
Plantar fascia rupture	Typically antecedent plantar fasciitis symptoms, with a pop or "crunch" during push-off or pivoting, then severe pain with subsequent inability to bear weight (or only with difficulty). Most commonly follows iatrogenic weaking of the fascia after cortisone injection.
Calcaneal stress fracture	Much more common in athletes and runners with overuse history and repetitive high-impact activity or osteoporotic elderly females with overuse in their walking or exercise regimen (e.g., 4 miles/day, 7 days/wk). Pain is **more diffuse** than plantar fasciitis, with a **positive squeeze test** (Fig. 5–22) rather than discrete, localized inferior heel pain. Bone scan is positive for linear fracture rather than increased tracer uptake at plantar fascia origin as in plantar fasciitis. Unless a calcaneal stress fracture is suspected, bone scanning is not part of routine work-up (Fig. 5–23).
Sever's disease (calcaneal apophysitis)	Symptoms almost identical to those of plantar fasciitis. Occurs only in skeletally immature patients with inflammation or apophysitis at the physis. Treatment is the same as for plantar fasciitis, except a well-padded UCBL orthotic is used.
Achilles tendinitis or rupture, Haglund's deformity	Pain is **posterior** rather than inferior. Haglund's deformity (pump bump) is tender over prominent bony deformity, and often rubs or is irritated by the heel counter of the shoe. Patients with a complete rupture of the Achilles tendon describe a feeling of being "shot" in the tendon while pushing off, and a positive Thompson squeeze test (see Fig. 5–39), and a lack of active plantar flexion except a small flicker from the long toe flexors.
Posterior tibial tendon (PTT) insufficiency	Pain is **medial** rather than inferior or posterior. Often, difficulty or inability to do a unilateral heel raise (see PTT section). Often, point tender and boggy along course of PTT medially.
Tarsal tunnel syndrome	Pain and numbness or tingling in medial ankle radiating into **plantar** aspect of foot only. No dorsal foot numbness or tingling (consider peripheral neuropathy if dorsal numbness present).

Table 5–2 (*Continued*)

Helpful Findings in Evaluating Etiologies of Heel Pain

Etiology	Findings
	Positive Tinel sign medially in tarsal tunnel. Electromyography is 90% accurate for identifying well-established tarsal tunnel syndrome.
	Decreased sensation in distribution of the medial plantar or lateral plantar nerve or both (plantar distribution only).
Reiter's syndrome, seronegative spondyloarthropathies	Bilateral plantar fasciitis in a young male is often one of the first symptoms of an inflammatory arthritis.
	Consider HLA-B27 test and rheumatoid profile if other joint involvement is noted.
Jogger's foot	Jogger's foot (as described by Rask) is a local nerve entrapment of the medial plantar nerve at the fibromuscular tunnel formed by the abductor hallucis muscle and its border with the navicular tuberosity. Most often associated with valgus hindfoot deformity (pronator) and long-distance running.
	Characterized by running-induced neuritic pain (medial arch) radiating into medial toes along distribution of medial plantar nerve. This distribution is medial and on plantar aspect of the foot.

Figure 5–22. Squeeze test of the calcaneus is positive when the patient has a stress fracture. Palpation of the calcaneal tuberosity is painful on squeeze testing.

Figure 5–23. Bone scan of the feet of a 40-year-old male runner demonstrates increased tracer uptake at the right medial calcaneal tuberosity (*arrow*) typical of acute plantar fasciitis. (From Batt T: Overuse injuries in athletes. Physician Sports Med 23[6]:63–69, 1995.)

Table 5–3

Palpatory Signs of Heel Pain Syndrome

Diagnosis	Anatomic Location of Pain
Plantar fasciitis	Origin of plantar aponeurosis at medial calcaneal tubercle
Fat pad syndrome	Plantar fat pad (bottom and sides)
Calcaneal periostitis	Diffuse plantar and medial and lateral calcaneal borders
Posterior tibial tendon disorders	Over medial midtarsal area at navicular, which may radiate proximally behind medial malleolus
Peroneal tendon disorders	Lateral calcaneus and peroneal tubercle
Tarsal tunnel syndrome	Diffuse plantar foot that may radiate distally with tingling, burning, and numbness in the bottom of foot only (not dorsal)
Medial calcaneal neuritis	Well localized to anterior half of medial plantar heel pad and medial side of heel; does not radiate into distal foot
Lateral calcaneal neuritis	Heel pain that radiates laterally, more poorly localized
Calcaneal stress fracture	Diffuse pain over entire calcaneus, positive squeeze test of calcaneal tuberosity
Calcaneal apophysitis	Generalized over posterior heel, especially the sides, in skeletally immature patients (apophysis)
Generalized arthritis	Poorly localized but generally over entire heel pad

Modified from Doxey GE: J Orthop Sports Phys Ther 9:30, 1987

Rehabilitation Protocol
Treatment of Plantar Fasciitis
Brotzman

General Principles

- Examine lower extremity for possible contributing factors: pes cavus (high arch), pes planus (flat arch), leg-length discrepancy, fat pad atrophy, signs of systemic inflammatory arthritis, etc.
- Review and question for possible training errors or overuse findings in runners and athletes (see Chapter 7, Special Topics).
- Identify poor shoe wear, hard walking or running surface, supinator- or pronator-like wear of running shoes.
- Treatment phases are progressively more aggressive, or more invasive measures are used if the first phase is unsuccessful in relieving symptoms.
- Repetitive daily plantar and Achilles tendon stretching has been shown to provide the **most effective relief** of plantar fasciitis (83% successful results). Stretching should be done each morning before ambulation and four or five times throughout the day. One to 2 mo of daily stretching may be required for significant pain relief.
- The key to successful treatment is **patient education** to convey that 95% of patients with plantar fasciitis eventually have resolution of symptoms in 6–12 mo with conservative treatment, despite the intense pain often encountered initially. We use a patient educational tape and handout from www.orthovid.com (Fig. 5–24).

Figure 5–24. The www.orthovid.com Plantar Fasciitis patient instructional video series (25 min) is utilized to give the patient all the background, anatomy, rehabilitation exercises, and other information that are difficult to cover in the office. These tapes were created in coordination with physicians from this text. (www.orthovid.com).

Phase 1

Plantar Fascia Stretching

- Done four or five times a day, 5 to 10 repetitions.
- Done before first steps in morning, before standing after long period of rest.
- Seated plantar fascia stretching
  - While sitting, grab all five toes and pull the toes back toward the knee (Fig. 5–25). Hold for 30 sec and repeat five times. An alternate method is to kneel with the toes curled (extension at the MTP joints) under the feet. Sit back on heels until tension is felt in plantar fascia origin (Fig. 5–26). Hold for 30 sec *without* bouncing. Repeat five times.
  - While seated, place the foot as shown in Figure 5–27, then begin applying downward pressure to the calf. Hold for 30 sec. Repeat five times.
- Plantar fascia stretches against the wall
  - Place the foot against the wall as shown in Figure 5–28. Gently lean forward slowly and hold for 30 sec. Repeat three to five times.

Runner's Stretches for the Achilles Tendon

- A tight Achilles tendon is often implicated as an exacerbating or causative factor in plantar fasciitis. For this reason, much attention is given to Achilles tendon stretching exercises.
- Soleus runner's stretch
  - Slowly stretch (no bobbing) the Achilles tendon by placing the affected leg back (Fig. 5–29) and slowly bending the knee into a flexed position. Hold for 30 sec and repeat five times.

Figure 5–25. Plantar fascia stretch. The patient sits with the knees bent and the heel flat on the floor. The tops of the toes are gently bent upward with the hand. With the ankle dorsiflexed, pull the toes toward the ankle. Hold the stretch in a sustained fashion for 10 sec, repeating 10 times a day. The stretch should be felt in the plantar fascia.

Rehabilitation Protocol
Treatment of Plantar Fasciitis *(Continued)*
Brotzman

Figure 5–26. Alternative plantar fascia stretches. The patient kneels with the toes curled up under the feet (MTP joint extension). The buttocks are gently lowered to the heels until a mild tension is felt in the bottom of the feet. Hold for 30 sec and repeat 5 times per session. Do not bounce.

Figure 5–27. Seated plantar fascia stretches. While seated, the patient places the MTP joints into hyperextension and gently presses the calf to further stretch the MTP joints. Hold for 30 sec. Repeat 5 times per session.

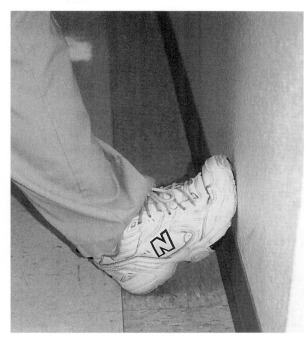

Figure 5–28. Plantar fascia stretch against the wall.

Figure 5–29. Bent-knee runner's stretch (soleus stretch).

continued

Rehabilitation Protocol
Treatment of Plantar Fasciitis *(Continued)*
Brotzman

- Gastrocnemius runner's stretch
  - Keep the knee straight and slowly stretch the affected leg for 30 sec (Fig. 5–30).
- Achilles stretching on incline board
  - Place the feet as shown in Figure 5–31 and hold for 30 sec, slowly leaning forward to stretch the Achilles tendon.

Relative Rest
- Discontinue running and walking for exercise until asymptomatic for 6 wk.
- Switch to low-impact exercise
  - Stationary bicycling.
  - Swimming.
  - Deep-water "running" with an aqua belt (see aquatic therapy section, Chapter 7).
- Weight loss.
- Modification of hard surfaces (cement) to soft surfacees (grass or cinder).

Cushioned Heel Inserts
- The American Orthopaedic Foot and Ankle Society (AOFAS) in a multicenter study found that inexpensive, over-the-counter cushioned heel inserts were **more effective** for plantar fasciitis than expensive, rigid, custom orthotics.

Figure 5–31. Runner's stretch on incline board. (From DeLee JC, Drez D Jr: Orthopaedic Sports Medicine: Principles and Practice. Philadelphia, WB Saunders, 1994.)

Figure 5–30. Runner's stretch (gastrocnemius).

Figure 5–32. Viscoheels. Soft cushions placed in and out of whatever shoe the patient is wearing (1-800-423-3405).

Rehabilitation Protocol
Treatment of Plantar Fasciitis (Continued)
Brotzman

- We typically use well-cushioned running shoes and Viscoheel inserts (Fig. 5–32) or PTT/Plastizote inserts (Alimed) first.
- Patients with abnormal biomechanics of the lower extremity, such as pes cavus or pes planus, may benefit from the eventual use of custom cushioned orthotics (see phase 2).

Shoewear Modification (Running Shoes)
- Flared, stable heel to help control heel stability.
- Firm heel counter to control the hindfoot.
- Soft cushioning of the heel, raising the heel 12–15 mm higher than the sole.
- Well-molded Achilles pad.
- Avoid rigid leather dress shoes that increase torque on the Achilles tendon.

Low-dye Taping
- Some patients obtain relief with low-dye taping, but from a practicality standpoint, daily taping is difficult to maintain.
- The science behind low-dye taping has not been effectively studied.

Ice Massage
- Ice to the area of inflammation for anti-inflammatory effect.
- Use ice in a paper or Styrofoam cup (peeled away) for 5–7 min; make sure to avoid frostbite.

Anti-inflammatories
- Oral anti-inflammatories have variable results. A brief trial of a cyclooxygenase (COX-2) inhibitor is tried. If response is not dramatic, this therapy is discontinued because of the possible side effects.

Phase 2
- If phase 1 measures fail to relieve symptoms after several months, phase 2 treatments are used.
- Before initiation of these measures, reevaluate the patient for other causes of heel pain
  - Consider a bone scan if calcaneal stress fracture is suspected.
  - HLA-B27 and rheumatoid/seronegative spondyloarthropathy laboratory work-up if other systemic signs or symptoms are evident.

Casting
- Casting has been shown to be helpful in about 50% of patients.
- A short-leg walking cast can be used for 1 mo, with the foot placed in neutral.
- A removable cast (cam boot) is used if the right foot is involved (to allow the patient to drive).
- Evaluate success at 1 mo, consider an additional month of removable cast wear if necessary.

- Complete second month of cast wear in removable boot to allow gradual transition from boot back into running shoes.

Orthotics
- Patients with very high or very low arches may benefit from orthotic inserts.
- A less rigid, accommodative insert is applicable to a more rigid cavus type of foot (high arch), which requires more cushion and less hindfoot control.
- A padded but rigid insert is indicated for a more unstable foot with compensatory pronation (pes planus or low arch), which requires more control.

Cortisone Injection (Fig. 5–33)
- Injection of cortisone into the area close to the plantar fascia often improves pain, but may weaken the plantar fascia and lead to rupture.
- The possible risks of injection (rupture, fat pad atrophy, infection) must be discussed with the patient and the possible long-term sequelae weighed against short-term benefits.
- One or possibly two steroid injections should be given in a 3- to 6-mo period, and only after failure of phase 1 treatment measures.

Night Splints
- A 5-degree dorsiflexion night splint has been reported to be beneficial. The splint holds the plantar fascia in a continuously tensed state. The theory behind the use of a night splint is to minimize the change of tension on the fascia that occurs with each day's new activities.

Figure 5–33. Technique for cortisone injection (plantar fasciitis).

continued

Rehabilitation Protocol
Treatment of Plantar Fasciitis *(Continued)*
Brotzman

Figure 5–34. Position of splint at night during patient use.

Figure 5–36. Deep friction massage of the plantar fascia.

Other night splints are placed at neutral (0 degrees); these are available through AliMed (1-800-225-2610) (Fig. 5–34).

Modalities
- Iontophoresis (see Chapter 10 for settings).
- Ultrasounds (Fig. 5–35).
- Deep friction massage (Fig. 5–36).
- Modalities may be beneficial for selected patients, but the literature on their efficiency is inconclusive.

Phase 3
- Patients in whom all phases 1 and 2 measures have failed may be candidates for surgical intervention (plantar fascia release).
- Because of the high complication rate from this surgery and the self-limited nature of plantar fasciitis in 90 to 95% of patients, we extend our operative indications to failure of all the phases 1 and 2 treatment for 18 mo. Much of the literature recommends 12 mo of conservative therapy.
- We **never** use endoscopic release because of the increased complication rate compared with that of open release and the inability to identify the nerve to the abductor digiti quinti.

Figure 5–35. Ultrasound of the plantar fascia.

Rupture of the Plantar Fascia

Background

Although not commonly reported in the literature, partial or complete plantar fascia ruptures may occur in jumping or running sports. Often, this is missed or misdiagnosed as an acute flare-up of plantar fasciitis. Complete rupture of the plantar fascia usually results in a permanent loss of the medial (longitudinal) arch of the foot. Such collapse is typically quite disabling for athletes.

Examination

Patients typically complain of a pop or crunch in the inferior heel area, with immediate pain and inability to continue play. This usually occurs during push-off, jumping, or initiation of a sprint. After an antecedent cortisone injection, the trauma may be much more minor (e.g., stepping off a curb).

Weight-bearing is very difficult, and swelling and ecchymosis in the plantar aspect of the foot occur fairly rapidly. Palpation along the plantar fascia elicits marked point tenderness. Dorsiflexion of the toes and foot often causes pain in the plantar fascia area.

Radiographic Evaluation

Diagnosis of a plantar fascia rupture is a clinical one. Pain radiographs are taken (three views of the foot) to

Figure 5–37. In this sagittal MRI of the right foot of a male college student basketball player, increased signal intensity and discontinuity of the plantar fascia *(arrows)* are consistent with edema, hemorrhage, and complete rupture. (Courtesy of the Radiology Department of the Medical College of Ohio at Toledo. From Kruse RJ: Diagnosing plantar fasciitis. Physician Sports Med 23[1]:117–126, 1995.)

rule out a fracture. MRI may be used but is not necessary for diagnosis (Fig. 5–37). MRI may miss the area of the actual rupture but does typically pick up the associated hemorrhage and swelling surrounding the rupture.

Rehabilitation Protocol
After Rupture of the Plantar Fascia
Brotzman

Phase 1: Days 0–14

- Immediate non–weight-bearing with crutches.
- Light compression wrap changed several times a day for 2–3 days.

- Ice therapy with ice massage of swollen/ecchymotic area several times a day.
- Maximal elevation on four or five pillows above the level of the heart for 72 hr, then elevation for 8–12 hr a day (sleeping with pillows under the foot).

continued

Rehabilitation Protocol
After Rupture of the Plantar Fascia *(Continued)*
Brotzman

A

B

C

- Non–weight-bearing, light, fiberglass cast on day 3, worn for 1–2 wk depending on resolution of pain.
- Nonsteroidal anti-inflammatory drugs (NSAIDs) (if not contraindicated) for 2–3 wk.
- Gentle active toe extension and flexion exercises while still in cast.

Phase 2: Weeks 2–3

- Removal of fiberglass cast.
- Use of $\frac{1}{8}$-inch felt pad placed from heel to heads of metatarsals (Fig. 5–38) and lightly wrapped with bandage (Coban, Unna boot, Ace bandage). We use a cotton sock or Coban to keep the felt in place.
- Foot and felt wrapping are placed in a removable walking cast, which allows the foot to be taken out daily for therapy and pool exercises.
- Weight-bearing is progressed from as tolerated in boot with crutches to weight-bearing in boot only. Pain is the guiding factor for progression of weight-bearing.
- Exercises are begun as pain allows
  - Swimming.
  - Deep-water running with Aquajogger.com flotation belt.
  - Stationary bicycling with no resistance.
  - Gentle Achilles stretches with towel looped around foot.

Phase 3: Weeks 3–8

- Proprioception exercises with BAPS board as pain allows.
- Removable cast and felt typically worn for 4–6 wk.
- Active ankle strengthening exercises are progressed.
- High-impact exercises are held until patient has been completely asymptomatic (with ambulation in tennis shoe) for 2–3 wk.
- Use of a custom orthotic layered with an overlying soft substance (such as Plastizote) is often helpful for eventual athletic participation.
- It is not uncommon to have permanent impairment in high-impact athletes who have suffered a plantar fascia rupture. For this reason, cortisone injections should rarely, if ever, be used in high-impact athletes.

Figure 5–38. Felt is placed under the foot for plantar fascia rupture. *A,* To allow mobility on a torn plantar fascia after the initial cast is removed, a $\frac{1}{8}$-inch felt pad is placed from the heel to the heads of the metatarsals. *B* and *C,* The pad is held in place with Coban or Unna boot dressing. (*A–C,* From Kruse RJ, McCoy RL, Erickson ATC: Diagnosing plantar fascia rupture. Physician Sports Med 23[1]:65, 1995.)

Achilles Tendon Dysfunction

Robert C. Greenberg, MD, and Charles L. Saltzman, MD

The Achilles tendon is the largest and strongest tendon in the body. The tendon has no true synovial sheath but is encased in a *paratenon* of varying thickness. The vascular supply to the tendon comes distally from intraosseous vessels from the calcaneus and proximally from intramuscular branches. There is a relative area of avascularity 2 to 6 cm from the calcaneal insertion that is more vulnerable to degeneration and injury. Achilles tendon injuries are commonly associated with repetitive impact loading due to running and jumping. *The primary factors resulting in damage of the Achilles tendon are training errors such as a sudden increase in activity, a sudden increase in training intensity (distance, frequency), resuming training after a long period of inactivity, and running on uneven or loose terrain.* Achilles dysfunction can also be related to postural problems (e.g., pronation), poor footwear (generally poor hindfoot support), and a tight gastrocsoleus complex.

Diagnosis—Achilles Tendinitis

Pain is typically located in the area of the distal Achilles tendon approximately 2 to 6 cm from the calcaneal insertion. With initial morning activity, pain is noted that is described as sharp or burning pain. The pain is initially present only with vigorous activity and progresses to pain with activities of daily living. Pain is typically relieved with rest.

> ## Differential Diagnosis of Achilles Tendinitis
>
> Partial rupture of Achilles tendon
>
> Retrocalcaneal bursitis (of retrocalcaneal bursa)
>
> Haglund's deformity (pump bump)
>
> Calcaneal apophysitis (skeletally immature—Sever's apophysitis)
>
> Calcaneal exostosis
>
> Calcaneal stress fracture (positive squeeze test)
>
> Calcaneal fracture (acute fall or MVA)
>
> PTT tendinitis (medial pain)
>
> Plantar fasciitis (inferior heel pain)

Examination

Examination is performed with the patient placed prone and the feet hanging off the edge of the table. Palpate the entire substance of the gastrocnemius-soleus myotendinous complex while the ankle is put through active and passive ROM. Evaluate for tenderness, warmth, swelling or fullness, nodularity, or substance defect. The **Thompson test** is performed to evaluate the continuity of the Achilles tendon (Fig. 5–39). A positive Thompson test (no plantar flexion of the foot with squeezing of the calf) indicates a complete rupture of the tendinoachilles. Note the resting position of the forefoot with the ankle and talonavicular joints held in the neutral position. Ankle and subtalar mobility may often be decreased. Calf atrophy is common in any Achilles tendon dysfunction.

Figure 5–39. Thompson squeeze test. This test evaluates the Achilles tendon for complete rupture. In the normal patient placed prone with the knee flexed at 90 degrees, squeezing the calf muscle will cause the foot to plantar flex *(arrow)* because the tendon is intact. In a *complete rupture* of the tendon, squeezing of the calf will *not* cause plantar flexion of the foot (i.e., a positive Thompson test indicates a complete rupture). This test is important because most patients with a completely ruptured Achilles tendon can still weakly plantar flex the foot, "cheating" with the long toe flexors, on request. (From Kovan JR, McKeag DB: Lower extremity overuse injuries in aerobic dancers. J Musculoskel Med 9[4]:43–52, 1992. Artist: Gwenn Alton-Bird.)

While seated on the exam table, the patient's foot shoud be passively dorsiflexed, first with the knee flexed and then with the knee fully extended. This will tell the examiner how tight the Achilles tendon is. Many females who have worn high heel shoes for years won't be able to dorsiflex the foot to neutral with the knee in full extension.

Classification of Achilles Tendon Problems

Achilles tendon problems generally are classified as paratenonitis, tendinosis, or rupture.

Imaging

Most Achilles problems can be diagnosed with a thorough history and physical examination. Imaging helps confirm the diagnosis, assist with surgical planning, or rule out other diagnoses.

- *Routine radiographs* are generally normal. Occasionally, calcification in the tendon or its insertion is noted. Inflammatory arthropathies (erosions), Haglund's deformity (pump bump) can be ruled out on radiographs.
- *Ultrasound* is inexpensive and fast and allows dynamic examination, but it requires substantial interpreter experience. It is the most reliable method for determining the thickness of the Achilles tendon and the size of a gap after a complete rupture.
- *MRI* is not used for dynamic assessment, but it is superior in the detection of partial tears and the evaluation of various stages of chronic degenerative changes, such as peritendinous thickening and inflammation. MRI can be used to monitor tendon healing when recurrent partial rupture is suspected and is the best modality for surgical planning (location, size).

Achilles Paratenonitis

Background

Inflammation is limited to the paratenon without associated Achilles tendinosis. Fluid often accumulates next to the tendon, the paratenon is thickened and adherent to normal tendon tissue. Achilles paratenonitis most commonly occurs in mature athletes involved in running and jumping activities. It generally does not progress to degeneration. Histology of paratenonitis shows inflammatory cells, and capillary and fibroblastic proliferation in the paratenon or peritendinous areolar tissue.

Clinical Signs and Symptoms

Pain starts with initial morning activity. The discomfort is well-localized tenderness and sharp, burning pain with activity. The discomfort is present 2 to 6 cm proximal to the insertion of the Achilles tendon into the calcaneus. Pain is primarily aggravated by activity and relieved by rest. Pain is present with single-heel raise and absent on the Thompson test. Significant heel cord contracture will exacerbate symptoms.

Swelling, local tenderness, warmth, and tendon thickening are common. Calf atrophy and weakness and

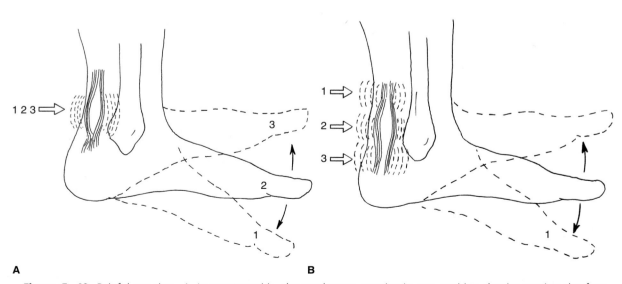

Figure 5–40. Painful arc sign. *A,* In peratenonitis, the tenderness remains in one position despite moving the foot from dorsiflexion to plantar flexion. *B,* In the case of partial tendon rupture or tendinitis, the point of tenderness *moves* as the foot goes from dorsiflexion to plantar flexion. (*A* and *B,* Redrawn from Williams JG: Achilles tendon lesions in sport. Sports Med 3:114, 1986.)

tendon nodularity can be present in chronic cases. Crepitation is rare.

Painful arc sign (Fig. 5–40) is negative in paratenonitis. It is important to localize the precise area of tenderness and fullness. In paratenonitis, the area of tenderness and fullness stays fixed with active ROM of ankle. The inflammation involves only the paratenon, which is a fixed structure, unlike pathology of the Achilles tendon itself, which migrates superiorly and inferiorly with ROM of the ankle.

In the acute setting, symptoms are typically transient, present only with activity, and last less than 2 weeks. Later, symptoms start at the beginning of exercising or at rest, and tenderness increases. The area of tenderness is well localized and reproducible by side-to-side squeezing of the involved region.

Partial rupture may be superimposed on chronic paratenonitis and can present as an acute episode of pain and swelling.

Rehabilitation Protocol
Treatment of Achilles Paratenonitis

Phase 1: 0–6 Weeks

- Rest and/or activity modification is required to reduce symptoms to a level that can achieve pain-free activity.
- If pain is severe, a walking boot or cast is worn for 3–8 wk to allow pain-free activities of daily living.
- Crutch-assisted ambulation added when there is persistent pain with boot or cast.
- Most patients have chronic pain that requires an initial period of complete rest until symptoms subside, followed by rehabilitation and gradual return to activities.
- NSAIDs and ice massage decrease pain and inflammation, particularly in the acute phase.
- A stretching program is essential. Gentle calf, Achilles, and hamstring stretching is done three to four times a day.
- Acute pain usually resolves in the first 2 wk.
- Footwear is changed or modified if overpronation or poor hindfoot support is present.
- Athletic activity
  - Gradual return to activity.
  - Adequate warm-up and cool-down periods.
  - Pre- and postexercise stretching of gastrocnemius and soleus complex.
  - Decrease duration and intensity.
  - Decrease training on hard surfaces.
  - Avoid hill and incline training.
  - Replace inadequate or worn-out footwear.
- Progress to gentle strengthening using low-impact exercises.

Phase 2: 6–12 Weeks

- Indicated for failed phase 1 or recurrent symptoms after previous resolution.
- Repeat or continue phase 1 immobilization and stretching.

- Add modalities
  - Contrast baths.
  - Ultrasound.
- Footwear
  - Small heel lift for severe pain.
  - Arch support orthotic if overpronation.
- Persistent heel cord tightness is treated with stretching exercises and use of a 5-degree dorsiflexion night AFO worn for 3 mo while sleeping.
- Staged cross-training program for most athletes, especially runners.
- Aqua-jogging and swimming, stationary cycling, exercise on stair-climbing and cross-country skiing machines. Avoid repetitive impact loading (e.g., running).

Phase 3: 3 Months and Beyond

- **Brisement** (only for paratenonitis)
  - Dilute local anesthetic and sterile saline injected into the paratenon sheath to break up adhesion between the inflamed paratenon and the Achilles tendon (preferable to steroid injection). Can be done with ultrasound to confirm correct placement.
- Corticosteroid injections
  - Generally avoided.
  - Rarely indicated, only for recalcitrant cases to inhibit inflammation and prevent scar formation.
  - Risk of adverse effects if injected into tendon or if overused is generally worse than any known benefit.

Operative Treatment for Paratenonitis

Operative treatment generally is indicated if 4 to 6 months of conservative treatment fails to relieve symptoms. Preoperative MRI usually is obtained primarily to evaluate for associated tendinosis and confirm diagnosis.

Technique

The patient is positioned prone and a thigh tourniquet is applied. A longitudinal incision is made posteromedially along the Achilles tendon. Full-thickness flaps are raised, with very gentle soft tissue handling.

The thickened paratenon and adhesions are removed posteriorly, medially, and laterally as needed. Anterior dissection is avoided because the blood supply of the tendon is primarily within the anterior mesotenon and fat pad. The tendon is inspected for thickening and degeneration (tendinosis); if noted intraoperatively or on MRI, surgical treatment is as described for tendinosis.

Postoperative Protocol

- Padded splint is applied in neutral position.
- Non–weight-bearing motion is initiated immediately, both active ROM and gentle passive dorsiflexion with rubber tubing.
- Crutch-assisted weight-bearing as tolerated after 7 to 10 days, when pain permits and swelling has decreased. If the wound is healing uneventfully at 2 to 3 weeks, ambulation is allowed as tolerated.
- Exercises are begun on a stationary bike and stair climber when the patient can walk without pain. Swimming and aqua jogging are allowed, as tolerated by the patient and when the wound is healed.
- Running can be resumed 6 to 10 weeks postoperative.
- Return to competition is allowed after 3 to 6 months; calf strength must be at least 80% of the normal side.

Achilles Tendinosis

Background

Achilles tendinosis is characterized by intratendinous or mucoid degeneration of the Achilles tendon without evidence of paratenonitis (inflammation). The process starts with interstitial microscopic failure, which leads to central tissue necrosis with subsequent mucoid degeneration Achilles tendinosis most commonly occurs in mature athletes as the result of accumulated repetitive microtrauma from training errors. It is associated with an increased risk of Achilles tendon rupture.

The histology generally is noninflammatory, showing decreased cellularity and fibrillation of collagen fibers within the tendon. Along with the collagen fiber disorganization, there is scattered vascular ingrowth and occasional areas of necrosis and rare calcification.

Initially, the paratenon sheath may become inflamed, and with overuse, the tendon itself becomes inflamed or hypovascular because of the restriction of blood flow through the scarred paratenon.

Clinical Signs and Symptoms

Achilles tendinosis is often asymptomatic and remains subclinical until it presents as a rupture. It may elicit low-grade discomfort related to activities, and a palpable painless mass or nodule may be present 2 to 6 cm proximal to the insertion of the tendon. This can progress to gradual thickening of the entire tendon substance.

The painful arc sign is positive in patients with Achilles tendinosis. The thickened portion of tendon **moves** with active plantar flexion and dorsiflexion of the ankle (in contrast to paratenonitis, in which the area of tenderness remains in one position despite dorsiflexion and plantar flexion of the foot).

Paratenonitis and tendinosis can coexist when inflammation involves both the paratenon and intratendinous focal degeneration. This gives the clinical appearance of paratenonitis because the symptoms associated with tendinosis are absent or very subtle. Most patients seek treatment for symptoms related to the paratenonitis, and usually, the tendinosis is unrecognized until both processes are noted on MRI or at surgery (most commonly after a rupture). Conservative treatment is the same as for paratenonitis. MRI is very useful in preoperative planning, which must consider both entities.

Treatment

The initial treatment of Achilles tendinosis is always conservative and progresses as described for paratenonitis. If symptoms are severe, initial treatment may include 1 to 2 weeks of immobilization and crutch ambulation, in addition to NSAIDs, ice, and heel cord stretching. Foot and leg alignment should be carefully evaluated, with orthotic correction if necessary. Conservative treatment is continued for 4 to 6 months; surgery is indicated if this fails to relieve symptoms.

Operative Treatment

MRI is used to confirm the diagnosis and plan the operative procedure.

Technique

The patient is placed prone with a thigh tourniquet and the foot hanging off the end of the table. The incision is placed posteromedially just off the edge of the tendon (avoids the sural nerve). Full-thickness flaps are created with very careful soft tissue handling. The paratenon is inspected and any hypertrophic paratenon adherent to the tendon is excised. A longitudinal incision is made within the body of the tendon over the thickened, nodular parts to expose areas of central tendon necrosis. Degenerative areas are excised (should correspond with MRI). Débridement is followed by side-to-side closure to repair any defect. If the defect is too large to be closed primarily or lacks adequate substance after débridement, the Achilles tendon is reconstructed using the plantaris tendon, flexor digitorum longus, or a turndown flap.

Rehabilitation Protocol
After Débridement of Achilles Tendinosis

- A padded splint is applied in neutral position.
- Gentle non–weight-bearing motion is begun in first week: active ROM and passive dorsiflexion with rubber tubing are done several times a day.
- A removable walking boot with an adjustable heel is used for 2–4 wk. Crutch-assisted ambulation for the first 10–14 days. At 2 wk, weight-bearing without crutches is allowed in the boot as tolerated.

- Stationary bicycling is begun when the patient is ambulating comfortably.
- Swimming and aqua jogging are started when the wound is completely healed.
- Running is typically allowed at 8–10 wk after surgery.
- Return to competition is allowed at 4–6 mo.
- If significant reconstruction is done along with débridement, rehabilitation must progress more slowly, similar to that after tendon repair after rupture.

Rehabilitation Protocol
General Guidelines for Achilles Tendinitis, Paratenonitis, and Tendinosis in High-impact Athletes
Brotzman

- Establish correct diagnosis.
- Correct underlying training and biomechanical problems
  - Stop rapid increase in mileage.
  - Stop hill running.
  - Correct improper intensity of training, duration, schedule, hard surface, poor shoewear.
  - Decrease mileage significantly and/or initiate cross-training (pool, bicycle) depending on severity of symptoms at presentation.

- Correction functional overpronation and resultant vascular wringing of the tendon (Fig. 5–41) with a custom orthotic that usually incorporates a medial rear foot post.
  - Stop interval training.
- Soften a hard heel counter or use shoe counter heel cushions (Fig. 5–42) to minimize posterior "rubbing" symptoms.

Region of relative avascularity

Foot strike   Mid stance

A   B   C

Figure 5–41. *A,* Correction of functional overpronation by a medial rearfoot post minimizes the potential for postulated vascular wringing. *B,* Whipping action of the Achilles tendon produced by overpronation. *C,* External tibial rotation produced by knee extension conflicting with internal tibial rotation produced by prolonged pronation. This results in "wringing out" of vessels in the zone of relative avascularity. (*A–C,* From Clement DB, Taunton JF, Smart GW: Achilles tendinitis and peritendinitis: etiology and treatment. Am J Sports Med 12[3]:181, 1984.)

continued

Rehabilitation Protocol
General Guidelines for Achilles Tendinitis, Paratenonitis, and Tendinosis in High-impact Athletes *(Continued)*
Brotzman

- Begin a runner's stretching program before and after exercises (see p. 519).
- Oral anti-inflammatories (over-the-counter or COX-2 inhibitors).
- **Avoid cortisone injection; this will cause weakening or rupture of the tendon.**
- Cryotherapy (ice massage) after exercise for anti-inflammatory effect.
- Correct leg-length discrepancy if noted. First try $1/4$-inch heel insert for a $1/2$-inch leg-length discrepancy; if not

improved, go to $1/2$-inch insert. "Overcorrection" (too rapid an orthotic correction of a leg-length discrepancy) may worsen symptoms.
- If symptoms persist after 4–6 wk of conservative measures, immobilization in a removable cam boot or cast may be required for 3–6 wk.
- Slow, painless progression to preinjury activities
  - Swimming.
  - Deep-water "running" with Aquajogger.com flotation belt.
  - Bicycling.
  - Walking.
  - Eccentric exercises for Achilles strengthening.
  - Light jogging.
- Eccentric strengthening of Achilles tendon should condition the tendon and make it less susceptible to overuse injuries; however, these exercises are not used until the patient is asymptomatic and painless for 2–3 wk
  - Toe raises in pool.
  - Plantar flexion against progressively harder Therabands.
  - Multiple sets of very light (20-pound) total gym or slider board exercises (Fig. 5–43).

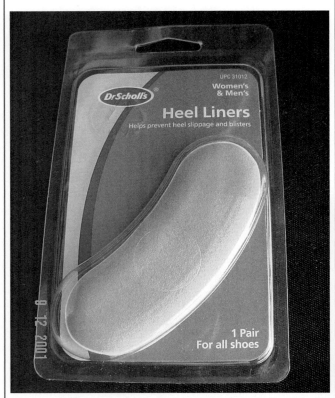

Figure 5–42. Use of soft heel counter inserts (Dr. Scholl's: www.DrScholls.com) to lessen rubbing of the posterior heel counter on the Achilles tendon.

Figure 5–43. Slider board or total gym exercises for Achilles tendon strengthening.

Achilles Tendon Rupture

Background

Complete ruptures tend to occur in middle-aged patients and those without preexisting complaints. Partial ruptures occur in well-trained athletes and involve the lateral aspect of the tendon. Acute ruptures commonly result from acute eccentric overload on a dorsiflexed ankle that has chronic tendinosis. Patients should be questioned about previous steroid injection and fluoroquinolones (possible association with tendon weakening and rupture).

Clinical Signs and Symptoms

Sharp pain and a pop heard at the time of complete rupture are commonly reported. Patients often describe a sensation of being kicked in the Achilles tendon. Most have an immediate inability to bear weight or return to activity. A palpable defect may be present in the tendon initially.

Partial rupture is associated with an acutely tender, localized swelling that occasionally involves an area of nodularity.

The Thompson test (see Fig. 5–39) is positive with complete Achilles tendon rupture. A positive test occurs when squeezing the calf fails to plantar flex the foot because of a lack of continuity of the tendon (rupture).

Thompson Test

The patient is placed prone, with both feet extended off the end of the table. Both calf muscles are squeezed by the examiner. If the tendon is intact, the foot will plantar flex when the calf is squeezed. If the tendon is ruptured, normal plantar flexion will not occur (a positive Thompson test).

In some patients, an accurate diagnosis of a complete rupture is difficult through physical examination alone. The tendon defect can be disguised by a large hematoma. A false-negative Thompson test can occur because of plantar flexion of the ankle caused by extrinsic foot flexors when the accessory ankle flexors are squeezed together with the contents at the superficial posterior leg compartment. It is important to critically compare the test with results in the normal side.

Partial ruptures are also difficult to accurately diagnose, and MRI should be used to confirm the diagnosis.

Treatment of Acute Rupture of the Achilles Tendon

Both conservative and operative treatments are commonly used to restore length and tension to the tendon to optimize strength and function. Both methods are reasonable, and treatment should be individualized based on operative candidacy. **High-level and competitive athletes usually undergo primary repair.** Operative repair is associated with lower re-rupture rates, quicker return to full activity, and a theoretically higher level of function. However, the difference in outcomes between conservative and operative treatment is variable. The main surgical risk is wound breakdown. Generally, surgery should be avoided in patients with poor wound healing potential (diabetics); smoking is a relative contraindication.

Regardless of definitive treatment, initial treatment is a short-leg splint in a comfortable position of plantar flexion, ice, elevation, and crutch ambulation.

Nonoperative treatment of complete Achilles tendon ruptures in a 20-degree plantar flexed cast is usually reserved for chronically ill patients, poor operative candidates, elderly patients, and low-demand patients. The re-rupture rate is much higher in patients treated nonoperatively (with a plantar flexed cast for 8 weeks of non–weight-bearing) than in those treated operatively. A review of multiple studies found an average re-rupture rate of 17.5% in nonoperative patients compared with 1.2% in operatively treated patients. However, major and minor complications were more frequent with operative treatment.

Nonoperative Treatment of Acute Achilles Tendon Rupture

Nonoperative treatment for poor operative candidates requires immobilization to allow hematoma consolidation. Ultrasound is used to confirm that tendon end apposition occurs with 20 degrees or less of plantar flexion. **Conservative treatment is best for small partial ruptures.** Surgical repair is indicated if a diastasis or gap remains with the leg placed in 20 degrees of plantar flexion.

A 20-degree non–weight-bearing plantar flexed short-leg cast (preference) or a removable boot (not to be removed by the patient) with an elevated heel is used for 8 weeks. **The patient remains non–weight-bearing in the cast for 8 weeks.**

At 6 to 8 weeks, plantar flexion of the cast is slowly decreased (most easily done in a commercial cam boot with adjustable ankle angle setting). An initial heel lift of 2 to 2.5 cm should be worn for 1 month when progressive weight-bearing is begun. Gentle non–weight-bearing active ROM exercises and gentle passive stretching with rubber tubing are begun. At 10 to 12 weeks, the heel lift is decreased to 1 cm and, over the next month, is progressively decreased so that the patient is walking without a heel lift by 3 months.

Progressive resistance exercises for the calf muscles should be started between 8 and 10 weeks. Running may be resumed after 4 to 6 months if strength is 70% of the uninvolved leg. Maximal plantar flexion power may not return for 12 months or more.

Operative Treatment for Complete Achilles Tendon Rupture

Operative treatment is generally preferred for young, athletic, and active patients. The incision and approach are the same as for paratenonitis and tendinosis. A medial approach is used to expose the tendon ends, and a modified Bunnell technique is used to repair the rupture.

Rehabilitation Protocol
After Surgical Repair of Acute Achilles Tendon Rupture in Athletes
Brotzman

- Well-padded 20-degrees equinus posterior splint with plaster *ankle stirrup* initially postoperative.
- Non–weight-bearing with crutches for 4 wk.
- Progress to partial weight-bearing with crutch-assisted ambulation in a short-leg fiberglass cast.

For High-level Compliant Athletes

- Initially use cam boot with 15–20 degrees of equinus (plantar flexion) dialed in, using a heel lift and ankle angle boot setting of 20 degrees of plantar flexion.
- Active non–weight-bearing ROM exercises can be started as early as 7 days after surgery. Incision must be well healed before initiation of exercises.
- Initial exercise consists of very gentle passive plantar flexion and active dorsiflexion limited to 20 degrees, two sets of five, three times a day.
- At 1 mo, start to slowly bring ankle toward neutral by decreasing the heel lift in the boot by 1 cm. Wean out of heel lift over 6- to 8-wk period.
- Use walking boot for 6–8 wk, then make the transition to normal shoes when using the smaller heel lifts.

- Stationary bicycling (no resistance) and swimming initiated at 6 wk.
- Gradual return to competition as in conservative treatment. Must have full strength (versus nonoperative side) and full endurance and have completed the running program.

For Lower-demand Athletes

- Use a short-leg non–weight-bearing gravity equinus cast for 6–8 wk followed by 1-cm heel lift in a removable boot for 1 mo.
- Progressive non–weight-bearing resistance exercises are started at 8–10 wk.
- Stationary bicycling and swimming at approximately 8 wk.
- Return to some athletic activity (light running) at 5–6 mo if strength is 70% of uninvolved leg.

Generally, return to full level takes 1 yr, can take up to 18 mo.

Posterior Tibial Tendon Insufficiency

S. Brent Brotzman, MD

PTT insufficiency is the most common cause of acquired flatfoot deformity in adults.

PTT injuries and/or insufficiency are some of the most commonly missed diagnoses in primary care and orthopaedics. Failure to perform an examination with the patient standing often results in the physician missing the collapse of the medial longitudinal arch, hindfoot valgus, and inability to perform a unilateral heel raise that usually characterize PTT injuries. This diagnosis must be remembered in the evaluation of medial ankle and foot pain and unilateral arch collapse with flatfoot deformity.

Anatomy and Pathophysiology

The PTT functions as a plantar flexor of the foot and as an inverter of the subtalar joint. It originates on the posterior aspect of the tibia, interosseous membrane, and fibula. It courses posteriorly along the medial ankle, adjacent and posterior to the medial malleolus. The PTT then inserts in the midfoot at the navicular tuberosity, sending bands that attach to the plantar aspect of the cuneiforms, the second, third, and fourth metatarsals, and the sustentaculum tali (Fig. 5–44).

The PTT and its opposing tendon, the peroneus brevis, function during the midstance phase of gait. The PTT is very large (cross-sectional area of 16.9 cm^2) in comparison with any of the available tendons that can be transferred to replace it (e.g., flexor digitorum longus is only 5.5 cm^2).

The loss of the PTT's force of inversion is evidenced in patients with PTT insufficiency by a limited ability or complete inability to perform a unilateral heel raise.

With progressive dysfunction of the PTT, the medial longitudinal arch of the foot collapses, the subtalar joint everts, the heel assumes a valgus position (Fig. 5–45A), and the foot eventually abducts (see Chapter 10) at the talonavicular joint (see Fig. 5–45B).

Figure 5–44. Posterior tibial tendon (PTT). (From Myburgh KH, Grobler N, Nockes TD: Factors associated with shin soreness in athletes. Physician Sports Med 16[4]:129–137, 1988.)

Figure 5–45. Hindfoot valgus and arch collapse of the foot as a result of PTT insufficiency. The forefoot is also "abducted" (pointing away from the midline) at the talonavicular joint. (From Mann RA, Coughlin MJ: Surgery of the Foot and Ankle. St. Louis, Mosby, 1993.)

Figure 5–46. Tenderness of the PTT proximal to its insertion onto the navicular tuberosity. FDL, flexor digitorum longus; FHL, flexor hallucis longus; PTT, posterior tibial tendon. (From Hunter-Griffin LY (ed): Athletic Training and Sports Med. Park Ridge, Ill., AAOS, 1991.)

Etiology

The etiology of PTT insufficiency ranges from inflammatory synovitis (leading to degeneration, lengthening, and rupture) to acute trauma. Holmes and Mann (1992) reported that 60% of those who suffered a PTT rupture had a history of obesity, diabetes, hypertension, previous surgery or trauma to the medial foot, or previous treatment with steroids. Acute traumatic PTT rupture is very rare. Most ruptures and insufficiency of the PTT are due to gradual failure or intrinsic abnormality rather than to extrinsic trauma.

Frey and coworkers (1990) demonstrated a zone of hypovascularity in the tendon beginning 1 to 1.5 cm distal to the medial malleolus and extending 1 cm farther. This area is where most ruptures and degenerative changes are found intraoperatively.

PTT dysfunction may be associated with seronegative inflammatory disorders, including ankylosing spondylitis, psoriasis, and Reiter's syndrome. Other conditions that may be associated with PTT dysfunction include rheumatoid arthritis and pes planus. Injection of steroids (cortisone) around the PTT appears to significantly increase the risk of rupture.

Injection of the PTT with cortisone is contraindicated because of the risk of weakening and rupture of the tendon.

Diagnosis

The diagnosis of PTT insufficiency is primarily a clinical one. MRI of the course of the tendon in the foot and ankle may be of some value if the diagnosis is uncertain. MRI is not routinely recommended and its clinical usefulness is questionable.

Signs and Symptoms

In the early stages of PTT insufficiency, most patients complain of fatigue, aching, and pain of the plantar-medial aspect of the foot and ankle just proximal to the tendon insertion onto the navicular tuberosity (Fig. 5–46). Discomfort is located medially along the course of the tendon. Swelling or bogginess along the tendon is common if the dysfunction is associated with tenosynovitis. Pain is exacerbated by activity, weight-bearing, and calf raises. The patient's ability to walk distances usually decreases.

Examination

Both feet should be examined with the patient standing and both lower extremities entirely visible. The feet should also be viewed from behind to appreciate hindfoot valgus on standing. The *too-many-toes sign* as described by Johnson (1983) should also be looked for from behind the patient: abduction of the forefoot relative to the hindfoot allows more of the lateral toes to be seen on the symptomatic foot than on the unaffected foot (Fig. 5–47).

Patients with early (stage 1) PTT insufficiency may have only swelling and tenderness medially. As the insufficiency progresses, the longitudinal arch collapses. Hindfoot valgus is initially flexible (hindfoot correctable to subtalar neutral) and eventually becomes fixed.

The single limb or "unilateral" heel raise should be attempted while the patient is standing (Fig. 5–48). This test is an excellent determinant of the function of the PTT. With support for balance by the examiner, the

Figure 5–47. The "too-many-toes" sign. More toes are visible lateral to the heel on the patient's right leg. The sign is found with PTT insufficiency and resultant collapse, forefoot abduction, and hindfoot valgus. (From DeLee JC, Drez D Jr: Orthopaedic Sports Medicine: Principles and Practice. Philadelphia, WB Saunders, 1994.)

Figure 5–48. Single-heel raise test. The affected (PTT-deficient) right heel does not assume a stable (varus) position (as seen on the left) when the patient attempts to stand on the toes (for details of the test, see text). (From DeLee JC, Drez D Jr: Orthopaedic Sports Medicine: Principles and Practice. Philadelphia, WB Saunders, 1994.)

patient is asked to first suspend the unaffected leg in the air, then attempt to perform a heel raise on the affected foot. With dysfunction of the PTT, inversion of the heel is weak, and the patient is unable to rise onto the forefoot or the heel remains in valgus rather than being swung into varus on heel raise.

While the patient is seated, the examiner should test PTT strength (inversion) against resistance. During the test, the hindfoot should first be positioned in plantar flexion and eversion and the forefoot in abduction (Fig. 5–49) to eliminate the synergistic action of the anterior tibial tendon, which would otherwise fire and mask a strength loss in the PTT. The patient is asked to invert the foot against the examiner's hand, and strength is graded. This test is less sensitive than the unilateral heel raise.

Areas of tenderness, swelling, and bogginess should be palpated. In the later stages of collapse, the patient may complain of lateral pain and tenderness in the sinus tarsi region (Fig. 5–50) as a result of impingement of the talus under the fibula. This is referred to as "sinus tarsi impingement."

The hindfoot (heel) should also be tested to see whether the subtalar joint can be reduced to neutral (flexible hindfoot) or not (fixed-deformity hindfoot). The Achilles tendon often becomes contracted or shortened in later states, and its passive ankle ROM in dorsiflexion should be compared with that of the other extremity.

Radiographic Evaluation

Radiographic evaluation should include four weight-bearing views: AP of both ankles, AP of both feet, lateral of both ankles, and lateral of both feet. On the weight-

Figure 5–49. PTT testing. The PTT is an inverter. During testing of a weak PTT, the anterior tibial tendon is often recruited. To test the "isolated" PTT, first bring the foot into plantar flexion and eversion (to eliminate the anterior tibial tendon). Then gauge the strength of inversion against the examiner's hand. (From McKeag DB, Dolan C: Overuse syndromes of the lower extremity. Physician Sports Med 17[2]:108–123, 1989.)

Figure 5–50. Sinus tarsi impingement. (From DeLee JC, Drez D Jr: Orthopaedic Sports Medicine: Principles and Practice. Philadelphia, WB Saunders, 1994.)

bearing lateral radiograph of the foot with longitudinal collapse, the talus inclines plantarward compared with the normal foot. AP foot films often reveal abduction of the midfoot by revealing an "uncovered" talar head at the talonavicular joint.

Classification of Posterior Tibial Tendon Insufficiency

Johnson and Strom (1989) described a classification of PTT insufficiency that is helpful in developing treatment algorithms, but does not consider the contracted gastrocnemius evident in some patients (shortened Achilles) (Table 5–4).

Table 5-4

Classification of Posterior Tibial Tendon Insufficiency

Stage 1	Absence of fixed foot or ankle deformity (except Achilles contracture). Normal foot alignment on standing. Pain, tenderness, or swelling medially along course of PTT.
Stage 2	Dynamic (correctable) hindfoot valgus deformity. Weakness of PTT on resistance testing. Too-many-toes sign. Inability to perform unilateral heel-rise. Relatively normal arc of subtalar motion.
Stage 3	Fixed hindfoot valgus deformity. Talonavicular joint cannot be reduced with hindfoot in fixed valgus position. Usually, fixed forefoot supination deformity compensating for hindfoot valgus to allow plantigrade foot. No obvious ankle deformities.
Stage 4	Stage 3 plus ankle deformity.

From Myerson MS: Adult aquired flat foot deformity: treatment of dysfunction of the posterior tibial tendon. Instr Course Lect. 46:393, 1997.

Treatment (Table 5–5)

The initial treatment for patients with any stage of PTT insufficiency is nonoperative, which includes relative rest (cast, splint, or orthotic) for 6 to 8 weeks, use of NSAIDs, and assessment of degree of improvement.

Table 5-5

Treatment of Dysfunction of the Posterior Tibial Tendon (PTT)

Stage	Characteristics	Nonoperative Treatment	Operative Treatment
Tenosynovitis	Acute medial pain and swelling Can perform heel-rise Seronegative inflammation Extensive tearing	NSAIDs Immobilization 6–8 wk If symptoms improve, ankle stirrup brace If symptoms do not improve, operative treatment	Tenosynovectomy Tenosynovectomy + calcaneal osteotomy Tenodesis of FDL to PTT
Stage I rupture	Medial pain and swelling Hindfoot correctable Can perform heel-rise	Medial heel-and-sole wedge Hinged AFO Orthortic arch supports	Débridement of PTT FDL transfer FDL transfer + calcaneal osteotomy
Stage II rupture	Valgus angulation of heel Lateral pain Hindfoot rigid (fixed) Cannot perform heel-rise	Medial heel-and-sole wedge Stiff orthotic support Hinged AFO Injection of steroids into sinus tarsi	FDL transfer + calcaneal osteotomy FDL transfer + bone-block arthrodesis at calcaneocuboid joint
Stage III rupture	Valgus angulation of heel Lateral pain Hindfoot rigid Cannot perform heel-rise	Rigid AFO	Triple arthrodesis
Stage IV rupture	Hindfoot rigid Valgus angulation of talus Ankle involvement	Rigid AFO	Tibiotalocalcaneal arthrodesis

AFO, ankle-foot orthosis; FDL, flexor digitorum longus; NSAIDs, nonsteroidal anti-inflammatory drugs.
From Myerson MS: Adult acquired flat foot deformity: treatment of dysfunction of the posterior tibial tendon. Instr Course Lect 46:393, 1997.

For **acute tenosynovitis,** a removable walking cast is worn for 6 to 8 weeks, with weight-bearing as tolerated with a cane or crutch. NSAIDs are given, and ice massage is applied to the tendon for 1 to 2 weeks. If improvements are noted in symptoms and on examination, the cast is removed and replaced with an orthotic with supportive medial longitudinal arch and stiff-sole shoe. Some authors recommend a stiff-sole shoe with a medial heel-and-sole wedge. Low-impact activities (swimming, cycling) are substituted for former high-impact activities (jogging, long-distance walking). If there is no improvement with nonoperative treatment, surgical tenosynovectomy is indicated (see later).

For **PTT insufficiency (stages 1–4),** a custom-molded ankle-foot orthosis (AFO), double upright brace with a medial T-strap (Fig. 5–51), or an ankle brace (Fig. 5–52) can help control deformity and alleviate symptoms. Sedentary or elderly patients can be treated with bracing if symptoms are tolerable in the brace. The brace will not "correct" the deformity, but acts as a stabilizer. If conservative measures fail, or the patient is unwilling to wear the bulky brace, operative treatment is indicated. Operative treatment often includes Achilles lengthening because the

Figure 5–52. Ankle brace.

Achilles is usually contracted and shortened in patients with PTT insufficiency. ∎

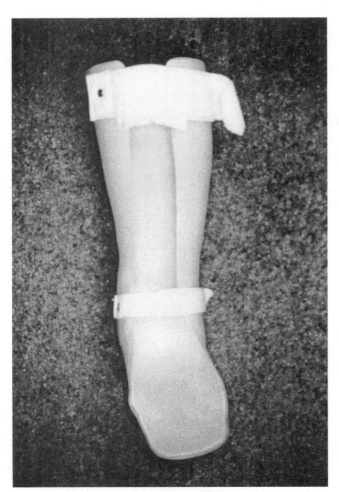

Figure 5–51. Polypropylene ankle-foot orthosis (AFO) with a molded Plastizote lining. (From Mann RA, Coughlin MJ: Surgery of the Foot and Ankle. St. Louis, Mosby, 1993.)

Metatarsalgia

Brett R. Fink, MD, and Mark S. Mizel, MD

Background

Metatarsalgia describes an assortment of conditions that cause plantar pain in the forefoot around the MTP joints.

Metatarsalgia is not, in itself, a diagnosis, but rather an anatomic description of where the patient is experiencing discomfort. *Successful treatment of this condition hinges on identifying the underlying cause.* A clear understanding of its etiologies and a systematic approach to examination are necessary to accomplish this. **Metatarsalgia is best characterized by pain under the metatarsal heads exacerbated by weight-bearing.**

The fatty cushion of the forefoot is a highly specialized tissue. Fibrous septae beneath the dermis compartmentalize the subcutaneous fat. When weight is applied, hydrostatic pressure builds within the compartments, dampening and dispersing forces on the plantar skin. This mechanism acts as a cushion, protecting the area from potentially damaging focal concentrations in pressure.

Inflammatory arthritis, trauma, or neuromuscular disorders can cause imbalances of flexion and extension forces around the small joints of the toes. Toe deformity is a consequence of this imbalance. Hyperextension at the MTP joint is a common component of these deformities and draws the fatty cushion of the forefoot distally and dorsally with the proximal phalanx (Fig. 5–53). When this occurs, the weight transferred through the metatarsal heads is applied to the thinner proximal skin without the intervening fatty cushion. Increases in local pressure result in a hyper-

Figure 5–53. With a claw toe, the MTP joint is hyperextended, essentially driving the metatarsal head into the ground. (From Coady CM, Gow MD, Stanish W: Foot problems in middle-aged patients: keeping active people up to speed. Physician Sports Med 26[5]:107–113, 1998.)

keratotic reaction of the plantar skin. This causes further increases in pressure, and eventually, a **painful intractable plantar keratosis (IPK)** forms (Fig. 5–54).

IPKs are often confused with plantar warts. Both cause hyperkerotic lesions of the plantar surface of the skin, which can be painful. However, plantar warts occur

A

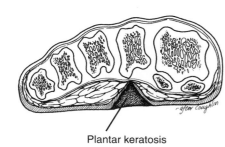

Plantar keratosis

B

Figure 5–54. *A,* Intractable plantar keratosis (IPK) under the second metatarsal head. *B,* Cross-section of the foot shows a discrete plantar keratosis beneath the prominent fibular condyle of a metatarsal head. (*A,* From Gould JS: Painful feet. In McCarthy DJ [ed]: Arthritis and Allied Conditions: A Textbook of Rheumatology, 11th ed. Philadelphia, Lea & Febiger, 1989, p. 1406; *B,* from Mizel MS, Yodlowski ML: Disorders of the lesser metatarsophalangeal joints. J Am Acad Orthop Surg 3:166–173, 1993.)

Figure 5–55. Synovitis leads to subluxation of the MTP joint. The fatty cushion is displaced dorsally with subluxation of the MTP joint. Pain occurs at the plantar aspect of the metatarsal. (From Mann RA, Coughlin MJ: Surgery of the Foot and Ankle, 6th ed. St. Louis, Mosby, 1993.)

as a result of infection of the epidermis with papillomavirus. Whereas the treatment of IPKs is mechanical (shaving, cushioning, relief pads), the treatment of symptomatic plantar warts is directed toward eradicating the infected tissue. Care should be used to ensure that the sometimes-caustic plantar wart preparations do not cause scarring of the plantar skin, which can be more painful than the initial wart. IPKs, unlike plantar warts, are almost always found directly below a weight-bearing area of the foot (e.g., metatarsal head). Plantar warts bleed with a characteristic "punctate" fashion when shaved, with multiple punctate areas of bleeding.

Synovitis and *instability* (Fig. 5–55) of the MTP joints can also cause pain along the metatarsal heads. Although **inflammatory arthritides** can incite this, the etiology *of the instability* is commonly mechanical. Chronic hyperextension of the MTP joints (claw toes) and flexion at the interphalangeal (IP) joints can occur in an attempt to accommodate a ***shoe toe box that is too small*** (Fig. 5–56). Eventually, this attenuates the plantar plate and collateral ligaments, leading to instability and subluxation

Callous from pressure of shoe

Callous (IPK)

Figure 5–56. IPK under the metatarsal head (plantar) and callosity at the proximal interphalangeal (PIP) joint (dorsally) from toe-box rub. A buckling effect may occur with concomitant hammertoe formation at the PIP joint and the development of an IPK beneath the second metatarsal head (cross-section of shoe). The same pressure that causes this callosity increases the pain under the metatarsal heads, or metatarsalgia. (From DeLee JC, Drez D Jr: Orthopaedic Sports Medicine: Principles and Practice. Philadelphia, WB Saunders, 1994.)

Figure 5–57. *A,* Medial deviation of the second toe (as a result of synovitis and subsequent alteration of the collateral ligaments and plantar plate) may be associated with development of acute pain in the second intermetatarsal space. *B,* Hyperextension of the second MTP joint may be associated with plantar capsular pain. (*A* and *B,* From Coughlin MJ: The crossover second toe deformity. Foot Ankle 8[1]:29–39, 1987.)

(Fig. 5–57). The toes can develop varus or valgus malalignment in relation because of this. Dorsal MTP joint dislocation is sometimes seen in severe cases.

Extra-articular cause of pain in the metatarsal region should also be considered. **Morton's neuroma** is a hypertrophy and subsequent irritation of the common interdigital nerve as it passes between the metatarsal heads. Inflammation of the intermetatarsal bursa and impingement by the intermetatarsal ligament are thought to contribute to the development of this condition. It most commonly affects the nerve of the third web space. It is often mistaken for synovitis (see Morton's neuroma section) and can coexist with it. It rarely involves more than one common digital nerve. The *tenderness* from a *stress fracture of the metatarsal* is typically in the metatarsal neck or shaft. These can be invisible on radiographs for several weeks *after onset.* Finally, pain from a herniated **lumbar disc, tarsal tunnel,** or other neurologic problem can be appreciated in the forefoot and is often mistaken for pain from a disorder *originating in the foot.*

History and Physical Examination

A careful history and physical examination are the most important tools for differentiating the etiologies of metatarsalgia. **This should begin with an evaluation of suitability of footwear in relation to the size of the foot.** Measure the patient's true shoe size and width, and then see what size shoe he or she wears into the office. A complete evaluation of the foot and ankle can disclose problems in other areas of the foot that may make the

forefoot painful. For instance, medial foot disorders can cause lateral forefoot pain because of lateral weight shifting. Weakness in the anterior tibial tendon can cause toe deformity through adaptive overuse of the extrinsic toe extensors, resulting in forefoot pain.

The **plantar skin** should be inspected for plantar keratoses. Paring these lesions is important, not only to decrease pressure but also to differentiate them from plantar warts. Plantar warts, unlike plantar keratoses, contain vessels within the keratinized tissue that are easily seen open and bleeding after paring. The interdigital spaces should also be inspected for soft corns. **Sensation** should be tested and **pulses** palpated. Careful palpation of the metatarsal heads and intermetatarsal spaces, localizing the exact area of tenderness, narrows the differential diagnosis.

Manual compression of the interspace (**Mulder's click**) can elicit crepitus, tenderness, and radiating pain from a Morton's neuroma (see Morton's neuroma section). A **drawer maneuver** of the MTP joint (Fig. 5–58) can detect articular stability problems. It is done by applying dorsally directed pressure to the plantar base of the proximal phalanx while stabilizing the metatarsal with the opposite hand.

The contralateral toes as well as the other toes on the ipsilateral foot should be evaluated to establish a baseline degree of normal translation on MTP joint drawer testing for each patient. MTP joint tenderness, swelling, and bogginess usually signify synovitis of the MTP joint, whereas pain with a relative increase in translation during MTP drawer testing usually signifies joint instability.

Figure 5–58. Drawer sign of the toe. *A,* The toe is grasped between the examiner's thumb and index finger. *B,* The toe is manipulated at the MTP joint in a plantar and dorsal direction. Instability is characterized by excess laxity (positive drawer) in the dorsal direction. (*A* and *B,* From DeLee JC, Drez D Jr: Orthopaedic Sports Medicine: Principles and Practice. Philadelphia, WB Saunders, 1994.)

Radiographic Evaluation

Radiographs are important to define forefoot deformities and identify neoplasms, fractures, dislocations, and arthritic joints that may contribute to pain in the metatarsal area. *The relative lengths of adjacent metatarsals should be compared, because discrepancies in metatarsal length can cause concentration of stress. Patients with significant shortening of the first metatarsal after a bunion operation sometimes develop pain under the second metatarsal (transfer metatarsalgia).* When combined with lead markers placed on the IPK skin, the radiographs help to identify prominent condyles or sesamoids under the metatarsal head that cause plantar keratoses. Isolated second metatarsal pain may be caused by **Freiberg's infraction** (Fig. 5–59).

Other imaging techniques, such as MRI and CT, are helpful only when specifically indicated and are not a routine part of the evaluation of metatarsalgia.

Although exercise and stretching offer little relief for most patients with metatarsalgia, **pedorthic management can figure prominently in the initial treatment.** For most patients who present with inappropriate (high heels) or tight shoewear, a discussion of the fit of the shoes should focus on the shape and room in the toe box for the toes. In addition, shoes with laces, stiff soles, and low heels help disperse and reduce the pressure on the forefoot. Occasionally, patients have severe fixed forefoot deformities that require prescription extradepth shoewear.

Full-length PPT and Plastizote or silicone insoles are very helpful in dispersing the pressure on tender areas in the forefoot. If this is unsuccessful, more sophisticated orthotic devices may be necessary. Soft metatarsal pads

Figure 5–59. Freiberg's infraction. This patient demonstrates deformity of the second metatarsal head. It is broadened, flattened, and somewhat sclerotic with osteophytes. Osteophytes have also developed at the base of the second proximal phalanx (degenerative changes superimposed on Freiberg's infraction). Note the thickened cortex of the shaft of the second metatarsal and the hallux valgus deformity. (From Brower A: Orthopaedic radiology. Orthop Clin North Am 14:112, 1983.)

made of felt or silicone (Fig. 5–60A) by themselves or added to a Spenco insert can be used to relieve pressure. Correct placement of the pad is crucial. *The crest of the pad* should be approximately 1 cm **proximal to the tender area** (see Fig. 5–60B). To help position the insert, lipstick or magic marker can be applied to the tender area on the foot and the patient asked to step on the insole, making apparent where to place the pad (1 cm proximal). A custom-molded accomodative insert can also be fabricated with a well-excavated well beneath the tender metatarsal to unload it (relief well).

Metatarsal bars can be built onto the shoe to unload the forefoot, but these tend to wear out quickly and encounter resistance from patients for cosmetic reasons. A rocker-bottom sole, along with a stiffener placed into the sole, helps reduce toe motion and disperse pressure away from the metatarsal heads.

Steroid injections combined with 1% lidocaine have a definite, but limited, role in diagnosing and treating pain due to synovitis or irritation of a Morton's neuroma from intermetatarsal bursitis.

Surgery is offered to patients in whom nonoperative treatment fails to relieve pain.

A

B

Figure 5–60. *A,* Felt Hapad (1-800-544-2733) should be placed 1 cm **proximal** to the metatarsal head(s) to "push" the metatarsal head(s) dorsally and decrease the pressure on them. We apply this pad on a full-length 1/8-inch PTT Plastizote insole or Spenco insole. *B,* Examples of felt supports that are extremely useful in alleviating areas of pressure beneath the metatarsal heads.

i   ii   iii   iv   v

C

Figure 5–60 *Continued. C,* Commonly used shoe pads for relief of painful conditions of the foot. *i,* Pad designed to relieve pressure on the sesamoids. *ii,* Pad to support various metatarsal heads (in this case, for treatment of Morton's neuroma). *iii,* Pad to support the short first metatarsal and relieve pressure on the lesser metatarsal heads. *iv,* Pad to support the longitudinal arch and relieve pressure on the metatarsal heads. *v,* Pad to relieve pressure on the metatarsal heads. (*B* and *C,* From Mann RA, Coughlin MJ: Surgery of the Foot and Ankle. St. Louis, Mosby, 1993.)

Differential Diagnosis of Metatarsalgia of the Foot
Brotzman

Metatarsalgia. Plantar pain under the lesser metatarsal heads exacerbated by weight-bearing. This may be exacerbated by hyperextension of the MTP joint (claw toe) driving the metatarsal head plantarward, fat pad atrophy, and the like. Transfer metatarsalgia occurs when a shortened metatarsal (e.g., iatrogenically or naturally "short" or incompetent first metatarsal [bunion]) does not allow well-distributed weight-bearing, and excess pressure is transferred laterally to the second, third, and possibly fourth and fifth metatarsals.

MTP joint synovitis. Inflammation of the MTP joints may occur (synovitis) with rheumatoid arthritis, cross-over toe deformity (see Fig. 5–57), and the like. This synovitis is typically boggy, swollen, and tender to palpation of the MTP joint both plantar **and dorsal.**

Arthritis of the MTP joints. This is confirmed on radiographs of the foot.

Morton's neuroma. Pain, numbness, burning, and tingling are localized to a discrete interspace (third or second) and not the MTP joint. Mulder's click and tenderness in the interspace are evident, *not* tender on palpation of the MTP joints (see section on Morton's neuroma).

Soft tissue tumor. Ganglion, synovial cyst, lipoma, neoplasm, rheumatoid nodule are examples.

IPK. A callosity is formed directly under a weight-bearing portion of the foot (e.g., metatarsal head). Usually a result of fat pad atrophy, claw toe, or excess pressure. The callosity (IPK) is formed by the body in response to repetitive excess pressure (see Fig. 5–54).

Abscess. This is usually hot, red, swollen, and fluctuant.

Stress fracture of the metatarsal(s). This may be confirmed by positive bone scan and/or eventual plain radiograph evidence of bone callous formation (≥2 wk postfracture).

Inflammatory arthritis may have multiple joint involvement, marker (HLA-B27), or systemic symptoms.

Neurogenic pain or burning

- Morton's neuroma.
- Tarsal tunnel—positive Tinel sign at the tibial nerve at the medial ankle and follows the medial and/or lateral plantar nerve distribution(s).
- Lumbar disc.
- Peripheral neuropathy.
- RSD.

Freiberg's infraction of second metatarsal. Pain occurs under the second metatarsal with radiographic findings compatible with Freiberg's (see Fig. 5–59).

Hallux Rigidus

Mark M. Casillas, MD, and Margaret Jacobs, PT

Clinical Background

The term **hallux rigidus** describes a limited arthrosis of the first MTP joint. The first MTP joint and the great toe (hallux) provide significant weight transfer from the foot to the ground as well as active push-off. An intact first MTP joint implies a complete and pain-free ROM, and full intrinsic and extrinsic motor strength.

The first MTP joint ROM is variable. The neutral position is described by 0 (or 180) degrees angulation between a line through the first metatarsal and a line through the hallux (Fig. 5–61). Dorsiflexion, the ROM

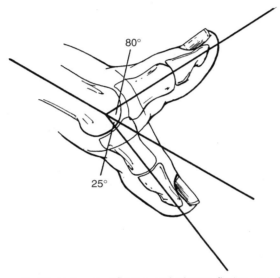

Figure 5–61. Hallux dorsiflexion and plantar flexion are determined by referencing the longitudinal axis of the first metatarsal. (From Coughlin MJ: Conditions of the forefoot. In DeLee JC, Drez D Jr: Orthopaedic Sports Medicine: Principles and Practice. Philadelphia, WB Saunders, 1994, p. 1861.)

above the neutral position, varies between 60 and 100 degrees (Fig. 5–62A). Plantar flexion, the ROM below the neutral position, varies between 10 and 40 degrees (see Fig. 5–62B). The ROM is noncrepitant and pain-free in the uninjured joint.

Two sesamoid bones (the medial, or tibial, sesamoid and the lateral, or fibular, sesamoid) provide mechanical advantage to the intrinsic plantar flexors by increasing the distance between the empirical center of the joint and the respective tendons.

Hallux rigidus is an arthritic condition limited to the dorsal aspect of the first MTP joint. Also known as a dorsal bunion or hallux limitus, the condition is most commonly idiopathic (but may be associated with post-traumatic OCD of the metatarsal head) and is characterized by an extensive dorsal osteophyte and dorsal third cartilage damage and loss. An associated synovitis may further aggravate the limited and painful ROM.

A foot with increased first ray ROM and increased pronation may be predisposed to the condition. Excessive flexibility of the shoe forefoot increases the potential for hyperdorsiflexion of the hallux MTP joint (Fig. 5–63). For this reason, this type of shoewear should be avoided.

Classification of Hallux Rigidus

A useful classification system grades clinical and radiographic findings from mild to end stage (Table 5–6).

Diagnosis

Clinical Examination

Patients with hallux rigidus complain of dorsal pain, swelling, and stiffness localized to the hallux MTP joint. The sitting examination may reveal decreased ROM in dorsiflexion and, to a lesser degree, in plantar flexion. The ROM becomes more and more painful as the condition advances. **Forced dorsiflexion reveals an abrupt**

A   **B**

Figure 5–62. Passive hallux dorsiflexion *(A)* and plantar flexion *(B)*.

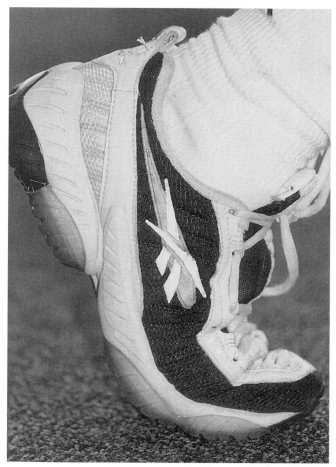

Figure 5–63. Excessive shoe flexibility at the forefoot increases the potential for hyperdorsiflexion of the hallux MTP.

Table 5–6

Hallux Rigidus Classification

Grade	Findings	Treatment
Mild	Near-normal ROM, pain with forced hyperdorsiflexion, tender dorsal joint, minimal dorsal osteophyte	Symptomatic
Moderate	Painful, limited dorsiflexion, tender dorsal joint, osteophyte on lateral radiograph	Symptomatic, consider early surgical repair
Severe	Painful, severely limited dorsiflexion, tender dorsal joint, large osteophyte on lateral radiograph, decreased joint space on AP radiograph	Symptomatic, consider surgical repair, dorsiflexion osteotomy
End-stage	Severe pain and limited motion, global arthrosis and osteophyte formation, with loss of joint space on all radiograph projections	Symptomatic, consider arthrodesis

ROM, range of motion.

Radiographic Evaluation

Standard radiographic evaluation includes AP and lateral views of the weight-bearing foot (Fig. 5–64). Bone scanning, CT, and MRI are capable of demonstrating the condition, but these are not part of a routine work-up.

The differential diagnosis of hallux rigidius is shown in Table 5–7.

Treatment

The treatment of hallux rigidus is symptom-based. ***Acute exacerbations*** are treated with the RICE (rest, ice, compression, and elevation) method followed by a gentle ROM program and protected weight-bearing. The ***chronic*** condition is treated with a ROM program and protected weight-bearing. The hallux MTP joint is

dorsal bony block associated with pain. Also, forced plantar flexion produces pain as the dorsal capsule and the extensor hallucis longus tendon are stretched across the dorsal osteophyte. The dorsal osteophyte is easily palpable and typically exquisitely tender.

A   **B**

Figure 5–64. Lateral views of foot preoperative (A) and postoperative (B) to excision of dorsal spur of the first metatarsal.

Table 5-7

Differential Diagnosis of First Ray Pain

Differential Diagnosis	Significant Findings
Hallux rigidus	Chronic condition **Limited dorsiflexion** **Dorsal osteophyte on lateral radiograph**
Hallux valgus (bunion)	Chronic condition Lateral deviation of great toe Tender medial eminence (not dorsal spur) Increased hallux valgus angle on radiograph
Hallux arthrosis (arthritic first MTP joint)	Chronic condition Painful and limited ROM **Loss of entire joint space on radiograph**
Gout	Acute severe pain Tenderness, erythema, joint irritability localized to first MTP Elevated uric acid Sodium urate crystals

MTP, metatarsophalangeal

Figure 5–65. Low-profile carbon plate shoe inserts increase shoe stiffness and decrease dorsiflexion of the first MTP joint.

supported by shoe modifications (e.g., rocker bottom sole), a rigid shoe insert (Fig. 5–65), a stiff-soled shoe, or various taping methods that resist forced dorsiflexion (Fig. 5–66). A soft upper and deep toe box reduce pressure over the dorsal osteophyte. The joint is also protected by reducing activity levels, increasing rest intervals and duration, and avoiding excessively firm play surfaces. Occasionally, a patient with excessive pronation will benefit

Figure 5–66. Dorsiflexion-limiting taping method: underwrap *(A)*, base or foundation *(B)*, 1-inch strips crossing on the plantar side of the joint *(C)*, and the circumferential cover to complete and secure the tape *(D)*.

A   B

Figure 5–67. Hallux MTP joint mobilization: gentle dorsal *(A)* and plantar *(B)* translation of the proximal phalanx relative to the metatarsal head.

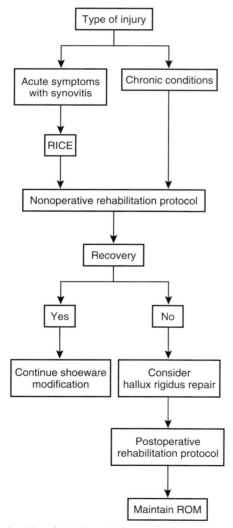

Figure 5–68. Treatment algorithm for hallux rigidus. RICE, rest, ice, compression, and elevation.

from an antipronation orthotic. NSAIDs and cold therapy are used to reduce swelling and inflammation. Occasionally, corticosteroid injection to the MTP joint is used as an adjunctive therapy.

Operative treatment is indicated for symptoms that fail to respond to a reasonable period of well-supervised conservative management (Fig. 5–67). Hallux MTP débridement and exostectomy are standard treatment for hallux rigidus. **Ideally, the intraoperative and postoperative passive ROM approaches 90 degrees of dorsiflexion.** If the arthrosis is extensive and this ROM not obtainable, **a dorsiflexion osteotomy** may be added to the surgical repair. The osteotomy is designed to place the functional ROM of the hallux within the newly established pain-free arc of motion. Patients with severe findings must be warned that outcomes become less predictable with advanced stages. CT images are useful in discriminating between severe hallux rigidus and frank degenerative joint disease. A hallux arthrodesis (fusion) is a more predictable reconstruction method for the most advanced cases of hallux rigidus. Pain relief is provided at the expense of permanent loss of joint motion.

Authors' Recommended Treatment (Figure 5–68)

The acutely swollen and painful hallux rigidus is treated with the RICE method for several days. For chronic conditions, a stiff-soled shoe with a soft upper is prescribed along with a rigid low-profile carbon insert. We often rocker-bottom the shoe. NSAIDs and ice are used as adjunct to reduce inflammation. Adequate rest and recovery are scheduled with increasing frequency and duration. If symptoms persist, or if the patient presents with moderate to severe findings, a hallux rigidus repair is considered. Adequate débridement and soft tissue release are done to achieve 90 degrees of intraoperative dorsiflexion. If the joint is globally affected (hallux arthrosis), a hallux arthrodesis is performed.

Nonoperative Rehabilitative Treatment of Hallux Rigidus

Occasionally, hallux rigidus is associated with a synovitis that is improved with nonoperative treatment. Fundamental to the protocol is the prevention of recurrent injury by limiting dorsiflexion of the hallux MTP with appropriate shoewear, rigid shoe inserts, or taping. Taping (by the trainer) is useful in athletic events, but is limited by time-related failure and the poor results with self-application. Off-the-shelf devices are readily available, and custom devices can be used for difficult sizes or specialty shoewear. The phases of rehabilitation are variable in length and depend completely on the reestablishment of ROM and resolution of pain. Flexibility is emphasized throughout the protocol.

Rehabilitation Protocol
Nonoperative Treatment of Hallux Rigidus
Casillas and Jacobs

Phase 1: Acute Phase—Days 0–6

- Rest, ice bath, contrast bath, whirlpool, and ultrasound for pain, inflammation, and joint stiffness.
- Joint mobilization (see Fig. 5–67), followed by gentle, passive, and active ROM.
- Isometrics around the MTP joint as pain allows.
- Isolated plantar fascia stretches with a can (Fig. 5–69) or golf ball.
- Cross-training activities, such as water activities and cycling, for aerobic fitness.
- Protective taping and shoe modifications for continued weight-bearing activities.

Phase 2: Subacute Phase—Weeks 1–6

- Modalities to decrease inflammation and joint stiffness.
- Emphasis on increasing flexibility and ROM, with both passive and active methods and joint mobilization.
- Plantar fascia stretching.
- Gastrocnemius stretching (Fig. 5–70).
- Progressive strengthening
  - Towel scrunches (Fig. 5–71).

Figure 5–69. Plantar fascia stretches are accomplished with a can rolled beneath the foot with varying amounts of force.

Rehabilitation Protocol
Nonoperative Treatment of Hallux Rigidus (Continued)
Casillas and Jacobs

A   B

Figure 5–70. *A,* Gastrocnemius stretching on an inclined box with the knee extended. *B,* The soleus is stretched more effectively by flexing the knee and relaxing the gastrocnemius muscle.

Figure 5–71. Towel scrunches. The towel is gathered by the toes.

- Toe pick-up activities (Fig. 5–72).
- Seated toe and ankle dorsiflexion with progression to standing (Fig. 5–73).
- Seated isolated toe dorsiflexion with progression to standing.
- Seated supination-pronation with progression to standing.
- Balance activities, with progression of difficulty to include BAPS board (Fig. 5–74).
- Cross-training activities (slide board, water running, cycling) to maintain aerobic fitness.

Phase 3: Return to Sport Phase—Week 7

- Continued use of protective inserts or taping.
- Continued ROM and strength exercises.
- Running, to progress within limits of a pain-free schedule.
- Monitored plyometric and cutting program, with progression of difficulty.

Care should be taken to avoid reinjury during these activities.

continued

Rehabilitation Protocol
Nonoperative Treatment of Hallux Rigidus (Continued)
Casillas and Jacobs

A

B

Figure 5–72. Toe pick-ups. A small object, in this case a ball of adhesive tape (A), is grasped by the toes (B).

Figure 5–73. Seated toe and ankle dorsiflexion.

Figure 5–74. Biomechanical Ankle Platform System (BAPS) board.

Rehabilitation Protocol
After Hallux Rigidus Cheilectomy (Removal of Dorsal Spur)
Casillas and Jacobs

General Principles
- Fundamental to postoperative rehabilitation is re-establishment of hallux MTP ROM in **dorsiflexion.**
- The surgical dressing is left undisturbed for 7–14 days.

- Full weight-bearing in a rigid postoperative shoe is allowed on the first postoperative day.
- Rehabilitation begins as soon as the wound appears stable, not necessarily before suture removal.

Rehabilitation Protocol
After Hallux Rigidus Cheilectomy (Removal of Dorsal Spur) *(Continued)*
Casillas and Jacobs

- The phases of rehabilitation are arbitrary in length and depend completely on the re-establishment of ROM and resolution of pain.
- Flexibility is emphasized throughout the protocol.

Phase 1: Acute Phase—Days 6–13

- Rest and ice for pain, inflammation, and joint stiffness.
- Joint mobilization followed by gentle, passive, and active ROM.
- Isometric around MTP joint as pain allows.
- Isolated plantar fascia stretches with can roll or frozen golf ball.
- Cross-training activities (such as cycling) to maintain aerobic fitness.
- Postoperative rigid shoe for continued weight-bearing for first 3 postoperative wk.

Phase 2: Subacute Phase—Weeks 2–6

- Ice, contrast bath, whirlpool, ultrasound to decrease inflammation and joint stiffness.
- Emphasis on increasing flexibility and ROM with both active and passive methods, with addition of joint and scar mobilization.
- Continued plantar fascia stretching.
- Gastrocsoleus stretching.

- Progressive strengthening
  - Towel scrunches.
  - Toe pick-up activities.
  - Manual resistive hallux MTP dorsiflexion and plantar flexion (Fig. 5–75).
  - Seated toe and ankle dorsiflexion, with progression to standing.
  - Seated isolated toe dorsiflexion, with progression to standing.
  - Seated supination-pronation, with progression to standing.
- Balance activities, with progression of difficulty to include BAPS board.
- Cross-training activities (slide board, water running, cycling) to maintain aerobic fitness.

Phase 3: Return to Sport Phase—Week 7

- Continued ROM and strength activities.
- Running, with progression within limits of pain-free schedule.
- Monitored plyometric and cutting program, with progression of difficulty.

Care must be taken to avoid exacerbation of postoperative pain and swelling.

A   B

Figure 5–75. Manual resistive hallux MTP dorsiflexion *(A)* and plantar flexion *(B)*.

First Metatarsophalangeal Joint Sprain (Turf Toe)

Mark M. Casillas, MD, and Margaret Jacobs, PT

Clinical Background

First MTP joint sprain (turf toe) is capable of producing significant impairment and disability in running athletes. Turf toe describes a range of injuries to the capsuloligamentous complex of the first MTP joint.

The first MTP joint ROM is variable. The neutral position is described by 0 (or 180) degrees angulation between a line through the first metatarsal and a line through the hallux (see Fig. 5–61). Dorsiflexion, the ROM above the neutral position, varies between 60 and 100 degrees. Plantar flexion, the ROM below the neutral position, varies between 10 and 40 degrees. The ROM is noncrepitant and pain-free in the uninjured joint.

The power to move the MTP joint is provided by both intrinsic (flexor hallucis brevis, extensor hallucis brevis, abductor hallucis, adductor hallucis) and extrinsic (flexor hallucis longus, extensor hallucis longus) muscle groups. Two sesamoid bones (medial, or tibial, sesamoid and lateral, or fibular, sesamoid) provide mechanical advantage to the intrinsic plantar flexors by increasing the distance between the empirical center of joint rotation and the respective tendons (Fig. 5–76). The sesamoid complex articulates with facets on the plantar aspect of the first metatarsal head and is stabilized by a plantar capsule (plantar plate) as well as a ridge (or crista) on the metatarsal head that separates the two sesamoids.

The mechanism of the first MTP joint sprain is forced dorsiflexion of the MTP joint (Fig. 5–77). The typical football-associated injury occurs when a player firmly plants his forefoot and is then struck from behind. The continued forward motion of the leg over the fixed forefoot produces hyperdorsiflexion of the first MTP joint and increased tension on the plantar plate and capsule. Taken to an extreme, these forces may continue and produce a dorsal impaction injury to the cartilage and bone of the metatarsal head.

The extreme motion required to produce an acute injury is more likely to occur in an **overly flexible shoe** as opposed to a relatively stiff-soled shoe (see Fig. 5–63). The **playing surface** has also been implicated as an asso-

ciated factor. The hard playing surface of an artificial turf field may result in an increased incidence first MTP joint sprain; hence, the term "turf toe." A chronic, cumulative injury mechanism is associated with similar risk factors.

The mechanism of injury for a first MTP joint sprain is by no means specific. A multitude of afflictions to the first MTP joint and its contiguous structures must be ruled out (Table 5–8).

Classification

Acute first MTP joint sprains are classified based on the degree of capsular injury (Clanton's classification) (Table 5–9).

Diagnosis

Signs and Symptoms

First MTP joint sprains are associated with acute localized pain, swelling, ecchymosis, and guarding. Increasing degrees of swelling, pain, and loss of joint motion are noted as the severity of the injury increases. An antalgic gait may be present as well a tendency to avoid loading of the first ray by foot supination.

Radiographic Evaluation

The standard radiographic evaluation includes AP and lateral views of the weight-bearing foot, as well as a sesamoid projection (Fig. 5–78). The diagnosis is confirmed on the MRI when capsular tears and associated edema are demonstrated. Bone scan, CT, and MRI may be used to rule out sesamoid avascular necrosis, sesamoid fracture, sesamoid stress injury, hallux MTP joint arthrosis, metatarsal-sesamoid arthrosis, or stenosing flexor tenosynovitis.

Treatment

The treatment of first MTP joint sprains is symptom based. ***Acute injuries*** are treated with the RICE (rest, ice, compression, elevation) method followed by a gentle ROM program and protected weight-bearing. ***Chronic injuries*** are treated with an ROM program and protected weight-bearing. The hallux MTP joint is supported by a variety of methods including walking cast, removable walking cast, rigid shoe modifications, rigid shoe inserts, stiff-soled shoes, and various taping methods (see Fig. 5–66). The joint is also protected by reducing activity levels, increasing rest intervals and duration, and avoiding rigid playing surfaces. Intra-articular steroids are of no benefit and may be detrimental to the joint.

Operative treatment is rare for isolated first MTP joint sprains. Occasionally, an associated condition is recognized and surgery becomes a treatment option (Table 5–10).

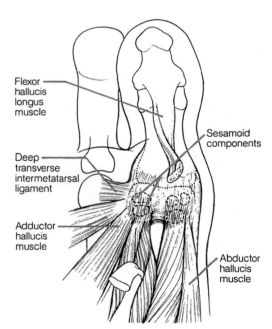

Figure 5–76. Anatomy of the MTP joint, which is affected in a turf toe injury. The tendons of the flexor hallucis brevis, adductor hallucis, and abductor hallucis muscles combine with the deep transverse metatarsal ligaments to form the fibrocartilaginous plate on the plantar aspect of the MTP joint capsule. The two sesamoid bones are contained within the fibrocartilaginous plate. (From Rodeo SA, O'Brien SJ, Warren RF, et al: Turf toe: diagnosis and treatment. Physician Sports Med 17[4]:132–140, 1989.)

Figure 5–77. *A,* The primary mechanism of **turf toe** occurs when the player's forefoot is fixed on the ground and the MTP joint is forced into hyperextension when another player falls across the dorsal surface of the first player's leg. *B,* A 0.51-mm spring steel shoe insert provides rigidity along the distal part of the shoe, preventing hyperextension of the MTP joint. The insert has a bilaminar construction. *C,* Disruption of the joint capsule in turf toe may result in separation of the components of a multipartite sesamoid. (*A–C,* From Rodeo SA, O'Brien SJ, Warren RF, et al: Turf toe: diagnosis and treatment. Physician Sports Med 17[4]:132–140, 1989.)

Prevention of turf toe includes the use of supportive footwear (with avoidance of overly flexible shoe forefoot) and firm inserts and avoidance of hard playing surfaces (e.g., Astroturf) when possible.

Authors' Recommended Treatment

The acute turf toe injury is treated with the RICE method for several days. This is followed by a secondary evaluation that allows a subacute staging to better delineate the location and degree of injury. For **low-grade injuries** that do not involve significant capsular tears, the patient is instructed to perform gentle ROM. Motion is limited during athletic activity by taping or shoe modification. For **moderate and severe injuries,** including severe capsular tears and dorsal articular fractures, the initial treatment is modified by a brief period of casting with a solid walking cast, or alternatively, a removable walking boot. Once the swelling and pain subside, attention is focused on re-establishing ROM. Activity is resumed once pain-free ROM is established.

Table 5-8

Pathology of the First Metatarsophalangeal Joint

Differential Diagnosis	Significant Findings	Differential Diagnosis	Significant Findings
First MTP joint sprain (turf toe)	Acute or chronic injury Tender MTP joint Limited motion		radiolucent line (cartilage) between the two ossicles, often mistaken for a fracture. Nontender to palpation, asymptomatic Comparison radiographs of the opposite foot may reveal a similar bipartile sesamoid. High incidence of bilaterality, so take a comparison radiograph to differentiate bipartite from a sesamoid fracture.
Hallux fracture	Acute injury Tenderness isolated to MTP or phalanx Fracture seen on radiograph, bone scan, CT, or MRI		
Hallux dislocation	Acute injury Severe deformity on examination, verified by radiograph		
Hallux rigidus	Chronic condition Limited dorsiflexion, painful ROM Dorsal osteophyte on lateral radiograph	Sesamoid arthrosis	Acute or chronic injury Painful ROM Tenderness isolated to sesamoid Arthrosis seen on radiograph, bone scan, CT, or MRI
Hallux arthrosis (arthritic first MTP joint)	Chronic condition Painful and limited ROM Loss of joint space on radiograph	Sesamoid avascular necrosis	Acute or chronic injury Tenderness isolated to sesamoid Fragmentation seen on radiograph, CT, or MRI
Sesamoid fracture	Acute injury Tenderness isolated to sesamoid Fracture seen on radiograph, bone scan, CT, or MRI	Stenosing flexor tenosynovitis	Overuse syndrome Trigger phenomenon Painful flexor hallucis longus (FHL) excursion Tenosynovitis seen on MRI
Sesamoid stress fracture	Chronic injury Tenderness isolated to sesamoid Stress fracture seen on radiograph, bone scan, CT, or MRI	Gout	Acute severe pain Tenderness, erythema, and joint irritability localized to first MTP Often elevated uric acid, sodium urate crystals on aspiration of joint
Sesamoid nonunion	Acute or chronic injury Tenderness isolated to sesamoid Nonunion seen on radiograph, bone scan, CT, or MRI		
Bipartite sesamoid	Congenital lack of fusion of the two ossicles of the sesamoid, leaving a		

Table 5-9

Classification of Metatarsophalangeal Joint Sprains (Turf Toe)—Clanton

Type	Objective Findings	Pathologic Condition	Treatment	Return to Sports
I	No ecchymosis Minimal or no swelling Localized plantar or medial tenderness	Stetching of capsulo-ligamentous complex	Ice/elevation NSAIDs Rigid insole Continued participation in athletics	Immediate
II	Diffuse tenderness Ecchymosis Pain, restriction of motion	Partial tear of capsuloligamentous complex	Same as type I Restriction of athletic activity for 7–145 days, depending on clinical course	1–14 days
III	Severe tenderness to palpation Considerable ecchymosis and swelling Marked restriction of motion	Tear of capsuloligamentous complex Compression injury of articular surface	Same as type II Crutches and limited weight-bearing If MTP dislocated, reduction and immobilization initially with case Restriction of athletic activity	3–6 wk

From Brotzman SB, Graves SG: Orthopaedic Knowledge Update: Sports Medicine, Griffin LY (ed.) Rosemont, Ill, American Academy of Orthopedic Surgeons, 1993.

Figure 5–78. Radiographic view of the sesamoid.

Table 5–10

Surgical Options for the First Metatarsophalangeal Joint

Injury	Surgical Treatment
Intra-articular loose body	Joint débridement
Hallux rigidus	Joint débridement and exostectomy (cheilectomy)
Hallux arthrosis	Arthroplasty (not silicone), Keller procedure, or MTP arthrodesis
Sesamoid nonunion	Bone graft
Sesamoid arthrosis	Sesamoid excision
Stenosing flexor tenosynovitis (FHL)	Flexor tunnel release
Hallux fracture or dislocation	Open reduction and internal fixation

Chronic turf toe is treated by activity and shoe modifications designed to limit ongoing injury. Shoe style, shoe inserts, playing surface, and taping are evaluated and adjusted to minimize pain and protect the MTP joint. NSAIDs and ice are used as adjuncts to reduce inflammation. Adequate rest and recovery must be scheduled with increased frequency and duration.

Rehabilitation for Turf Toe

Fundamental to the protocol is the prevention of recurrent injury by limiting hallux MTP dorsiflexion with appropriate shoe wear, taping, or rigid shoe inserts. Taping is useful but is limited by time-related failure and the poor results associated with self-application. Off-the-shelf devices, such a steel leaf plates and low-profile carbon fiber inserts, are readily available. Custom devices may be used for difficult sizes or specialty shoewear. The phases of rehabilitation are variable in length and depend completely on the re-establishment of ROM and resolution of pain. Flexibility is emphasized throughout the protocol.

Rehabilitation Protocol
Treatment of Turf Toe
Casillas and Jacobs

Phase 1: Acute Phase—Days 0–5

- Rest, ice bath, contrast bath, whirlpool, and ultrasound for pain, inflammation, and joint stiffness.
- Joint mobilization (see Fig. 5–67), followed by gentle, passive, and active ROM.
- Isometrics around the MTP joint as pain allows.
- Cross-training activities, such as water activities and cycling, for aerobic fitness.
- Protective taping and shoe modifications for continued weight-bearing activities.

Phase 2: Subacute Phase—Weeks 1–6

- Modalities to decrease inflammation and joint stiffness.
- Emphasis on increasing flexibility and ROM, with both passive and active methods and joint mobilization.
- Progressive strengthening
  - Towel scrunches (see Fig. 5–71).
  - Toe pick-up activities (see Fig. 5–72).
  - Manual resistive hallux MTP dorsiflexion and plantar flexion (see Fig. 5–75).

continued

Rehabilitation Protocol
Treatment of Turf Toe *(Continued)*
Casillas and Jacobs

- Seated toe and ankle dorsiflexion with progression to standing (see Fig. 5–73).
- Seated isolated toe dorsiflexion with progression to standing.
- Seated supination-pronation with progression to standing.
- Balance activities, with progression of difficulty to include BAPS (see Fig. 5–74).
- Cross-training activities (slide board, water running, cycling) to maintain aerobic fitness.

Phase 3: Return to Sport Phase—Week 7

- Continued use of protective inserts or taping.
- Continued ROM and strength exercises.
- Running, to progress within limits of a pain-free schedule.
- Monitored plyometric and cutting program, with progression of difficulty.

Care should be taken to avoid reinjury during these activities.

Ventral view

A

B

Figure 5–79. *A,* **Morton's neuroma** represents a proliferation of fibrous tissue surrounding the plantar nerve where the medial and lateral plantar branches approximate in the area between the third and the fourth metatarsal heads. The nerve is tethered proximally by the flexor digitorum brevis tendon and is stretched around the transverse metatarsal ligament as the toes naturally dorsiflex during ambulation. This repetitive trauma causes localized inflammation and irritation in the area of the third and fourth web space. *B,* Typical distribution of sensation affected by Morton's neuroma in the third interspace (although this has some variability). (*A,* From Mann RA, Coughlin MJ: Surgery of the Foot and Ankle, 6th ed. St. Louis, Mosby, 1993, p.560.)

Morton's Neuroma (Interdigital Neuroma)

Presentation

The most common presentation of an interdigital (Morton's) neuroma is pain located between the third and the fourth metatarsal heads (in the third interspace) (Fig. 5–79) that radiates into the third and fourth toes. Patients often describe this as a burning pain that intermittently "moves around." Usually, the pain is exacerbated by tight-fitting and/or high-heeled shoes or increased activity on the foot. The pain is often relieved by removing the shoe and rubbing the forefoot. Occasionally, these symptoms occur in the second interspace with radiation into the second and third toes. Seldom do neuromas occur in both interspaces simultaneously.

Table 5–11 presents a list of the preoperative symptoms given by patients (percentage) with an interdigital neuroma in Mann's series (1997).

Anatomy and Pathophysiology

The "classic" Morton neuroma is a lesion of the common digital nerve that supplies the third and fourth toes (see Fig. 5–79). This is not a true neuroma, but rather an irritated perineural fibrosis where the nerve passes plantar to the transverse metatarsal ligament (Fig. 5–80).

It has been speculated that because the common digital nerve to the third interspace has branches from the medial *and* lateral plantar nerves (and thus *increased thickness*) that this accounts for the third interspace being the one most commonly involved. The occasional involvement of the second interspace may be a result of anatomic variation in the distribution of the common digital nerves.

The incidence of interdigital neuromas is 8 to 10 times more common in females.

Table 5–11	
Percentage of Preoperative Symptoms Noted by Patients with Morton's Neuroma	
Symptom	**Incidence (%)**
Plantar pain increased by walking	91
Relief of pain by resting	89
Plantar pain	77
Relief of pain by removing shoes	70
Pain radiating into toes	62
Burning pain	54
Aching or sharp pain	40
Numbness in toes or foot	40
Pain radiating up foot or leg	34
Cramping sensation	34

From Mann R, Coughlin M: Surgery of the Foot and Ankle. St. Louis, Mosby, 1997.

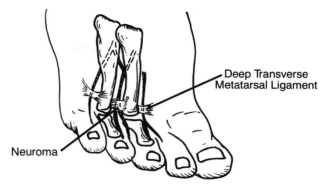

Figure 5–80. Interdigital neuroma. (From Mann RA, Coughlin MJ: Surgery of the Foot and Ankle, 6th ed. St. Louis, Mosby, 1993.)

The mechanism is probably chronic hyperextension of the MTP joints (in high heels) with tethering and irritation of the nerve across the transverse metatarsal ligament. This results in an entrapment neuropathy.

Diagnosis

The diagnosis of a Morton neuroma is clinical. There are no useful radiographic or electrodiagnostic tests. Serial examinations may be necessary to establish the correct diagnosis.

Examination

Direct palpation and palpation with a stripping motion (Fig. 5–81) of the interspace will usually reproduce the patient's pain. This maneuver, called **"Mulder's sign,"** often reproduces a clicking or popping sensation and pain

Figure 5–81. Mulder sign. The examiner places the index finger and thumb proximal to the metatarsals in the interspace, and while pushing firmly, strips the interspace distally. A pop or click reproducing the patient's pain should be elicited. (From Coughlin MJ, Pinsonneault T: Operative treatment of Interdigital neuroma. J Bone Joint Surg 83A[9]:1321–1328, 2001.)

in the third (or second) interspace. The examiner places the index finger and thumb proximal to the metatarsal heads in the interspace, and while pushing firmly into the interspace, "strips" distally to the end of the interspace, often feeling a click or pop that elicits pain (Mulder's click).

Widening of the involved (third and fourth) toes may be noted on occasion as a result of the neuroma mass in the interspace. Subjective numbness of the involved toes is often noted, but sensory examination may reveal partial, complete, or no sensory deficit in the nerve's distribution (see Fig. 5–79).

The patient with a Morton neuroma does not have pain over the metatarsal heads.

Occasionally, the examination will be positive only after a vigorous workout or tight shoewear. Often, the patient's physical examination is inconclusive and requires several serial examinations and a ruling out of related pathology.

A

B

Figure 5–82. *A,* Distribution of the medial and lateral plantar nerves on the bottom of the foot. *B,* Distribution of symptoms (numbness) on the plantar aspect (bottom *only*) of the foot associated with tarsal tunnel syndrome. (*A, Left,* Gray H: Anatomy: Descriptive and Surgical. Philadelphia, Henry C Tea, 1870, p. 660 *Right.* Modified from Mann RA, Coughlin MJ: Foot and Ankle Surgery, 6th ed. St. Louis, Mosby, 1993. *B,* from Chapman MW: Operative Orthopaedics. Philadelphia, JB Lippincott, 1988.)

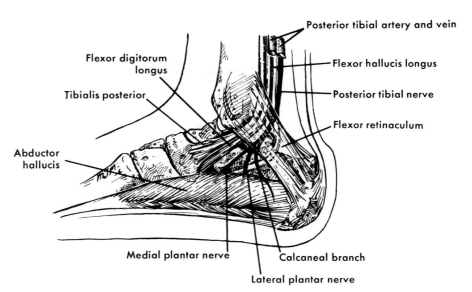

Figure 5–83. Tarsal tunnel syndrome.
A Tinel sign reproduces the pain and/or paresthesias on palpation of the tibial nerve of the medial ankle. The paresthesias occur in the distribution of the tibial nerve (plantar skin). This may involve the medial plantar nerve, the lateral plantar nerve, or both. (From Mann RA, Coughlin MJ: Surgery of the Foot and Ankle. St. Louis, Mosby, 1993, p. 554.)

Differential Diagnosis

Morton's neuroma may be mimicked by a number of other conditions. The following differential diagnoses should be considered to rule out an incorrect diagnosis of a Morton neuroma.

1. Neurogenic pain, tingling, or numbness
   - *Peripheral neuropathy* typically has more global numbness (entire foot or glove and stocking rather than in the interspace and its two toes) and is numb (not painful) unless early in the onset of neuropathy.
   - *Degenerative disc disease* often has accompanying motor, sensory, and reflex changes rather than numbness in a single interspace and its corresponding two toes.
   - *Tarsal tunnel syndrome* has a positive Tinel sign over the tarsal tunnel (medial ankle) and numbness limited to the **plantar** aspect of the foot (no dorsal foot numbness) (Figs. 5–82 and 5–83).
   - Lesions of the medial or lateral plantar nerves (see above).

2. MTP joint pathology
   - *Synovitis of the lesser MTP joint(s)* from rheumatoid arthritis or nonspecific synovitis has tenderness over the metatarsal head or MTP joint rather than the interspace (see Fig. 5–55).
   - *Fat pad atrophy* or degeneration of the plantar fat pad or capsule has tenderness over the metatarsal head or MTP joint rather than the interspace.
   - *Subluxation or dislocation* of the lesser MTP joints has tenderness over the metatarsal head or MTP joint rather than the interspace.
   - *Arthritis of the MTP joint* has tenderness over the metatarsal head or MTP joint rather than the interspace.

3. Plantar foot lesions
   - *Synovial cysts* is usually a tender mass but no numbness or tingling.
   - *Soft tissue tumors of the interspace*: ganglion, synovial cyst, lipoma, soft tissue neoplasm; usually a tender mass but no numbness or tingling.
   - *Abscess.* Plantar abscess foot. Usually, a tender mass but no numbness or tingling.

Treatment

Rehabilitation Protocol
After Morton's Neuroma Excision
Brotzman

- Maximal elevation of foot as much as possible for 72 hr.
- Light, compressive, well-padded forefoot dressing in a wooden shoe for approximately 3 wk.
- Weight-bearing as tolerated with crutches for 1–14 days postoperative.

- Work on ankle active ROM exercises and stretching to avoid stiffening of the ankle.
- At 3–4 wk, begin using a wide, soft, comfortable loosely laced tennis shoe, low-impact activities (e.g., bicycling).

Rehabilitation Protocol
Initial Nonoperative Treatment of Morton's Neuroma (Interdigital Neuroma)
Brotzman

Shoe Modification

- Use soft, wide comfortable shoe with a *wide* toe box, allowing the foot to spread out and relieve metatarsal pressure on the nerve. Women should go to men's tennis shoes because of the increased width in men's shoes.
- Employ low heels to avoid hyperextension of the metatarsophalangeal joints associated with high heels.
- Change the lacing pattern on shoes to avoid pressure across the forefoot.

Pads in the Shoe

- A metatarsal pad (Hapad) placed proximal to the involved metatarsal may relieve some pressure on the inflamed area. We put the Hapad in the right place (proximal to the metatarsal heads) by using a Magic Marker to mark the balls of the foot (Fig. 5–84) then place the pad just proximal to the ink marks left by the metatarsal heads.

Injection of the Interspace

- Injection of a small amount of 1% lidocaine *without* epinephrine (2–3ml) and 1ml of cortisone may be a useful diagnostic tool (Fig. 5–85). Relief of symptoms often indicates a painful neuroma. The physician should inject the medicine in the affected interspace.
- The use of injected corticosteroids is helpful. Greenfield and associates noted that 80% of injected neuromas had relief that lasted more than two yr.

Many physicians use NSAIDs for two wk in an attempt to decrease inflammation.

If the patient has continued symptoms despite shoe wear modification, padding, and cortisone injection, surgical resection of the Morton neuroma is indicated.

Figure 5–84. With the heel in the correct position in the orthotic, mark the metatarsal heads you wish to pad (e.g., third and fourth) with marker; then lower the foot onto the insert. This leaves a dark black circle on the insert. Place the Hapad just proximal to these circles.

Figure 5–85. Area of injection of 1 ml of cortisone (e.g., 40 mg of Depo-Medrol) and 1 ml of 1% lidocaine without epinephrine to decrease the size and irritation of the Morton neuroma.

Bibliography

Plantar Fasciitis (Heel Pain)

Baxter DE, Thigpen CM: Heel pain: operative results. Foot Ankle Int 5:16, 1984.

Berman DL: Diagnosing and treating heel injuries in runners. Phys Asst 3(3):331, 1986.

Campbell JW, Inman VT: Treatment of plantar fascitis with UCBL insert. Clin Orthop 103:57, 1974.

DeMaio M, Paine R, Mangine RE, Drez D Jr: Plantar fascitits. Orthopedics 10:1153, Review 1993.

Doxey GE: Calcaneal pain: a review of various disorders. J Orthop Sports Phys Ther 9:925, 1987.

Dreeban SM, Mann RA: Heel pain: sorting through the differential diagnosis. J Musculoskel Med 9:21, 1992.

Graham CE: Painful heel syndrome. J Musculoskel Med 3:42, 1986.

Jahss MH, et al: Investigations into the fat pads of the sole of the foot: anatomy and histology. Foot Ankle Int 13:233, 1992.

James SL, Bates BT, Osternig LR: Injuries to runners. Am J Sports Med 6:40, 1978.

Kosmahl EM, Kosmahl HE: Painful plantar heel, plantar fasciitis, and calcaneal spur: etiology and treatment. J Orthop Sports Phys Ther 9:17, 1987.

Leach RE, Schepsis A: When hindfoot pain slows the athlete. J Musculoskel Med 9:82, 1992.

Leach RE, Seavey MS, Salter DK: Results of surgery in athletes with plantar fasciitis. Foot Ankle Int 7:156, 1986.

Noyes FE, DeMaio M, Mangine RE: Heel pain. Orthopedics 16:1154, 1993.

Rask MR: Medial plantar neuropraxia (joggers's foot): report of 3 cases. Clin Orthop 134:193, 1987.

Schepsis AA, Leach RE, Goryzca J: Plantar fasciitis. Clin Orthop 266:185, 1991.

Tanner SM, Harvey JS: How we manage plantar fasciitis. Physician Sports Med 16(8):39, 1988.

Tanz SS: Heel pain. Clin Orthop 28:169.

Wapner KL, Sharkey PF: The use of night splints for treatment of recalcitrant plantar fasciitis. Foot Ankle Int 12:135, 1991.

Chronic Lateral Instability

Hamilton WG: Foot and ankle injuries in dancers. Clin Sports Med 1:143, Review 1988.

Hamilton WG, Thompson FM, Snow SW: The modified Brostrom procedure for lateral instability. Foot Ankle 1:1, 1993.

Posterior Tibial Tendon Insufficiency

Frey C, Shereff M, Greenidge N: Vascularity of the posterior tibial tendon. J Bone Joint Surg Am 6:884, 1990.

Holmes GB Jr, Mann RA: Possible epidemiological factors associated with rupture of the posterior tibial tendon. Foot and Ankle 2:70, 1992.

Johnson K: Tibialis posterior tendon rupture. Clin Orthop 177:140, 1983.

Johnson KA, Strom DE: Tibialis posterior tendon dysfunction. Clin Orthop 239:206, 1989.

Hallux Rigidus

Bingold AC, Collins DH: Hallux rigidus. J Bone Joint Surg 32B:214, 1950.

Mann RA, Clanton TO: Hallux rigidus treatment by cheilectomy. J Bone Joint Surg 70A:400, 1988.

Mann RA, Coughlin MJ, DuVries HL: Hallux rigidus: a review of the literature and a method of treatment. Clin Orthop 142:57, 1979.

McMaster MJ: The pathogenesis of hallux rigidus. J Bone Joint Surg 60B:82, 1978.

Moberg E: A simple operation for hallux rigidus. Clin Orthop 142:55, 1979.

First Metatarsophalangeal Joint Pain (Turf Toe)

Bowers KD Jr, Martin RB: Turf-toe: a shoe-surface related football injury. Med Sci Sports Exerc 8:81, 1976.

Clanton TO: Athletic injuries to the soft tissues of the foot and ankle. In Coughlin MJ, Mann RA (eds). Surgery of the Foot and Ankle. St. Louis, Mosby, 1999, p. 1184.

Clanton TO, Butler JE, Eggert A: Injuries to the metatarsophalangeal joint in athletes. Foot Ankle 7:162, 1986.

Coker TP, Arnold JA, Weber DL: Traumatic lesions to the metatarsophalangeal joint of the great toe in athletes. Am J Sports Med 6:326, 1978.

Mortor's Neuroma

Greenfield J, Rea J Jr, Ilfeld FW: Morton's interdigital neuroma: indications for treatment by local injections versus surgery. Clin Orthop 185:142, 1984.

Mann RA, Coughlin MJ: Surgery of the Foot and Ankle, 6th ed. St. Louis, Mosby, 1993.

Chapter 6
The Arthritic Lower Extremity

Hugh Cameron, MD, and S. Brent Brotzman, MD

Osteoarthritis is the most prevalent joint disease in the United States, afflicting an estimated 43 million people. A report by the Centers for Disease Control and Prevention indicated that patients with arthritis have substantially worse health-related quality of life than those without it.

The Arthritic Hip

Clinical Background

Arthritis of the hip can result from many causes, such as childhood sepsis, slipped capital epiphysis, and rheumatoid arthritis. About 30% of all patients with hip arthritis have a mild form of acetabular dysplasia (a shallow socket), and 30% have a retroverted socket. Both of these conditions **reduce the contact area** of the femoral head in the acetabulum, which increases the pressure and makes wear more likely. Approximately 30% of patients have no obvious risk factors.

Disorders of the Hip Joint for Which Total Hip Arthoplasty May Be Indicated

Arthritis
  Rheumatoid
  Juvenile rheumatoid (Still's disease)
  Pyogenic—resolved infection

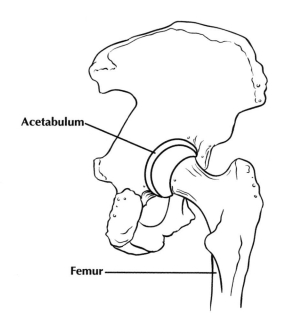

Acetabulum

Femur

Arthritis of the hip is marked by progressive loss of articular cartilage with joint space narrowing and pain. **Stiffness** encourages development of osteophyte formation (bone spurs), which in turn lead to further stiffness, making it difficult for the patient to put on socks and shoes. This eventually leads to the general picture of shortening, adduction deformity, and external rotation of the hip, often with a fixed flexion contracture. Bone loss usually occurs slowly, but in AVN occasionally it occurs precipitously.

General Features of Osteoarthritis*

- A heterogeneous group of conditions that share common pathologic and radiographic features.
- Focal loss of articular cartilage in part of a synovial joint is accompanied by hypertrophic reaction in the subchondral bone and joint margin.
- Radiographic changes of joint space narrowing, subchondral sclerosis, cyst formation, and marginal osteophytes.
- Common and age-related, with identified patterns of involvement targeting the hands, hips, knees, and apophyseal joints of the spine.
- Clinical findings often include joint pain with use, stiffness of joints after a period of inactivity, and lost range of motion (ROM).

Primary Symptoms and Signs of Osteoarthritis*

Symptoms

- Pain during activity
- Stiffness after inactivity (stiffness usually lasts less than 30 min)
- Loss of movement (difficulty with certain tasks)
- Feelings of insecurity or instability
- Functional limitations and handicap

Signs

- Tender spots around joint margin
- Firm swellings of the joint margin
- Coarse crepitus (creaking or locking)
- Mild inflammation (cool effusions)
- Restricted, painful movements
- Joint "tightness"
- Instability (obvious bone or joint destruction)

Disorders of the Hip Joint for Which Total Hip Arthoplasty May Be Indicated *(Continued)*

Ankylosing spondylitis
Avascular necrosis (AVN)
　Postfracture or dislocation
　Idiopathic
Bone tumor
Cassion's disease
Degenerative joint disease
　Osteoarthritis (OA)
Developmental dysplasia of the hip (DDH)
Failed hip reconstruction
　Cup arthroplasty
　Femoral head prosthesis
　Girdlestone procedure
　Resurfacing arthroplasty
　Total hip replacement
Fracture or dislocation
　Acetabulum
　Proximal femur
Fusion or pseudarthrosis of hip
Gaucher's disease
Hemoglobinopathies (sickle cell disease)
Hemophilia
Hereditary disorders
Legg-Calvé-Perthes disease (LCPD)
Osteomyelitis (remote, not active)
　Hematogeneous
　Postoperative osteotomy
Renal disease
　Cortisone-induced
　Alcoholism
Slipped capital femoral epiphysis (SCFE)
Tuberculosis

*From Dieppe P: Osteoarthritis: Are we asking the wrong questions? Br J Rheumatol Aug 23(3):161, 1984.

Findings in Common Conditions of the Pelvis, Hip, and Thigh

Osteoarthritis of the Hip

- ***Pain reproduced by passive internal rotation of the hip.***
- Tenderness over the anterior hip capsule (variable).
- Restricted ROM (rotation is usually affected first).
- Pain reproduced by Stinchfield test.
- Abductor limp (with severe involvement).
- Functional leg-length discrepancy (if abduction contracture has developed).

Posterior Hip Dislocation

- MVA or history of major trauma.
- Hip held in position of flexion, internal rotation, and adduction.
- Possible concomitant sciatic nerve injury (weakness of dorsiflexion and plantar flexion of the ankle).

Anterior Hip Dislocation

- MVA or history of major trauma.
- Hip held in position of mild flexion, abduction, and external rotation.
- Possible associated femoral nerve injury (quadriceps weakness).

Hip Fracture

- Tenderness over the anterior hip capsule or the intertrochanteric region.
- Limb externally rotated and shortened (displaced fracture).
- Stinchfield test painful or cannot be done.

Pelvic Fracture or Disruption

- Tenderness of pubic symphysis, iliac crest, or sacroiliac joint.
- Pain in response to pelvic compression tests (lateral and anteroposterior [AP] pelvic compression tests, pubic symphysis stress test).
- Pain with Patrick test or Gaenslen test (especially in fractures of the sacroiliac joint).

Sacroiliac Joint Dysfunction

- Tenderness over the sacroiliac joint.
- Pain with Patrick test or Gaenslen test (especially in the sacroiliac joint).

Entrapment of the Lateral Femoral Cutaneous Nerve (Meralgia Paresthetica)

- Altered sensation over the anterolateral thigh.
- Symptoms reproduced by pressure or percussion of the nerve just medial to the anterior superior iliac spine.

Piriformis Tendinitis

- Tenderness to deep palpation near the hook of the greater trochanter.
- Pain reproduced by piriformis test.

Gluteus Maximus Tendinitis

- Tenderness at the gluteal fold at the inferior aspect of the gluteus maximus.
- Pain reproduced by Yeoman test.

Gluteus Minimus Tendinitis

- Tenderness just proximal to the greater trochanter.
- Pain reproduced by resisted abduction of the hip.

Trochanteric Bursitis

- Tenderness over the lateral aspect of the greater trochanter.
- Popping or crepitation felt with flexion-extension of the hip (occasionally).
- Tight iliotibial tract revealed by Ober test (variable).

Quadriceps Strain or Contusion

- Tenderness and swelling of the involved area of the quadriceps.
- Weakness of quadriceps contraction.

continued

Findings in Common Conditions of the Pelvis, Hip, and Thigh (Continued)

- Restriction of knee flexion, especially when the hip is extended.
- Palpable divot in the quadriceps (more severe injuries).
- Warmth and firmness in quadriceps (impending myositis ossificans).

Hamstring Strain

- Localized tenderness and swelling at the site of injury.
- Ecchymosis (frequently).
- Restricted knee extension and straight leg raises (SLR) from posterior hamstring pain.
- Palpable divot in the injured hamstring (more severe injuries).
- Abnormal tripod sign.

Modified from Reider B: The Orthopaedic Physical Examination. Philadelphia, WB Saunders, 1999.

Classification of Hip Arthritis

The radiographic appearance of OA can be classified as (1) **concentric,** in which there is uniform loss of articular cartilage, (2) **downward and medial migration** of the femoral head, or (3) **upward migration** and **superolateral migration** of the femoral head. This is important if a corrective osteotomy is considered, but is otherwise of no significance.

Diagnosis of Hip Arthritis

Hip pain can be simulated by referred pain from the spine, L3–4 sciatica, and stenosis of the internal iliac artery. Causes of referred pain must be ruled out. *The classic clinical test for hip arthritis is internal rotation of the hip in flexion.* With hip arthritis, this internal rotation will be limited and painful. **Differential diagnoses** include hip dislocation, hip fracture, pelvic fracture or disruption, entrapment of the lateral femoral cutaneous nerve, tendinitis of the piriformis or gluteus maximus or minimus tendons, trochanteric bursitis, L3–4 sciatica, spine referred pain, internal iliac artery stenosis, and strain or contusion of the quadriceps or hamstring muscles.

Radiographic examination includes an AP view of the pelvis and AP and lateral views of the hip. **The lateral view must be a modified frog-leg lateral or Lauenstein.** A shoot-through lateral is of no value to the surgeon because it gives a distorted picture of the femur. Serologic investigations are seldom required. The only indication for further imaging studies such as bone scanning and MRI is suspected AVN in the absence of radiologic findings.

Treatment of Hip Arthritis

Anti-inflammatories and analgesics are of some value (albeit limited). In general, nonsteroidal anti-inflammatory drugs (NSAIDs) act by reversibly inhibiting the cyclo-oxygenase or lipo-oxygenase side of arachidonic acid metabolism. This effectively blocks the production of proinflammation agents such as prostaglandins and leukotrienes. Also inhibited are the beneficial effects of prostaglandins, including protective effects on the gastric mucosal lining, renal blood flow, and sodium balance. Unlike aspirin, which has an irreversible anti-platelet effect persisting for the life of the platelet (10 to 12 days), NSAID bleeding times usually correct within 24 hours of their discontinuation.

Dyspepsia (GI upset) is the most common side effect of NSAIDs. Other potential side effects include gastrointestinal ulceration, renal toxicity, hepatotoxicity, and cardiac failure.

Contraindications to the use of NSAIDs include history of GI disease, renal disease, hepatic disease, or simultaneous anticoagulation therapy. The American College of Rheumatology recommends annual CBC, liver function, and creatinine testing in patients on a course of prolonged NSAID use. Hemograms and fecal occult blood testing are recommended both before initiating NSAIDs and regularly thereafter.

Because of its favorable side-effect profile and equivalent efficacy in pain relief (Bradley, Brandt, Katz, et al 1991), Tylenol has become accepted as a first-line analgesic agent by the orthopaedic and rheumatologic communities. The recommended dosage of acetaminophen is 650 mg every 4 to 6 hours prn, to a maximum dosage of 4,000 mg per day. A dose of 1000 mg three times a day is usually sufficient. **Neutraceuticals** such as chondroitin sulfate and glucosamine are popular but unproven.

Glucosamine and chondroitin sulfate are synergistic endogenous molecules in articular cartilage. Glucosamine is thought to stimulate chondrocyte and synoviocyte metabolism, and chondroitin sulfate is believed to inhibit degredative enzymes and prevent formation of fibrin thrombi in periarticular tissues (Ghosh, Smith and Wells, 1992).

A minimum of 1 gram of glucosamine and 1,200 mg of chondroitin sulfate per day are the standard recommended doses. The average cost of this oral therapy is 50 dollars per month.

A **cane** in the opposite hand helps to unload the hip significantly (Fig. 6–1). A properly fitted cane should reach the top of the patient's greater trochanter of the hip while wearing shoes. **Stretching** and strengthening exercises or joining a yoga class can be of surprising value in terms of regaining ROM because it may be stiffness (e.g., the inability to put on shoes and socks) rather than pain that makes surgery necessary.

Hip abductors

Figure 6–1. Use of a cane redirects the force across the hip. Without the cane, the resultant force across the hip is about three times body weight because the force of the abductors acts on the greater trochanter to offset body weight and levels the pelvis in single stance. (From Kyle RF: Fractures of the hip. In Gustilo RB, Kyle RF, Templeton D [eds]: Fractures and Dislocations. St. Louis, Mosby, 1993.)

Exercises for the Arthritic Hip (NOT after Total Hip Replacement)

We use exercises that strengthen and stretch the muscles and capsule of the arthritic hip, incorporating motion and strength needed by the patient for daily functioning. **These exercises are for the arthritic hip, *not after hip replacement.***

Leg Rotations (Fig. 6–2)

1. Lying on your back, straighten your right leg and bend your left knee to take strain off your back.
2. Point your toes (right foot) up to the ceiling; then rotate the leg clockwise and hold 10 sec. Then rotate the foot counterclockwise, pointing again at the ceiling; then point inward toward the left side of the body.

Number of repetitions: repeat for each leg, 10 times a set.

Number of sets: 2 a day.

Figure 6–2. Leg rotations. The patient internally and externally rotates the hip while lying supine. (From Patient handout. Women's Health Orthop Ed 2[4]:62, Aug-Sept 1999.)

continued

Exercises for the Arthritic Hip (NOT after Total Hip Replacement) (Continued)

Leg Raises (Fig. 6–3)

1. Stand next to a chair and lean on it for support.
2. Raise your left leg to the front as far as you can, keeping it straight.
3. Lower your left leg and repeat the exercise with your right leg.
4. Face the chair, and leaning on it for support, lift your left leg out to the side as far as you comfortably can.
5. Lower your left leg and repeat the exercise with your right leg.

Number of repetitions: 10–15.

Number of sets: 2 a day.

Figure 6–3. Leg raises. (From Patient handout. Women's Health Orthop Ed 2[4]:62, Aug-Sept 1999.)

Knee Cross-Overs (Fig. 6–4)

1. Lie on your right side on a bed or floor, resting your head on your right arm. For support, bend your left arm in front of your chest. Straighten your legs.
2. Bend your left knee and pull it toward your chest. Your left foot should have moved close to your right knee.
3. Cross your left knee over your right leg and down toward the bed or floor.
4. Keeping your left foot on your right knee, lift the left knee and return it to its starting position in step 2.
5. Roll onto your left side and repeat the exercise with your right leg.

Number of repetitions: 10–15.

Number of sets: 2 a day.

Figure 6–4. Knee cross-overs. (From Patient handout. Women's Health Orthop Ed 2[4]:62, Aug-Sept 1999.)

Strengthening Exercises

Leg Scissors against Resistance (Fig. 6–5)

1. Loop elastic tubing over your ankles, calves, or thighs.
2. Lie on your back on a bed or floor and extend your legs straight in front of you. Let your arms rest at your sides.
3. Spread your legs as far apart as you can, moving them against the resistance of the elastic tubing, and then bring them back together. (If your doctor permits, you may raise your legs slightly off the bed or floor before spreading them.)

Number of repetitions: 5–10.

Number of sets: 2–3 a day.

Figure 6–5. Leg scissors against resistance. (From Patient handout. Women's Health Orthop Ed 2[4]:62, Aug-Sept 1999.)

Exercises for the Arthritic Hip (NOT after Total Hip Replacement) *(Continued)*

Straight Leg Lifts (Fig. 6–6)

1. Lie on your back. Keep both knees bent and your feet flat on the floor or bed. Let your arms rest at your sides.
2. Straighten your right leg, and then, while keeping your knee straight, lift it as high as you can.
3. Lower your leg slowly to the floor and bend your knee, returning to your starting position.
4. Repeat the exercise with your left leg.

Number of repetitions: 10–15.

Number of sets: 2 a day.

Figure 6–6. Straight leg raises. (From Patient handout. Women's Health Orthop Ed 2[4]:62, Aug-Sept 1999.)

Knee-to-Chest Lifts (Fig. 6–7)

1. Lie on your back. Keep both knees bent and your feet flat on the floor or bed. Let your arms rest at your sides.
2. Bend your right leg at the hip, bringing your knee as close to your chest as you can.
3. Lower your leg slowly to its starting position, and relax.
4. Repeat the exercise with your left leg.

Number of repetitions: 10.

Number of sets: 2–3 a day.

Figure 6–7. Knee-to-chest lifts. (From Patient handout. Women's Health Orthop Ed 2[4]:62, Aug-Sept 1999.)

Side Kicks (Fig. 6–8)

1. Lie on your right side, resting your head on your right arm. For support, bend your left arm in front of your chest and bend your right knee.
2. Keeping your upper (left) leg straight and in line with your body, lift it as high as you can. Make sure that your toes remain pointing forward.
3. Hold the position for a few seconds; then lower your leg slowly.
4. Turn on your left side and perform the side kicks with your right leg.

Number of repetitions: 10–15.

Number of sets: 2 a day.

Figure 6–8. Side kicks. (From Patient handout. Women's Health Orthop Ed 2[4]:62, Aug-Sept 1999.)

continued

Exercises for the Arthritic Hip (NOT after Total Hip Replacement) *(Continued)*

Minimal Sit-Downs (Flexing the Knees Only 30 Degrees)
(Fig. 6–9)

1. Stand in front of a chair or up against the wall. Let your arms rest at your sides.
2. Bend your hips and knees and begin to lower yourself into a sitting position.
3. Stop when you are halfway into the chair, or 30 degrees of bend, and return to a standing position. Do not use your hands and arms to help lower and raise yourself. Do *not* bend the knees deeply. This should barely bend the knees (have your therapist show you 30 degrees of knee flexion).

Number of repetitions: 10–15.

Number of sets: 2 a day.

Figure 6–9. A 30–degree mini-squat with the patient standing over a chair.

Note: Do not lower yourself to the point where you cannot stand up using your leg muscles or so far that your knees hurt.
From Eichner ER: Patient handout for the arthritic hip. Women's Health Orthop Edition 2(4):1, Aug–Sept, 1999.

Table 6–1

Suggested Exercise Plan for Patients with Osteoarthritis of the Hips*

Mild Symptoms	Moderate to Severe Symptoms (Pain on Range of Motion)
Active ROM exercises.	Active-assisted ROM exercises.
Stretches for hip flexor, adductor, iliotibial band, and gastrocnemius muscles and for hamstring tendons.	Stretches.
	Isometric strengthening only when ROM is less painful.
Strengthening (belt exercises, leg lifts, closed kinetic chain, standing on one foot, walking).	Physical therapy modalities as needed.
Aerobic conditioning (preferably walk 1 hr five times a week).	Unloaded ambulation (**Aquasizer, pool,** grocery cart, cane, walker). Start at comfortable duration (1 min if necessary), once to several times a day, gradually increasing to 45 min. Then gradually reload (shallower water, less pressure on cane) until fully loaded for 1 hour three to five times a week.
Aquatic therapy in warm water (not a hot tub) to "unload."	

*Patients with mild symptoms receive one or two physical therapy visits. Patients with moderate to severe symptoms see a therapist daily for 1–2 wk, then three times a week for 1–2 mo, then once a week for 1–4 wk, then once a month for a total of approximately 6 mo until they are advancing independently.
OA, osteoarthritis; ROM, range of motion.
From Ike RW, Lampman RM, Castor CW: Arthritis and aerobic exercise: a review. Phys Sports Med 17(2):27–31, 1989.

Table 6–2

Exercise Devices Suitable for Patients with Arthritis

	Joints Stressed				
	Hip	Knee	Ankle	Shoulder	Spine
Stationary bicycle	+ +	+ +	+	−	+
Arm-crank ergometer	−	−	−	+ +	+ +
Rowing machine	−	−	−	+ +	+ +
Cross-country skiing machine	+	±	±	±	+
Climbing machine	+ +	+ +	+ +	+	+
Water-running with limited-buoyancy vest	−	−	−	±	±

+ +, greatly stressed; +, stressed; ±, somewhat stressed; −, not stressed.
From Ike W, Lampman RM, Castor W: Arthritis and aerobic exercise: a review. Physician Sports Med 17(2):27–31, 1989.

Table 6–3

Aerobic Conditioning Protocol for Patients with Arthritis (Low to Moderate Intensity on Bicycle Ergometer)

Frequency	Three times a week
Workload	Resistance that attains 70% of maximal heart rate at 50 rpm in a stable class 1 or 2 patient
Structure	Five exercise sessions separated by one-min rest periods
Progression of *exercise time* initially	2 min (low intensity) 15 min (moderate intensity)
Rate of increase	2 minutes every 2 wk
Maximum	15 min/session (low intensity) 35 min/session (moderate intensity)

From Ike RW, Lampman RM, Castor CW: Arthritis and aerobic exercise: a review. Physician Sports Med 17(2):27–31, 1989.

Figure 6–10. Total hip replacement. (From Howmedica Instructional Handout. Salt Lake City, Howmedica Press, 1993, p2.)

Operative Options for Hip Arthritis

Osteotomies, such as pelvic and intertrochanteric osteotomies, were popular in the past, and they still may have a limited role in selected situation. **Fusion** still does have a role but in very early childhood only. **The mainstay of surgical treatment is total hip replacement** (Fig. 6–10). In general, for elderly patients with low activity demands, both the acetabular and the stem components can be cemented. For young, high-demand patients, the current trend is to use noncemented implants. These are only general guidelines. In revisions with poor-quality bone, the surgeon makes fixation choices based on intra-operative findings.

Weight-bearing restrictions are very different after arthroplasty with cemented and cementless hip devices. **Cement** is as strong as it will ever be 15 minutes after insertion. Some surgeons believe that some weight-bearing protection should be provided until the bone at the interface with the cement (which has been damaged by mechanical and thermal trauma) has reconstituted with the development of a peri-implant bone plate. This phenomenon takes 6 weeks. **Most surgeons, however, believe that the initial stability achieved with cement fixation is adequate to allow immediate full weight-bearing with a cane or walker.**

With a **noncemented hip prosthesis,** the initial fixation is press-fit, and maximal implant fixation is unlikely to be achieved until some tissue ongrowth or ingrowth into the implant has been established. Stability is usually adequate by 6 weeks. **However, maximal stability is probably not achieved until approximately 6 months with noncemented prostheses.** For these reasons, many surgeons advocate **toe-touch weight-bearing for the first 6 weeks.** Some believe that the initial stability achieved is adequate to allow weight-bearing as tolerated immediately after surgery.

Straight-leg raises (SLR) can produce very large out-of-plane loads on the hip and should be avoided. Side-leg-lifting in the lying position also produces large loads on the hip. Even vigorous isometric contractions of the hip abductors should be practiced with caution, especially if a trochanteric osteotomy has been done.

Initial rotational resistance of a noncemented hip may be low, and it may be **preferable to protect the hip from large rotational forces for 6 weeks or more.** The most common rotational load comes when arising from a sitting position, so pushing with hands from a chair is strongly recommended.

After full weight-bearing is established, it is essential that the patient continue to use a cane in the contralateral hand until the limp stops. This helps prevent the development of **a Trendelenburg gait,** which may be difficult to eradicate at a later date. In some difficult revisions in which implant or bone stability has been difficult to establish, a patient may be advised to continue to use a cane indefinitely. In general, when a patient gets up and walks away, forgetting about the cane, this is an indicator that the cane may be safely discarded.

Contraindications to Total Hip Arthroplasty

Absolute Contraindications

1. Active infection in the joint, unless carrying out a revision as either an immediate exchange or an interval procedure.
2. Systemic infection or sepsis.
3. Neuropathic joint.
4. Malignant tumors that do not allow adequate fixation of the components.

Relative Contraindications

1. Localized infection, especially bladder, skin, chest, or other local regions.
2. Absent or relative insufficiency of the abductor musculature.
3. Progressive neurologic deficit.
4. Any process rapidly destroying bone.
5. Patients requiring extensive dental or urologic procedures, such as transurethral resection of the prostate, should have this performed before total joint replacement.

Rehabilitation after Total Hip Replacement

The protocols outlined here for rehabilitation after total hip replacement are general and should be tailored to specific patients. For example, **weight-bearing should be limited to toe-touch if an osteotomy of the femur has been done for any reason.** Osteotomies can be required for **alignment correction**, either **angular** or **rotational; shortening**, such as a calcar episiotomy or subtrochanteric shortening; or **exposure**, such as a trochanteric osteotomy or slide, extended trochanteric osteotomy or slide, or a window. **Expansion osteotomies** allow the insertion of a larger prosthesis, and **reduction osteotomies** allow narrowing of the proximal femur. In patients with any of these osteotomies, weight-bearing should be delayed until some union is present. This is obviously the decision of an operating surgeon. **These patients should also avoid SLR and side-leg-lifting until, in the opinion of the surgeon, it is safe to do so.**

Treatment may also have to be adjusted because of difficulty of **initial fixation.** In revision surgery, a stable press-fit of the acetabular component may be difficult to achieve and multiple-screw fixation may be required. Under these circumstances, caution should be exercised in rehabilitation.

Treatment might also have to be adjusted because of **stability.** Revision of recurrent dislocations may require the use of an abduction brace to prevent adduction and flexion of more than 80 degrees for varying periods of time, up to 6 months. Similarly, leg shortening through a hip at the time of revision with or without a constrained socket should be protected for several months with an abduction brace until the soft tissues tighten up.

These considerations should be reviewed and integrated into a specific rehabilitation protocol tailored to the individual patient.

Postoperative Precautions after Total Hip Replacement

To avoid prosthesis dislocation (posteriorly with our posterior surgical approach), we give our patients this handout and instruct them in the office on motions to avoid.

Patient Instructions after Total Hip Replacement (Posterior Surgical Approach)

Do Not Bend Over Too Far
Do not let your hand pass your knee. Use your reacher (Fig. 6–11).

Figure 6–11.

Do Not Lean Over to Get Up
Instead, slide hips forward first, then come to standing (Fig. 6–12).

Figure 6–12.

Patient Instructions after Total Hip Replacement (Posterior Surgical Approach) *(Continued)*

Do Not Pull Blankets Up Like This
Use your reacher (Fig. 6–13).

Figure 6–13.

Do Not Sit Low on Toilet or Chair
You must use a raised toilet seat.
Build up a low chair with pillows (Fig. 6–14).

Figure 6–14.

Do Not Stand with Toes Turned In
Do not let knees roll inward while sitting (Fig. 6–15).

Figure 6–15.

Do Not Cross Your Legs
While sitting, standing, or lying down (Fig. 6–16).

Figure 6–16.

Do Not Lie Down without a Pillow between Legs
You do not want to cross or turn your legs inward (Fig. 6–17).

Figure 6–17.

You have been instructed to **avoid:**
1. Crossing your legs or bringing them together—adduction.
2. Bringing the knee too close to your chest—extreme hip flexion (you can bend until your hand gets to your knee).
3. Turning the foot in toward the other leg (internal rotation).

Listed below are several positions that could occur during your everyday activities. Remember to apply the above precautions.

1. When sitting, sit with knees comfortably apart.
2. Avoid sitting in low chairs and, especially, overstuffed sofas or chairs.
3. Do not lie on the involved side until cleared by your doctor.
4. When lying on the uninvolved side, always have a large pillow or two small pillows between your knees. Have the knees in a slightly bent position.
5. Continue to use your elevated commode seat after you have been discharged from the hospital, until cleared by the doctor (usually around 6–10 wk).
6. Do not cross legs while walking, especially when turning.
7. Avoid bending past 80 degrees (e.g., touching your feet, pulling up pants, picking up something off the floor, pulling up blankets while in bed).

continued

Patient Instructions after Total Hip Replacement (Posterior Surgical Approach) *(Continued)*

8. Sit in a slightly reclined position—avoid leaning forward when sitting on the commode. Do not let your shoulders get ahead of your hips when sitting or getting up.
9. Avoid raising knee higher than hip when sitting in a chair.
10. Do not try to get into a bathtub for a bath, unless using a tub chair.
11. *Going up and down stairs:*
    Up—step up with uninvolved leg, keeping crutches on the step below until both feet are on the step above, and then bring both crutches on the step.
    Down—place crutches on the step below, step down with the involved leg, and then with the uninvolved leg.
12. Continue to use your crutches or walker until you return to see your doctor.
13. Avoid prolonged sitting for longer than 1 hr before standing and stretching.
14. You can return to driving 6 wk after surgery only if you have good control over the involved leg and can move your extremity from accelerator to brake with little effort.
15. Place nightstand on the same side of the bed as the uninvolved leg. Avoid twisting the trunk toward the involved side, which would be the same as turning the leg inward.
16. Try to lie flat in bed at least 15–30 min per day to prevent tightness in the front part of the hip.
17. If you find you have increased swelling in the involved leg after going home, try propping foot up (remembering to lean back)—if swelling persists, contact your doctor. Also contact your doctor if you develop calf tenderness. Remember that as long as you are touch weight-bearing only, the muscles are not acting to pump blood up the leg, so the leg is likely to swell somewhat until full weight-bearing is established. This swelling usually disappears during the night.

This precaution sheet is borrowed with permission from the www.orthovid.com patient instructional video series on postoperative total joint rehabilitation.

Rehabilitation Protocol
Postoperative Total Hip Replacement—Posterior Approach
Cameron and Brotzman

Goals
- Guard against dislocation of the implant.
- Gain functional strength.
- Strengthen hip and knee musculature.
- Prevent bedrest hazards (e.g., thrombophlebitis, pulmonary embolism, decubiti, pneumonia).
- Teach independent transfers and ambulation with assistive devices.
- Obtain pain-free ROM within precaution limits.

Rehabilitation Considerations in Cemented and Cementless Techniques
- Cemented total hip
  - Weight-bearing to tolerance (WBTT) with walker immediately after surgery.

Preoperative Instructions
- Instruct on precautions for hip dislocation (handout).
- Transfer instructions
  - In and out of bed.
  - Chair
    - Depth-of-chair restrictions: avoid deep chairs. We also instruct patients to look at the ceiling as they sit down to minimize trunk flexion.
    - Sitting: avoid crossing legs.
    - Rising from chair: scoot to edge of the chair, then rise.
  - Use of elevated commode seat: elevated seat is placed on commode at a slant, with higher part at the back, to aid in rising. Have elevated seat sent to house prior to surgery for installation.
- Ambulation: instruct on use of anticipated assistive device (walker).
- Exercises: demonstrate day 1 exercises (see following).

Postoperative Regimen
- Out of bed in stroke chair twice a day with assistance 1 or 2 days postoperative. DO **NOT** use a low chair.
- Begin ambulation with assistive device twice a day (walker) 1 or 2 days postoperative with assistance from therapist.

Weight-bearing Status
Cemented prosthesis: weight-bearing as tolerated with walker for at least 6 wk, then use a cane in the contralateral hand for 4–6 mo. *Cementless technique:* touch-down weight-bearing with walker for 6–8 wk (some authors recommend 12 wk), then use a cane in the contralateral hand for 4–6 mo. A wheelchair may be used for long distances with careful avoidance of excessive hip flexion of more than 80 degrees while in the wheelchair. Therapist must check to ensure that the foot rests are long enough. Place a triangular cushion in the wheelchair seat with the highest cushion point posterior, to avoid excessive hip flexion.

Rehabilitation Protocol
Postoperative Total Hip Replacement—Posterior Approach *(Continued)*
Cameron and Brotzman

Isometric Exercises (Review Restrictions)

- SLR (if not contraindicated): tighten knee and lift leg off bed, keeping the knee straight. Flex the opposite knee to aid this exercise. SLRs are more important after total knee arthroplasty than after total hip arthroplasty. Surgeon may desire holding SLR depending on construct.
- Quadriceps sets: tighten quadriceps by pushing knee down and holding for a count of 4.
- Gluteal sets: squeeze buttocks together and hold for a count of 4.
- Ankle pumps: pump ankle up and down repeatedly.
- Isometric hip abduction with self-resistance while lying. Later, wrap a Theraband around the knees and perform abduction against the Theraband.
- Four-point exercise
  - Bend knee up while standing.
  - Straighten knee.
  - Bend knee back.
  - Return foot to starting position.
- Hip abduction-adduction (hold initially if patient had a trochanteric osteotomy):
  - Supine position: abduct (slide the leg out to the side) and back, keeping the toes pointed up. Make sure the leg is not externally rotated or the gluteus medius will not be strengthened.
  - Standing position: move the leg out to the side and back. Do not lean over to the side.
  - Side-lying position (probably 5–6 wk postoperative): Lying on side, the patient abducts the leg against gravity (Fig. 6–18). The patient should be turned 30 degrees toward prone to utilize the gluteus maximus and medius muscles. Most patients would otherwise tend to rotate toward the supine position, thus abducting with the tensor fascia femoris.

Cameron (1999) emphasizes that hip abductor strengthening is the most important single exercise that will allow the patient to return to ambulation without a limp. The type of surgical approach (e.g., trochanteric osteotomy) and implant fixation (e.g., cement) dictate the timing of initiating hip abduction exercises (see pp. 449 and 450).

ROM and Stretching Exercises

- 1 or 2 days postoperative, begin daily *Thomas stretch* to avoid flexion contracture of the hip. Pull the **uninvolved** knee up to the chest while lying supine in bed. At the same time, **push the postoperative leg into extension against the bed.** The hip extension stretches the anterior capsule and hip flexors of the involved hip and aids with previous flexion contracture and avoidance of postoperative contracture. Perform this stretch five to six times per session, six times a day (Fig. 6–19).
- May begin stationary exercise bicycling with a high seat 4–7 days postoperative. To mount the bicycle, the patient stands facing the side of the bicycle and places one hand on the center of the handle bars and the other on

Figure 6–19. Thomas stretch. The patient lies supine in bed, holding the uninvolved knee flexed to the chest, with the postoperative (left) leg perfectly straight, pressing down on the bed.

Figure 6–18. Side-lying hip abduction. Postoperatively, lying on the side, the patient lifts the involved extremity 8–10 inches away from the floor. The patient should turn the body 30 degrees toward prone. Hold these until the surgeon requests. There is a potential loss of fixation of trochanteric osteotomy with this exercise.

continued

Rehabilitation Protocol
Postoperative Total Hip Replacement—Posterior Approach (Continued)
Cameron and Brotzman

the seat. Place the uninvolved leg over the bar and onto the floor so that the seat is straddled. Protect the involved leg from full weight-bearing by putting pressure on the hands. With both hands on the handle bars and partial weight on the involved leg, place the uninvolved leg on the pedal. Stand on the uninvolved leg to sit on the seat. Then turn the pedals so that the involved leg can be placed on the pedal at the bottom of the arc.

Until successful completion of a full arc on the bicycle, the seat should be set as high as possible. Initially, most patients find it easier to pedal backward until they can complete a revolution. The seat may be progressively lowered to increase hip flexion within safe parameters.

Initially, the patient should ride the bicycle with minimal tension at 15 mph, two to four times a day. We leave a stationary bicycle on the hospital floor for use in the room. By 6–8 wk, may increase the tension until fatigue occurs after approximately 10–15 min of riding.

- May also perform extension stretching of the anterior capsule (to avoid hip flexion contracture) by extending the involved leg while the uninvolved leg is mildly flexed at the hip and knee, supported by a walker (**the therapist stabilizes the walker**). Slowly thrust the pelvis forward and the shoulders backward for a sustained stretch of the anterior capsule (Fig. 6–20).
- Observe and correct gait faults, because many of these faults involve the patient's avoidance of stretching the anterior structures of the hip secondary to pain (p. 456).

Figure 6–20. Extension stretch of the anterior capsule while the patient is standing. The therapist *must* stabilize the walker during stretching.

Abduction Pillow

- Keep an abduction pillow between the legs while in bed.

Note: Many surgeons also use a knee immobilizer on the ipsilateral knee during the first week to avoid possible prosthesis dislocation. The knee immobilizer does not allow excessive hip or knee flexion. Use the abductor pillow while asleep or resting in bed for 5–6 wk; it may then be safely discontinued.

Bathroom Rehabilitation

- Permit bathroom privileges with assistance and an elevated commode seat.
- Teach bathroom transfers when the patient is ambulating 10–20 feet outside of room.
- Use elevated commode seat at all times.

Assistive Devices

Occupational therapist brings these and instructs patient on assisted activities of daily living:

- "Reacher" or "grabber" to help retrieve objects on the floor or assist with socks or stockings. Do not bend to put on slippers.
- Shoe horn and loosely fitting shoes or loafers.

Transfer Instructions

- Bed to chair
  - Avoid leaning forward to get out of chair or off bed.
  - Slide hips forward to the edge of the chair first, then come to standing.
  - Do not cross legs when pivoting from supine to bedside position.
  - Nurse or therapist assists until able to perform safe, secure transfers.
- Bathroom
  - Use elevated toilet seat with assistance.
  - Continue assistance until able to perform safe, secure transfers.

Transfer to Home

- Instruct patient to travel in the back seat of a four-door sedan, sitting or reclining lengthwise across the seat, leaning on one or two pillows under the head and shoulders to avoid sitting in a deep seat.
- Avoid sitting in conventional fashion (hip flexed more than 90 degrees) to avoid posterior dislocation in the event of a sudden stop.
- Urge those without a four-door sedan to sit on two pillows with the seat reclined (minimize flexion of hip).
- Adhere to these principles for 6 wk until soft tissue stabilization is achieved (Steinberg and associates [1988]).
- May begin driving 6 wk postoperative.
- Review hip precautions and instructions with patient (see boxes).

Rehabilitation Protocol
Postoperative Total Hip Replacement—Posterior Approach *(Continued)*
Cameron and Brotzman

Exercise Progression

- Hip abduction: progress exercises from isometric abduction against self-resistance to Thera-band wrapped around the knees. At 5–6 wk, begin standing hip abduction exercises with pulleys, sports cord, or weights. Also may perform side-stepping with a sports cord around the hips, as well as lateral step-ups with a low step, if clinically safe.

Progress hip abduction exercises until the patient exhibits a normal gait with good abductor strength. Our progression for a postoperative cemented prosthesis with *no trochanteric osteotomy* generally follows the outline below.

1. Supine isometric abduction against hand or bedrail (2 or 3 days).
2. Supine abduction, sliding the involved leg out and back.
3. Side-lying abduction with the involved leg on top and abduction against gravity.

Figure 6–22. Prone-lying extension exercises of the hip are performed to strengthen the gluteus maximus. Lying prone, the patient lifts the leg 8–10 inches from the floor, keeping the knee locked.

4. Standing abduction, moving the leg out to the side and back (Fig. 6–21).
5. Theraband exercises, sports cord, and step-ups (5–6 wk).

Perform *prone-lying extension exercises* of the hip to strengthen the gluteus maximus (Fig. 6–22). These may be performed with the knee flexed (to isolate the hamstrings and gluteus maximus) and with the knee extended to strengthen the hamstrings and gluteus maximus.

Note: This exercise progression is slower in certain patients (see pp. 449 and 450).

Initiate general strengthening exercises: develop endurance, perform cardiovascular exercise, and general strengthening of all extremities.

Instructions for Home

- Continue previous exercises (pp. 453 and 454) and ambulation activities.
- Continue to observe hip precautions.
- Install elevated toilet seat in home.
- Supply walker for home.
- Review rehabilitation specific to home situation (e.g., steps, stairwells, narrow doorways).
- Ensure home physical therapy and/or home nursing care has been arranged.
- Orient family to patient's needs, abilities, and limitations, and **review hip precautions with family members.**
- Reiterate avoidance of driving for 6 wk (most cars have very low seats).
- Give patient a prescription for prophylactic antibiotics that may be needed eventually for dental or urologic procedure.

Figure 6–21. Standing abduction, moving the leg out to the side and back.

Managing Problems after Total Hip Replacement

1. **Trendelenburg gait** (weak hip abductors)
   - Concentrate on hip abduction exercises to strengthen abductors.
   - Evaluate leg-length discrepancy.
   - Have patient stand on involved leg while flexing opposite (uninvolved) knee 30 degrees. If opposite hip drops, have patient try to lift and hold in an effort to reeducate and work gluteus medius muscle (hip abductor).
2. **Flexion contracture** of the hip
   - **AVOID** placing pillows under the knee after surgery.
   - Walking backward helps stretch flexion contracture. Perform a Thomas stretch (p. 453) of 30 stretches a day (five stretches six times per day). Pull the uninvolved knee to the chest while supine. Push the involved (postoperative) leg into extension against the bed. This stretches the anterior capsule and hip flexors of the involved leg.

Gait Faults

Gait faults should be watched for and corrected. Chandler (1982) points out that most gait faults either are caused by or contribute to flexion deformities at the hip.

The **first** and **most common gait fault** occurs when the patient takes a large step with the involved leg and a short step with the uninvolved leg. The patient does this to avoid extension of the involved leg, which causes a stretching discomfort in the groin. The patient should be taught to **concentrate on taking longer strides with the uninvolved extremity.**

A **second common gait fault** occurs when the patient breaks the knee in late stance phase. Again, this is done to avoid extension of the hip. It is associated with flexion of the knee and early and excessive heel rise at late stance phase. The patient should be instructed to keep the heel on the ground in late stance phase.

A **third common gait fault** occurs when the patient flexes forward at the waist in mid and late stance. Once again, the patient is attempting to avoid hip extension. To correct this, teach the patient to thrust the pelvis forward and the shoulders backward during mid and late stance phase of gait.

One additional fault, a limp, occasionally arises simply as a habit that can be difficult to break. A full-length mirror is a useful adjunct in gait training because it allows patients to observe themselves while walking toward it.

All of these gaits faults are corrected with observation and teaching.

Position of Postoperative Total Hip Instability (Cameron)

- Posterior dislocation: flexion, adduction, and internal rotation will cause dislocation.
- Anterior dislocation: extension, adduction, and external rotation will cause dislocation.

Important Rehabilitation Points

- **Going up stairs:** step up first with the uninvolved leg, keeping crutches on the step below until both feet are on the step above, then bring both crutches up on the step. If available, hold the handrail.
- **Going down stairs:** place crutches on the step below, then step down with the involved leg, and then with the uninvolved leg. If possible, hold the rail.
- Stretching of the anterior hip structures can be gently achieved by having the patient hang the involved leg laterally off the table as the therapist stabilizes the pelvis (Fig. 6–23).

Figure 6–23. Therapist stretching the anterior hip structures.

Stair Training

The good go up to Heaven: "good" extremity goes first upstairs.

The bad go down to Hell: "bad" or involved extremity goes first downstairs.

Restraints of Home Environment and Activities of Daily Living

- Assess home environment and activities of daily living for unique rehabilitation problems
  - Assess home equipment needs.
  - Assess unique barriers to mobility.
  - Institute a home exercise program that may be realistically performed.

Cane

We also advocate the long-term use of a cane in the contralateral hand to minimize daily forces across the hip arthroplasty and, it is hoped, to prolong implant longevity (see Fig. 6–1).

Deep Vein Thrombosis Prophylaxis for Total Joint Replacement

Thromboembolic disease is the most common cause of serious complications after total hip arthroplasty. The mortality caused by emboli in total hip arthroplasty patients who do not receive prophylactic medication is reported to be five times greater than that after abdominal and thoracic surgery. ***It is the most common cause of death occurring within 3 mo of surgery.*** Kakkar and colleagues (1985) found 29% of thrombi developed before postoperative day 12, and 23% between 12 and 24 days after surgery. ***Thus, the risk of deep vein thrombosis (DVT) appears to be highest during the first 3 wk after surgery.***

Numerous studies have shown clotting in the calf or thigh veins in up to 50% of patients after elective surgery; 80 to 90% of the thromboses occur in the limb that has undergone surgery. Calf thrombi alone are unlikely to produce clinically apparent pulmonary emboli; these typically arise from larger, more proximal veins. From 5 to 23% of calf vein DVTs propagate proximally.

Several factors increase the risk of thrombolism:

- Prior episode of thromboembolism.
- Prior venous surgery and varicose veins.
- Previous orthopaedic surgery.
- Advanced age.
- Malignancy.
- Congestive heart failure and chronic lower extremity swelling.
- Immobilization.
- Obesity.
- Oral contraceptives and hormones.
- Excessive blood loss and transfusion.

Spinal and epidural anesthesia carry a lower risk of DVT than does general anesthesia (13% versus 27%).

The best method of prophylaxis remains controversial. Much of the literature is difficult to interpret because of variability in reporting calf or thigh thrombi, clinical methods used to detect pulmonary embolism and DVT, and a large variation in pharmacologic protocol. Multiple pharmacologic agents are available for prophylaxis. The data from comparison studies vary widely. The most commonly used agents are low-dose warfarin, low-dose heparin, adjusted-dose herapin, dextran, and aspirin. Duration of therapy is also a source of disagreement in the literature.

Most authors recommend early ambulation, leg elevation, and the use of graded-pressure stockings, but the effectiveness of these stockings is not well documented. External sequential pneumatic compression devices may decrease the overall incidence of DVT, but are less effective in reducing the formation of the more proximal thrombi. The choice of anticoagulation therapy is the physician's and is beyond the scope of this rehabilitation text.

Antibiotic Regimens Suggested for Prophylaxis of High-risk Dental Patients with Total Joint Replacements

Prophylactic Antibiotics for Future Dental and Genitourinary Procedures (See p. 458)

To avoid possible hematogenous seeding of joint prostheses after transient bacteremias caused by invasive dental procedures or urologic procedures, most orthopaedists recommend antibiotic prophylaxis. No conclusive research data have established the true risk of infection of joint replacements after dental bacteremias. Significant disagreement exists in the dental literature. Because of catastrophic nature of a total joint infection, we advocate prophylactic antibiotic use for dental procedures, genitourinary procedures, or purulent skin infections. Potentially high-risk patients should have concomitant gingival sulcus irrigation and mouth rinsing with chlorhexidine solution before periodontal procedures or extractions.

continued

Antibiotic Regimens Suggested for Prophylaxis of High-risk Dental Patients with Total Joint Replacements (*Continued*)

Standard Regimens

- Cephradine (Anspor or Velosef)
  1 g orally 1 hr prior to dental procedure
- Cephalexin (Keflex)
  1 g orally 1 hr prior, 500 mg 6 hr later
- Cephalexin (Keflex)
  2 g orally 1 hr prior, 1 g 6 hr later
- Cephalexin (Keflex)
  1 g orally 1 hr prior, 500 mg 4 hr later

Allergic to Penicillin or Cephalosporins

- Clindamycin
  600 mg orally 1 hr prior to dental procedure
- Clindamycin
  300 mg orally 1 hr prior to dental procedure
- Clindamycin
  600 mg orally 1 hr before dental procedure, 600 mg 6 hr later
- Erythromycin
  500 mg orally 1 hr prior to dental procedure, 500 mg 4 hr later

From Little JW: Managing dental patients with joint prostheses. J Am Dent Assoc 125:1376, 1994.

Patients with Increased Risk of Postoperative Infection following Total Joint Replacement

Predisposing Conditions

- Rheumatoid arthritis
- Steroid use
- Use of other agents causing immunosuppression
- Insulin-dependent diabetes
- Hemophilia
- Hemoglobinopathies such as sickle cell disease

Local Factors

- Complications associated with joint prosthesis
  - Replacement of prosthesis
  - Loose prosthesis
- History of previous infection

Acute Infection Located at Distant Sites

- Skin
- Other

Modified from Little JW: Managing dental patients with joint prostheses. J Am Dent Assoc 125:1376, 1994.

Table 6-4

Risk Factors for Osteoarthritis of the Knee

Established	Controversial
Obesity	Physical activity
Age	Genetics
Osteoarthritis at other sites	Smoking
Previous knee trauma or injury	Estrogen deficiency
Previous knee surgery	
Sex (female)	

---

ment). **Patellofemoral arthritis** is common in an arthritic knee but is surprisingly seldom a source of symptoms.

Articular surface damage has been variously classified, but the most useful categories are **minimal,** in which there is no radiologic narrowing; **mild,** in which there is loss of one third of the joint space; **moderate,** in which two thirds of the joint space has been lost; and **severe,** in which there is bone-on-bone contact.

Diagnosis

To examine for arthritis of the knee, move the joint under load (e.g., to examine the medial compartment, a varus strain is applied to the knee and the knee is moved). Crepitus will be felt under the hand applying the varus strain and pain will be produced. Similarly, a valgus strain and load are applied to the lateral joint. The knee should be examined for laxity of the collateral ligaments and, to some extent, the cruciate ligaments, although this is less important. The presence of any fixed flexion deformity (e.g., lack of passive extension of the knee) should be noted. The patellar position (central or subluxed) is important, as is the presence of a rotatory deformity of the tibia. When the patient stands, note any genu varum (bow-legged) or genu valgum (knock-kneed).

By the end of our history and exam of the arthritic knee we have obtained the following information:

1. Symptom location
   - Isolated (medial, lateral, or patellofemoral)
   - Diffuse

The Arthritic Knee

Clinical Background

Arthritis of the knee can be due to many causes, including congenital deformities (such as axial and rotatory deformity), trauma, and rheumatoid arthritis (Table 6–4). Eighty percent of patients develop medial compartment OA, and as the bone wears away, they develop a **varus** or "bow-legged" deformity. Five to ten percent develop a lateral compartment OA of the knee resulting in a **valgus** or "knock-kneed" deformity. A small percentage of patients have rotatory deformities of the tibia that cause significant patellar maltracking or subluxation.

Classification

Arthritic deformity of the knee is classified as varus or valgus (with or without symptomatic patellar involve-

2. Type of symptoms
   - Swelling
   - Giving way, instability (ligament tear or weak quadriceps)
   - Diminished ROM
   - Mechanical (crepitance, locking, catching, pseudolocking)
3. Timing of onset
   - Acute
   - Insidious
4. Duration
5. Exacerbating factors
6. Prior intervention (e.g., NSAIDs, surgery) and the patient's response

Radiographic Evaluation of the Arthritic Knee (Table 6–5)

Evaluation should always include a standing (weight-bearing) AP view of the knee. If surgery is contemplated, there should be a full-limb (three-foot) view to detect any deformities or problems above and below the standard radiographic views (e.g., a valgus deformity of the ankle). A lateral radiograph is required, as is a skyline view of the patella. **If the problem is on the lateral side of the joint, a standing posteroanterior view must be** obtained with the knee in 30 degrees of flexion. The reason for this is that the articular cartilage loss in the medial compartment is in the distal femur and central tibia, but articular cartilage loss in the lateral compartment is in the posterior femur and posterior tibia.

Treatment of Knee Arthritis
(see Rehabilitation Protocol)

Nonoperative

Treatment of early OA of the knee may be very effective if conscientiously carried out. **Weight loss** should be strongly encouraged but not expected immediately. **Quadriceps strengthening** makes a surprising difference. Very strong quadriceps can considerably delay the necessity for surgery. If the patella is painful, extension exercises should be carried out only over the last 20 degrees of extension. Activities such as deep squatting, kneeling, and stair climbing that increase the patellofemoral joint reaction forces (PFJRFs) increase pain. Those activities should be avoided. If the patient starts with extremely weak muscles, electric stimulation may be used to begin the process. **Modalities** other than heat or cold have not been shown to be of value. **Hyaluronic acid injections** into the knee are of limited value. They appear to work best *before* there is bone-on-bone crepitus. Studies by independent researchers have found hyaluronic acid injections to be of "equal benefit" to nonsteroidal anti-inflammatory drugs (NSAIDs) (naproxyn [Naprosyn]). Patrella (2002) purports that hyaluronic acid intra-articular injection was of benefit. Careful review of the study actually reveals that injection of hyaluronate sodium (Synvisc, Provise, and Suplasyn) to be no better than placebo. Similarly, **intra-articular steroid injections** have a very temporary and limited role.

Keating (1993) found that of 85 patients with medial compartment arthritis of the knee, more than 75% had statistical improvement on their Hospital for Special Surgery pain scores at 12 months with the use of a lateral wedged insole in their shoe. For example, a 0.25 inch soft wedge or a 5 degree wedged insole placed laterally will reduce medial joint reactive forces from the medial joint line.

Table 6–5		
Findings Indicating the Presence of Knee Osteoarthritis		
Symptoms	**Signs**	**Radiography**
Pain with activity	Joint line or condylar tenderness	Subchondral sclerosis Intra-articular osseous debris (loose bodies or joint mice)
Stiffness	Effusion	Joint narrowing (unicompartmental)
	Crepitation	Joint irregularity
	Decreased ROM	Subchondral cysts
	Angular deformity	Osteophytosis ("central or marginal")

Rehabilitation Protocol
Nonoperative and Operative Treatment Algorithm for Patients with Arthritis of the Lower Extremity (Hip or Knee)
Brotzman

Tier 1: Nonoperative Options
- Weight loss!—successful weight loss (difficult) dramatically improves pain in lower extremity arthritics and prolongs total joint arthroplasty longevity after arthro-

plasty has been performed. Physician must be proactive and implement low-impact aerobic exercise (water aerobics, cycling, swimming) and direct the patient to a reputable weight-loss center (e.g., Weight Watchers).

continued

Rehabilitation Protocol
Nonoperative and Operative Treatment Algorithm for Patients with Arthritis of the Lower Extremity (Hip or Knee) *(Continued)*
Brotzman

Table 6–6

Suggested Exercise Plan for Patients with Osteoarthritis of the Knee

Mild Symptoms*	Moderate to Severe Symptoms
Active ROM exercises for the hip, knee, and ankle.	Active-assisted ROM exercises for hip, knee, and ankle.
Physical therapy modalities as needed.	Physical therapy modalities as needed.
Knee sleeve if comfortable.	Stretching for quadriceps, hamstrings, adductors (Fig. 6–24), gastrocnemius; may use ultrasound for hamstrings if there is contraction.
Quadriceps sets for vastus medialis obliques, especially if there is a prominent patellofemoral component to symptoms.	Quadriceps sets for vastus medialis obliques; start supine if there is a hamstring contracture and gradually work up to a sitting position.
Advance to isometric progressive resistive exercises for quadriceps, hamstrings, and hip adductors and abductors.	Unloaded aerobic conditioning (pool, walker, grocery cart, cane); advance as described for hip.
Low-impact conditioning exercises. Avoid high patellofemoral compressive forces.	Advance strengthening to isometric closed–kinetic chain exercises, such as wall-sitting (not "slide," because this word implies repetitions, which usually are not well tolerated).
Authors are strong proponents of aquatic (unloading) exercise for mild, moderate, and severe arthritis (see Chapter 7).	Hip adductor and abductor strengthening.
	Later, add straight leg raising progressive resistance exercise (2 pounds on the thigh).
	Later still, try lunges; however, lunges require great strength and excellent balance and coordination, and few patients are strong enough or can understand the importance of positioning; lunges can therefore aggravate symptoms.

*The program for mild symptoms is given in one or two physical therapy visits.
OA, osteoarthritis; ROM, range of motion.
From Baum AL, Baum J: Coming to grips with depression in rheumatoid arthritis. J Musculoskel Med 15:36, 1998.

Figure 6–24. Stretching exercises help preserve or increase joint range of motion (ROM). *A,* In this example of a hip adductor stretch, the patient lies supine on a firm surface, with the hips and knees bent and the feet flat. The patient then lets the knees fall apart, keeping the soles of the feet together, until an inner thigh stretch is felt. *B,* To stretch the hamstrings, the patient lies on the floor near a doorway, with one leg extending into the doorway. The patient slides forward while gently raising the other leg with the foot flat against the wall until a gentle stretch is felt behind the knee. (*A* and *B,* From Hicks JE: Rehabilitation strategies for patients with rheumatoid arthritis. J Musculoskel Med 17:191, 2000.)

Rehabilitation Protocol
Nonoperative and Operative Treatment Algorithm for Patients with Arthritis of the Lower Extremity (Hip or Knee) (Continued)
Brotzman

- Activity modification (Table 6–6)
  - Discontinue high-impact sports (e.g., running, tennis, basketball), change to low-impact **water-based** sports or cycling.
  - Avoid stair-climbing, kneeling, squatting, low chairs if patellofemoral arthritis exists.
  - Change hard surface at work to soft if possible, sit more than previously, and so on.
  - Water aerobics in a warm pool (*not* a hot tub) for aerobic exercise or strengthening.
- NSAIDs
  - We typically employ cyclooxygenase-2 (COX-2) inhibitors (Vioxx, Celebrex) for their improved *safety profile* (no difference in efficacy).
  - Employ the *minimal* effective dose, intermittent use if possible.
  - *Significant* potential long-term *complication rate* makes these less attractive
    - Peptic ulcer disease.
    - Renal effects.
    - Gastrointestinal bleed.
- *Cane* in the *opposite* hand (see Fig. 6–1)
  - Greatly decreases stress on arthritic joint, but for cosmesis considerations, many "young" or female arthritics will not use a cane.
- Viscosupplementation of the knee (e.g., hylan G-F 20 [Synvisc], hylauronate sodium [Hyalgan])
  - Although some patients do respond well to serial injections, studies have shown efficacy only comparable with taking Naprosyn.
- "Unloading" graphite braces for knee arthritis (not hip)
  - If the patient has unicompartmental knee involvement (e.g., medial), she or he may derive some benefit from a custom "unloader" brace
    - Very expensive.
    - Most patients quit wearing quickly secondary to bulkiness, inconvenience.
- Knee sleeve for proprioception (knee arthritis)
  - Some patients derive benefit from a light Neoprene knee sleeve, which may improve proprioceptive feedback (indications are soft, but the braces are inexpensive with little if any possible complication).
- Chondroitin sulfate/glucosamine
  - Moderately expensive ($40 a mo).
  - No multi-center studies confirming or denying efficacy.
  - No side effects or complications. If patients wish to try and derive great benefit (? placebo), we have them continue. Otherwise, patient instructed to discontinue at 3 mo if no benefit.
- Physical therapy
  - A brief course of therapy to teach home program of hamstring and quadricep strengthening, flexibility,

ROM exercises, and aquatic therapy is *very* useful if good patient compliance. Have follow-up visits to monitor compliance and progression.
- Intra-articular cortisone (knee *not* hip)
  - Response to aspiration and injection is highly variable (2 wk–6 mo).
  - Injections should be limited to three per year (potential articular cartilage softening/AVN). Warn patients of potential corticosteroid-related flare. Application of ice that evening can help avoid this.
- Topical therapy
  - We have found topical therapy to be largely ineffective.

The Arthritis Foundation offers the following exercise programs for arthritic patients:

- Aquatics—heated pool, 6–10 wk, minimal joint stress, increased ROM.
- Joint efforts—6–8 wk, for patients with very limited mobility or elderly.
- PACE (People with Arthritis Can Exercise)—6–8 wk, two levels of classes.
- PEP (Pool Exercise Program)—45-min video that increases flexibility, strength, and endurance.

Multiple brochures on arthritis information are available. Call Arthritis Foundation 1-800-283-7800 or www.arthritis.org.

Tier 2: Operative Options for Patients with Symptomatic Arthritic Knees
Arthroscopy
- With OA, degenerating articular cartilage and synovial tissue release proinflammatory cytokines that induce chondrocytes to release lytic enzymes leading to degradation of type 2 collagen and proteoglycans.
- The "lavaging" effect of arthroscopy may dilute or "wash out" these inflammatory mediators, **although the effect is temporary.**
- Patients often have unrealistic expectations of arthroscopy for arthritis, so counseling on the palliative or temporary effect is needed.
- Microfracture may or may not offer some pain benefit. Drilling and abrasion chondroplasty seem to offer little benefit.
- Patients who benefit most from arthroscopy have mechanical symptoms (locking meniscus) of short duration (<6 mo) with mild arthritis on radiographs.
- Patients with 3–6 mo of unsuccessful supervised nonsurgical management with normal mechanical alignment and mild to moderate arthritis on weight-bearing films are considered candidates for arthroscopic débridements.

continued

Rehabilitation Protocol
Nonoperative and Operative Treatment Algorithm for Patients with Arthritis of the Lower Extremity (Hip or Knee) (Continued)
Brotzman

Table 6-7

Prognostic Factors for Arthroscopic Débridement of the Arthritic Knee

History	Physical Examination	Radiographic Findings	Arthroscopic Findings
Good Prognosis			
Short duration	Medial tenderness	Unicompartmental	Outbridge I or II changes
Associated trauma	Effusion	Normal alignment	Meniscal flap tear
First arthroscopy	Normal alignment	Minimal Fairbank's changes	Chondral fracture or flap
Mechanical symptoms	Ligaments stable	Loose bodies	Loose bodies
		Relevant osteophytes	Osteophytes at symptom site
Poor Prognosis			
Long duration	Lateral tenderness	Bi- or tri-compartmental	Outbridge III or IV changes
Insidious onset	No effusion	Malalignment	Degenerative meniscus
Multiple procedures	Malalignment	Significant Fairbank's changes	Diffuse chondrosis
	Varus > 10 degrees		
	Valgus > 15 degrees		
Pain at rest	Ligaments unstable	Irrelevant osteophytes	Osteophyte away from symptom site
Litigation			
Work-related			

From Di Nubile N: Osteoarthritis of the knee—a special report. Physician Sports Med May: 2000.

- Patients with tibial spine pain, osteophyte formation, and lack of extension (flexion deformity) may benefit from arthroscopic notch plasty and osteophyte removal.
- Table 6–7 reviews the prognostic factors for arthroscopic débridement of an arthritic knee.
- Arthroscopic management of the arthritic knee should be considered palliative, temporary, and most effective in the patient with concomitant mechanical findings (e.g., bucket-handle meniscal tear with a positive McMurray examination).

Surgery for Focal Cartilage Defects of the Femur (Cartilage Transfer or Chondrocyte Implantation) (Table 6–8)

Table 6-8

Surgical Treatment Options for Symptomatic Focal Cartilage Defects of the Femur*

Lesion	Treatment	Rehabilitation†	Comments
	Primary		
<2 cm²	Débridement and lavage.	Straightforward.	Provides short-term symptomatic relief.
	Marrow stimulation techniques.	Significant.	Ideal for smaller lesions located on femoral condyle; provides intermediate short-term relief; low cost.
	Osteochondral autograft.	Moderate.	Relatively new procedure; probably as good as, if not better than, marrow stimulation techniques; provides potentially long-term relief.
>2 cm²	Débridement and lavage.	Straightforward.	Provides short-term symptomatic relief.
	Marrow stimulation techniques.	Significant.	Has lower success rate for larger lesions; good choice for symptomatic relief in low-demand individuals; intermediate-term relief is possible; low cost.

Rehabilitation Protocol
Nonoperative and Operative Treatment Algorithm for Patients with Arthritis of the Lower Extremity (Hip or Knee) *(Continued)*
Brotzman

Table 6–8 *(Continued)*

Surgical Treatment Options for Symptomatic Focal Cartilage Defects of the Femur*

Lesion	Treatment	Rehabilitation[†]	Comments
	Cartilage biopsy for future autologous chondrocyte implantation.	Straightforward.	Staged procedure.
	Osteochondral autograft.	Significant.	With larger lesions, potential for donor site morbidity exists; results are variable.
	Osteochondral allograft.	Significant.	Useful for larger lesions with significant bone stock loss; small concern for disease transmission and allograft availability; provides potentially long-term relief.
	Secondary		
<2 cm²	Osteochondral autograft.[‡]	Moderate.	Relatively new procedure; probably as good as, if not better than, marrow stimulation techniques; provides potentially long-term relief.
	Autologous chondrocyte implantation.	Significant.	High success rate for return to activities; potentially long-term relief; relatively high cost.
>2 cm²	Osteochondral autograft.	Significant.	With larger lesions, potential for donor site morbidity exists; results are variable.
	Osteochondral allograft.	Significant.	Useful for larger lesions with significant bone stock loss; small concern for disease transmission and allograft availability; provides potentially long-term relief.
	Autologous chondrocyte implantation.	Significant.	High success rate for return to activities; potentially long-term relief; relatively high cost.

*Procedure selection depends on patient's age, expectations, demand, activity level, coexisting pathology, and extent and location of disease. For rehabilitation after articular defect surgery, please see Chapter 4, Knee Injuries.
[†]Straightforward, early weight-bearing and return to activities within 4 wk; moderate, short-term protected weight-bearing and return to activities within 12 wk; significant, prolonged protected weight-bearing and significant delay until return to activities (6–8 mo).
[‡]Follows failed primary treatment.
From Cole BJ: Arthritis of the knee—a special report, Physician Sports Med 28(5):1–15, 2000.

Osteotomy
- *Varus* malalignment of the knee (bow-legged) in a younger, active patient with medial compartment arthritis is addressed with a valgus-producing, high tibial osteotomy.
- Mild *valgus* malalignment (<10 degrees of valgus) may be treated with a medial, high tibial closing wedge osteotomy. Patients with greater than 10 degrees of valgus undergo femoral osteotomy.
- Supracondylar femoral osteotomies do not interfere with subsequent total knee replacements. However, tibial osteotomies compromise total knee replacement results. For this reason, osteotomies are seldom performed in the United States. New opening-wedge osteotomy techniques for the tibia purport not to alter the joint line for later total knee replacement.

Unicompartmental Knee Replacement
- More controversial, *patient selection is critical*.
- Ideal candidate is
  - Older than 60 yr.
  - Low-demand (sedentary).
  - Thin.
  - Isolated unicompartmental arthritic involvement (Table 6–9).

Tier 3: Options for the Symptomatic Arthritic Knee

TOTAL Joint Replacement
- Total joint replacements work best in thin sedentary patients older than 65 yr.
- A proportion of replacements "wear out" with time (osteolysis), requiring revision. This revision rate is increased with obesity, high-impact activity, overuse, and so on.

continued

Rehabilitation Protocol
Nonoperative and Operative Treatment Algorithm for Patients with Arthritis of the Lower Extremity (Hip or Knee) *(Continued)*
Brotzman

Table 6-9

Treatment Criteria for Unicompartmental Knee Athritis

	Unicompartmental Knee Arthroplasty	High Tibial Osteotomy	Total Knee Arthroplasty
History	>60 yr old Sedentary Pain with weight-bearing	<60 yr old, ideally 50s Laborer Activity-related pain	>65 yr old Sedentary Degenerative traumatic or inflammatory arthritis
	Noninflammatory arthritis No patellofemoral symptoms	Noninflammatory arthritis No patellofemoral symptoms	
Exam	ROM 5–90 degrees or better <15 degrees coronal deformity	Flexion > 90 degrees Flexion contracture < 15 degrees	Joint line tenderness Altered ROM
	Intact ACL (controversial) Intact collateral ligaments <200 pounds (90 kg)	Competent MCL Heavier patients	Varus or valgus deformity
X-rays	Isolated unicompartmental disease	Mild to moderate osteoarthritis	Multicompartmental disease
	Asymptomatic patellofemoral disease Acceptable No tibial or femoral bowing	Varus alignment	Varus or valgus alignment
Intraoperative Findings	Contralateral compartment without eburnated bone and has normal meniscus	Inspection of articular surface prior to osteotomy of no prognostic value	Multicompartmental articular degeneration
	No evidence of inflammatory process		Bony defects
Contraindications	Inflammatory arthritis Limited ROM Advanced patellofemoral disease or contralateral compartment disease Chondrocalcinosis (controversial) ACL deficiency (controversial)	Inflammatory arthritis Limited ROM Advanced patellofemoral disease Varus > 10 degrees	Acute infection Extensor mechanism disruption Severe recurvatum deformity Severe vascular disease

ACL, anterior collateral ligament; MCL, medial collateral ligament; ROM, range of motion.
From Seigel JA, Marwin SE: The role of unicompartmental knee arthroplasty. Orthopaedics Special Ed 5(2):62, 1999.

Operative—Arthritic Knee

Arthroscopic débridement is of temporary value, simply cleaning out the tags and meniscal tears and flushing from the joint fluid that contains pain-producing peptides. Cole and Harners' (1999) article on the evaluation and management of knee arthritis provides an ex-

cellent overview on arthroscopy in patients with knee arthritis.

Livesley et al (1991) compared the results in 37 painful arthritic knees treated with arthroscopic lavage by one surgeon against those in 24 knees treated with physical therapy alone by a second surgeon. The results suggested that there was better pain relief in the lavage group at 1 year. Edelson et al (1995) reported that lavage alone had good or excellent results in 86% of their patients at 1 year and in 81% at 2 years using the Hospital for Special Surgery scale.

Jackson and Rouse (1982) reported on the results of arthroscopic lavage alone versus lavage combined with debridement, with 3-year follow-up. Of the 65 patients treated with lavage alone, 80% had initial improvement but only 45% maintained improvement at follow-up. Of the 137 patients treated with lavage plus debridement, 88% showed initial improvement, and 68% maintained improvement at follow-up. Gibson et al (1992) demonstrated no statistically significant improvement with either method, even in the short term. Patients who present with flexion deformities associated with pain or discomfort and osteophyte formation around the tibial spines may benefit from osteophyte removal and notchplasty, as demonstrated by Puddu et al (1994).

The efficacy of lavage with or without debridement is controversial, and randomized prospective controlled trials have not been performed. The literature suggests that arthroscopic lavage and debridement, when performed for appropriate indications, will provide improvement in pain relief for 50% to 70% of patients, with relief lasting from several months to several years. Drilling and abrasion arthroplasty do not appear to offer additional benefit. Arthroscopy is also a sensitive way to evaluate cartilage when contemplating osteotomy or unicompartmental knee arthroplasty, as plain radiography and magnetic resonance imaging often underestimate the extent of osteoarthritis.

Several factors determine prognosis after lavage and debridement. **Those who benefit most** present with a history of mechanical symptoms, symptoms of short duration (<6 months), normal alignment, and only mild to moderate radiographic evidence of osteoarthritis. It is not uncommon for patients to have unrealistic expectations after arthroscopic debridement. Thus, it is important to counsel patients about the limited indications and palliative results.

Osteotomy of the Knee

This is a mechanical load-shifting procedure. The mechanical axis of the knee is "shifted" from the worn compartment (usually medial) to the good compartment. Closing wedge osteotomies have an inherent disadvantage in that the tibiofibular joint must be disrupted with some degree of shortening and joint-line alteration. *Because the joint line must remain "horizontal," in OA with a valgus deformity, the osteotomy is done through the supracondylar region of the femur; and for varus deformity, it is done through the proximal tibia.* Contraindications to tibial osteotomy include panarthrosis (tricompartmental involvement), severe patellofemoral disease, severely restricted ROM (loss of more than 15 to 20 degrees of extension, or flexion less than 90 degrees), and inflammatory arthritis. There are very few contraindications to a varus osteotomy other than damage to the medial compartment. There are many **contraindications for a tibial osteotomy.** Outcome after a valgus osteotomy depends on the varus thrust force. This force, however, can be detected only by the use of a very sophisticated force plate analysis, of which there are very few available worldwide, and other indications must be used. **Strength-to-weight ratio** is extremely important, meaning that the older the patient and the heavier they are, the less the indication. A straight tibial diaphysis will result in an oblique joint line. A pagoda-shaped or sloping surface of the tibial plateaus usually produces a bad result. Lateral subluxation of the tibia on the femur and flexion contracture of more than 7 degrees also produce a bad result.

No osteotomy will last indefinitely. **Supracondylar femoral osteotomies do not interfere with subsequent total knee replacement because the osteotomy is done above the level of the collateral ligaments. Tibial osteotomy will produce an inferior result with a total knee replacement because the osteotomy is done inside the collateral ligaments and patellar tendons and may produce a patella baja deformity.** Eventually, a total knee replacement will be required in these patients. For this reason, osteotomies are seldom done in the United States, although they remain moderately popular in many places in the world. New "opening wedge" techniques with Puddu plate type fixation are currently being evaluated. Their purported value is that the open wedge does not adversely affect the joint line in subsequent total knee replacement.

Total Knee Arthroplasty

Many surgeons use identical routines after total knee replacement, whether the implants are cemented or noncemented. *Their rationale is that the initial fixation of noncemented femoral and tibial components is in general so good that loosening is very uncommon.* The tibia is largely loaded in compression. The stability achieved with pegs, screws, and stems on modern implants is now adequate to allow full weight-bearing. However, if the bone is exquisitely soft, weight-bearing should be delayed. The progression to weight-bearing, therefore, must be based solely on the surgeon's discretion and intraoperative observations.

The guidelines for rehabilitation given here are general guidelines and should be tailored to individual patients. *Concomitant osteotomies and significant structural bone grafting are indications for limited weight-bearing until healing has been achieved.* Similarly, if the bone is extremely osteoporotic, full weight-bearing is delayed until the peri-implant bone plate develops. Exposure problems requiring a tibial tubercle osteotomy or a quadriceps tendon division may require that SLR be avoided until adequate healing has occurred, which typically takes 6 to 8 weeks.

Component design, fixation methods, bone quality, and operative techniques all affect perioperative rehabilitation. The implant choice no longer determines rehabilitation methods. It does not or should not make much difference whether the implant is unconstrained, semiconstrained, or fully constrained.

Postoperative return of 90 degrees of knee flexion is generally considered the minimal requirement for activities of daily living with an involvement of one knee. However, if both knees are replaced, it is essential that one knee reach more than 105 degrees of knee bend to allow the patient to rise from a normal low toilet seat.

Continuous passive motion (CPM) may be used after surgery, but there is a certain increase in wound problems with it. Furthermore, if the patient is left on it for long periods of time, a fixed flexion contracture of the knee tends to develop. If CPM is to be used, therefore, the patient must come off the machine for part of the day and work at achieving full extension. We limit aggressive or prolonged CPM use in patients with the potential for wound problems (such as those with diabetes or obesity).

Immediately after surgery, patients frequently have a flexion contracture because of hemarthrosis and irritation of the joint. These flexion contractures generally resolve with time and appropriate rehabilitation. However, patients who have been left with a fixed flexion contracture at the time of the surgery frequently are unable to achieve full extension. *It is important, therefore, that full extension be achieved in the operating room.*

Manipulation under anesthesia may occasionally be required. This is a very individual decision on the part of the surgeon. The author's (HUC) preference is to carry out a full manipulation under anesthesia using muscle relaxant if the patient has not achieved greater than 70 degrees of flexion by 1 week. **The usual area at which adhesions develop is the suprapatellar pouch.** Many surgeons rarely perform any manipulations under anesthesia and believe that the patient will be able to work through the motion loss. Late manipulation under anesthesia (after 4 weeks) requires great force and risks serious injury to the knee. Alternatively, arthroscopic lysis of adhesions in the suprapatellar pouch can be done with an arthroscopy obturator or a small periosteal elevator.

Reflex sympathetic dystrophy (RSD) of the knee is uncommon after total knee replacement and is usually diagnosed late. The hallmarks are chronic pain that is present 24 hours a day and allodynia or skin tenderness. Such patients usually fail to achieve a reasonable ROM and usually also develop a flexion contracture. If this suspected, a lumbar sympathetic block may be of not only diagnostic but also therapeutic value and should be carried out as soon as possible.

Total Knee Arthroplasty: Indications and Contraindications

Indications for total knee arthroplasty include disabling knee pain with functional impairment and radiographic evidence of significant arthritic involvement, and failed conservative measures; including ambulatory aids (cane), NSAIDs, and lifestyle modification (see p. 461).

Contraindications for Total Knee Arthroplasty

Absolute

- Recent or current joint infection—unless carrying out an infected revision.
- Sepsis or systemic infection.
- Neuropathic arthropathy.
- Painful solid knee fusion (painful healed knee fusions are usually due to RSD. RSD is not helped by additional surgery).

Relative Contraindications

- Severe osteoporosis.
- Debilitated poor health.
- Nonfunctioning extensor mechanism.
- Painless, well-functioning arthrodesis.
- Significant peripheral vascular disease.

Classification of Tricompartmental Total Knee Implants

Constraint

Unconstrained (Fig. 6–25)

- Relies heavily on soft tissue integrity to provide joint stability.
- Rarely used in total knee arthroplasty.

Semiconstrained

- Most knee prostheses fall into this group.
- With judicious soft tissue releases and proper implant selection, flexion contractures up to 45 degrees and angular deformities up to 25 degrees can be corrected.

Fully Constrained

- Fully constrained in one or more planes of motion.
- Because of restriction of motion in one or more planes of motion, implant stresses are very high, with potentially higher incidence of loosening, excessive wear, and breakage.
- Reserved for severe instability and severe deformity too large for semiconstrained implants.

Figure 6–25. Total knee arthroplasty. (From Howmedica Instructional Handout. Salt Lake City, Howmedica Press, 1993, p2.)

Rehabilitation of Patients with "Hybrid" Ingrowth Implants versus Those with Cemented Total Knee Implants

Cemented Total Knee Arthroplasty

- Ability for weight-bearing as tolerated with walker from 1 day postoperative.

"Hybrid" or Ingrowth Total Knee Arthroplasty

- Touch-down weight-bearing (TDWB) only with walker for first 6 wk.
- Next 6 wk, begin crutch walking with weight-bearing as tolerated.

Note: Surgeon's preference may be different. Many believe that because of compression with weight-bearing and good stability of the tibial implant, weight-bearing as tolerated with a walker is allowed immediately after surgery.

Posterior Cruciate Ligament—Sacrifice or Retain

Advantages of Preserving the Posterior Cruciate Ligament

- Potentially restores more normal knee kinematics, resulting in a more normal stair-climbing ability compared with those with PCL-sacrificing knees.

Disadvantages of Preserving the Posterior Cruciate Ligament

- Excessive rollback of the femur on the tibia if too tight.
- Preoperative joint line must be reproduced.
- More difficult collateral ligament balancing.
- More difficulty in correcting large flexion contractures.

Fixation Method for Total Knee Implants

Cemented

- Used for older, more sedentary patients.

Porous Ingrowth

- Theoretically, porous ingrowth fixation should not deteriorate with time (unlike cemented fixation) and is thus the ideal choice for younger or more active candidates.

Hybrid Technique

- Noncemented "ingrowth" femoral and patellar component with a cemented tibial component.
- Frequently used because of failure to achieve fixation with some of the original porous-coated tibial components reported in the literature.

Goals of Rehabilitation after Total Knee Arthroplasty

- Prevent hazards of bedrest (e.g., DVT, pulmonary embolism, pressure ulcers).
- Assist with adequate and functional ROM
  - Strengthen knee musculature.
  - Assist patient in achieving functional independent activities of daily living.
- Independent ambulation with an assistive device.

Perioperative Rehabilitation Considerations

Component design, fixation method, bone quality, and operative technique (osteotomy, extensor mechanism technique) will all affect perioperative rehabilitation. Implants can be posterior cruciate ligament (PCL)–sacrificing, PCL-sacrificing with substitution, or PCL-retaining. See the box for advantages and disadvantages of these component designs.

Continuous Passive Motion

There is conflicting data on the long-term effects of CPM on ROM, DVT, PE, and pain relief. Several studies have shown a shorter period of hospitalization with the use of CPM by shortening the length of time required to achieve 90 degrees of flexion. However, an increased incidence of wound complications has also been reported. Reports vary on whether there is any long-term (1 year) improvement of postoperative flexion in patients using CPM versus those who do not.

Transcutaneous oxygen tension of the skin near the incision for total knee replacement has been shown to decrease significantly after the knee is flexed more than 40 degrees. Therefore, a CPM rate of 1 cycle per minute and a maximal flexion limited to 40 degrees for the first 3 days is recommended.

If a CPM unit is used, the leg seldom comes out into full extension. Such a device must be removed several times a day so that the patient can work to prevent the development of a fixed flexion deformity.

Patient-related Risk Factors for Postoperative Complications

- Chronic use of corticosteroids
- Smoker
- Obesity
- Malnutrition (albumin < 3.5 and lymphocyte count < 1500)
- Diabetes mellitus
- Immunosuppressive use (e.g., methotrexate)
- Hypovolemia
- Peripheral vascular disease

Deep Vein Thrombosis Prophylaxis

The incidence of DVT after total knee arthroplasty is much higher than originally suspected. Based on clinical detection, the DVT rate after total knee arthroplasty ranges from 1 to 10%. However, more sensitive techniques (radioactive fibrinogen scans) have revealed a much higher incidence (50 to 70%). Prophylactic treatment is indicated (p. 457).

Total Knee Arthroplasty Rehabilitation Outline

Preoperative Physical Therapy

- Review transfers with patient
  - Bed-to-chair transfers.
  - Bathroom transfers.
  - Tub transfers with tub chair at home.
- Teach postoperative knee exercises and give patient handout.
- Teach ambulation with assistive device (walker): TDWB or WBAT for total knee arthroplasty at the discretion of the surgeon.
- Review precautions
  - To prevent possible dislocation, avoid hamstring exercises in a sitting position when using a posterior stabilized prosthesis (cruciate-sacrificing).

Inpatient Rehabilitation Goals

- 0–90 degrees ROM in the first 2 wk before discharge from an inpatient (hospital or rehabilitation unit) setting.
- Rapid return of quadriceps control and strength to enable patient to ambulate without knee immobilizer.
- Safety during ambulation with walker and transfers.
- Rapid mobilization to minimize risks of bedrest.

Because of tradeoffs between early restoration of knee ROM (especially flexion) and wound stability in the early postoperative period, different protocols are used, according to surgeon preference.

Rehabilitation Protocol
Total Knee Arthroplasty—"Accelerated" Postoperative Rehabilitation Protocol
Cameron and Brotzman

Day 1

- Initiate isometric exercises (p. 447)
  - SLR.
  - Quad sets.
- Ambulate twice a day with knee immobilizer, assistance, and walker.

NOTE: Use knee immobilizer during ambulation until patient is able to perform three SLR in succession out of the immobilizer.

- Cemented prosthesis: Weight-bearing as tolerated (WBAT) with walker.
- Noncemented prosthesis: TDWB with walker.

Rehabilitation Protocol
Total Knee Arthroplasty—"Accelerated" Postoperative Rehabilitation Protocol *(Continued)*
Cameron and Brotzman

- Transfer out of bed and into chair twice a day with leg in full extension on stool or another chair.
- **CPM machine**
  - Do not allow more than 40 degrees of flexion on settings until after 3 days.
  - Usually 1 cycle per min.
  - Progress 5–10 degrees a day as tolerated.
  - Do not record passive ROM measurements from CPM machine, but rather from patient because these may differ 5–10 degrees.
- Initiate active ROM and active-assisted ROM exerises.
- During sleep, replace the knee immobilizer and place a pillow under the ankle to help passive knee extension.

2 Days–2 Weeks

- Continue isometric exercises throughout rehabilitation.
- Use vastus medialis oblique (VMO) biofeedback if patient is having difficult with quadriceps strengthening or control.
- Begin gentle passive ROM exercises for knee
  - Knee extension (Fig. 6–26).
  - Knee flexion.
  - Heel slides.
  - Wall slides.
- Begin patellar mobilization techniques when incision stable (postoperative days 3–5) to avoid contracture.
- Perform active hip abduction and adduction exercises.
- Continue active and active-assisted knee ROM exercises.
- Continue and progress these exercises until 6 wk after surgery. Give home exercises with outpatient physical therapist following patient two to three times per week.

- Provide discharge instructions. Plan discharge when ROM of involved knee is from 0–90 degrees and patient can independently execute transfers and ambulation.

10 Days–3 Weeks

- Continue previous exercises.
- Continue use of walker until otherwise instructed by physician.
- Ensure that home physical therapy and/or home nursing care has been arranged.
- Prescribe prophylactic antibiotics for possible eventual dental or urologic procedures.
- Do not permit driving for 4–6 wk. Patient must have regained functional ROM, good quad control, and pass physical therapy functional testing.
- Provide walker for home and equipment and supplies as needed.
- Orient family to patient's needs, abilities, and limitations.
- Review tub transfers
  - Many patients lack sufficient strength, ROM, or agility to step over tub for showering.
  - Place tub chair as far back in tub as possible, facing the faucets. Patient backs up to the tub, sits on the chair, and then lifts the leg over.
  - Tub mats and nonslip stickers for tub floor traction also are recommended.

6 Weeks

- Begin weight-bearing as tolerated with ambulatory aid, if this has not already begun.
- Perform wall slides; progress to lunges.

Figure 6–26. Passive ROM exercises for knee extension. The patient places a towel under the foot. Use a slow, sustained push with the hands downward on the quadriceps.

continued

Rehabilitation Protocol
Total Knee Arthroplasty—"Accelerated" Postoperative Rehabilitation Protocol *(Continued)*
Cameron and Brotzman

Figure 6–27. Four-inch-high step-ups for quadriceps strengthening.

Figure 6–28. Lap-stool exercises for hamstring strengthening.

- Perform quadriceps dips or step-ups (Fig. 6–27).
- Begin closed-chain knee exercises on total gym and progress over 4–5 wk
  - Bilateral lower extremities.
  - Single-leg exercises.
  - Incline.
- Progress stationary bicycling.
- Perform lap-stool exercises (hamstring strengthening) (Fig. 6–28).
- Cone-walking: progress from 4- to 6- to 8-inch cones.

- Use McConnell taping of patella to unload patellofemoral stress if patellofemoral symptoms occur with exercise.
- Continue home physical therapy exercises.

Rehabilitation Protocol
After Total Knee Arthroplasty
Wilk

Phase 1: Immediate Postoperative Phase—Days 1–10

Goals
- Active quadriceps muscle contraction.
- Safe (isometric control), independent ambulation.
- *Passive knee extension to 0 degrees.*

- Knee flexion to 90 degrees or greater.
- Control of swelling, inflammation, and bleeding.

Days 1–2
Weight-bearing
- Walker/two crutches WBAT.

Rehabilitation Protocol
After Total Knee Arthroplasty *(Continued)*
Wilk

Continuous Passive Motion
- 0–40 degrees as tolerated if stable wound, and no contraindications. Take knee out of CPM several times a day and place in a knee immobilizer with pillows under the ankle (not the knee) to encourage passive knee extension (see p. 469).

Cryotherapy
- Commerical unit used.

Deep Vein Thrombosis Prophylaxis
- Per physician.

Exercises
- Ankle pumps with leg elevation.
- Passive knee extension exercise.
- SLR if not contraindicated (see p. 447).
- Quad sets.
- Knee extension exercise 90–30 degrees.
- Knee flexion exercises (gentle).

Days 4–10
Weight-bearing
- As tolerated.

Continuous Passive Motion
- 0–90 degrees as tolerated.

Exercises
- Ankle pumps with leg elevation.
- Passive knee extension stretch.
- Active-assisted ROM knee flexion.
- Quad sets.
- SLR.
- Hip abduction-adduction.
- Knee extension exercise 90–0 degrees.
- Continue use of cryotherapy.

Gait Training
- Continue safe ambulation.
- Instruct in transfers.

Phase 2: Motion Phase—Weeks 2–6

Criteria for Progression to Phase 2
- Leg control, able to perform SLRs.
- Active ROM 0–90 degrees.
- Minimal pain and swelling.
- Independent ambulation and transfers.

Goals
- Improve ROM.
- Enhance muscular strength and endurance.
- Dynamic joint stability.
- Diminish swelling and inflammation.
- Establish return to functional activities.
- Improve general health.

Weeks 2–4
Weight-bearing
- WBAT with assistive device.

Exercises
- Quad sets.
- Knee extension exercise 90–0 degrees.
- Terminal knee extension 45–0 degrees.
- SLR (flexion-extension).
- Hip abduction-adduction.
- Hamstring curls.
- Squats.
- Stretching
  - Hamstrings, gastrocnemius, soleus, quads.
- Bicycle ROM stimulus.
- Continue passive knee extension stretch.
- Continue use of cryotherapy.
- Discontinue use of TED hose at 2–3 wk (with physician's approval).

Weeks 4–6
Exercises
- Continue all exercises listed above.
- Initiate
  - Front and lateral step-ups (minimal height).
  - Front lunge.
  - Pool program.
  - Continue compression, ice, and elevation for swelling.

Phase 3: Intermediate Phase—Weeks 7–12

Criteria for Progression to Phase 3
- ROM 0–110 degrees.
- Voluntary quadriceps muscle control.
- Independent ambulation.
- Minimal pain and inflammation.

Goals
- Progression of ROM (0–115 degrees and greater).
- Enhancement of strength and endurance.
- Eccentric-concentric control of the limb.
- Cardiovascular fitness.
- Functional activity performance.

Weeks 7–10
Exercises
- Continue all exercises listed in phase 2.
- Initiate progressive walking program.
- Initiate endurance pool program.
- Return to functional activities.
- Lunges, squats, step-ups (small 2-inch step to start).
- Emphasize eccentric-concentric knee control.

Phase 4: Advanced Activity Phase—Weeks 14–26

Criteria for Progression to Phase 4
- Full, nonpainful ROM (0–115 degrees).
- Strength of 4+/5 or 85% of contralateral limb.
- Minimal or no pain and swelling.
- Satisfactory clinical examination.

continued

Rehabilitation Protocol
After Total Knee Arthroplasty (Continued)
Wilk

Goals
- Allow selected patients to return to advanced level of function (recreational sports).
- Maintain and improve strength and endurance of lower extremity.
- Return to normal lifestyle.

Exercises
- Quad sets.
- SLR (flexion-extension).
- Hip abduction-adduction

- Squats.
- Lateral step-ups.
- Knee extension exercise 90–0 degrees.
- Bicycle for ROM stimulus and endurance.
- Stretching
  - Knee extension to 0 degrees.
  - Knee flexion to 105 degrees.
- Initiate gradual golf, tennis, swimming, bicycle, walking program.

Recommended Long-term Activities after Total Joint Replacement

DeAndrade (1993) developed an evaluation scale of the activities for patients with total joint replacements. Stress on the joint replacement should be minimized to avoid excessive wear and tear that would reduce the longevity of the implant. Intensity of the exercise should be adjusted so that it is painless, but still promotes cardiovascular fitness. Running and jumping should be avoided, and shoes should be well cushioned in the heel and insole. Joints should not be placed at the extremes of motion. Activity time should be built up gradually, with frequent rest periods between activity periods. Correct use of walking aids is encouraged to minimize stress on the joint replacement. The first long-term activity undertaken should be walking (Table 6–10).

Management of Rehabilitation Problems after Total Knee Arthroplasty

Recalcitrant Flexion Contracture (Difficulty Obtaining Full Knee Extension)
- Initiate backward walking.
- Perform passive extension with the patient lying prone with the knee off the table, with and without weight placed across the ankle (see Fig. 4–24). This should be avoided if contraindicated by the PCL status of the arthroplasty.

Table 6–10

Recommended Long-term Activities after Total Replacement of the Hip or Knee

Very Good, Highly Recommended	Good, Recommended	Needs Some Skill, Prior Significant Expertise	With Care, Ask Your Doctor	AVOID
Stationary bicycling	Bowling	Bicycling (street)	Aerobic exercise	Baseball
Ballroom dancing	Fencing	Canoeing	Calisthenics	Basketball
Square dancing	Rowing	Horseback riding	Jazz dancing	Football
Golf	Speed walking	Rock climbing		Softball
Stationary (Nordic-Track) skiing	Table tennis	Inline skating		Handball
	Cross-country skiing	Nautilus exercises		Jogging
Swimming		Ice skating		Racquetball/squash
Walking			Downhill skiing	
	Weight-lifting		Tennis—doubles	Lacrosse
			Step machines (for patients with hip replacements; not for those with knee replacements)	Soccer
				Tennis—singles
				Volleyball

From De Andrade RJ: Activities after replacement of the hip or knee. Orthop Special Ed 2(6):8, 1993.

- Eccentric extension. The therapist passively extends the leg and then holds the leg as the patient attempts to lower it slowly.
- With the patient standing, flex and extend the involved knee. Sports cord or rubber bands can be used for resistance.
- Use electric stimulation and VMO biofeedback for muscle re-education if problem is active extension.
- Passive extension is also performed with a towel roll placed under the ankle and the patient pushing downward on the femur (or with weight on top of the femur) (see Fig. 6–26).

Delayed Knee Flexion
- Passive stretching into flexion by therapist.
- Wall slides for gravity assistance.
- Stationary bicycle. If patient lacks enough motion to bicycle with saddle high, then begin cycling backward, then forward, until able to make a revolution. Typically, this can be done first in a backward fashion.

Bibliography

Hip Arthritis

Brady LP: Hip pain: don't throw away the cane. Postgrad Med 83(8):89, 1988.

Cameron HU: The Cameron anterior osteotomy. In: Bono JV et al (ed): Total Hip Arthroplasty. New York, Springer-Verlag, 1999.

Centers for Disease Control and Prevention: Health-related quality of life among adults with arthritis: behavioral risk factor surveillance system. MMWR Morb Mortal Wkly Rep 49(17):366, 2000.

Chandler DR, Glousman R, Hull D, McGuire PJ, Kim IS, Clarke IC, Sarmiento A: Prosthetic hip range of motion and impingement: the effects of head and neck geometry. Clin Orthop June (166):284, 1982.

Collis DK: Total joint arthroplasty. In Frymoyer JW (ed): Orthopedic Knowledge Update, No. 4. Rosemont, Ill, American Academy of Orthopedic Surgeons, 1993.

DeAndrade RJ: Activities after replacement of the hip or knee. Orthop Special Ed 2(6):8, 1993.

Horne G, Rutherford A, Schemitsch E: Evaluation of hip pain following cemented total hip arthroplasty. Orthopedics 3(4):415, 1990.

Johnson R, Green JR, Charnley J: Pulmonary embolism and its prophylaxis following Charnley total hip replacement. J Arthroplasty Suppl 5:21, 1990.

Kakkar VV, Fok PJ, Murray WJ: Heparin and dihydroergotamine prophylaxis against thrombo-embolism of the hip arthroplasty. J Bone Joint Surg Aug; 67(4):538, 1985.

Little JW: Managing dental patients with joint prostheses. J Am Dent Assoc 125:1374, 1994.

Pellicci PM: Total joint arthroplasty. In Daniel DW, Pellicci PM, Winquist RA (eds): Orthopedic Knowledge Update, No. 3, Rosemont, Ill, American Academy of Orthopedic Surgeons, 1990.

Steinberg ME, Lotke PA: Postoperative management of total joint replacements. Orthop Clin North Am 19(4):19, 1988.

Knee Arthritis

Bradley JD, Brandt KD, Katz BP, et al: Comparison of an anti-inflammatory dose of ibuprofen, an analgesic dose of ibuprofen, and acetaminophen in the treatment of patients with osteoarthritis of the knee. N Engl J Med 325:87, 1991.

Chen PQ, Cheng CK, Shang HC, Wu JJ: Gait analysis after total knee replacement for degenerative arthritis. J Formos Med Assoc Feb; 90(2):160, 1991.

Cole BJ, Harner CD: Degenerative arthritis of the knee in active patients: evaluation and management. J AAOS 7(6):389, 1999.

Colwell CW, Morris BA: The influence of continuous passive motion on the results of total knee arthroplasty. Clin Orthop 276:225, 1992.

Corsbie WJ, Nichol AC: Aided gait in rheumatoid arthritis following knee arthroplasty. Arch Phys Med Rehabil 71:191, 1990.

DeAndrade RJ: Activities after replacement of the hip or knee. Orthop Spec Ed 2(6):8, 1993.

Edelson R, Burks RT, Bloebaum RD: Short-term effects of knee washout for osteoarthritis. Am J Sports Med 23:345, 1995.

Fox JL, Poss P: The role of manipulation following total knee replacement. J Bone Joint Surg 63A:357, 1981.

Ghosh P, Smith M, Wells C: Second-line agents in osteoarthritis. In Dixon JS, Furst DE (ed): Second-Line Agents in the Treatment of Rheumatic Diseases. New York: Marcel Dekker, 363, 1992.

Gibson JN, White MD, Chapman VM, Strachan RK: Arthroscopic lavage and debridement for osteoarthritis of the knee. J Bone Joint Surg 74:534, 1992.

Jackson RW, Rouse DW: The results of partial arthroscopic meniscectomy in patients over 40 years of age. J Bone Joint Surg Br 64:481, 1982.

Keating EM, Faris PM, Ritter MA, Kane J: Use of lateral heel and sole wedges in the treatment of medial osteoarthritis of the knee. Orthop Rev 22:921, 1993.

Kozzin SC, Scott R: Current concepts: unicondylar knee arthroplasty. J Bone Joint Surg 71A:145, 1989.

Livesley PJ, Doherty M, Needoff M, Moulton A: Arthroscopic lavage of osteoarthritic knees. J Bone Joint Surg Br 73:922, 1991.

Maloney WJ, Schurman DJ, Hangen D: The influence of continuous passive motion on outcome in total knee arthroplasty. Clin Orthop Jul; 256:162, 1990.

McInnes J, Larson MG, Daltroy LH: A controlled evaluation of continuous passive motion in patients undergoing total knee arthroplasty. JAMA Sep 16; 268(11):1423, 1992.

Morrey BF: Primary osteoarthritis of the knee: a stepwise management plan. J Musculoskel Med 79:(3), 1992.

Puddu G, Cipolla M, Cerullo C, Scala A: Arthroscopic treatment of the flexed arthritic knee in active middle-aged patients. Knee Surg Sports Traumatol Arthrosc 73, 1994.

Ritter MA, Campbell ED: Effect of range of motion on the success of a total knee arthroplasty. J Arthroplasty 2:95, 1987.

Ritter MA, Stringer EA: Predictive range of motion after total knee arthroplasty. Clin Orthop 143:115, 1979.

Shoji H, Solomoni WM, Yoshino S: Factors affecting postoperative flexion in total knee arthroplasty. Orthopedics June; 13:643, 1990.

Steinberg ME, Lotke PA: Postoperative management of total joint replacements. Orthop Clin North Am 19(4):19, 1988.

VanBaar ME, Assendelft WJ, Dekker J: Effectiveness of exercise therapy in patients with osteoarthritis of the hip or knee: a systematic review of randomized clinical trials. Arthritis Rheum 42(7):1361, 1999.

Chapter 7
Special Topics

Thomas Clanton, MD, Stan L. James, MD,
and S. Brent Brotzman, MD

Hamstring Injuries in Athletes

Thomas Clanton, MD, Kevin J. Coupe, MD, S. Brent Brotzman,
MD, and Anna Williams, BS, MSPT

Clinical Background

Hamstring injuries are common in athletes and often become a troublesome chronic condition. The hamstring muscle group consists of three muscles: **the semimembranosus, the semitendinosus, and the biceps femoris** (long and short heads). These three muscles function during the early stance phase for knee support, during the late stance phase for propulsion of the limb, and during mid swing to control momentum of the extremity. Injury to the hamstrings, whether partial or complete, typically occurs at the myotendinous junction where the eccentric force is concentrated.

Hamstring injuries are also notorious for reinjury, often because of inadequate rehabilitation and premature return to competition before complete recovery of the hamstring muscle group.

Anatomy

The three muscles of the hamstring group, the semimembranosus, semitendinosus, and biceps femoris (long and short heads) (Fig. 7–1), originate as a tendinous mass from the ischial tuberosity of the pelvis, with the exception of the short head of the biceps femoris.

Figure 7–1. Origins of the hamstring tendons *(left)* and muscles of the hamstring group *(right)*. (From Clanton TO, Coupe KJ: Hamstring strains in athletes: diagnosis and treatment. © 1998 American Academy of Orthopaedic Surgeons. Reprinted from the Journal of the American Academy of Orthopaedic Surgeons, Volume 6 (4), pp. 237–248, with permission.)

- The ischial tuberosity acts as a common point of attachment and thus may occasionally result in an avulsion fracture.
- This short head of the biceps femoris originates from the linea aspera along the distal femur. This is the only hamstring muscle with a dual innervation.
- The semimembranosus, semitendinosus, and the long head of the biceps femoris are innervated by the tib-

ial branch of the sciatic nerve. The short head of the biceps femoris is innervated by the peroneal portion of the sciatic nerve.
- The semimembranosus and semitendinosus muscles course along the medial aspect of the femur to their separate medial attachments (Fig. 7–2). The semimembranosus exerts multiple insertions at the posterior medial corner of the knee, acting as a significant

Figure 7–2. *Left,* Attachment of the semitendinosus with the pes anserinus at the proximal medial aspect of the tibia. *Right,* Insertions of the gracilis (G), sartorius (S), semimembranosus (SM), and semitendinosus (ST). (From Clanton TO, Coupe KJ: Hamstring strains in athletes: diagnosis and treatment. © 1998 American Academy of Orthopaedic Surgeons. Reprinted from the Journal of the American Academy of Orthopaedic Surgeons, Volume 6 (4), pp. 237–248, with permission.)

Figure 7–3. Insertions of the long and short heads of the biceps femoris at the lateral aspect of the knee. (From Clanton TO, Coupe KJ: Hamstring strains in athletes: diagnosis and treatment. © 1998 American Academy of Orthopaedic Surgeons. Reprinted from the Journal of the American Academy of Orthopaedic Surgeons, Volume 6 (4), pp. 237–248, with permission.)

contributor to knee stability. The semitendinosus joints with the gracilis and sartorius to form the pes anserinus attachment to the medial tibial metaphysis in close proximity to the distal insertion of the medial collateral ligament of the knee.

- The biceps femoris attaches laterally as shown in Figure 7–3.
- The hamstring group is a two-joint muscle group, which means the muscle crosses two joints. This is believed to make this group more susceptible to strain. Clanton and Coupe (1998) describe the mechanism for injury as increased force generated during eccentric action of the muscle as opposed to a concentric contraction. In the running cycle, the hamstring becomes vulnerable when the muscle group decelerates the extending knee during forward swing and also at take-off, owing to the sudden change in function of the muscle from stabilizing the knee in flexion to having to assist in paradoxical extension of the knee.

The most common site of injury to the hamstrings is the myotendinous junction, as are most indirect muscle injuries.

Mechanism of Injury

The two most common factors in hamstring injury are lack of adequate flexibility and strength imbalances in the hamstrings (flexor-to-extensor and right-to-left).

An imbalance may exist in the muscle strength of the hamstrings between the patient's limbs, and there may also be a decreased ratio between the flexor (hamstring) and the extensor (quadriceps) groups. A flexor-to-extensor strength ratio of less than 0.6 or a strength imbalance of 10% or more between the right and the left hamstrings has been proposed as a causative factor in hamstring injury. Numerous studies have used isokinetic dynamometry to suggest appropriate flexor-to-extensor ratios, extension torque ratios, and flexion torque ratios. Initially, a flexion-to-extension ratio of 0.5 to 0.6 was considered a standard for a number of years. It has become apparent that these ratios actually vary between male and female athletes as well as among athletes in different sports and playing different positions in the same sport.

Right-to-left hamstring strength imbalances appear to increase the likelihood of hamstring injury in the lower extremity. Also, a ratio of 50 to 65% for hamstring strength compared with quadriceps strength (flexor-to-extensor ratio) is recommended to decrease the chance of hamstring injury.

Other controllable factors such as lack of adequate warm-up, lack of flexibility, overall conditioning, and muscle fatigue should all be corrected to minimize the chance of hamstring injury.

Prevention

Because strength imbalance, lack of adequate flexibility, lack of adequate warm-up, and overall conditioning play varying roles in the etiology of hamstring injuries, a prevention regimen addressing these factors is very important. A preparticipation hamstring stretching regimen and warm-up algorithm follows (see p. 480).

Clinical Findings

Hamstring injuries are common in all athletes, especially those who participate in kicking, running, and jumping. Typically, an injury occurs during sprinting or high-speed exercises (e.g., the lead leg for a hurdler, a jumper's take-off leg). Avulsion fractures of the ischial tuberosity may also occur in other sports including water skiing, weight-lifting, dancing, and ice skating.

Most hamstring injuries occur acutely when the athlete experiences sudden onset of pain in the posterior aspect of the thigh during strenuous exercises. This most commonly occurs during sprinting. Often, the history of inadequate warm-up or fatigue may be elicited.

The participant may describe an audible pop and pain, which would not allow continued participation in the sport. In more severe injuries, the patient may describe falling to the ground. Milder injuries are often described as a pull or tightness in the posterior aspect of the thigh during exercise that did not limit participation but subsequently "tightened up."

Avulsion fractures of the ischial tuberosity typically result from severe hip flexion while the knee is maintained in full extension.

Clinical Examination

A minor hamstring strain may produce no physical findings, whereas a severe tear may produce extensive bruising, swelling, tenderness, and possibly a palpable defect.

With an acute injury, the athlete may be lying on the ground grabbing the back of the thigh. This is not pathognomonic but is highly suggestive for a hamstring injury.

The entire length of the hamstring muscles should be palpated by the examiner. This is typically done with the patient lying prone and with the knee flexed to 90 degrees (Fig. 7–4). Any extension of the knee may cause cramping or increased pain, which will limit the scope of the examination. The muscle is palpated fully relaxed and then with mild tension. Palpation should also be

A

B

C

Figure 7–4. *A,* Examination of the hamstring with the knee flexed 90 degrees. *B,* Athlete with a large tear of the hamstring muscle group. *C,* Radiograph demonstrates an avulsion injury *(arrowhead)* of the common hamstring tendon. (*B* and *C,* From Clanton TO, Coupe KJ: Hamstring strains in athletes: diagnosis and treatment. © 1998 American Academy of Orthopaedic Surgeons. Reprinted from the *Journal of the American Academy of Orthopaedic Surgeons,* Volume 6 (4), pp. 237–248, with permission.)

Figure 7–5. Measurement of restriction of passive knee extension after hamstring injury. (From DeLee JC, Drez D Jr: Orthopaedic Sports Medicine: Principles and Practice. Philadelphia, WB Saunders, 1994.)

done at the ischial tuberosity for any possible palpable bony avulsion. The position of maximal tolerance for straight leg raise (SLR) should be documented because this is a useful guide to determining the initial severity of the injury and the likely response to rehabilitation.

Another useful guideline is a restriction of passive extension of the knee with the hip flexed to 90 degrees (Fig. 7–5). In this position, active knee flexion will serve as an indicator of the amount of tension that can be generated before pain when compared with the contralateral, uninvolved leg.

Rarely, the injury is dramatic and there is a large defect with an impressive palpable wad of muscle appearing in the posterior thigh during contraction of the hamstrings.

Classification

Hamstring injuries are classified in three groups: mild (grade I), moderate (grade II), and severe (grade III) (Table 7–1).

- **Grade I** strain or "pulled muscle" signifies an overstretching of the muscle resulting in disruption of less than 5% of the structural integrity of the musculotendinous unit.
- **Grade II** represents a partial tear with a more significant injury but an incomplete rupture of the musculotendinous unit.
- **Grade III** represents a complete rupture of the muscle with severely torn, frayed ends similar to those seen in an Achilles tendon rupture.

Avulsion fractures may occur at the ischial tuberosity proximally or at the distal insertion at the knee.

Kujala and Orava (1993) have further classified injuries of the *ischial apophysis* (growth plate). This classification includes apophysitis, adult tug lesions, painful unfused apophysis, and acute and chronic avulsions of the apophysis. Very young patients have a much lower frequency of hamstring strains. This may be due in part to the much greater flexibility of this age group and to the susceptibility to injury of the apophyseal attachment of the hamstring, which is greater rather than that of the myotendinous junction. Surgery is considered in cases with dislocation of the apophysis (bony avulsion) of more than 2 cm.

Radiographic Studies

Currently, there is *little indication* for detailed radiographic studies of acute hamstring injuries.

The information provided by an MRI typically does not change the course of treatment.

MRI should be infrequently used. On MRI, acute injuries typically show up as high signal intensity on T2-

Table 7-1		

Signs and Symptoms of Muscle Strains

Severity	Symptoms	Signs
Mild (first-degree)	Local pain, mild pain on passive stretch and active contraction of the involved muscle; minor disability.	Mild spasm, swelling, ecchymosis; local tenderness; minor loss of function and strength.
Moderate (second-degree)	Local pain, moderate pain on passive stretch and active contraction of the involved muscle, moderate disability.	Moderate spasm, swelling, ecchymosis, local tenderness; impaired muscle function and strength.
Severe (third-degree)	Severe pain, disability.	Severe spasm, swelling, ecchymosis, hematoma, tenderness, loss of muscle function; palpable defect may be present.

From Andrews JR, Harrelson GL: Physical Rehabilitation of the Injured Athlete, 1st ed. Philadelphia, WB Saunders, 1991, p. 344.

weighted images as a result of hemorrhage or edema within the muscle belly. Chronic muscle injuries are less predictable in appearance.

Plain radiographs are of little value unless an avulsion fracture of the ischial tuberosity is suspected. Because *bony avulsions with more than 2 cm of displacement are surgically repaired*, plain films of the pelvis (anteroposterior view of the pelvis that includes the ischial tuberosity) should be taken if an avulsion fracture of the ischial tuberosity is suspected.

Chronic myositis ossificans may be shown on plain radiographs but is very uncommon. The discovery of calcification or ossification of the soft tissues of the thigh on plain radiographs should raise the examiner's suspicion for other pathology (e.g., neoplasm) and initiate a more extensive investigation and work-up.

Prevention of Hamstring Injuries

Because of the chronicity of hamstring injuries, emphasis at our institution is placed on prevention of the injury. Because the most common factors cited in hamstring injury are *lack of flexibility* and *strength imbalance* (hamstring-to-quadriceps; right-to-left leg), we emphasize these areas in our exercises.

In collegiate and high school athletes, prepractice regimens, the following stretches are used.

Hamstring Stretching Regimen

Single-Leg Hamstring Stretch

Lie supine with both legs flat on the table. Loop a towel around the foot and hold the ends of the towel with your hands. Keep the knee straight and the foot in dorsiflexion (pointing toward the ceiling). Pull the leg up toward the ceiling. Pull until you feel a stretch in back of the leg and sustain the stretch for 30 seconds. Relax the leg and repeat (Fig. 7–6).

Figure 7–7. Straddle groin and hamstring stretch.

Straddle Groin and Hamstring Stretch

Sit on the floor with both legs straddled (Fig. 7–7). Keep knees straight with the kneecap facing the ceiling and the feet in dorsiflexion (pointing toward the ceiling). Be sure to keep your back straight and bend forward at the hips. First reach straight forward until you feel a stretch in the hamstring and sustain the stretch for 30 seconds. Relax and reach to the right until a stretch is felt and hold for 30 seconds. Relax and reach to the left.

Side-Straddle and Hamstring Stretch

Sit on the floor with the injured leg straight, keeping the kneecap facing the ceiling and the foot pointing toward the ceiling. The uninvolved leg is relaxed with the knee bent. Bend forward at the hips, keeping your back straight. Reach for the injured leg's ankle until a hamstring stretch is felt and then sustain the stretch for 30 seconds (Fig. 7–8). Relax and repeat.

Figure 7–6. Single-leg hamstring stretch.

Figure 7–8. Side-straddle groin and hamstring stretch.

Figure 7–9. Hamstring stretch with anterior pelvic tilt.

Figure 7–10. Isometric hamstring exercise. The patient pushes down against the bed with the left (involved) leg.

Pelvic-Tilt Hamstring Stretch

Sit on the edge of the chair with the injured leg resting straight. The uninjured leg is bent at 90 degrees (Fig. 7–9). With your back straight, bend forward at the hips. Rest your hands on your thighs for support. Lean forward until you feel a stretch and then hold for 30 seconds. Relax and repeat.

Hamstring Strengthening Regimen for Injury Prevention

Hamstring strengthening exercises are also used to improve the quadricep-to-hamstring ratio and any asymmetry between the hamstrings of the right and left legs. Strong, symmetrical hamstrings should be less prone to injury.

Isometric Hamstring Curls

Sit on the floor with the uninjured leg straight. The involved leg is bent with the heel on the floor. Push the heel into the floor and then pull toward the buttocks to tighten the hamstring muscle (Fig. 7–10). Hold the contraction for 5 seconds. Relax. Begin with one set of 12 to 15 and progress to perform two to three sets of 12 to 15 repetitions.

Prone Hamstring Curls

Place an ankle weight on the involved leg. Lie prone, placing a pillow under the involved knee if needed. With the foot in position, as shown in the photo, bring the heel toward the buttocks in a slow, controlled manner. Begin with one set of 12 to 15 repetitions and progress to two to three sets of 12 to 15 repetitions (Fig. 7–11).

Standing Hamstring Curls

Place an ankle weight on the involved leg. Stand with your feet shoulder-width apart. Holding on to a support, curl the heel toward the buttocks in a slow, con-

A

B

Figure 7–11. *A* and *B,* Prone hamstring curls with weight.

Figure 7–12. Standing hamstring curls.

Figure 7–13. Seated walking on a stool with wheels.

trolled manner. Be sure to maintain proper knee alignment with the uninvolved leg. Begin with one set of 12 to 15 repetitions and progress to two to three sets of 12 to 15 repetitions (Fig. 7–12).

Hamstring Curl Machine

The exercise can be performed on a prone or a standing hamstring machine. The weight will be at the ankle. Curl the leg against resistance by bringing the heel toward the buttocks. Begin with one set of 12 to 15 repetitions and progress to two to three sets of 12 to 15 repetitions.

Seated Walking

Sit on a rolling stool with wheels. Begin walking forward while sitting on the stool (Fig. 7–13).

Treatment of Hamstring Injuries

Treatment of hamstring injuries is directed toward restoration of strength and flexibility of the muscle group. This is critical for appropriate muscle regeneration and prevention of reinjury. A shortened, scarred, hamstring muscle is more susceptible to strain.

Days 1 through 5 after Hamstring Injury

For the first 3 to 5 days after injury, the main goal of treatment is control of hemorrhage, swelling, and pain. The familiar RICE (rest, ice, compression elevation) regimen is used during this period. Any range of motion (ROM) is gently increased and strengthening exercises are gradually progressed with the resumption of activities. This may take several days to weeks depending on the extent of injury, the level of competition, and the upcoming activities anticipated for the athlete. The two competing processes that the physician has to manage are

muscle regeneration and production of connective scar tissue.

The goal is to maximize muscle regeneration and minimize dense, restrictive scar formation.

- **Rest.** Jarvinen and Lehto (1993) have shown that a *relatively short period* of *immobilization is advantageous* in limiting the extent of dense connective tissue scar at the site of injury. The absolute optimal time of mobilization has not been defined but *less than 1 week of relative immobilization is typically recommended* in the literature.

  Early controlled mobilization guided by pain tolerance is begun after 1 to 5 days of immobilization. This will allow better regeneration and alignment of the injured muscle fiber.

  In the laboratory setting, weakened muscle is able to regain its normal capacity for energy absorption around 7 days. Until this time is reached, it is more susceptible for further injury.

  Acutely, crutches or occasionally bedrest may be warranted for a severe grade II or grade III hamstring injuries, but *complete immobilization* of the knee or hip *is not indicated.* Crutches are weaned from two crutches to one crutch and then discontinued when the patient is able to ambulate without a limp or alteration in gait. Early motion is important, but is progressed in a controlled fashion.

- **Ice.** Ice should be applied to the hamstring immediately in an effort to delay and decrease inflammation and edema. The physiologic effects of ice are beneficial in the healing process and allow more rapid return to athletics.

  Ice should be applied to the hamstring in a plastic bag and wrapped directly over the posterior thigh with an Ace bandage. We typically employ this for 20 to 30 minutes for application and reapply the ice two to four times a day or as frequently as every 2 hours for the first 48 to 72 hours.

- **Compression.** Gentle compression is used with a firm compressive bandage placed around the thigh. No studies document any efficacy of compression alone as a treatment for muscle injury.
- **Elevation.** In an effort to reduce edema and allow return of fluid to the heart, the athlete elevates the extremity *above the heart* two to three times a day whenever possible. We do not use bedrest for hamstring injuries.
- **Anti-inflammatory medication.** The only controversy with regard to the use of anti-inflammatories is the timing of administration. Almekinders (1993) recommends the use of anti-inflammatories immediately after injury and discontinuation after 3 to 5 days. Other research indicates that anti-inflammatories interfere with chemotaxis of cells necessary for laying down new muscle fibers, therefore, possibly inhibiting the healing response. These studies suggest delaying the administration of anti-inflammatories for 2 to 4 days.

We use anti-inflammatories beginning on day 3 and discontinue on day 6.

General Treatment and Rehabilitation Goals

Treatment is directed toward restoration of both strength and flexibility to this muscle unit. Even in the early period after injury, attention is turned to initiating gentle muscle action to prevent atrophy and promote healing.

- Because motion is initially limited and painful, *isometric exercises* are initiated first, using submaximal isometric contraction (example: two to three sets of 5 repetitions, 5-second contraction, varying by 15- to 20-degree increments). Care should be taken to limit tension to the injured muscle to avoid reinjury during this period.
- With improvement in motion and pain, the isometric exercises are replaced by *isotonic exercise with light weights.* These can be increased daily in 1-pound increments. This program uses concentric contractions

with no pain. Eccentric muscle activity is avoided to prevent increased tension in the muscle unit.

- When the athlete is pain-free throughout the prone hamstring exercise program, a *high-speed, low-resistance isokinetic exercise program* is begun. Machines that create only concentric contractions are used. Isokinetic exercises are advanced as tolerated to include higher resistance and slower speeds.
- Pool walking and stationary bicycle with no resistance are also used in the early stages because they allow pain-free motion with controlled resistance. Hamstring curls in the water are also beneficial in the early postinjury phase. This is eventually progressed to running in place in the water with a supportive vest in the deep end of the pool as well as swimming with a gentle flutter kick employing a kick board.
- Well-leg exercise and upper body exercises are also used throughout for aerobic conditioning.
- When the patient has a normal gait with minimal tenderness and improved muscle strength, a walking program on the track is employed with eventual progression to a walk/jog program.
- Isokinetic testing is used to gain useful information on strength, balance, and degree of persistent deficit in hamstring strength. The final decision is based on clinical parameters and the athlete's progress and functional activities.

Stretching after Injury

Stretching to avoid loss of flexibility is an important component of the postinjury treatment regimen. Gentle active stretching is used initially with progression to passive static stretching as pain allows. Worrell (1994) emphasized the advantage of hamstring stretching in an anterior pelvic tilt (see Fig. 7–9) and minimized the advantage of proprioceptive neuromuscular facilitation (PNF) stretching over static stretching. The former generally requires an assistant trained in a technique, such as a therapist or athletic trainer. Others prefer this method for gaining and maintaining flexibility.

Rehabilitation Protocol
Treatment for Hamstring Strain
Modified Clanton, Coupe, Williams, and Brotzman Protocol

	Time Frame	Goals	Treatment
Phase 1: Acute	3–5 days 1–5 days	• Control pain and edema. • Limit hemorrhage and Inflammation.	• RICE regimen. • Immobilization (brief in extension), NSAIDs.

continued

Rehabilitation Protocol
Treatment for Hamstring Strain *(Continued)*
Modified Clanton, Coupe, Williams, and Brotzman Protocol

Time Frame	Goals	Treatment
After 5 days	• Prevent muscle fiber adhesions.	• *Pain-free passive ROM* (gentle stretching). Sit on a firm surface with a sock on the foot. Place a towel around the foot as if the foot were in a sling. Gently pull the towel to bring the heel toward the buttocks. Hold for 3–5 sec and slowly return to the starting position (Fig. 7–14). • *Heel slides.* Sit on a firm surface with a sock on the foot or a towel under the heel. Gently flex the knee with the foot approaching the buttocks, then return to the starting position (Fig. 7–15). • *Wall slides.* Lie on a firm surface with the feet resting on the wall. Slowly begin to walk the feet down the wall, gently increasing knee flexion. At the end-range, slowly begin returning to the starting position (Fig. 7–16).

Figure 7–14. Pain-free passive range of motion (ROM) (gentle stretching) of the hamstrings.

Figure 7–15. Heel slides on a table.

Rehabilitation Protocol
Treatment for Hamstring Strain *(Continued)*
Modified Clanton, Coupe, Williams, and Brotzman Protocol

	Time Frame	Goals	Treatment
			• *Hamstring stretch.* Sit on a firm surface with a small bolster or towel roll under the ankle. Place a 3- to 5-pound weight on the top of the thigh to allow a passive stretch of the hamstring muscle (Fig. 7–17).
	Up to 1 wk	• Normal gait.	• Crutches.
Phase 2: Subacute	Day 3–>3 wk	• Control pain and edema.	• Ice, compression, and electric stimulation.
		• Full active ROM.	• Pain-free pool activities.
		• Alignment of collagen.	• Pain-free passive and active ROM.
		• Increase collagen strength.	• *Pain-free submaximal isometrics.* Sit on a firm surface with the involved leg in slight flexion and the heel on the mat. Push the heel into the firm surface and then pull toward the buttocks (Fig. 7–18). It is important to note that no actual movement of the extremity occurs—only a hamstring muscle contraction. Hold the contraction for 5 sec and then relax. Also perform stationary bicycle.

Figure 7–16. Wall slides.

Figure 7–17. Hamstring stretch.

continued

Rehabilitation Protocol
Treatment for Hamstring Strain (Continued)
Modified Clanton, Coupe, Williams, and Brotzman Protocol

Figure 7–18. Pain-free submaximal isometric hamstring exercise.

Figure 7–19. Prone concentric isotonic exercise.

	Time Frame	Goals	Treatment
		• Maintain cardiovascular conditioning.	• Well-leg stationary bike, swimming with pull buoys, upper body exercise.
Phase 3: Remodeling	1–6 wk	• Achieve phase II goals. • Control pain and edema. • Increase collagen strength.	• Ice and compression. • Ice and electric stimulation. • *Prone concentric isotonic exercises.* Lie prone on a firm surface with a pillow under the hips to increase hip flexion. Place a cuff weight on the involved leg and flex the leg to bring the heel toward the buttocks. Perform the flexion movement slowly, then return the leg to the starting position (Fig. 7–19). • *Standing concentric isotonic exercises.* Stand near a table or wall for support. Place a cuff weight on the involved leg. Keeping the knees aligned, flex the involved leg to bring the heel toward the buttocks in a slow, controlled manner. Return the leg to the starting position (Fig. 7–20).

Rehabilitation Protocol
Treatment for Hamstring Strain *(Continued)*
Modified Clanton, Coupe, Williams, and Brotzman Protocol

Figure 7–20. Standing concentric isotonic hamstring exercise.

Figure 7–22. Seated walking on a stool with wheels.

Time Frame	Goals	Treatment
		• *Isokinetic exercise.* Must be performed at a facility with the proper equipment. Lie prone on the table with a stabilizing strap placed across the hips. The involved leg will also have a stabilizing strap placed across the thigh. The ankle is strapped into the movable arm. The therapist then programs the computer to perform the movement at a certain speed and angle* (Fig. 7–21).

Figure 7–21. Isokinetic exercise for the hamstring. (From Andrews JR, Harrelson GL, Wilk KE, : Physical Rehabilitation of the Injured Athlete, 2nd ed. Philadelphia, WB Saunders, 1998.)

continued

Rehabilitation Protocol
Treatment for Hamstring Strain *(Continued)*
Modified Clanton, Coupe, Williams, and Brotzman Protocol

	Time Frame	Goals	Treatment
			• *Rolling stool.* Sit on a rolling stool and propel forward. Begin by using both legs simultaneously, progressing to alternating the lower extremities. To further advance, propel using only one extremity (Fig. 7–22).
		• Increase hamstring flexibility.	• Moist heat or exercise prior to pelvis-tilt hamstring stretching.
		• Increase eccentric loading.	• *Prone eccentric exercises.* Performed same as concentric, except quickly flex the lower extremity and return to the starting position, a very slow, controlled manner. Also jump rope (Fig. 7–23).
			• *Standing eccentric isotonic exercise.* Same as standing concentric exercise, except flex the lower extremity *quickly* and return to the starting position in a very slow, controlled manner.
Phase 4: Functional	2 wk–6 mo	• Return to sport without reinjury.	• Walk/jog, jog/sprint, sport-specific skills and drills (slideboard, lateral drills).

Figure 7–23. Jump rope.

Figure 7–24. Pelvic-tilt hamstring stretch.

Rehabilitation Protocol
Treatment for Hamstring Strain *(Continued)*
Modified Clanton, Coupe, Williams, and Brotzman Protocol

	Time Frame	Goals	Treatment
		• Increase hamstring flexibility.	• *Pelvic-tilt hamstring stretching.* Sit on the edge of the chair with spine in neutral position. The involved leg is straight, with the heel resting on the floor and the toes in dorsiflexion. The uninvolved leg is resting in a comfortable position with the hip and knee flexed at 90 degrees. Keeping the spine straight, lean forward, bending at the hips. A stretch will be felt along the posterior aspect of the leg (Fig. 7–24).
			• *Supine hamstring stretch.* Sit on a firm surface. Place a towel around the sole of the foot. Keeping the knee straight and toes dorsiflexed, pull the towel toward the chest. The foot will raise as if doing an SLR. Hold the stretch for 30 sec. Return to the starting position (Fig. 7–25).
		• Increase hamstring strength. • Control pain.	• *Prone concentric and eccentric exercises.* Heat, ice, and modalities; NSAIDs as needed.
Phase 5: Return to Competition	3 wk–6 mo	• Avoid reinjury.	• Maintenance stretching and strengthening.

Figure 7–25. Supine hamstring stretch.

NSAIDs, nonsteroidal anti-inflammatory drugs.
*Concentric high speeds at first, proceeding to eccentric low speeds.

Operative Indications

Surgery is typically considered only after a complete hamstring avulsion from the ischial tuberosity with a bony avulsion displacement of 2 cm or more.

Distal hamstring injuries are typically present in combination with more serious injuries such as biceps femoris tendon ruptures associated with posterolateral corner knee injuries.

Distal avulsions are treated like proximal avulsions when these occur in isolation (rarely occur).

Readiness for Return to Competition

Isokinetic testing is used to confirm restoration of muscle strength imbalances to appropriate ratios. ■

Quadriceps Strains and Contusions

Steven J. Meyers, MD, and S. Brent Brotzman, MD

Important Rehabilitation Points for Quadriceps Injuries

- Acute injuries to the thigh are common and represent approximately 10% of all sports injuries.
- Differentiating between a quadriceps **strain** or **tear** (indirect mechanism) and a **contusion** (direct trauma mechanism) is important for appropriate treatment.
- **Quadriceps contusions** result from a **direct blow** to the anterior thigh from a knee or helmet.

- **Quadriceps tears or strains** are typically caused by **indirect trauma.** The patient complains of a feeling of a "pulled" muscle, and the mechanism often occurs by the patient missing a soccer ball and striking the ground violently with forced stretching of the contracting quadriceps muscle.

Quadriceps Strain or Tear (Indirect Mechanism)

- **Risk factors** for quadriceps strains (or tears) include inadequate stretching, inadequate warm-up before vigorous exercise, and muscle imbalance of the lower extremity.
- **Prevention** of quadriceps injuries employs preactivity quadriceps stretching (Fig. 7–26) and institution of proper warm-up before vigorous play. Muscle imbalances (e.g., large quadriceps and atrophic hamstrings) are corrected in off-season training.
- The patient typically complains of a "pulled" thigh.
- Examination typically reveals tenderness on palpation of the rectus femoris (strain) or defect (tear). This is usually found in the muscle belly.
- Because the rectus femoris is the only quadriceps that crosses the hip joint, extending the hip with the knee flexed causes more discomfort than flexing the hip with the knee extended. This **extended hip maneuver** causes pain because of its isolation of the rectus femoris.
- Look for a muscle defect (tear) on this maneuver or on quadriceps contraction.

Figure 7–26. *A,* Standing quadriceps stretch. *B,* Single-leg quadriceps stretch. A towel is used to stretch the quadriceps muscle gradually. In later stages of rehabilitation, the proprioceptive neuromuscular facilitation contract-relax technique can be used to increase ROM.

A   B

Rehabilitation Protocol
Treatment of Quadriceps Strains (or Tears)

Acute Phase

- RICE.
- NSAIDs if not contraindicated.
- Crutches in a touch-down or partial weight-bearing (painless) fashion.
- Hold all lower extremity athletic participation.
- *Avoid SLR in early rehabilitation because of increased stress on the torn rectus femoris.*

Intermediate Phase (Usually 3–10 Days Postinjury)

Goals
- Regain normal gait.
- Regain normal knee and hip motion.
- Usually intermediate phase begins 3–10 days postinjury, depending on severity of injury.

Exercises
- Initiate a *gentle* quadriceps (see Fig. 7–26) and hamstring (Fig. 7–27) stretching program.
- PNF patterns.
- Aquatic rehabilitation program in deep water with flotation belt.
- Cycling with no resistance.

Return of Function Phase

- Terminal knee extension exercises.
- Increase aquatic program (deep-water running [DWR]).
- Begin knee extension with light weights, progress.
- SLR, quad sets progressing to PRE (progressive resistance exercises) with 1- to 5-pound weight on the ankle.
- Increase low-impact exercises to progress endurance and strength
  - Progress bicycle resistance and intensity of workout.
  - Elliptical trainer.
  - Thera-bands for hip flexion, extension, abduction, adduction.
  - Walking progression to jogging (painless).
  - 30-degree mini-squats (painless).

Figure 7–27. Single hamstring stretch.

- Initiate sport-specific drills and agility training.
- Isokinetic equipment (at higher speeds) with patient supine.

Note: Even quadricep tears with palpable defects typically respond to this conservative regimen. Persistent defects are common, but rarely, if ever, require surgery or cause loss of function.

Employ preactivity quad stretching program and appropriate warm-up regimen with return to sports.

Criteria for Return to Play

- Quadriceps flexibility equal bilaterally.
- Asymptomatic with functional drills at full effort.
- Quadricep strength 85 to 90% (via isokinetic testing) of contralateral quadricep.

Quadriceps Contusions (Direct Blow [Helmet] Mechanism)

- Severity ranges from mild bruise to large, deep hematoma requiring months to heal.
- Rarely, compartment syndrome of thigh or artery injury (be aware).
- Attempt to avoid development of myositis ossificans.
- Jackson and Feagin (1973) functionally classify thigh contusions into **mild, moderate, or severe.** The classification is designated **24 to 48 hours** after the in-jury to observe the edema and hematoma, which should have stabilized at that point (Table 7–2).
- **Cryotherapy (icing) to reduce edema and bleeding is key in the early stages of this injury** (Table 7–3).
- **Normal knee flexion is typically the slowest parameter to return after thigh contusions. For this reason, Jackson and Feagin's protocol recommends placing the knee and hip in flexion (120 degrees at the knee) for the first 24 hours only** (Fig. 7–28).

Table 7–2

Clinical Grading of Severity of Quadriceps Contusion*

Contusion Severity	Knee Range of Motion	Gait	Physical Findings	Can Do Deep Knee Bend?
Mild	>90 degrees	Normal	Mild tenderness	Yes
Moderate	45–90 degrees	Antalgic	Enlarged, tender thigh	No
Severe	<45 degrees	Severe limp	Greatly swollen thigh, pain with quadriceps contraction	No

*Severity is graded 24–48 hr postinjury.
From Kaeding CC, Sanka WA, Fisher RA: Quadriceps strains and contusions: decisions that promote rapid recovery. Physician Sports Med 23(1):59, 1995.

Table 7–3

Management of Quadriceps Contusions Immediately after Injury

Time after Injury	Treatment
Immediately	Knee immobilization in 120 degrees of flexion
First 24 hr	Knee bracing in 120 degrees of flexion, crutches, then discontinue brace
After 24 hr	Crutches, high-voltage galvanic stimulation, ice, quadriceps stretching exercises
Return to play	Protective pad over injury site for rest of season

Figure 7–28. After acute quadriceps contusion, the athlete's knee is passively flexed and immobilized in 120 degrees of flexion using an elastic wrap.

A

B

Figure 7–29. Special pad worn after a quadriceps contusion can help prevent reinjury in patients who play contact sports. *A,* An appropriate thigh pad consists of a rigid, foam-covered plastic shell with a thick, ring-shaped foam pad *(arrow)* inside it. It should be of an appropriate size and shape to cover and protect the injured site and comfortable for athletic participation. *B,* The injured area should be centered in the ring-shaped pad, and the pad must be secured to the thigh so that it does not migrate. (*A* and *B,* From Kaeding CC, Sanko WA, Fisher RA: Quadriceps strains and contusions: decisions that promote rapid recovery. Physician Sports Med 23[1]:59–64, 1995.)

Rehabilitation Protocol
Quadriceps Contusion

	Phase 1	Phase 2	Phase 3
Purpose	• Limit the hemorrhage.	• Restoration of pain-free motion.	• Functional rehabilitation; strength and endurance.
Modalities	• High-voltage galvanic stimulation. • *Rest:* weight-bearing to tolerance, *crutch ambulation* if limp present; frequent ice; ice massage for 10 min; cold pack/cool whirlpool, 20 min. • *Compression:* elastic wrap entire thigh (occasional use: long-leg support hose, confirm taping). • *Elevation:* in class and in barracks, hip and knee flexed to tolerance; isometric quadriceps contracture <10 repetitions; immobilize the knee in 120 degrees of flexion for 24 hr (hinged leg brace).	• Ice or cool whirlpool, 15–20 min; pain-free isometric quadriceps exercises, 15–20 min; supine and prone active flexion; well-leg gravity-assisted motion; static cycling, minimum resistance; *discard:* (1) crutches when ROM >90 degrees, no limp, good quadriceps control, and pain-free with flexed weight-bearing gait; (2) elastic wrap when thigh girth reduced to equivalent of uninjured thigh; initiate pain-free quadriceps stretching several times a day (see Fig. 7–26).	• Always pain-free: static cycling with increasing resistance; Cybex; swim; walk; jog (pool and surface); run.
Advance to Next Phase When	• Comfortable; pain-free at rest; stabilized thigh girth.	• >120 degrees pain-free active motion; equal thigh girth bilaterally.	• Full active ROM; full squat; pain-free all activities; wear with **thick thigh pad** 3–6 mo for all contact sports.

Modified from Ryan JB, Wheeler JH, Hopinkson WJ, et al: Quadriceps contusions: West Point update. Am J Sports Med 19(3):299–304, 1991.

• Aronen (1990) places the knee in immediate passive knee flexion to 120 degrees with icing within 10 minutes of the injury and maintains this for 24 hours. This flexion places the quadriceps under tension and may lessen intramuscular bleeding. This maximizes stretching of the quadricep and decreases flexion loss.

• Other authors use simultaneous cryotherapy with frequent 20-minute intervals of knee flexion.

• *Do not* aspirate or inject cortisone or enzymes.

• **Avoid heat, massage, or ultrasound of thigh contusions initially, which intensifies swelling and the inflammatory reaction.**

• A special thigh pad manufactured from foam-covered plastic is worn when contact sport patients return to play. The pad is secured to the thigh to avoid migration (Fig. 7–29).

Criteria for Return to Play after Thigh Contusion

• Injured area is appropriately protected in contact sports (thigh pad).

• Full, symmetrical quadriceps flexibility.

• Eighty-five to 90% strength, power, and time to peak torque on isokinetic and dynamometer testing compared with uninvolved quadriceps.

• Nontender to palpation of injured quadriceps. ■

Groin Pain

S. Brent Brotzman, MD

Background

• Groin pain is a broad, confusing "garbage-can" type of term that means different things to different people. Patients may describe "I pulled my groin" (groin

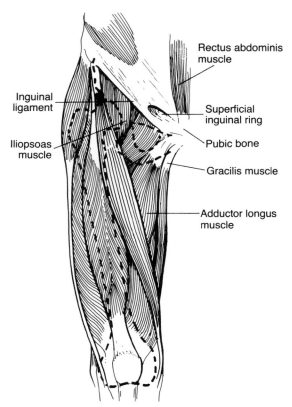

Rectus abdominis muscle

Inguinal ligament

Superficial inguinal ring

Iliopsoas muscle

Pubic bone

Gracilis muscle

Adductor longus muscle

Figure 7–30. Among the musculotendinous injuries of the thigh that can cause groin pain, adductor longus muscle injuries are most common. Any injury to the iliopsoas, rectus femoris, sartorius, or gracilis muscle can also produce groin pain. (From DeLee JC, Drez D Jr: Orthopaedic Sports Medicine: Principles and Practice. Philadelphia, WB Saunders, 1994.)

strain), or "I got kicked in the groin" (testicle), or "I have a lump in my groin" (lower abdominal wall).

- The key to this diagnostically challenging problem is a very thorough history-taking and examination.
- In our institution, we first try to establish accurately if this is an **acute injury** (usually musculoskeletal) or a **chronic** symptom (often nonmusculoskeletal in origin).
- Second, we attempt to establish the correct **anatomic area** being described as the groin (e.g., hip adductors [medial], hip, testicle, lower abdominal wall).
- The commonly accepted **definition of a groin strain** focuses on injury to the hip adductors and includes the iliopsoas, rectus femoris, and sartorius musculotendinous units (Fig. 7–30). An accurate area of anatomic pain must be delineated by the examiner (e.g., adductor origin or testicular pain with radiation).

Differential Diagnosis of Groin Pain: Using a "How to Approach Groin Pain" Mnemonic

How	**H**ip/pelvis
To	**T**high
Approach	**A**bdomen
Groin	**G**enitalia
Pain	**P**ain (referred)

Differential Diagnosis of Groin Pain: Using a "How to Approach Groin Pain" Mnemonic *(Continued)*

Hip/Pelvis

Stress fracture of the femoral neck*

Pubic ramus fracture*

Osteitis pubis*

Legg-Calvé-Perthes disease*

Slipped capital femoral epiphysis*

Avulsion fracture about the pelvis*

Snapping hip*

Acetabular labral tear*

Bursitis (iliopectineal,* trochanteric)

Avascular necrosis

Osteoarthritis

Synovitis or capsulitis

Thigh

Muscle strains

Adductor longus*

Rectus femoris*

Iliopsoas*

Sartorius*

Gracilis*

Femoral hernia

Lymphadenopathy

Abdomen

Lower Abdominal Wall

Strain of the rectus abdominis*

Inguinal hernia*

Ilioinguinal nerve entrapment*

Sports hernia (hockey player's syndrome)*

Abdominal Organ Conditions

Abdominal aortic aneurysm

Appendicitis

Diverticulosis, diverticulitis

Inflammatory bowel disease

Pelvic inflammatory disease

Ovarian cyst

Ectopic pregnancy

Genitalia

Prostatitis

Epididymitis

Hydrocele/varicocele

Testicular torsion

Testicular neoplasm

Urinary tract infection

History

Careful history-taking is required to avoid missing a potentially catastrophic problem (e.g., stress fracture of the femoral neck).

Acute (Traumatic) Injuries

- Mechanism of injury (e.g., change of direction, pivoting).
- Hear or feel a pop?
- Swelling or bruising noted? If so, location?
- Previous groin injury?
- Recent change in training regimen?

Chronic Injuries or Those with No Clear-cut Traumatic, Musculoskeletal Mechanism

- Pain at rest or at night (neoplasm possible).
- Does the pain radiate (e.g., to the back, thigh, hip, scrotum, or perineum)?
- What alleviates pain (e.g., physical therapy, rest, NSAIDs)?

- Associated numbness (look for a dermatomal pattern emanating from the back).
- Pain on coughing or sneezing, which increases intra-abdominal pressure (hernia or low back disc).
- Can patient reproduce pain with exertion or certain movements?
- Fever or chills (possible infection or neoplasm).
- Activities that cause the pain.
- Recent weight loss (neoplasm).
- Urinary symptoms such as dysuria, urgency, frequency, hematuria (possible sexually transmitted disease, urinary tract infection, stones).
- Bowel symptoms such as blood in stool, mucus, diarrhea (Crohn's disease, ulcerative colitis).

Risk Factors for Groin Injuries

Contact sports

Obesity

Poor muscle conditioning

Inflexibility

Sports that require quick starts

Examination

- Examination should include the groin, hip area, back, genitourinary, and lower abdominal wall.
- See Tables 7–4 and 7–5 for examination and potential causes of groin pain.
- If the patient's complaint is anatomically hip pain rather than groin, differential diagnosis can include a number of possible causes of hip pain in athletes.

Table 7-4

Physical Examination of the Groin (Fig. 7–31)

Patient's Position	Procedure	Details
Standing	Observe posture, gait, limb alignment, muscle wasting, ability to sit and stand up, swelling.	Have the patient point to the area of pain and the pattern of radiation. Have the patient reproduce painful movements.
	Examine the low back: active ROM.	Forward flexion, side bending, extension.
	Examine the hip: active ROM.	Trendelenburg's sign (hip adductor strength), ability to squat and duck-walk.
	Examine the hernia.	Palpate the inguinal region (have the patient cough or strain down).
Supine	Examine the abdomen.	Palpate for abdominal aortic aneurysm, pain, rebound, guarding, hernia, pulses, nodes. Test for costovertebral angle tenderness (renal area). When appropriate, perform a rectal examination to palpate the prostate and rule out occult blood.
	Examine male genitalia.	Palpate for a testicular mass, varicocele, or tender epididymis.
	Pelvic examination in women, if appropriate.	Look for purulent vaginal discharge of pelvic inflammatory disease and bluish cervix of pregnancy (ectopic). Palpate for tender cervix or adnexa, ovarian mass.
	Examine low back, sciatic nerve roots.	Perform SLR, test for Lasègue sign and Bragard sign (dorsiflexion of ankle).
	Examine hip motion.	Evaluate flexion, external rotation, **internal rotation,** abduction, adduction, joint play, quadrant tests, **any groin pain with internal rotation?** Perform passive SLR, Thomas, and rectus femoris stretch tests.
	Palpate pelvic structures.	Palpate symphysis, pubic rami, iliac crests, adductor insertions, ASIS, PSIS, ischial tuberosities.

Table 7-4 *(Continued)*

Physical Examination of the Groin

Patient's Position	Procedure	Details
	Examine sacroiliac joints.	Perform Patrick (flexion, abduction, external rotation, extension [FABERE]) test, palpate sacroiliac joint.
	Look for leg-length discrepancy.	Verify grossly and determine true length by measuring from ASIS to lateral malleoli.
Prone	Examine hip motion.	Evaluate extension as well as internal and external rotation. Perform Ely and femoral nerve stretch tests.
Side-lying	Examine iliotibial band.	Perform Ober test
Sitting	Evaluate muscle strength.	Test hip flexion (L2, L3), hip extension (L5, S1, S2), abduction (L4, L5, S1), adduction (L3, L4).
	Test reflexes.	Assess patellar tendon (L4).
	Test sensation.	Asses lower abdomen (T12), groin (L1), medial thigh (L2), anterior quadriceps (L3).

ASIS, anterior superior iliac spine; PSIS, posterior superior iliac spine; ROM, range of motion; SLR, straight-leg raises.
From Lacroix VJ: A complete approach to groin pain. Physician Sports Med 28(1):66, 2000

A

B

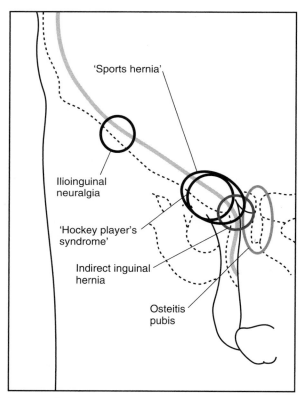

Figure 7–31. *A,* Direct trauma, intense abdominal muscle training, or inflammatory conditions can lead to entrapment of the ilioinguinal nerve, which innervates the lowest portions of the transversus abdominis and internal oblique muscles and the skin overlying the inguinal ligament. The nerve transmits sensation from the base of the penis, scrotum (or labium major), and part of the medial thigh. Patients describe a burning or shooting pain in these areas. Hip hyperextension may exacerbate it. Treatment usually consists of injecting anesthetics or corticosteroids. *B,* Typical sites of pain in the "sports hernia," "hockey player's syndrome," and other conditions that cause pain in the same general anatomic region. *C,* Anterior *(i, ii),* superior *(iii),* and posterior *(iv)* views of the pelvis depict anatomy relevant to various sports-related causes of groin pain. *D,* Locations of several major muscle origins and insertions of the pelvis and proximal femur. Avulsion injuries have been reported at each of these sites. (*A* and *B,* From Lacroix VJ: A complete approach to groin pain. Physician Sports Med 28[1]:32–37, 2000; *C,* from Swain R, Snodgrass S: Managing groin pain even when the cause is not obvious. Physician Sports Med 23[1]:54–62, 1995; *D,* from Anderson K, Strickland SM, Warren R: Hip and groin injuries in athletes. Am J Sports Med 29[4]:521–533, 2001.)

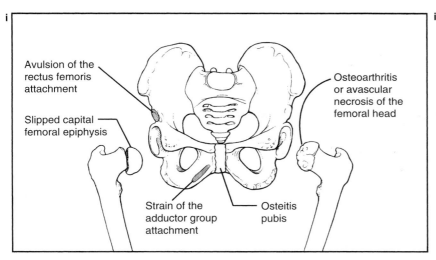

i

Avulsion of the rectus femoris attachment

Slipped capital femoral epiphysis

Osteoarthritis or avascular necrosis of the femoral head

Strain of the adductor group attachment

Osteitis pubis

ii

Iliopectineal bursitis

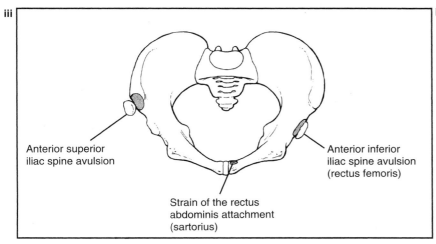

iii

Anterior superior iliac spine avulsion

Anterior inferior iliac spine avulsion (rectus femoris)

Strain of the rectus abdominis attachment (sartorius)

iv

Trochanteric bursitis

C

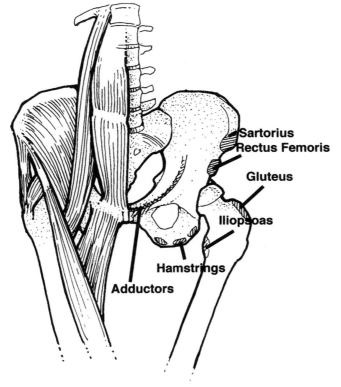

Sartorius
Rectus Femoris

Gluteus

Iliopsoas

Hamstrings

Adductors

D

Figure 7–31. *Continued*

Table 7-5

Potential Causes of Groin Pain: Key Features and Treatments

Causes	Key Features	Treatment Options
Musculoskeletal		
Abdominal muscle tear	Localized tenderness to palpation; pain with activation of rectus abdominis	Relative rest, analgesics
Adductor tendinitis	Tenderness over involved tendon, pain with resisted adduction of lower extremity	NSAIDs, rest, physical therapy
Avascular necrosis of the femoral head	Radiation of pain into the groin with internal rotation of hip; decreased hip ROM	Recommend MRI *Mild*: conservative measures, possible core decompression; *severe*: total hip replacement, **needs orthopaedic hip specialty consult**
Avulsion fracture	Pain on palpation of injury site; pain with stretch of involved muscle, x-ray positive, felt a pop when "turning on speed"	Relative rest; ice; NSAIDs; possibly crutches, evaluate for ORIF of fragment if > 1 cm displacement
Bursitis	Pain over site of bursa	Injection of cortisone, anesthetic, or both; avoid injections around nerves (e.g., sciatic)
Conjoined tendon dehiscence	Pain with Valsalva's maneuver	Surgical referral (general surgeon)
Herniated nucleus pulposus	Positive dural or sciatic tension signs	Physical therapy or appropriate referral (spine specialist)
Legg-Calvé-Perthes disease	Irritable hip with pain on rotation, positive x-rays, pediatric (usually ages 5–8 yr)	Pediatric orthopaedic surgeon referral
Muscle strain	Acute pain over proximal muscles of medial thigh region; swelling; occasional bruising	Rest; avoidance of aggravating activities; initial ice, with heat after 48 hr; hip Spica wrap; NSAIDs for 7–10 days See section on treatment
Myositis ossificans	Pain and decreased ROM in involved muscle; palpable mass within substance of muscle, x-ray shows calcification, often history of blow (helmet) to area	Moderately aggressive active or passive ROM exercises; wrap thigh with knee in maximum flexion for first 24 hr; NSAIDs used sparingly for 2 days after trauma
Nerve entrapment	Burning or shooting pain in distribution of nerve; altered light-touch sensation in medial groin; pain exacerbated by hyperextension at hip joint, possibly radiating; tenderness near superior iliac spine	Possible infiltration of site with local anesthetic; topical cream (e.g., capsaicin)
Osteitis pubis	Pain around abdomen, groin, hip, or thigh, increased by resisted adduction of thigh, tender on palpation of pubis symphysis, x-ray positive for sclerosis irregularity, osteolysis at the pubis symphysis, bone scan positive	Relative rest; initial ice and NSAIDs; possibly crutches; later, stretching exercises
Osteoarthritis	Groin pain with hip motion, especially internal rotation	Non-narcotic analgesics or NSAIDs; hip replacement for intractable pain See Chapter 6, The Arthritic Lower Extremity
Pubic instability	Excess motion at pubic symphysis; pain in pubis, groin, or lower abdomen	Physical therapy, NSAIDs; compression shorts
Referred pain from knee or spine	Hip ROM and palpation response normal	Identify true source of referred pain
Seronegative spondyloarthropathy	Signs of systemic illness, other joint involvement	Refer to rheumatologist
Slipped capital femoral epiphysis†	Inguinal pain with hip movement; insidious development in ages 8–15 yr; walking with limp, holding leg in external rotation	Discontinue athletic activity; refer to orthopaedic surgeon for probable pinning, crutches TDWB
Stress fracture		
Pubic ramus	Chronic ache or pain in groin, buttock, and thighs	Relative rest; avoid aggravating activities, crutches PWB
Femoral neck†	Chronic ache or pain in groin, buttock, and thighs, or pain with decreased hip ROM (internal rotation in flexion)	Refer to orthopaedist if radiographs or bone scan show lesion; TDWB crutches and cessation of all weight-bearing activities until orthopaedic consult

Table 7–5 (Continued)

Potential Causes of Groin Pain: Key Features and Treatments

Causes	Key Features	Treatment Options
Nonmusculoskeletal		
Genital swelling or inflammation		
Epididymitis	Tenderness over superior aspect of testes	Antibiotics if appropriate, or refer to urologist
Hydrocele	Pain in lower spermatic cord region	Refer to urologist
Varicocele	Rubbery, elongated mass around spermatic cord	Refer to urologist
Hernia	Recurrent episodes of pain; palpable mass made more prominent with coughing or straining; discomfort elicited by abdominal wall tension	Refer for surgical evaluation and treatment (general surgeon)
Lymphadenopathy	Palpable lymph nodes just below inguinal ligaments; fever, chills, discharge	Antibiotics, work-up, also rule out underlying sexually transmitted disease
Ovarian cyst	Groin or perineal pain	Refer to gynecologist
PID	Fever, chills, purulent discharge + chandelier sign, "PID shuffle"	Refer to gynecologist
Postpartum symphysis separation	Recent vaginal delivery with no prior history of groin pain	Physical therapy, relative rest, analgesics
Prostatitis	Dysuria, purulent discharge	Antibiotics, NSAIDs
Renal lithiasis	Intense pain that radiates to scrotum	Pain control, increased fluids until stone passes; hospitalization sometimes necessary
Testicular neoplasm	Hard mass palpated on the testicle; may not be tender	Refer to urologist
Testicular torsion or rupture*	Severe pain in the scrotum; nausea, vomiting; testes hard on palpation or not palpable	Refer immediately to urologist
Urinary tract infection	Burning with urination; itching; frequent urination	Short course of antibiotics

*Emergent immediate referral.
†Non–weight bearing until orthopaedic evaluation to avoid fracture.
NSAIDs, nonsteroidal anti-inflammatory drugs; ORIF, open reduction and internal fixation; PID, pelvic inflammatory disease; PWB, partial weight-bearing; TDWB, touch-down weight-bearing.
Modified from Ruane JJ, Rossi TA: When groin pain is more than just a strain. Physician Sports Med 26(4):78, 1998.

Differential Diagnosis of Hip Pain in Athletes

Hip dislocation
Hip subluxation with or without acetabulum or labrum injury
Osteochodritis dissecans
Acetabulum or pelvis fracture or stress fracture
Femoral neck fracture or stress fracture
Anterior superior iliac spine avulsion (sartorius or rectus femoris origin)
Iliac spine contusion (hip pointer)
Adductor muscle strain
Osteitis pubis
Inguinal hernia
Lateral femoral cutaneous nerve entrapment or injury (meralgia paresthica)
Femoral artery or nerve injury

Differential Diagnosis of Hip Pain in Athletes (Continued)

Idiopathic avascular necrosis of the femoral head
Idiopathic chondrolysis
Slipped capital femoral epiphysis
Legg-Calvé-Perthes disease
Metabolic disorders
Sickle cell disease
Inflammatory disease
Lumbar disc disease
Neoplastic abnormalities of the pelvis, acetabulum, or femur
Piriformis syndrome

From Lacroix VJ: A complete approach to groin pain. Physician Sports Med 28(1):66–86, 2000.

Urgent Hip/Groin Diagnoses That Require Immediate Attention and Appropriate Treatment

- Hip dislocation
- Neurovascular injury (Fig. 7–32)
- Hip fracture
  - Acetabulum
  - Femoral neck
  - Femur
- Septic hip (infected)
- Slipped capital femoral epiphysis
- Sickle cell crisis

- Testicular torsion or rupture
- Incarcerated hernia

Special attention should be given to

- Legg-Calvé-Perthes disease
- Neoplasm
- Avascular necrosis
- Idiopathic chondrolysis
- Femoral neck stress fracture

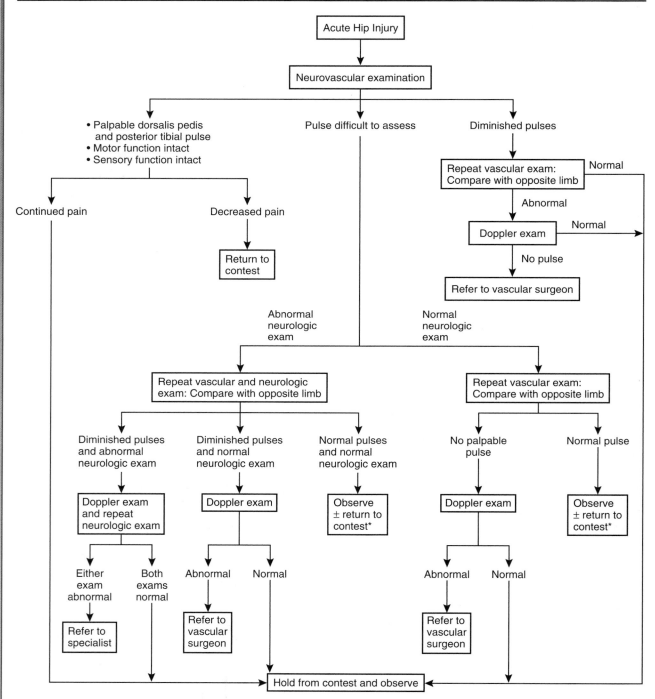

* The on-field physician decides whether the athlete should return to competition based on the athlete's symptoms.

Figure 7–32. Neurovascular evaluation for the athlete who has hip pain during an athletic event. (From Lacroix VJ: A complete approach to groin pain. Physician Sports Med 28(1):32–37, 2000.)

Rehabilitation Protocol
After Groin (Adductor) Strain
Brotzman

Phase 1: Immediate Postinjury Phase

Activity
- Relative rest from athletic injury until patient is asymptomatic and rehabilitation protocol complete.
- Avoid lateral movements, pivoting, twisting, reverse of direction.
- Initiate PRICE regimen (protection, rest, ice, compression, elevation above heart).

Crutches
- Employ crutches weight-bearing as tolerated until patient walks with a normal, nonantalgic gait.

Modalities
- Cryotherapy postexercise.
- Pulsed ultrasound.
- Electric stimulation.

Exercises
- Aquatic deep-water pool running.
- Stationary bicycling with no resistance.
- Active ROM exercises of hip
  - Flexion, extension, abduction, gentle adduction.
- Isometric exercises
  - Hip adduction.
  - Hip abduction.
  - Hip flexion.
  - Hip extension.
- SLR, quad sets.

Phase 2: Intermediate Phase

Criteria for Progression to Phase 2
- Minimal to no pain on gentle groin stretching.
- Good, painless gait.
- Swelling minimal.

Progressive Resistance Exercises (1- to 5-pound weight)
- Hip abduction, adduction, flexion, extension.
- SLR.

Continue modalities (ultrasound, moist heat).

Proprioceptive exercises.

Initiate *gentle* groin stretches

- Wall groin stretch (Fig. 7–33).
- Groin stretch (Fig. 7–34).
- Straddle groin and hamstring stretch (see Fig. 7–7).
- Side-straddle groin/hamstring stretch (see Fig. 7–8). (*Note:* long 10- to 15-sec stretches with no bobbing.)
- Hamstring stretches.
- Passive rectus femoris stretch (Fig. 7–35).
- Passive hip flexor stretch (Fig. 7–36)
  - Progress stationary bicycling resistance.
  - DWR in pool (see section on Aquatic Therapy).
  - PNF patterns.

Figure 7–33. Wall groin stretch.

Phase 3: Advanced Phase

- Continue stretches above.
- Concentric and eccentric hip abduction and adduction with Thera-band.
- Function drills after warmed up and full stretch
  - Cariocas.
  - Slide board.

Figure 7–34. Groin stretch.

continued

Rehabilitation Protocol
After Groin (Adductor) Strain *(Continued)*
Brotzman

A

B

Figure 7–35. *A,* Passive rectus femoris stretch. The amount of passive stretch can be modified by the amount of hip extension, which is based on the athlete's tolerance to stretch. It can be used in conjunction with cryotherapy techniques. *B,* Manual rectus femoris stretch can be used to stretch the muscle and also to determine its length. (*B,* From Andrews JR, Harrelson GL, Wilk KE: Physical Rehabilitation of the Injured Athlete, 2nd ed. Philadelphia, WB Saunders, 1998.)

- Jogging/running.
- Box drill.
- Protective wrapping or commercial hip Spica–type protection (Fig. 7–37).

Criteria for Return to Sports
- Equal muscular strength of adductors, abductors, flexors, extensors on manual muscle testing.

- Full, pain-free ROM.
- Ability to perform all sport-specific functional drills at full speed without pain.
- Athlete must develop a rigorous pre– and post–sporting activity groin stretching program for the remainder of the season.

Rehabilitation Protocol
After Groin (Adductor) Strain *(Continued)*
Brotzman

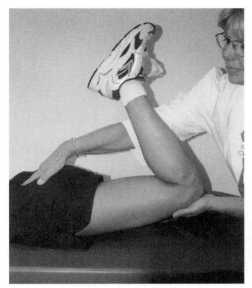

Figure 7–36. Passive hip flexor stretch.

Figure 7–37. Commercial hip Spica brace for groin injury. (From Kinetic Innovation, 1-887-272-2376.)

Modified from Andrews JR, Harrelson GL, Wilk KE: Physical Rehabilitation of the Injured Athlete. Philadelphia, WB Saunders, 1998.

Aquatic Therapy for the Injured Athlete

Teresa Triche, M Ed

Important Rehabilitation Points for Aquatic Therapy Training

- As athletes train harder, compete more often, and take less time to taper (at advancing ages), overuse injuries have become more frequent.
- Elite athletes are under time constraints (often self-imposed) for injury rehabilitation.
- Research has demonstrated that 6 weeks of inactivity may result in significant loss of cardiovascular fitness (as much as 14 to 16% of maximal oxygen consumption). Even 3 weeks of inactivity causes significant cardiovascular fitness loss.
- Aquatic therapy allows "active rest" that avoids high impact to the injured extremity (e.g., stress fractures of the foot) yet maintains
  - Cardiovascular fitness.
  - Flexibility.
  - Speed.
  - Balance and proprioception.
  - Coordination.
  - Strength.
- Exercises performed against the water's resistance almost always elicit concentric muscle contractions. Eccentric contractions may be elicited for the lower extremity if the water is shallow enough to minimize buoyancy (e.g., lunges in hip-deep water elicits eccentric quadriceps contraction).

In general, heart rates during deep water exercise will be approximately 17 beats per minute (bpm) lower than comparable exercise on land. Training heart rates should be established in the water rather than applying land-based heart rates. Because of the physiologic changes incurred while immersed, it is recommended that the athlete train at a heart rate 17 to 20 bpm lower than on land.

- The rate of perceived exertion (RPE) by the athlete is often unreliable because of the effects of skill and comfort on perceived exertion.
- Warm-up and cool-down are essential and should be done in the pool.
- The fundament guidelines for cardiovascular training should be incorporated into the program design: 25 minutes five times per week at a minimum, with longer training periods for elite athletes.

- Exercises should *not* be done in hot tub temperatures (100 to 103°F).
- Therapy pools serving an orthopaedic population are typically 90 to 94°F. The Arthritis Foundation requires pool temperature for its approved courses be at least 84 to 86°F.
- Thein and Brody (1998) recommend elite athletes undergoing intense training should train in water between 26 and 28°C to prevent heat-related complications. Warm water increases cardiovascular demands above those of the exercise done. The athlete should be kept well hydrated.
- Before resuming land-based impact activities, the athlete is placed through a battery of sport-specific tests in shallow water to assess readiness for impact. Athletes should be able to complete the test without pain, swelling, or significant soreness.
- On initiation of a land-based impact program, the water-based program is continued on alternate days.
- We typically use Aqua Jogger equipment (e.g., flotation belt, dumbbells, Aquarunners). These are available at www.aquajogger.com or 1-800-922-9544.
- VO_{2max}, referred to in the following section, is the maximal amount of oxygen that can be taken in by the body, delivered to the muscles, and used.

Deep-Water Running (DWR)—Background

Individuals who perform land-based training exercises, such as running or jogging, may be required to discontinue that activity if an injury occurs. One treatment for running-related injuries is to simply decrease or discontinue running for 4 to 6 weeks. Runners fear that such a break will lead to a decrease in fitness or an increase in body weight, and few are willing to endure long periods of inactivity. It is well known that the cessation of activity results in a significant loss of functional capacity. A 4- to 6-week period of inactivity will lead to a 14 to 16% reduction in VO_{2max} over the 4- to 6-week period. Thus, we use aquatic-based therapy for "active-rest" from an injury. The goal is to maintain cardiovascular endurance, mobility, strength, and flexibility while "resting" the injury.

Many athletic organizations today, from those in high schools to those representing the professional athlete, are recognizing the benefits of including an aquatic rehabilitation component when an injury is sustained. **DWR** has become the newest form of aquatic therapy for injured athletes. It has been accepted as a popular and effective form of cardiovascular conditioning for both rehabilitation and training. It is becoming popular among runners as a training exercise during periods of injury because there is less musculoskeletal stress than normal running. Runners are also replacing part of their existing training program with DWR to re-

duce overuse injuries. DWR enables the athlete to continue in an activity that is specific to running without incurring the possible harmful effects of weight-bearing work.

DWR consists of simulated running in the deep end of the pool aided by a flotation device (vest or belt) that maintains the head above the water. The athlete may be held in one location by a tether cord, essentially running in place, or may actually run through the water the length or width of the pool.

- During DWR, the body is tilted slightly forward approximately 5 degrees past the vertical, with the spine in neutral position. The bend should occur at the hips, not the waist.
- The head is held comfortably out of the water, facing forward; avoid neck extension.
- The arm action is the same as for land running, with the primary movement occurring at the shoulder and with the hands relaxed but lightly closed.
- Ankles should perform both dorsiflexion and plantar flexion.
- Hip flexion should reach about 60 to 80 degrees.
- No contact is made with the bottom of the pool, thus eliminating impact.
- This form of running in the water closely follows the pattern used on land. However, the center of gravity on land is at the hips. In water, the center of buoyancy is at the lungs. To get used to this change, the athlete must retrain the body to use the abdominal muscles to maintain the correct vertical posture.

The athletic community has been attracted to DWR as a way to maintain cardiovascular conditioning while recovering from injury. The literature has shown that DWR can duplicate the sport-specific of running, and with 4 to 6 weeks of DWR, there is a drop in VO_{2max} of 5 to 7%. DWR allows runners to put in miles without incurring the impact of land-based training. Also, land-based runners who water-train maximize speed gains—and these gains can transfer to land performance.

Water's buoyancy virtually eliminates the effects of gravity—supporting 90% of the body's weight in deep water reduces impact and creates greater flexibility. Water acts as a cushion for the body's weight-bearing joints, reducing stress on muscles, tendons, and ligaments. The depth of the water directly affects the amount of impact transferred through the musculoskeletal system. Moving deeper in the water decreases the impact for a given exercise. Moving to the shallower end of the pool increases the load on the body. Using variable depths is very useful when recovering from an injury or after a hard training session or to partially unload the body.

Exercise intensity is an important part in any program. Conventional exercise prescription for DWR has relied on heart rate and subjective rating of perceived exertion. *Three methods are useful for grading exercise intensity* and maximizing physiologic responses during deep water exercise: *heart rate, RPE, and cadence. The American College of Sports Medicine: Guidelines for Graded Exercise Testing and Exercise Prescription (1986) suggests that, for a training effect, one should exercise at a level between 55 and 90% of one's maximal heart rate.* This method is most applicable when one wishes to train at a constant rate, that is, the target heart rate. Most authors suggest that it is important for alternative training to be conducted at or close to actual training intensities.

Heart Rates

In the aquatic environment, heart rate can be affected by the water's temperature, compression, reduced gravity, partial pressure, and the dive reflex. It is recommended that a 6-second heart rate count be used in the water. Heart rate levels in the water tend to be lower than those attained on land. If an aquatic exercise heart rate is to be used to measure intensity, a 13 or 17 bpm should be taken from the minimal and maximal training thresholds. The physiologic changes that occur when the athlete is submerged up to the neck in water will cause the heart rate to be from 10 to 15% lower than for similar effort on land.

In other words, because of the physiologic changes incurred while immersed in water, it is recommended that the athlete train at a heart rate that is 17 to 20 bpm lower than they do on land. The RPE is often unreliable owing to the effects of skill and comfort on perceived exertion.

Table 7-6

Borg Scale of Perceived Exertion

6	
7	Very, very light
8	
9	Very light
10	
11	Fairly light
12	
13	Somewhat hard
14	
15	Hard
16	
17	Very hard
18	
19	Very, very hard
20	

Rate of Perceived Exertion

The most commonly used scale of perceived exertion is the **Borg scale,** a 15-point scale with verbal descriptions ranging from very, very light to very, very hard (Table 7–6). In DWR, though, the **Brennan scale** is very popular (Table 7–7). It is a 5-point scale designed for DWR, with verbal descriptions ranging from very light to very hard. Intensity level is subjectively determined by the participant in this method. The Brennan scale facilitates the incorporation of both speed and distance work into the athlete's workout.

Table 7-7

How Hard Are You Working in the Pool? Brennan Rate of Perceived Exertion

	Rate of Perceived Exertion				
	1	2	3	4	5
	Very light	Light	Somewhat hard	Hard	Very hard
Cadence (cycles/min)	60	60–70	70–80	80–90	90+
Dry-land Equivalent	Brisk walk	Easy jog	Brisk jog	Race pace	Track

Level 1   (very light): a light jog or recovery run
Level 2   (light): a long steady run
Level 3   (somewhat hard): a 5–10-K road race pace
Level 4   (hard): a 400–800-m track speed
Level 5   (very hard): sprinting (a 100–200-m track speed)

Note: The cycles/min are approximate numbers for a well-conditioned athlete. Substitute the cadence numbers that are appropriate for your training level.

Table 7–8

Deep-water Running Cadence Chart

RPE	Water Tempo (CPM)	Land-based Equivalent (min/mile)
1	Very light (50)	Slow walk (>21)
2	Light (50–60)	Medium-paced walk (15–20)
3	Somewhat hard (60–75)	Fast walk/jog (<15)
4	Hard (75–85)	Run (5–10)
5	Very hard (>85)	Very hard run (<5)

CPM, cycles per min; double the number of times your right knee comes forward and up. This count is taken on the last 30 sec of each interval; RPE, rating of perceived exertion.

Cadence

Another form of monitoring intensity is counting cadence (Table 7–8). Brennan (1997) has the athlete count the number of times the right knee comes forward and up. That count is taken on the last 30 seconds of each interval. Doubling the count gives the cycles per minute (cpm).

Wilder and associates (1993b and c) discovered a high correlation between cadence, an environment-specific measure, and heart rate during DWR. In their study, they found a quantitative, objective measure (cadence) could be used to predict a cardiovascular response to a particular workout for DWR and concluded that cadence can be used as a measure for exercise prescription for DWR.

Heart rates are used primarily during long runs, prolonged periods of exercise at a specific rate (target heart rate). RPE exertion and cadence are most often used for interval sessions. RPE is most useful in group settings, whereas cadence is most appropriate for individual sessions (Wilder and Brennan, 1993b).

David Brennan, M.Ed, assistant clinical professor in the department of physical medicine and rehabilitation at Baylor College of Medicine in Houston, recommends that people new to aquatic running should be initially taught at low speeds, for example, under 65 cpm. Participants can then increase speed gradually. Most distance runners tend to peak to at 85 to 95 cpm.

Patients with lower extremity injuries start in deep water. A 6-week program includes DWR, incorporating all the training methods used in a land-based program. Long runs, interval training, and strength runs can be incorporated into a training schedule. Resistive equipment can be introduced about week 3.

After 6 weeks, the athlete can be moved from deep water to chest level, which is about 25% loading. After several weeks, the athlete can be moved to waist level, which is about 50% loading. The belt is kept on to further reduce the impact. To begin progressing to land, the belt is removed to increase the loading effect and transfer to land.

Indications for Aquatic Therapy

An athlete presenting with any of (but not limited to) the following conditions may benefit from aquatic therapy:

- Inability to train for a specific sport on land in a normal training environment
- Poor proximal stability and core weakness
- Weakness and deconditioning
- Pain
- Limited ROM
- Muscle spasm
- Limited weight-bearing or non–weight-bearing
- Gait deviations
- Limited functional ability
- Abnormal tone
- Impaired sensation
- Decreased lung capacity
- Spatial-perceptual problems
- Uncoordination
- Decreased aerobic fitness
- Weight reduction
- Depression
- Impaired circulation
- Edema (especially in the extremities)
- Decreased ability to relax
- Decreased self-image secondary to being unable to perform normal activities

From Harvey G: "Why Water?" Sports Med Update. HealthSouth Patient Education Handout. Birmingham, Alabama, HealthSouth, 1996.

Aquatic Therapy for Orthopaedic Patients

Orthopaedic patients who may benefit from aquatic therapy include, but are not limited to:

- Sports injuries: non– or partial weight-bearing sport-specific training and rehabilitation
- Muscle and connective tissue injuries: e.g., sprains, strains, contusions, and tears, tendinitis, bursitis
- Multiple traumatic injuries
- Joint injuries: presurgical, postsurgical, and nonsurgical
- Joint replacements: total hip, total knee, and total shoulder
- Fractures: open reduction and internal fixation (ORIF), external fixation, nonrepaired fractures, casted fractures (removable casts or casts that can be covered), instrumentation removal, and bone grafts
- Spine injuries (cervical, thoracic, or lumbar): acute injury, chronic injury, exacerbation, strain, sprain, spasm, herniated discs, stenosis, spondylosis, spondylolisthesis, fracture and compression fracture, conservative care (nonsurgical or presurgical), and postsurgical (e.g., fusion, discectomy, laminectomy)
- Arthritis
- Fibromyalgia
- Lupus
- Ankylosing spondylitis
- Reflex sympathetic dystrophy
- Parkinson's disease
- Spina bifida
- Guillain-Barré syndrome
- Upper motor neuron lesions
- Peripheral neuropathy

From Harvey G: "Why Water?" Sports Med Update. HealthSouth Patient Education Handout. Birmingham, Alabama, HealthSouth, 1996.

Precautions for Aquatic Therapy

- Medically controlled seizure disorders.
- Diabetes. (Determine the severity, method of control, and related symptoms. Instruct the patient to take medication properly and to eat and hydrate before exercising in the pool.)
- Cardiac involvement. (Determine the type of involvement and if medically controlled. Instruct the patient to take medication as prescribed. If the patient carries nitroglycerine or other emergency medication, it should be accessible in the pool area.)
- Pulmonary problems or disorders (e.g., chronic obstructive pulmonary disease, asthma). (A portable oxygen unit can be used poolside when necessary. Inhalers should be readily accessible from poolside.)
- Neurologic deficits or problems. (Patients may require hands-on treatment.)
- Fear or apprehension of the water. (Determine the patient's swimming ability and comfort level in water. If the patient is fearful, make a special effort to slowly progress, give extra attention, and do not enter deep water. Keep the patient next to the edge of the pool, and stay with him or her in the water. Either assist the patient or avoid activities that require the feet to float off of the bottom of the pool. **Monitor closely.**)
- Lung capacity of 1.5 L or less. (The patient may have to be treated in shallow water or in the supine position, gradually immersing the lungs over a period of time to build up tolerance to hydrostatic pressure.)
- Autonomic dysreflexia. (The patient may require hands-on treatment and additional staff.)
- Behavioral problems (depression, magnified pain behavior, combative behavior, inappropriate sexual behavior, or other disruptive behaviors). (The patient may require special scheduling or additional staff.)
- Tracheotomies. (If proper precautions can be taken so that no water enters the stoma, the patient may be treated.)
- Open wounds, surgical incisions, or skin conditions. (If a wound, incision, or skin lesion is not actively bleeding or oozing, it may be covered with an occlusive dressing to avoid contact with the water. Warm water increases circulation and will exacerbate bleeding, oozing, blistering, or boils.)
- External fixators. (If the pin holes are not oozing or bleeding, the patient can get into the pool. The pin hole sites can be covered with an occlusive dressing, but this is usually unnecessary if proper pin care is done before and after aquatic therapy.)
- Colostomy stomas. (Caps or plugs are available to fit a stoma, preventing water contamination. If the patient does not have a cap or plug, the stoma can be covered with an occlusive dressing.)
- Indwelling catheters. (The bag can be emptied, clamped, and taped to the patient's leg.)
- Subclavian catheters and heparin locks. (These can also be covered with an occlusive dressing, and they cannot leak. Use a sterile cotton applicator to apply a generous painting of tincture of benzene onto the skin where the edges of the dressing meet the skin. Apply the dressing so that benzene is underneath it and extends beyond all edges as well. Also, smaller pieces of dressing overlapping each other are more adhesive and create a tighter seal. If an edge is peeling up, it will leak. Reapply and cut a strip of occlusive dressing to reinforce the edge. This same technique works well to cover incisions or anything with the dressing.)
- Incontinence of bowel or urine. (If the patient is on a successful bowel program and is able to eliminate on a regulated basis, she or he may be successfully treated in the pool without accident. However, the patient must successfully eliminate before each pool session to ensure that an accident does not occur. Waterproof adult diapers may be purchased as a precaution.)
- Orthostatic hypotension. (Monitor all patients exiting the pool and hot tub. A healthy, young person can experience orthostatic hypotension and fall unconscious without much warning.)
- Hypersensitivity—tactile or temperature. (Water increases tactile stimulation. This can often be used to desensitize the athlete, but monitor the patient closely for nontolerance.)
- Medically controlled hypertension. (Obtain the results of the last blood pressure reading from the patient. If the patient is unsure of the reading, a resting test may reveal that the blood pressure is not under control. If the resting blood pressure remains higher than 165/95 after three tests, the patient should be referred back to the physician treating the hypertension and not be allowed to exercise in warm water until the blood pressure is brought within reasonable limits.)
- Low blood pressure. (There are no standards to limit participation; however, monitor closely, especially for orthostatic hypotension.)

From Harvey G: "Why Water?" Sports Med Update. HealthSouth Patient Education Handout. Birmingham, Alabama, HealthSouth, 1996.

Contraindications for Aquatic Therapy

The following contraindicate safe treatment for the athlete or for other patients in the pool:

- Fever (exercise in warm water will increase fever).
- Incontinence of bowel (and possibly urine).
- Open wounds, incisions, or skin lesions that are oozing or bleeding and cannot be covered with an occlusive dressing.
- Blistering.
- Boils close to rupture.
- Infectious processes such as hepatitis A (fecal-oral–contracted diseases), strep throat and other communica-

Contraindications for Aquatic Therapy
(Continued)

ble diseases, vaginal or urinary infection untreated by antibiotic or treated for less than 24 hr, staphylococcus infection that will be exposed through a wound or other infectious processes where skin lesions are present. (Blood-borne pathogens cannot be spread through the water unless blood contaminates the water.)
- Skin infections.
- Uncontrolled seizure disorder (the light, reflection, and acoustics in a pool can trigger auras).

continued

Contraindications for Aquatic Therapy
(Continued)

- Uncorrected cardiac problems.
- Impaired vital capacity with intolerance to the water pressure even in modified positions.
- Acute lung infection (tuberculosis).
- Catheters or intravenous lines that cannot be clamped or covered with an occlusive dressing.
- Tracheotomies.

Contraindications for Aquatic Therapy
(Continued)

- No internal protection during menstrual cycle.
- Excessively high or low blood pressure.
- Extreme fear.
- Inappropriate or disruptive behavior.

From Harvey G: "Why Water?" Sports Med Update. HealthSouth Patient Education Handout. Birmingham, Alabama, HealthSouth, 1996.

Rehabilitation Protocol
Deep-water Training for the Athlete with a Lower Extremity Injury
Triche

Week 1

Goals

- Introduce DWR to the athlete.
- Maintain cardiovascular fitness.
- Specific exercises in relation to the injury.
- Proceed as tolerated.

Begin by introducing the athlete to the correct form used in DWR (Figs. 7–38 and 7–39).

20–40 min at a steady-pace RPE at 1 or 2 (see Tables 2 and 3) begin with three or four times a week.

Employ ROM exercises in relation to the injury.

Example: ankle injury:

- Ankle flexion and extension.
- Foot circles, inversion, and eversion.

Weeks 2–3

Goals

- Introduce the athlete to "cadence" with interval training (see Aquatic Therapy section).
- Maintain cardiovascular fitness.
- Increase sets and repetitions of ROM exercises in relation to injury.
- Proceed as tolerated; if not well tolerated, repeat week 1.

Correct body alignment

Incorrect body alignment

Figure 7–38. Correct posture for deep-water running (DWR). The key to any safe, effective exercise or movement is correct body alignment. Initially, as you adjust to the buoyancy, you may find yourself hunching over in the water. It is common when you first get in the water to lean forward at the waist as you adjust to a new center of gravity. To adapt to this new environment and attain correct body position, lean back slightly and try a small flutter kick with your feet directly under you. Checklist for vertical body alignment:
- Head up.
- Chest lifted.
- Shoulders positioned directly above hips.
- Abdominals tight (do not hold your breath).
- Buttocks squeezed together and slightly tucked under (pelvic tilt).
(From Aquajogger Handbook: The New Wave of Fitness. Eugene, Oregon, Excel Sports Science Inc, 1998.)

Rehabilitation Protocol
Deep-water Training for the Athlete with a Lower Extremity Injury *(Continued)*
Triche

Figure 7–39. Correct form for DWR. The desired running form in water is almost identical to the running form on land. Maintain vertical posture with your head tall and your chest lifted; coordinate arm and leg movements as in running.
- Push down with a flat foot as if you are stomping on grapes, then lift your heel toward your buttocks as you cycle through.
- Cup your hands and swing your arm from the shoulder in a relaxed, pendulum-like action with the elbow about 3 inches out from your side.
- Avoid hunching your shoulders, bending at the hips, or reaching out too far in front of the body with your lower leg.

(From Aquajogger Handbook: The New Wave of Fitness. Eugene, Oregon, Excel Sports Science Inc, 1998.)

Teach the athlete how to count "cadence."

Begin with 2 days/wk of intervals

- Repeats of 2- to 4-min RPE of 3–4 with a 30-sec recovery (depending on fitness level of athlete; (increase recovery time if needed).
- 2 days/wk of easy running at an RPE of 2 (30–45 min).

ROM Exercises
- *Example*: stress fracture.

Week 4
Goals
- Add resistive equipment as tolerated (gloves, delta bells, aquarunners).
- Maintain cardiovascular fitness.

Athlete continues with interval training (specific to the sport and fitness level) two times a week.

Example: training sprinters is different from marathon runners—marathon runners might perform low-intensity, long-duration cardiovascular exercise, maintaining the workload at 70 to 80% maximal oxygen consumption. A sprinter would work at peak oxygen consumption, with intermittent jogging for recovery.

- Sprinters: 1–2 min (10 ×) RPE 4–5 (15–30 sec rest).
- Marathoners: 3–5 min (6–8 ×) RPE 4 (30–60 sec rest).

Two times a week easy running (30–45 min) with resistive equipment (as tolerated).

Example: I add aquarunners (foot flotation) to my athletes with stress fractures. This increases the workload.

Continue with ROM exercise.

Weeks 5–6
Goals
- Sport-specific training.
- Increase cardiovascular conditioning.
- Resistive equipment continued (as tolerated).

Athlete is trained in the water specifically to their sport.

Example: marathoners:

1 day/wk: long run; run in the water at RPE of 2–3 for 1–2 hrs (depending on the fitness level and timing of the training).

1 day/wk: interval training at RPE of 4–5 with 30-sec recovery.

1 day/wk: strength run; a steady run of 20–40 min at RPE of 3 (can also do 2 × 20-min runs with a 1-min rest between).

2 days/wk: easy running in the water; 30–60 min at RPE of 2

Use the easy days between the hard training sessions. It gives the body a chance to recover. The hard-easy system of training works best.

Introduction to Land Exercises: Loading

After 6 wk of DWR, there are two options for introduction to loading.

Option 1
The athlete starts with 1 day/wk on land, starting with a slow, easy jog on a soft surface (10–15 min) as tolerated. The other days are a continuation of weeks 5–6.

continued

Rehabilitation Protocol
Deep-water Training for the Athlete with a Lower Extremity Injury *(Continued)*
Triche

Figure 7–40. Cross-country ski position for DWR. Scissor straight arms and legs forward and back. Keep your limbs fairly straight and work out of the shoulders and hips. Your trunk should remain stable and the abdominals and buttocks tight.
- Cup your hands and point your toes for increased resistance.
- Work both sides of the body with equal force.
(From Aquajogger Handbook: The New Wave of Fitness. Eugene, Oregon, Excel Sports Science Inc, 1998.)

Figure 7–42. Sit kicks for deep-water exercise. Visualize sitting in a chair with your legs resting on the seat and your spine against the back of the chair. Keep your thighs level with your hips. Kick out from the knee, then pull your heel back to your bottom. Breast-stroke, scull, or scoop the water in toward your chest.
- Point toes to increase resistance.
- Stay tall and keep your abdominal muscles tight.
(From Aquajogger Handbook: The New Wave of Fitness. Eugene, Oregon, Excel Sports Science Inc, 1998.)

Figure 7–41. Sumo wrestler position for deep-water exercise. Stand tall and outwardly rotate your hips with your legs turned out and your feet flexed. Alternate pushing each leg down, using a flat foot for maximum surface area. Breast-stroke with your arms.
- Make sure that you maintain a strong neutral spine, meaning that your back and neck are vertical and relaxed.
- Sumo legs will work well with many different arm moves; experiment with a variety of upper body exercises.
(From Aquajogger Handbook: The New Wave of Fitness. Eugene, Oregon, Excel Sports Science Inc, 1998.)

Figure 7–43. Flutter kick for deep-water exercise. Stand tall and flutter your legs, focusing on pushing your thighs forward and keeping your ankles and knees relaxed. This is a small but strengthening exercise, which is great for toning the buttocks.
- Flutter kick is an excellent leg exercise to mix and match with different arm movements. Try biceps curls, figure-of-8s at your side, or breast-stroke.
- Keep your kicks small and powerful.
(From Aquajogger Handbook: The New Wave of Fitness. Eugene, Oregon, Excel Sports Science Inc, 1998.)

Rehabilitation Protocol
Deep-water Training for the Athlete with a Lower Extremity Injury *(Continued)*
Triche

Progression of Land Exercises

Each week, add another day of land running; can increase the time by 5 min. Continue all interval training in the water.

Continue until the athlete is back running, then keep the athlete in the water 1–2 days/wk until the end of the season, so that injury does not recur.

Option 2

One or 2 days/wk bring the athlete to chest-deep water. Keep the flotation belt on. Have the athlete run in the water for 10–15 min (as tolerated). Continue the DWR on the other days.

Other commonly used water aerobic exercises are illustrated in Figures 7–40 to 7–43. ∎

Running Injuries

Stan L. James, MD

Background Information (Table 7–9)

The incidence of injuries among serious runners (over 20 miles a week) in a given year is approximately 34 to 65%. ***The most common causes of running injuries are training errors.*** The most significant training errors are in duration (high mileage), frequency, and intensity along with rapid changes or transitions in the program. Anatomic and biomechanical factors, shoes, surfaces, gender, age, experience, and running terrain are also contributory factors. The history of previous injury is also a significant risk factor for reinjury. It is interesting that through the years no correlation has been established between a specific anatomic or biomechanical variation and a specific running injury.

The most frequent injuries in runners include

- Anterior knee pain with extensor mechanism problems (Fig. 7–44).

Table 7–9

Risk Factors in Running Injuries

Characteristics of Runners	Characteristics of Running	Characteristics of Running Environment
Age	Distance	Terrain
Gender	Speed	Surface
Structural abnormalities	Stability of pattern	Climate
Body build	Form	Time of day
Experience	Stretching, weight training, warm-up, cool-down	Shoes
Individual susceptibility		
Past injury		

- Iliotibial band syndrome (Fig. 7–45).
- Achilles tendon tendinopathy.
- Medial tibial stress syndrome.
- Plantar fasciitis.
- Stress fractures (Table 7–10).

Tissues in these areas are all subjected to repetitive forces several times body weight while running and therefore are more susceptible to injury. In distance running, the injuries are generally due to excessive, repetitive usage of various tissues exceeding their stress/strain characteristics for sustained use, resulting in a degenerative process or chronic overuse syndrome. The musculoskeletal system is tremendously adaptable to changes in stress but does require time to accommodate. Its response to stress is either a desirable physiologic, anabolic, regenerative response or an undesirable, pathologic, catabolic, degenerative response, depending on the level and duration of stress. Training within the physiologic window of stress or subthreshold level with small incremental increases in stress (training) results in increased tissue strength with a desirable training effect and avoids injury. To achieve this goal, a carefully designed training program becomes essential.

Treatment of Runners' Injuries

This treatment protocol is applicable to virtually all running injuries and provides a logical, consistent guide for the treating physician.

The Training Program

Most running injuries are related to the training program, and therefore, analysis of training is essential. Experienced runners are as likely to make the same mistakes as beginning runners. ***The most common errors*** are high mileage and a sudden change or transition in the program. To a lesser extent, shoes, surfaces, terrain, and anatomic factors play a role. An optimal program, doing the least training while maximizing the runner's capability, is ideal. A training program should consist of hard, or quality, days with interspersed easy days essential for recovery. A hard, or quality, day is one of appropriate in-

Quadriceps
tendinosis

Patellar
instability

Plica

Patellar
tendinosis

Medical collateral
ligament
instability

Voschel's
bursitis

Pes anserine
bursitis

Stress
fracture

Excessive
lateral
pressure
syndrome

Fibular
collateral
ligament
instability

Anterior View

ITB
friction
syndrome

Excessive
lateral
pressure
syndrome

Osteoarthritis

Anterior
cruciate
ligament
instability

Meniscal lesion

Popliteal
tenosynovitis

Fibular
collateral
ligament
instability

Lateral View

Figure 7–44. Sites in the knee frequently affected in runners. ITB, iliotibial band. (From James SL: Running injuries of the knee. J Am Acad Orthop Surg 3[6]:312, 1995.)

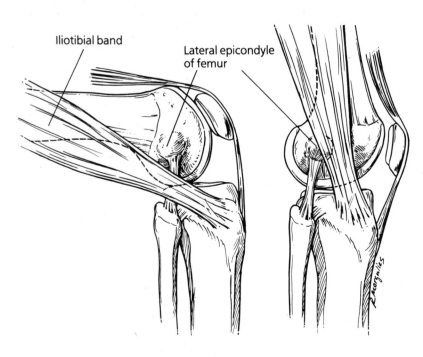

Iliotibial band

Lateral epicondyle
of femur

Figure 7–45. As the knee moves from flexion to extension, the iliotibial band (ITB) passes from behind to in front of the lateral femoral epicondyle. The pain experienced by runners with ITB friction syndrome is caused by the tight band rubbing over the bony prominence of the lateral epicondyle. This pain presents as lateral pain and tenderness palpated at the ITB insertion just distal to the lateral joint line. (From Dugas R: Causes and treatment of common overuse injuries in runners. J Musculoskel Med 17[2]:72–79, 1991.)

Table 7-10

Most Common Problems in Runners (N = 232)

Knee pain	29%
Shin splints	13%
Achilles tendinitis	11%
Plantar fascitis	7%
Stress fractures	6%
Iliotibial tract tendinitis	5%

From James SL, Bates BT, Oslering LR: Injuries to runners. Am J Sports Med 6:40, 1978.

cremental increase, whereas an easy day is one that does not detract from the training benefits of a quality day. Most runners can safely tolerate 3 quality days in a 7- to 10-day period. Increase in weekly mileage should be no more than 5 to 10%. Maximal training benefits for distance running can be achieved at approximately 80 to 90 kilometers a week. *It is better to be slightly "under-trained" and running than injured from overtraining.*

A customized training program for an individual runner at a level below "the line" at which injury or illness becomes a serious risk is desirable. This is where good coaching, appropriate goals, and common sense become essential. Too often, injury occurs when emphasis is placed on training the aerobic system while disregarding the ability of the musculoskeletal system to accommodate to the imposed repetitive stress, resulting in injury and disrupting training.

If injury occurs, reducing training is more acceptable than ceasing training, although that may be necessary in some circumstances. Aerobic conditioning should be maintained by cross-training with no- or low-impact activities such as running in water with a flotation device (see Aquatic Therapy section), biking, steppers, and elliptical trainers.

Biomechanical and Anatomic Factors

No specific anatomic or biomechanical variation correlates with a specific condition or injury, but biomechanics do play a role. *The most important aspect of the examination is to evaluate the entire lower extremity and not just concentrate on the area of injury.* The lower extremity functions as a kinetic chain, and disruption at any given area can affect function throughout.

The running stride is divided into an active and passive absorption phase and a generation phase (Fig. 7–46). The purpose of the **active absorption phase** is initially to decelerate the rapidly forward-swinging recovery leg with eccentric hamstring activity, first absorbing and then transferring the energy to the extend-

ing hip, placing the hamstrings under considerable stress. **Passive absorption** begins at foot-strike with absorption of the shock of ground reaction force (GRF) resulting in a force 2.5 to 3 times body weight (BW) and up to 10 times BW running downhill. This initial shock is attenuated by the surface, the shoe, and the heel pad but not to a great extent. Subsequently, the GRF is actively absorbed by muscles and tendons as it increases to midsupport with a relative shortening of the extremity. This is accomplished by hip and knee flexion, ankle dorsiflexion, and subtalar pronation accompanied by eccentric contraction of the hip abductors, quadriceps, and gastrocsoleus muscles along with stretching of the quadriceps and patellar tendon, Achilles tendon, and plantar fascia. *At this point, the GRF with running may be as much as 5 times BW.* The stretched tendons absorb energy, store it as potential energy, and then return 90% of it later in the generation or propulsive phase as kinetic energy, with the remaining 10% creating heat in the tendon.

During the **generation phase** in the second half of support, there is a relative lengthening of the extremity with concentric muscle contraction and joint extension, with return of stored potential energy as kinetic energy from the tendons significantly assisting the now concentrically contracting muscles. Peak forces maximize at the sites of chronic injury (Scott and Winter, 1990). Forces in the patellofemoral joint estimated at 7 to 11.1 times BW, 4.7 to 6.9 times BW in the patellar tendon, 6 to 8 times BW in the Achilles tendon, and 1.3 to 2.9 times BW in the plantar fascia predispose the tissues to potential injury from repetitive overuse—particularly if combined with even a minor anatomic or functional variation.

Examination of the entire lower extremity becomes essential (Fig. 7–47) when the extremity is viewed as a kinetic chain whose normal function is dependent on the proper sequential function of each segment. Therefore, concentrating on only the area of complaint may overlook the underlying cause of the problem (e.g., anterior knee pain related to compensatory foot pronation).

The examination evaluates (Fig. 7–48)

- Bilateral lower extremity length.
- Extremity alignment in the frontal and sagittal planes.
- Hip motion.
- Muscle strength and flexibility.
- Extensor mechanism dynamics.
- Leg-heel alignment.
- Heel-forefoot alignment.
- Subtalar motion.
- Shoe inspection.

A basic video analysis of the runner's gait is also helpful and can be accomplished with an inexpensive camcorder in the office.

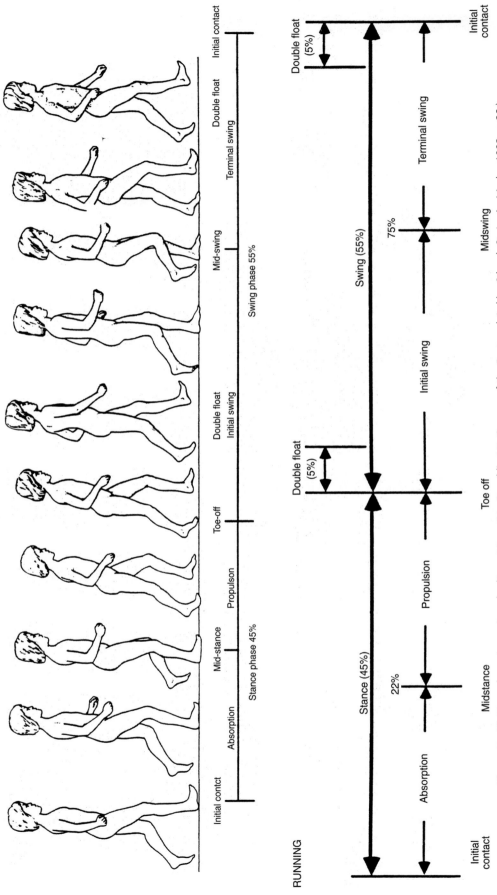

Figure 7–46. Normal running gait cycle. (From Mann RA, Coughlin MJ: Surgery of the Foot and Ankle, 6th ed. St. Louis, Mosby, 1993, p 28.)

RUNNER ENCOUNTER SHEET

Name_____   Date _____

Age_____ Sex_____ Weight_____ Height_____

1. Decribe how your injury occurred and where you are hurting.
   _____
   _____
   _____

2. How long ago did you notice your first symptoms?
   _____
   _____

3. Pain is present
   ____ At all times
   ____ During running
   ____ During walking
   ____ After running
   ____ At rest

4. If pain during running starts:
   ____ Midrun
   ____ Late run
   ____ After run
   ____ Start of run

5. Pain is ____improving ____ worsening ____unchanged

6. Present running mileage
   ____ miles per day
   ____ miles per week

7. How many days a week do you run?_____

8. Mileage before injury
   ____ miles per day
   ____ miles per week

9. What surface do you run on?
   ____ Grass   ____ Indoor track
   ____ Concrete ____ Hills
   ____ Asphalt   ____ Street with slope or pitch
   ____ Cinder   ____ Other

10. Have you recently
    ____ Increased your distance   ____ Increased hill running   ____ Increased workout intensity
    ____ Gained significant weight ____ Changed shoes   ____ Started interval training
    ____ Changed surfaces

11. Do you stretch
    ____ Before run
    ____ After run

12. List and describe other running injuries in the past year
    _____
    _____

Figure 7–47. Runner's encounter form.

13. Describe pain
    ____ Burning   ____ Sharp
    ____ Aching   ____ Dull
    ____ Cramping   ____ Pins and needles

14. On a scale of 1 to 10 (10 worst pain you've ever had)
    rate your pain ____   ____ at rest   during activity

15. How many miles do you run on each pair of shoes before changing? (approximate)

16. Do your shoes wear out in more than one area
    ____ inner toe
    ____ outer toe
    ____ inner heel
    ____ outer heel
    ____ other   Describe _____

Other notes:

Figure 7–47. *Continued*

RUNNER EXAM SHEET

Standing exam
Increased Q angle _____
Genu valgum _____
Genu varum _____
Normal knee align _____
Tibial torsion _____
Foot Pronation _____
 (pes planus) _____
Foot Supination _____
 (pes cavus) _____
Pelvic obliquity _____
Scoliosis _____
Obesity _____

Sitting exam
Patellar maltracking _____
Patellar crepitance _____
Motor strength _____
Hip extension _____
 flexion _____
Knee flexion _____
 extension _____
Ankle _____
 inversion _____
eversion _____
DF _____
PF _____
Muscle imbalance(s) _____
_____
_____
forefoot alignment _____
hindfoot alignment _____

Supine exam
Leg length
discrepancy of _____
shorter leg is L or R _____
ROM
hip _____
knee _____
ankle _____
subtalar _____
INFLEXIBILITY
Hip _____
Hamstring _____
Quad _____
Iliotibial band (Ober s) _____

meniscal
pathology _____
patellofemoral _____

Gait assessment
Antalgic gait _____
Pronator _____ Supinator _____

Asymetric arm motion _____
Excessive pelvic tilt _____
neutral _____

Areas of point tenderness
_____
_____
_____
Shoes
_____ new _____ very worn
type of shoe _____
wear pattern
_____ medial toe box
_____ lateral toe box
_____ medial hindfoot
_____ lateral hindfoot

Miscellaneous
pathology _____
_____
knee effusion _____
ligament
exam knee _____
Generalized
ligamentous
laxity _____
forefoot alignment _____
hindfoot alignment _____
excess callosities _____
_____
_____
_____

_____
_____
_____
_____
_____

Figure 7–48. Runner's examination sheet.

Shoes

Most shoe manufacturers have three general classifications of running shoes: (1) motion control for control of compensatory pronation, (2) support for a "normal"-type foot, and (3) cushion for the more rigid, higher-arched foot. These are merely general guidelines with selection still largely a factor of what fits, feels good, and has worked in the past. Much emphasis has been placed on the role of shoes for shock absorption at foot-strike, and shoes are of some benefit but provide little, if any, force attenuation when the forces are maximal at midsupport. This does not mean shoes are of no importance in protecting the runner, perhaps just not as much as was once thought.

Shoes can be modified for certain specific conditions such as leg-length discrepancies; a difference in configuration, function, or size between feet; and decompressing areas of pressure by changing the upper configuration or midsole and heel wedge stiffness.

Inspect the runner's shoes that have been worn for running for a while for excessive wear or distortion, particularly the heel wedge and heel counters.

Patterns of Wear for Running Shoes

Severe compensatory pronation frequently overruns (i.e., wears down) the heel counter medially, and cavus-type feet distort (i.e., wear down) the heel counter laterally.

Distorted shoes must be replaced as needed. A poorly padded heel counter may apply pressure to the Achilles insertion site. Outsole wear patterns may indicate an anatomic or functional problem with the area of wear indicating abnormal force application (e.g., a plantar flexed first ray will display wear under the first metatarsophalangeal joint). Temperature changes may affect the midsole and heel wedge stiffness, altering shoe function.

A relatively inflexible midsole in a shoe may be associated with Achilles tendinopathy by functionally increasing the forefoot lever arm with more stress applied to the Achilles tendon.

A shoe that still "looks good" may have lost many of its protective qualities, with most midsole material having a life of approximately 300 miles.

We recommend new shoes in the serious runner every 300 miles.

A running shoe should possess an adequate toe box; a well-molded, substantial, properly aligned and padded heel counter; protection from the laces; a flexible midsole with appropriate cushion; and adequate heel height in relation to the midsole.

Orthotics

Orthotic inserts have been used for a number of running-related conditions with reportedly satisfactory results, but significant data on their efficacy and precise function are soft. Theoretically, the purpose of orthotic inserts is to promote more normal, efficient subtalar and midtarsal motion, which in turn, will result in more normal function of the proximal kinetic segments of the lower extremity, reducing injury. Empirically, a well-fabricated orthotic insert does appear useful in many conditions. I have found orthotics to be most successful for plantar fasciitis (consider a lateral forefoot post with plantar fasciitis) and medial tibial stress syndrome. Other conditions reportedly helped by orthotics are patellofemoral disorders, Achilles tendinopathy, and

leg-length discrepancy. The past few years have seen a plethora of orthotic inserts on the market, ranging from a variety of off-the-shelf inserts to expensive "customized" types mostly of the semirigid variety. ***Theoretically, a less rigid, accommodative insert is applicable to the more rigid cavus-type (high arch) foot, which requires more cushion and less control, whereas a more rigid insert is indicated for the more unstable foot with compensatory pronation benefiting from more control.***

A trial of a less expensive off-the-shelf insert to see whether there is a benefit may be a reasonable approach before prescribing a more expensive custom insert. When prescribing a custom orthotic, be certain to understand and fulfill the fabricator's requests for measurements and cast molds. A poorly fabricated orthotic is a waste of time and money. The insert should be as light as possible. The foot of a runner is the worst location to apply additional weight.

Medications

Medications such as aspirin, acetaminophen, and NSAIDs are useful in reducing minor pain and inflammation, but do not substitute for ceasing the abusive activity or taking steps to correct the offending condition. The use of narcotics to continue running or the injection of analgesics cannot be condoned. Excessive or prolonged use of NSAIDs can have significant side effects, even at the recommended reduced dose when purchased over the counter.

The literature cautions against indiscriminate use of oral or injectable steroids. One condition in which steroid injection may have reasonable success is acute iliotibial band friction syndrome with injection deep to the iliotibial band over the prominence of the lateral femoral condyle. Injection directly into tendons should be avoided and into the peritendinous tissues administered with caution.

NEVER inject cortisone in or around the Achilles tendon or posterior tibial tendon. This will result in weakening and probable rupture of the tendon.

Surgery

An earnest, conservative rehabilitation program is generally effective for most running-related conditions. Surgery should be considered only after failure of a conservative program; however, this does not mean unnecessary delay for well-indicated surgery, but many serious runners can be impetuous in electing surgery as an anticipated "quick fix." The indications for surgery are the same as for any athletically active person. If surgery is elected, all the options should be explained in detail, and with some conditions, the patient should be cautioned that in spite of well-planned and executed surgery, there may not be good odds for return to running.

Physical Therapy and Rehabilitation

The treatment of runners must be a coordinated effort on the part of the physician, therapist/trainer, coach, and runner.

The goal of a rehabilitation program for runners after injury or surgery is restoration of flexibility, ROM, muscle strength, balance, and endurance of the entire lower extremity with return to uninterrupted running.

As a general rule, closed-chain exercise including concentric and eccentric muscle activity is preferable for runners. Isolated, concentric, open-chain exercises may induce strength changes in ROM not present in running

as well as muscle imbalance. Specific rehabilitation regimens for a given condition are covered elsewhere in the book under the condition.

Stretching for flexibility (Figs. 7–49 and 7–50) should be an integral part not only of a rehabilitation program but also of the daily training program (see each section). Although important for all runners regardless of age, it becomes even more significant with aging as tendons become less extensible and joints tend to lose flexibility.

The vague complaint of the extremity "not feeling right" may be due to muscle imbalance secondary to weakness or contracture. Runners frequently have chronic hamstring and gastrocnemius-soleus muscle contractures resulting in recurrent or chronic muscle or tendon strains

RUNNER'S FLEXIBILITY PROGRAM

 1. Back stretch: Lie on your back with both knees bent. Pull one or both knees up to your chest and hold for 5 seconds. Repeat.

 2. Hip abductor stretch: Stand with your feet together. Move your hips sideways, while your torso moves in the opposite direction. You will feel a stretch on the outside of your hip. Hold for 5 seconds. Place your hands on your hips or grasp a stationary object for support.

 3. Iliotibial band stretch: Cross one leg over in front of the other leg. Bend the knee of the back leg slightly. Move your hips sideways toward the side with the bent knee. You will feel a stretch on the outside of the bent knee. Hold for 5 seconds.

 4. Hamstring stretch: Sit on the floor with your legs straight in front of you. Reach for your toes until you feel a stretch in the back of your thighs. Hold for 5 seconds.

 5. Quad stretch: Stand facing a stationary object for support. Bend one knee as far as possible, reach back, and grasp the foot. Pull the heel toward your butocks until you feel a stretch in the front of the thigh. Hold this position for 5 seconds. *Do not arch back.*

 6. Heel cord stretch: Stand facing a stationary object with your feet apart and your toes turned in slightly. Place your hands on the object and lean forward until you feel a stretch in the calf of your leg. Hold for 5 seconds. *Do not bend your knees or allow your heels to come off the floor.*

 7. Soleus stretch: Assume the same position as in number 6. Place one foot in front of the other foot and and bend both knees. Lean forward, keeping the heel of the front foot on the ground. You should feel a stretch in the lower calf of the front leg. Hold for 5 seconds.

Figure 7–49. Runner's flexibility program.

ILIOTIBIAL BAND STRETCHING PROGRAM

Each exercise is to be done _____ times per day, _____ repetitions of each exercise. *Hold all stretches for 5 seconds.*

1. HIP ABDUCTOR STRETCH

Stand with legs straight, feet together. Bend at waist toward side opposite leg to be stretched. Unaffected knee may be bent.

2. ILIOTIBIAL BAND STRETCH

Stand with knees straight; cross leg to be stretched behind other as far as possible. Stretch to side of leg in front.

3. ILIOTIBIAL BAND STRETCH

Same stance as exercise number 2. Slightly bend back knee. Move trunk toward unaffected side and hips toward affected side. Stretch will be felt along outside of bent knee.

4. ILIOTIBIAL BAND/HAMSTRING STRETCH

Stand with knees straight. Cross legs so that affected knee rests against back of unaffected leg. Turn trunk away from affected side as far as possible, reaching and attempting to touch heel of affected leg.

5. ILIOTIBIAL BAND STRETCH

Lie on unaffected side with your back a few inches from table edge. Bend unaffected hip to maintain balance. Straighten affected knee and place leg over edge of table so leg hangs straight. Let gravity pull leg down, causing the stretch.

6. ILIOTIBIAL BAND STRETCH

Lie on affected side with knee locked and leg in a straight line with trunk; bend upper knee with your hands placed directly under shoulders to bear the weight of the trunk. Push up, extending your arms as far as possible. Affected leg must be kept straight to get maximum stretch in hip.

Figure 7–50. ITB stretching program. (Modified from Lutter LD: Form used in Physical Therapy Department at St. Anthony Orthopaedic Clinic and University of Minnesota, St. Paul, Minn.)

with imbalance. This can lead to alterations in stride, predisposing tissues to excessive stress.

A tip for hamstring strains, chronic or acute, is to run uphill or up stairs, which places less strain on the hamstrings just before foot-strike when the hamstrings are simultaneously decelerating the forward-swinging leg and extending the hip.

A program should be designed to simulate as close as possible the normal muscle and joint function of running. Often, so much emphasis is placed on the injured area that the rest of the body is ignored. Total body fitness should be included and cross-training techniques like running in water can be beneficial as well as reconditioning the injured area.

Once the runner is ready to return to running after missing training, the following guidelines may be helpful. If left to their own judgment, most will return too fast and either delay recovery or be reinjured.

Return to Running

This program is a "guide" for return to running after a significant **absence from training of 4 weeks or more** (Table 7–11). The purpose is to condition the musculoskeletal system and is not intended to be a significant aerobic conditioning program, which can be accomplished with low- or no-impact cross-training. The running pace should be no faster than 7 minutes per mile and the walking done briskly. The program is based on time, not distance. A rest day should be scheduled every 7 to 10 days. The schedule can be varied to meet individual situations. If need be, the runner may hold at a given level longer, drop back a level, or in some instances, skip a level if progressing well. Discomfort may be experienced, but it should be transient and certainly not accumulate. Include general strength training, specific prescribed exercises for rehabilitation, and stretching for flexibility.

Table 7–11

Runner's Guide for Return to Running after Absence from Training of Four Weeks or More

Week	Schedule
1	Walk 30 min, alternating 1 min normal and 1 min fast.
2	Walk 30 min, alternating 1.5 min normal and 1.5 min fast. If doing well, jog easily instead of walking fast.
3	Alternate walking 1 min and jogging 2 min × 7. The next day, run easy 5 min and walk 1 min × 3.
4	Alternate walking 1 min and jogging 3 min × 7. The next day, run 5 min and walk 1 min × 4.
5	Run continuously 20 min. The next day, run 5 min and walk 1 min × 5.
6	Run continuously 20 min. The next day, run 10 min and walk 1 min × 3.
7	Run continuously 20 min one day and 35 min the next.
8	Run continuously 20 min one day and 40 min the next.
9	If doing well, resume a training schedule, increasing the duration, intensity, and frequency appropriately. The key is to avoid reinjury.

From James SL, Bates BT, Oslering LR: Injuries to runners. Am J Sports Med 6:40, 1978.

Rehabilitation Protocol
For Return to Running after Missed Training
James

The following protocol is a conservative guide that can be varied depending on individual situations.

Absence from training for

- 1 wk or less—reduce training 60% for 3 days, 30% for the next 3 days, and then resume normal training but monitor closely.
- 1–2 wk—reduce training 60% the first 5 days, 30% the second 5 days, and then resume appropriate training.
- 2–3 wk—reduce training 60% the first 5 days, 40% the second 5 days, 20% the third 5 days, and then resume appropriate training.
- 4 wk or more—see Table 7–11.

Nirschl Pain Phase Scale for Athletes' Overuse Injuries

Phase 1. Stiffness or mild soreness after activity. Pain is usually gone within 24 hr.

Phase 2. Stiffness or mild soreness before activity that is relieved by warm-up. Symptoms are not present during activity but return after, lasting up to 48 hr.

Phase 3. Stiffness or mild soreness before specific sport or occupational activity. Pain is partially relieved by warm-up. It is minimally present during activity but does not cause athlete to alter activity.

Phase 4. Similar to but more intense than phase 3 pain. Phase 4 pain causes athlete to alter performance of the activity. Mild pain may also be noticed with activities of daily living.

Phase 5. Significant (moderate or greater) pain before, during, and after activity, causing alteration of activity. Pain occurs with activities of daily living but does not cause a major change in them.

Phase 6. Phase 5 pain that persists even with complete rest. Phase 6 pain disrupts simple activities of daily living and prohibits doing household chores.

Phase 7. Phase 6 pain that also consistently disrupts sleep. Pain is aching in nature and intensifies with activity.

From O'Connor FG, Nirschl RP: Five step treatment for overuse injuries. Physician Sports Med 20(10):128, 1992.

General Treatment Guidelines for Overuse Injuries in Runners
Brotzman

First, establish correct diagnosis and pathoanatomy.

1. Discontinue or decrease running, depending on severity.
2. Cross-train with nonimpact cardiovascular exercise (DWR exercise with Aquajogger belt [www.aquajogger.com], bicycling, swimming, elliptical trainer).
3. Ice.
4. NSAIDs.
5. Initiate stretching exercises for area of tightness (e.g., iliotibial band, hamstrings, quadriceps).
6. Patient education on avoiding training errors in future (e.g., too rapid a progression).
7. Conservative correction of underlying biomechanical malalignment (e.g., orthotics for pronators, McConnell taping or Palumbo bracing for patellofemoral malalignment, heel-lift for leg-length discrepancy).
8. Education for appropriate running shoe and less than 300 miles per pair.
9. Address and treat any underlying metabolic contributors to overuse injury (e.g., address amenorrhea, obesity, calcium or protein deficiency, osteoporosis, eating disorders).
10. Surgery only as a last resort for injuries failing conservative measures and time.
11. Gradual resumption of running as described by James (p. 521) rather than the overzealous return attempted by all runners if not supervised.
12. Alteration of surface to grass, cinder, or cushioned track. Avoid running on road with a slope; avoid hill running.
13. No cortisone injections except for iliotibial band tendinitis.
14. Improve overall fitness and resistance to breakdown or overuse by sport-specific agility, speed, and skill drills such as plyometrics, eccentric strengthening, and coordinating and strengthening antagonistic muscles and supporting muscles.

Shin Splints in Runners

Mark M. Casillas, MD, and Margaret Jacobs, PT

Shin splints is a nonspecific term typically used to describe exertional leg pain. Although common in runners, this condition probably is overdiagnosed. A number of specific conditions are known to also cause exercise-induced leg pain. It is appropriate to identify a specific etiology whenever possible.

Relevant Anatomy

The leg bones (tibia and fibula) serve as the origin for the extrinsic muscles of the foot and ankle. The muscles of the leg are surrounded and divided by the crural fascia.

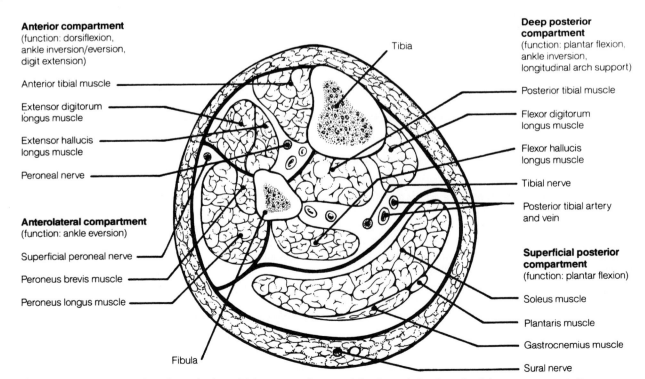

Anterior compartment
(function: dorsiflexion, ankle inversion/eversion, digit extension)

Anterior tibial muscle

Extensor digitorum longus muscle

Extensor hallucis longus muscle

Peroneal nerve

Anterolateral compartment
(function: ankle eversion)

Superficial peroneal nerve

Peroneus brevis muscle

Peroneus longus muscle

Fibula

Tibia

Deep posterior compartment
(function: plantar flexion, ankle inversion, longitudinal arch support)

Posterior tibial muscle

Flexor digitorum longus muscle

Flexor hallucis longus muscle

Tibial nerve

Posterior tibial artery and vein

Superficial posterior compartment
(function: plantar flexion)

Soleus muscle

Plantaris muscle

Gastrocnemius muscle

Sural nerve

Figure 7–51. Cross-section through the mid leg. Note the crural fascia and the four fascial compartments. (From McKeag DB, Dolan C: Overuse syndromes of the lower extremity. Physician Sports Med 17[7]:108–123, 1989.)

The resulting compartments (anterior, lateral, superficial posterior, and deep posterior) are unyielding with regard to volume and are prone to develop increased pressure (Fig. 7–51). The anterior compartment contains the extensor muscles, including the anterior tibial, the extensor digitorum longus, and the extensor hallucis longus muscles. The posterior medial tibia serves as the origin for the posterior tibial muscle, the flexor digitorum longus muscle, the soleus muscle, and the deep crural fascia.

Etiology

Anterior shin splints are related to dysfunction of the anterior leg compartment or its contiguous structures. **Medial tibial stress syndrome** is the clinical entity that most likely represents medial shin splints. The exercise-induced pain associated with medial tibial stress syndrome tends to involve the distal two thirds of the leg. The etiology of anterior shin splints is not completely understood; overuse or chronic injury of the anterior compartment muscles, fascia, and bony and periosteal attachments is most commonly implicated. The most likely cause of medial tibial stress syndrome is a traction periostitis of the soleus or flexor digitorum longus muscle origins. Increased heel eversion is a suggested risk factor.

Diagnosis (Table 7–12)

A diagnosis of shin splints is suggested by a history of exercise-induced pain at the distal two thirds of the leg. **The pain is localized to the anterior compartment in anterior shin splints and to the distal two thirds of the posterior medial tibial border in medial tibial stress syndrome** (Fig. 7–52). The pain is brought on by activity such as prolonged walking or running, and it is relieved by decreased activity. The condition is never associated with neurologic or vascular symptoms or findings.

Radiographic Examination

Radiographs are negative in this condition, but it should be remembered that they are also negative for the first weeks of a developing stress fracture. Therefore, a bone scan is used to differentiate between a stress fracture and shin splints. A longitudinal uptake along the posterior medial border of the distal tibia is consistent with medial tibial stress syndrome. This is in contrast to a focal or linear uptake that is diagnostic for a stress fracture (Fig. 7–53). Compartment syndrome, spinal claudication, vascular claudication, anomalous muscle, infection, and tumor must be ruled out.

Treatment

Perhaps the most efficient approach to managing shin splints is prevention. Lower-impact conditioning and

Table 7–12

Differential Diagnosis of Shin Splints

Differential Diagnosis	Significant Findings
Anterior shin splints	Exercise-induced leg pain, tender at anterior compartment, normal radiograph and bone scan
Medial tibial stress syndrome (medial shin splints)	Exercise-induced leg pain, tender at posterior-medial tibial border, normal radiograph, linear uptake on bone scan
Tibial stress fracture	Exertional pain at tibia; point-tender tibia; pain with three-point stress; abnormal radiograph, fusiform uptake on bone scan, abnormal CT or MRI
Fibular stress fracture	Exertional pain at fibula; pronation or valgus alignment; point-tender fibula; abnormal radiograph, bone scan, CT, or MRI
Acute compartment syndrome	Leg pain secondary to trauma, tender compartments, pain with passive motion, decreased sensation, elevated compartment pressures, paresthesias
Chronic exertional compartment syndrome	Exertional leg pain, no acute trauma, tender compartments, muscle herniation, decreased sensation after exertion, elevated postexertion compartment pressures, paresthesias
Congenital anomaly	Exertional leg pain, no acute trauma, anomalous muscle such as accessory soleus, symptoms similar to chronic exertional compartment syndrome, accessory muscle identified on MRI
Tumor	Night pain, abnormal radiograph, bone scan, CT, or MRI

cross-training appear to reduce the incidence of shin splints.

The acute exertional pain associated with shin splints is treated with the RICE regimen until symptoms subside. Increasing rest intervals and duration are also beneficial to both types of shin splints. Running is prohibited until the patient is pain-free.

Anterior shin splints are treated with aggressive warm-up and stretching, with particular attention to the gastrosoleus–Achilles tendon complex (Fig. 7–54). Anterior symptoms may also respond to decreased shoe weight and level running surfaces. **Medial tibial stress syndrome** is treated in a similar fashion. Medial symptoms may also respond to antipronation taping and or-

Figure 7–52. *A*, Pain is localized to the anterior compartment for anterior shin splints *(left)* or to the distal two thirds of the posterior medial tibial border for medial tibial stress syndrome *(right)*. *B*, Posterior views of the attachments of the posterior tibial muscle *(left)* and the soleus muscle *(right)*. (*A*, From Fick DS, Albright JP, Murray BP: Relieving painful "shin splints." Physician Sports Med 20[12]:105-111, 1992; *B*, from McKeag DB, Dolan C: Overuse syndromes of the lower extremity. Physician Sports Med 17[7]:108–112, 1989.)

thotics (Figs. 7–55 and 7–56) and running on a non-banked, firm surface.

Surgery is never indicated for anterior shin splints. For recalcitrant medial tibial stress syndrome, deep posterior compartment fasciotomy and release of the soleus muscle origin off the posterior medial tibial cortex have been suggested.

The most important aspect of treatment is appropriate diagnosis. Radiographs and bone scans are obtained of all patients to rule out stress fracture. Once the diagnosis of shin splints is established, running is stopped until the exercise-related pain has resolved. Stretching and conditioning are emphasized throughout a comprehensive reha-

bilitation program. Antipronation orthotics are fitted if taping reduces symptoms. Any underlying biomechanical, anatomic, or nutritional precipitating causes should also be treated.

Fundamental to the rehabilitation protocol is the patient's self-discipline to avoid running until the exercise-related pain has completely resolved. The phases of rehabilitation are variable in length and depend completely on the resolution of pain with weight-bearing and eventually with running. Flexibility is emphasized throughout the protocol, with particular attention to the gastroc-soleus–Achilles tendon complex for anterior shin splints and the soleus for medial tibial stress syndrome.

A   B   C

Figure 7–53. *A* and *B,* Bone scans diagnostic of a right-sided posteromedial stress fracture. *C,* Lateral plain film of the tibia reveals an ominous focal transverse radiolucent line (stress fracture). (*A* and *B,* From Hutchinson MR, Cahoon S, Atkins T: Chronic leg pain. Physician Sports Med 26[7]:37-46, 1998; *C,* from Mann RA, Coughlin MJ: Surgery of the Foot and Ankle. St. Louis, Mosby, 1999.)

Rehabilitation Protocol
Shin Splints
Casillas and Jacobs

0–3 Days: Acute Phase

This phase is defined by the initial date of treatment through the resolution of weight-bearing pain. Relative rest (no running), ice massage, and whirlpool are used for acute pain.

- Ultrasound therapy is considered if the bone scan demonstrates no bony involvement.
- Nonimpact activities are begun and are advanced as pain allows
  - Gastrocnemius and soleus stretching.
  - Isometrics.
  - Seated towel scrunches.
  - Cycling.
  - Water activities (DWR) with an Aquajogger belt and swimming.

Day 4–Week 6: Subacute Phase

This phase begins with the resolution of weight-bearing pain and ends with the resolution of activity-related pain.

- Modalities to decrease inflammation are continued.
- Emphasis remains on improving flexibility.
- Isometrics are progressed to Thera-band exercises.
- Towel scrunches are progressed from a seated to a standing position.
- Balance activities are begun with progression of difficulty to include the biomechanical ankle platform system (BAPS).
- Aerobic fitness is maintained with cross-training activities such as slideboard, water running, and cycling.

Week 7: Return to Sport Phase

- Running commences once all activity-related pain has resolved.
- Warm-up and stretching are emphasized.
- Running is allowed to progress within the limits of a pain-free schedule. See James' protocol for gradual return to running (p. 521).
- Patients are to initially avoid running on uneven surfaces.

Rehabilitation Protocol
Shin Splints (Continued)
Casillas and Jacobs

- If the patient is using an oval track, each direction should be used in an equal fashion (i.e., change direction).
- Attention is directed to first reestablishing distance, followed by reestablishing speed.

- Antipronation orthotics are fitted for patients with medial tibial stress syndrome or if warranted by a successful trial of low dye taping.

A

B

Figure 7–54. *A,* Gastrocnemius stretching on an inclined box with the knee extended. *B,* The soleus is stretched more effectively by flexing the knee and relaxing the gastrocnemius muscle.

A   B   C   D

Figure 7–55. *A–D,* Antipronation taping.

Figure 7-56. Orthotics for correction of pes planus. Pes planus feet have decreased "shock absorption" at the subtalar joint during high-impact activities because the subtalar joint is already everted at heel-strike. This precludes the usual shock absorption of the normal subtalar joint. Orthotics place the foot in a more subtalar neutral position.

Sideline Neurologic Evaluation for a Concussion

History

- Mechanism or description of how injury occurred.
- Loss of consciousness? Duration?
- Amnesia? Duration?
- Headache? Duration?
- Associated symptoms? Duration?
- Sensation intact?
- Numbness?
- Extremity movement?
- Neck pain?

Physical Examination

- Appearance (alert, dazed, unconscious).
- Mental status (person, place, time).
- Eyes (pupils, visual fields, equal ocular movements, fundi—if ophthalmoscope available).
- Cranial nerves.
- Sensation (light touch, sharp).
- Motor (strength, movement).
- Reflexes.
- Cognition (serial 7s, score, school, president).
- Arm extension.
- Toe signs.
- Cerebellar function (finger-to-nose, Romberg).
- Gait.

Functional Tests before Return to Play

- Running, jumping, cutting.
- Sport-specific skills.

Return to Play after a Concussion

S. Brent Brotzman, MD, Jenna Deacon Costella, MA, ATC, and Mark Bohling, MS, ATC

Background

A **concussion** is a clinical syndrome characterized by the immediate and transient impairment of neural function. This includes alteration of consciousness, disturbance of vision, and loss of equilibrium owing to mechanical injury.

- Fewer than 10% of concussions result in a loss of consciousness (Cantu 1996).
- Common symptoms of concussions include headache, dizziness, confusion, tinnitus, blurred vision, and nausea.
- Simple neuropsychological tests are routinely used to assess an athlete suspected of having a concussion. The athlete is asked orientation questions such as
  - What field are we playing on?
  - Which team scored last?
  - What quarter is it?
  - Did our team win last week?
  - What team did we play last week?

- Return to play criteria after a concussion is a controversial topic. The goal is to avoid exposing the athlete to an increased risk of injury.
- **The prevention of second-impact syndrome is of utmost importance.**
- **Second impact syndrome** occurs when a player sustains a (minor) second head injury before the symptoms of a previous concussion have cleared. This syndrome results in brain swelling, which follows vascular engorgement caused by autoregulation of cerebral blood flow (Fig. 7–57). This vascular engorgement leads to a massive increase in intracranial pressure. **Death frequently follows.**
- Whether it takes days, weeks, or months to reach the asymptomatic state, the athlete must *never* be allowed to practice or compete while postconcussion syndrome is present.
- Because of additive effects of repeated head blows manifesting in boxing's "punch-drunk syndrome," the number of concussions an athlete is allowed to sustain should be very limited. The athlete should be

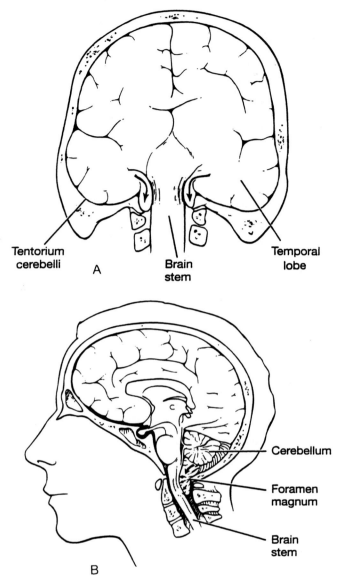

A
Tentorium cerebelli — Brain stem — Temporal lobe

B
Cerebellum
Foramen magnum
Brain stem

Figure 7–57. In second-impact syndrome, vascular engorgement within the cranium increases intracranial pressure, leading to herniation of the uncus of the temporal lobe *(arrows)* below the tentorium in this frontal section *(A)* or to herniation of the cerebellar tonsils *(arrows)* through the foramen magnum in this midsagittal section *(B)*. These changes compromise the brain stem, and coma and respiratory failure rapidly develop. The *shaded areas* of the brain stem represent the areas of compression. (*A* and *B*, From Cantu RC: Neurologic athletic injuries. Clin Sports Med 17[1]:37–45, 1998.)

rapidly, safely disqualified from further competition in high-risk sports.

- Football, hockey, soccer players, and wrestlers are at greatest risk of concussion. High school football play-

ers face a 20% risk each season, high school hockey players a 10% risk.

- Cantu (1986) uses a scale that applies loss of consciousness (LOC) *duration* and post-traumatic amnesia (PTA) to differentiate mild, moderate, and severe concussions (Table 7–13). Other commonly used scales include the Colorado Guidelines for Management of Concussion in Sports (Table 7–14) and the American Academy of Neurology (AAN) guidelines.
- We use the Colorado Guidelines or the AAN in our practice because "up to 5 minutes of loss of consciousness" in Cantu's classification is considered only a grade 2 injury. We consider this a grade 3 injury.
- **Evaluation and treatment of a concussion** should include survey of the **ABCs** (airway, breathing, circulation). If the patient has any neck pain or neurocervical symptoms, perform transportation with cervical spine precautions. If the patient is unconscious, assume a cervical spine injury and use cervical spine precautions.
- *Do not remove the helmet if a cervical spine injury is suspected. Instead, cut (detach) the plastic mounting clips on facemask with trainer's angels.*
- Airway protection should take precedence.
- When assessing an athlete with a suspected concussion, the examiner should consider and document
  - Time and place of injury.
  - Mechanism of injury
  - Presence of duration of LOC.
  - Postinjury behavior.
  - Presence or convulsions after injury.
  - Past medical history.
  - Medication use.

Sideline Evaluation after Concussion

- ABCs (Airway, Breathing and Circulation).
- Evaluate for loss of consciousness.
- Cervical spine assessment.
- Assess cranial nerves, coordination, and motor function.
- Assess cognitive function.
- Evaluate short-term and long-term memory (e.g., detailed questions about recent events, three-word memory, Serial 7's).
- Frequent reassessment of the injured player to determine if continuation or deterioration of symptoms is noted.
- Any loss of consciousness should result in transport of the athlete to a hospital for further evaluation and work-up (CT scan, neurological consult).

Table 7-13

Concussion Classification Systems and Return to Play Recommendations
Cantu

Severity	First Concussion	Second Concussion	Third Concussion
Grade 1 (mild) No loss of consciousness: Post-traumatic amnesia <30 min	May return to play if asymptomatic	May return in 2 wk if asymptomatic at that time for 1 wk	Terminate season; may return next year if asymptomatic
Grade 2 (moderate) Loss of consciousness <5 min or post-traumatic amnesia >30 min	Return after asymptomatic for 1 wk	Wait at least 1 mo; may return then if asymptomatic for 1 wk; consider terminating season	Terminate season; may return next year if asymptomatic
Grade 3 (severe) Loss of consciousness >5 min or post-traumatic amnesia >24 hr	Wait at least 1 mo; may return then if asymptomatic for 1 wk	Terminate season; may return next year if asymptomatic	

From Cantu RC: Guidelines for return to sports after cerebral concussion. Physican Sports Med 14(10):75, 1986.

Table 7-14

Colorado Guidelines to Return to Contact Sports after Cerebral Concussion (Authors' Choice)

Severity	First Concussion	Second Concussion	Third Concussion
Grade 1 (mild) Confusion without amnesia; no loss of consciousness	May return to play if asymptomatic for at least 20 min	Terminate contest or practice for the day	Terminate season; may return in 3 mo if asymptomatic
Grade 2 (moderate) Confusion with amnesia; no loss of consciousness	Terminate contest/practice; may return if asymptomatic for at least 1 wk	Consider terminating season, buy may return if asymptomatic for 1 mo	Terminate season; may return to play next season if asymptomatic
Grade 3 (severe) Loss of consciousness	May return after 1 mo if asymptomatic for 2 wk at that time; may resume conditioning sooner if asymptomatic for 2 wk	Terminate season; discourage any return to contact sports	

Roos R: Guidelines for managing concussion in sports: a persistent headache. 24(2):67, 1996.

- A prolonged loss of consciousness should also result in immediate transport to the hospital using cervical spine precautions. Perform CT scan or MRI to rule out an acute epidural or subdural hemorrhage.
- **Athletes who are symptomatic after a head injury are not to participate in collision or contact sports until *all* cerebral symptoms have *subsided* for *at least 1 week.***
- Athletes who have sustained a concussion should be reevaluated by a physician in a clinical setting within a few days of injury and again before they are allowed to return to participation.
- If an athlete with a concussion is sent home after the game, it should be in the care of a responsible adult provided with instruction and a head injury instruction sheet (Fig. 7-58).

HEAD INJURY INSTRUCTION SHEET

Date: _____

_____ has suffered a head injury. Although the athlete is currently alert, conscious and shows no signs or symptoms of serious brain injury, a potentially catastrophic result can still occur, leading to permanent neurological deficit or even death. Occassionly, following even the mildest head injuries, blood will slowly accumulate, causing compression of the brain hours or even days after the initial injury. Thus, the following guidelines should be followed in conjunction with the physician's or the athletic trainer's advice.

1. The injured athlete should never be alone for the first 24 hours after the injury.
2. The athlete should be awakened every two hours in the evening to establish arousability and alertness.
3. The following signs mandate immediate emergency room evaluation:

   - Blood or watery fluid emanating (coming out) from ears or nose
   - Unequal or dilated pupils
   - Weakness or clumsiness in arms or legs
   - Slurred or garbled speech
   - Asymmetry of the face
   - Increased swelling along the scalp
   - Hard to arouse, irritable or stuporous (reduced sensibilty)

4. The following symptoms (complaints) mandate immediate emergency room evaluation

   - Change in mental status (inability to concentrate or understand directions, alteration of alertness or consciousness)
   - Double or blurred vision
   - Severe headache
   - Increased incoordination (clumsiness) or weakness
   - Vomiting
   - Loss of memory
   - Difficulty with speech

Please realize the above are only guidelines to assist you. If a sign or symptom develops that is new and is not mentioned above, err on the side of safety and have the athlete evaluated by a physician immediately.

Figure 7–58. Head injury instruction sheet.

Osteoporosis: Evaluation, Management, and Exercise

S. Brent Brotzman, MD

Background

- In the United States, 20 million people, predominantly postmenopausal women, have osteoporosis.
- Osteoporosis leads to more than 1.5 million fractures each year.
- One of every two women older than 50 years will have an osteoporosis-related fracture.
- One in every three men older than 75 years will be affected by osteoporosis.
- *The current goal for patient management in women at risk for osteoporosis, or who have osteoporosis, is the prevention of fracture by preventing bone loss and increasing bone mass.*

Definition of Osteoporosis

- Osteoporosis is a disease characterized by **low bone mass,** microarchitectural deterioration of bone tissue leading to bone fragility, and consequent increase in fracture risk.
- Osteoporosis reflects inadequate accumulation of bone tissue during growth and maturation, excessive losses thereafter, or both.
- Fractures of the wrist, spine, and hip are most commonly involved. Fractures of the ribs, humerus, and pelvis are not uncommon.
- Two categories of osteoporosis exist: **primary** and **secondary** osteoporosis.

Primary Osteoporosis

- The most common form of osteoporosis.
- Includes postmenopausal osteoporosis (**type 1**) and age-associated osteoporosis (**type 2**), formerly termed *senile* osteoporosis.

Secondary Osteoporosis
- Loss of bone is caused by an identifiable agent or disease process such as an inflammatory disorder, bone marrow cellularity disorder, and corticosteroid use.

> **Possible Secondary Causes of Osteoporosis**
> - Long-term use of corticosteroids
> - Antiseizure medication (e.g., phenytoin)
> - Gonadotropin hormones (for treatment of endometriosis)
> - Excessive use of aluminum-containing antacids
> - Excessive thyroid hormone medication
> - Certain anticancer drugs
> - Inflammatory disorders treated with steroids (rheumatoid arthritis, asthma, and lupus)
> - Hypogonadism (inadequate function of the gonads)
> - Hyperparathyroidism
> - Cushing's syndrome (overactive adrenal glands)
> - Turner's or Kleinfelter's syndrome
> - Low sex hormone levels
>   - In women: a result of excessive exercise (amenorrhea) or eating disorders that decrease estrogen production, or premature menopause
>   - In men: a result of decreased testosterone production
> - Blood or bone marrow disorders (myeloma)
> - Organ transplantation (immunosuppressives such as cyclosporine or steroids)
> - Chronic kidney, liver, lung, or gastrointestinal disorders
> - Breast or prostate cancer (if treatment lowers estrogen)
> - Spinal cord injury with paralysis of the lower limbs
> - Multiple sclerosis (if steroids used or walking impaired)

Risk Factors for Developing Osteoporosis

> **National Osteoporosis Foundation Physician Guidelines for Risk Factors for Osteoporotic Fracture**
> - Current cigarette smoking
> - Low body weight (<127 pounds)
> - Alcoholism
> - Estrogen deficiency
>   - Prolonged amenorrhea (>1 yr)
>   - Early menopause (<45 yr) or bilateral ovariectomy
> - Lifelong low calcium intake
> - Recurrent falls
> - Poor health/fragility
> - Inadequate physical activity
> - Impaired eyesight

Prevention of Osteoporosis
- Prevention of osteoporosis begins in childhood with adequate calcium and vitamin D intake and continues throughout life (Fig. 7-59).
- Prevention is of great importance because of limited therapeutic alternatives for reversing the loss of bone mass.

- **Osteomalacia,** which may masquerade as osteoporosis, must be excluded if risk factors exist.

> **Preventative Measures**
> - Adequate weight-bearing physical activity for 3-4 hr a wk.
> - Avoid low body weight or excessive thinness (<127 pounds).
> - Avoid excess alcohol intake.
> - Lifelong appropriate calcium and vitamin D intake.
> - Avoidance of bone-leaching medicines if possible.
> - Maximal accumulation of bone during skeletal growth and maturation and reducing or eliminating bone loss after skeleton matures.

Evaluation and Treatment of Osteoporosis
- Patients at increased risk for fracture may be identified on the basis of **clinical factors** (e.g., previous fracture, smoker) and through **bone mineral density (BMD) testing** (Table 7-15).
- The National Osteoporosis Foundation has identified the following **key risk factors** for osteoporosis (with a **recommendation that BMD** *tests be done on these patients*).
  - History of a fracture as an adult.
  - History of a fracture in first-degree relative.
  - Current cigarette smoking.
  - Low body weight or thin (<127 pounds).
- Drug therapy is considered if BMD T-score is below -1.5 if concomitant risk factors are present (e.g., smoker).
- Patients with a BMD T-score below -2 should undergo drug therapy treatment.
- Because of the strong correlation between BMD testing and fracture risk, the World Health Organization (WHO) diagnostic categories are based on BMD measurements.

> **Bone Mineral Density (BMD) Parameters for Osteoporosis**
> *Normal:* bone density on BMD no lower than 1 standard deviation (SD) below the mean for "young normal" adult women (T-score above -1).
> *Low bone mass (osteopenia):* bone density on BMD between 1 and 2.5 SD below the mean for "young normal" adult women (T-score between -1 and -2.5).
> *Osteoporosis:* bone density on BMD 2.5 SD below the "young normal" adult mean (T-score is -2.5 or below); women in this group who have already experienced one or more fractures are deemed to have severe or "established" osteoporosis; as a general rule, for every SD below the normal, the fracture risk doubles.

PATIENT EDUCATION HANDOUT

RISK FACTORS YOU CAN CHANGE

HORMONE LEVELS
Early menopause, occurring naturally or surgically (for example, surgical removal of the ovaries), can increase a woman's likelihood of developing osteoporosis. If you fall into this category, hormone supplements are available. It is important to discuss your bone health and hormone therapy with your physician.

DIET
Inadequate calcium and vitamin D intake is harmful to bone health. Excessive consumption of other nutrients, such as protein and sodium, can decrease calcium absorption.

EXERCISE
Maintaining a physically active lifestyle throughout life is important. Individuals who are inactive, immobilized, or bedridden for a long time, are at risk for osteoporosis.

LIFESTYLE CHOICES
Smoking and excessive alcohol consumption are bad for the skeleton. Women who smoke have lower estrogen levels than non-smokers and go through menopause earlier. Excessive alcohol use increases the risk of bone loss and fractures, due to both poor nutrition and increased risk of falling.

RISK FACTORS YOU CANNOT CHANGE

GENDER
Women are more likely to develop osteoporosis than men, because they have lighter, thinner bones, and lose bone mass rapidly after menopause.

AGE
The longer you live, the greater the likelihood of developing osteoporosis. Although all of us lose some bone tissue as we age, the amount and rate of loss varies widely in different individuals.

HEREDITY
Susceptibility to osteoporosis is in part due to heredity. Young women whose mothers and fathers have had fractures tend to have lower bone mass.

BODY SIZE
Small-boned, thin women and men are more at risk than larger, big-boned persons, but bigger bone size is no guarantee that you will not get osteoporosis.

ETHNICITY
Caucasians and those of Asian descent are at higher risk of developing osteoporosis than individuals of African-American descent, however, anyone may be at risk.

Figure 7–59. Patient education handout for osteoporosis. (From Brown EF, Evans RM, Cole HM, Coble YE (ed): Managing Osteoporosis: Part 3, AMA Continuing Medical Education Program. Chicago, AMA Press, 2000.)

Vitamins and Medications for Osteoporosis

Calcium

Patient Education Handout on Calcium

- **Calcium supplements.** Although food sources of calcium are preferred, sometimes it is necessary to use a calcium supplement to meet your daily calcium re-

quirement. The amount of supplement you need depends on how much calcium is in your diet (Table 7–16).

Many brands of calcium supplements are on the shelves in supermarkets, health food stores, and pharmacies (Table 7–17). The most expensive brand is not necessarily the best. The most common calcium

Table 7-15

Bone Mineral Density Testing Recommendations

Who Should Get a BMD Test?	Main Risk Factors
Postmenopausal women younger than 65 yr with one or more risk factors	Low BMD (T-score < −1.5)
All postmenopausal women older than 65 yr	History of fracture—personal or first-degree relative
Postmenopausal women who present with fractures	Cigarette smoker
Women considering therapy for osteoporosis	Low body weight (<127 pounds)

BMD, bone mineral density.
Recommendations based on National Osteoporosis Foundation—"Guide to Prevention and Treatment of Osteoporosis." For more information contact the NOF at 202-223-2226 or at http://www.nof.org. Guidelines are based on data for Caucasian postmenopausal females.

Table 7-16

Adequate Calcium Intake Guidelines

Life-stage Group	Estimated Adequate Daily Calcium Intake (mg)
Infants (birth–6 mo)	210
(6–12 mo)	270
Young children (1–3 yr)	500
Older children (4–8 yr)	800
Adolescents and young adults (9–18 yr)	1300
Men and women (19–50 yr)	1000
(51 yr and older)	1200

Note: Pregnancy and lactation needs are the same as for nonpregnant women (i.e., 1300 mg for adolescent/young adult and 1000 mg for age 19 and older).
Adapted from Standing Committee on the Scientific Evaluation of Dietary Reference Intakes. Food and Nutrition Board, Institute of Medicine. Washington, DC, National Academy Press, 1997.

supplements are calcium carbonate and calcium citrate (there are others). **Calcium carbonate,** the most popular calcium supplement, has the highest percentage of calcium and the lowest unit cost. Both calcium carbonate and **calcium citrate** are easily absorbed and used by the body. Calcium carbonate should be taken with meals, whereas calcium citrate can be taken with or without.

- **Tips on taking calcium supplements**
  - Look for the amount of "elemental" calcium the supplement provides (this can be found by reading the label on the calcium supplement package). **Elemental refers to the amount of usable calcium in the mineral.** Figure out how much you will need to take in order to reach your daily requirement.

- The supplement must meet **"dissolution" requirements,** which means that it will dissolve in the stomach (necessary for absorption). Look for labels that say "passed dissolution test" or "USP dissolution tested." If you are not sure about your supplement, you can test it yourself by placing the tablet in a small glass of vinegar or warm water. Stir it occasionally; after 30 minutes the tablet should dissolve. If not, it is probably not dissolving in your stomach either, and is not being absorbed.

- **Avoid calcium from unrefined oyster shell, bone meal, or dolomite.** These forms may contain higher amounts of lead, and may contain other toxic metals. Also, **avoid** using aluminum-containing antacids, which contain no calcium.

Table 7-17

Some Commonly Used Calcium Supplements

Type	Trade Name	Strength per Tablet (mg)	Elemental Calcium (mg)*
Calcium carbonate	Alka-Mints	850	340
	Caltrate	1600	600
	Os-Cal	625 or 1250	250 or 500
	Rolaids	550	220
	Titralac	420	168
	Titralac Liquid	1000	400
	Tums/Tums E-X	500 or 750	200 or 300
	Tums Ultra/Tums 500	1000 or 1250	400 or 500
Calcium citrate	Citracal Liquitabs	2376	500
	Citracal	950	200
	Citracal Caplets + D	1500	315 + 200 IU vitamin D

*Amount of usable calcium.

- Calcium is absorbed better if 500 mg or less is taken at any one time.
- Certain calcium preparations may cause side effects, such as constipation or gas. It may help to drink more fluids and eat more fiber. You may need to try different calcium supplements until you find one that works for you.
- *Do not take more than 2000 mg of elemental calcium per day.*
- Individuals with a personal or family history of kidney stones should talk to their physician before increasing their calcium intake. Calcium rarely causes kidney stones in people with normal kidney function.
- Talk to your physician or pharmacist about possible interactions between calcium supplements and prescription and over-the-counter medications. For example, when calcium is taken with the antibiotic tetracycline, the absorption of the tetracycline is reduced.
- Because calcium can interfere with iron absorption, *iron supplements should not be taken at the same time as calcium carbonate supplements.* This does not happen if the iron supplement is taken with vitamin C or calcium citrate.

Vitamin D

- Recommend daily intake: 400 to 800 IU daily.
- Avoid higher doses to avoid vitamin D toxicity.
- The elderly may benefit from higher calcium intake (1200 mg) and higher vitamin D intake (up to 800 IU daily).

Patient Education Handout on Vitamin D

- Vitamin D plays a major role in calcium absorption and bone health. Vitamin D has been called the "key" that opens the intestinal wall "door," so that calcium can leave the intestine and enter the blood stream. Vitamin D also helps absorb calcium in the kidneys that might otherwise be lost in the urine.
- Vitamin D is formed naturally in the body after skin exposure to *sunlight.* Fifteen minutes of sun each day is plenty of time for you to make and store all the vitamin D you need. Remember that sunscreen will block the body's ability to manufacture vitamin D.
- The ability to make vitamin D in the skin decreases with age, so an older person may have to take a vitamin D supplement.
- Studies have shown that the elderly benefit from higher vitamin D (up to 800 IU) and calcium intakes (1200 mg) daily.
- *Food sources* of vitamin D are vitamin D–fortified dairy products, egg yolks, saltwater fish, and liver. Some calcium supplements and many multivitamins contain vitamin D.

- Experts recommend a daily intake of 400 to 800 IU of vitamin D for bone health. Do not take more than 800 IU unless your physician prescribes it. Massive doses of vitamin D can be harmful.

Table 7–18

Osteoporosis Treatment Options

Option	Comments
Calcium.	Increases spine BMD and reduces the risk of fractures (vertebral and nonvertebral). Recommended intake for adults, 1000–1500 mg/day. Preferred sources are dietary; supplements should have USP designation.
Vitamin D.	Essential for calcium absorption. Maximally effective dosage is thought to be 400–1000 IU/day.
Exercise.	Resistance and impact exercises are likely the most beneficial to bone. May promote attainment of high peak bone mass during childhood and adolescence. May slow down decline in BMD if performed later in life, provided calcium and vitamin D intakes are adequate.
Bisphosphonates (etidronate, alendronate, [Fosamax] risedronate [Actonel]).	Increase BMD at the spine and hip; reduce the risk of vertebral fractures by 30 to 50%. Reduce the risk of nonvertebral osteoporotic fractures, including those due to glucocorticoid-induced osteoporosis (alendronate and risedronate). Safety in children and young adults has not been evaluated.
Hormone replacement therapy (including SERMs).	Established treatment for osteoporosis. Observational data point to reduced hip fracture risk. Trial data indicate reduced risk of vertebral fracture. Approved by the FDA for the treatment and prevention of osteoporosis; reduces vertebral fracture risk by 36% (raloxifene, a SERM). Maintains bone mass in postmenopausal women; effect on fracture risk unclear (tamoxifen, a SERM).
Salmon calcitonin.	Has positive effects on BMD at the lumbar spine. Fracture risk data unclear.
Phytoestrogens.	Have weak estrogen-like effects. Have positive effects on BMD at the lumbar spine.
Other interventions.	Physical therapy helps strengthen and improve balance. Hip protectors may absorb or deflect impact of a fall.

BMD, bone mineral density; FDA, U.S. Food and Drug Administration; SERM, selective estrogen receptor modulator; USP, *United States Pharmacopeia.*
From Brown EF, Evans RM, Cole HM, Coble YE (eds): Managing Osteoporosis: Part 3, AMA Continuing Medical Education Program. Chicago, AMA Press, 2000.

ALGORITHM FOR EVALUATION OF OSTEOPOROTIC FRACTURE RISK

Figure 7-60. Algorithm for evaluation of osteoporotic fracture risk. (Modified from National Osteoporosis Foundation: Physician's Guide to Prevention and Treatment of Osteoporosis. Copyright 1998 National Osteoporosis Foundation, Washington, DC. For information on ordering single or bulk copies of the NOF guidelines, contact the National Osteoporosis Foundation, Professional Education Order Fulfillment, 1150 17th Street, NW, Suite 500, Washington, DC 20036.)

Osteoporosis Treatment Considerations
(Fig. 7-60; Tables 7-18 to 7-21)

A suggested algorithm for the evaluation and management of osteoporotic fracture risk is shown in Figure 7-60.

Secondary Osteoporosis

- Possible causes of secondary osteoporosis (p. 531) should be considered in newly diagnosed patients
- A *z-score* may be helpful in determining this. A *z-score* is similar in concept to the *T-score* (p. 531),

except in a z-score the BMD is compared with an **age-matched control group,** *not* to a young healthy control group. A **low z-score** may reflect bone loss not attributable to age alone, and suggests the possibility of secondary osteoporosis. **A z-score of −1.5 should arouse clinical suspension of secondary osteoporosis.**

- National Osteoporosis Foundation guidelines suggest that women suspected of having **secondary osteoporosis** should undergo **initial laboratory evaluation** of a CBC, *chemistry profile,* and *urinary calcium* test. After clinical evaluation, additional tests may be required, including

- Serum thyrotropin.
- Protein electrophoresis.
- Parathyroid hormone.
- Urine cortisol.
- Vitamin D metabolites.

Serial Bone Mineral Density Measurements

- **Measurements from peripheral skeletal sites are *not* useful for serial BMD measurements.**
- For technical reasons, BMD measurements should be, whenever possible, done on the same machine.
- Usual intervals for serial BMD measurements are every 1 to 2 years. However, some situations dictate more frequent intervals (e.g., significant BMD loss owing to steroid therapy may be detected within 6 months).

Prevention of Falls in Osteoporotic Patients

Elimination of environmental hazards is an easily modifiable risk factor for geriatric patients. The American College of Rheumotology recommends:

- Night lights in bathrooms and hallways.
- Nonskid soles for shoes.
- Nonslip mats under rugs.
- Equip tub, shower, and toilet areas with grab bars.
- Rise cautiously from a supine position.
- Ensure stairway rails are sturdy.
- Keep a flashlight by the bedside.

Exercise Treatment for Patients with Osteoporosis

How Exercise Builds Bone

Although the evidence that exercise prevents and combats osteoporosis is substantial, how it does so is far from clear. Both mechanical and hormonal processes appear to be involved. One explanation of the way bone responds to exercise is the "error strain distribution hypothesis."

According to this theory, bone cells sense the mechanical strain induced by weight-bearing or resistance exercise. The cells then communicate load imbalances with each other on a local level. In vitro, mechanical strain causes a cellular influx of calcium ions, followed by production of prostaglandin and nitric oxide, increased enzyme activity, and the release of growth hormones; these changes may trigger bone remodeling. The theory suggests that such changes also occur in vivo.

Table 7–19

Pharmacologic Options for Managing Osteoporosis

Drug	Indications	Daily Dose	Comments
HRT	Prevention and treatment.	Conjugated equine estrogen, 0.625 mg; estropipate, 0.625 mg; micronized estradiol, 0.5 mg; transdermal estradiol, 0.05 mg.	First-line therapy; benefits of cardioprotection and reduction of hot flushes must be weighed against the risk of a modest increase in breast cancer risk and DVT; combining estrogen with progesterone reduces the problem of cyclic bleeding.
Alendronate (Fosamax)	Prevention and treatment.	5 mg for prevention; 10 mg for treatment.	A bisphosphonate that specifically inhibits osteoclast-mediated bone resorption; an alternative for women who are not candidates for HRT or in whom HRT is ineffective; reduces the incidence of fracture at the spine, hip, and wrist by 50%; esophageal irritation can be reduced by taking the drug with a full glass of water on rising in the morning and avoiding the supine position and other medicine, food, and beverages for a half hour afterward.
Calcitonin	Treatment.	200 IU.	A polypeptide hormone that down-regulates osteoclastic activity; an alternative for women in whom HRT is unsuitable or in whom HRT or alendronate has been ineffective; less effective than these other agents; delivered as a nasal spray (a subcutaneous form is available but used rarely).
Raloxifene (Evista)	Prevention.	60 mg.	A selective estrogen receptor modulator; reduces the incidence of vertebral fracture by 40 to 50%; cannot be used to treat menopausal symptoms; incidence of DVT similar to that observed with estrogen; no estrogenic effect on uterus.

DVT, deep venous thrombosis; HRT, hormone replacement therapy.
Brown EF, Evans RM, Cole HM, Coble YE (eds): Managing Osteoporosis: Part 3, AMA Continuing Medical Education Program.

Table 7-20

Summary of Risks and Benefits of Osteoporosis Therapy

	Estrogen	Raloxifene	Intranasal Calcitonin	Alendronate	Risedronate
Evidence supports reduction of spinal fractures	Yes	Yes	Yes	Yes	Yes
Evidence supports reduction of nonspinal fractures	Yes	No	No	Yes	Yes
Experience with long-term use	Large epidemiologic studies over decades	Randomized trial 3 yr	Randomized trial 5 yr	Randomized trial 4 yr	Randomized trial 3 yr
Administration	Orally: once daily any time Transdermally: weekly patches	Orally: once daily any time	Intranasally: once daily, any time	Once daily in AM, 30 min before eating, with water, while upright	Once daily in AM, 30–60 min before eating, with water, while upright
Specific adverse effects	Breast tenderness vaginal bleeding, thromboembolic disorders	Increased risk of venuous thrombosis, hot flushes, leg cramps	Nasal irritation	Dyspepsia; esophagitis; avoid in patients with esophageal disorders	Dyspepsia
Effect on cardiovascular mortality	Possibly decreased; unconfirmed by randomized trials	No final outcome data	None	None	None
Breast cancer	Increased, but probably very small increase in cancer risk	Possibly decreased risk of estrogen receptor–positive breast cancer	None	None	None
Endometrial cancer	Increased if unopposed estrogen used	None	None	None	None
Dementia; Alzheimer's disease	Epidemiologic studies suggest decreased incidence	Maybe	None	None	None

From Brown EF, Evans RM, Cole HM, Coble YE (ed): Managing Osteoporsis: Part 3, AMA Continuing Medical Education Program. Chicago, AMA Press, 2000.

Exercise Prescription (Impact Training)
- For general health reasons, walking or weight-bearing exercise should raise the heart rate enough to prove aerobic conditioning.
- Patients should walk (or perform comparable exercise) 15 to 20 minutes three to four times a week. No available studies have shown that longer duration or increased frequency improves the effect on osteoporosis. Overuse injuries (e.g., stress fractures) can occur with overtraining and lack of appropriate rest intervals.
- Patients should increase their exercise gradually—1 minute every other session—until they reach their target length of workout.
- Brisk walking is almost always the weight-bearing exercise of choice for osteoporosis unless contraindicated (e.g., arthritic lower extremities, cardiovascular limitations).
- *Do not* use the incline on the treadmill.

- Low-impact aerobics may be suitable for most patients, but high-impact aerobic exercises place too much stress on already weakened bone and should be avoided.
- **Avoid running** (five times body weight at heel-strike) in patients with osteoporosis.
- **Avoid rowing machines,** which cause **vertebral compression fractures** in those at risk.
- Patients who do not have osteoporosis (or medical contraindications) may perform some high-impact exercises to help avoid osteoporosis.
- Counsel young female patients that excessive exercise and consuming fewer calories than required for vigorous training will cause significant bone loss (**athletic amenorrhea**).
- The **"female athlete triad"** describes the complex, deleterious interplay of menstrual irregularity (amenorrhea), eating disorder, and premature osteoporosis seen in some vigorous female athletes.

Table 7–21

Preparations of Estrogen and Progestin for Estrogen Therapy

Trade Name	Generic Name	Minimum Dose for Preventative Therapy (mg)	Upper-end Dose (mg)	FDA-approved Labeling for Prevention of Osteoporosis	Comments
Premarin Cenestin	Conjugated equine estrogens	0.3 0.625	1.25 0.625–0.9	Prevention	Usual dose 0.625 mg, but 2.5 mg sometimes necessary to control hot flushes in young women
Ogen Ortho-Est	Estropipate	0.625	1.25	Prevention	2.5 mg sometimes necessary to control hot flushes in young women
Estratab	Esterified estrogen (estrone, equilin)	0.3	2.5	Prevention	Derived from plant sterol precursors
Estratest H.S. Estratest	Esterified estrogens and methyltestos-terone	0.625–1.25 1.25/2.5	1.25–2.5	No indication for osteoporosis	Contains androgens
Estrace	Micronized estradiol	0.5	2.0	Prevention	0.5 mg effective for bone preservation
Transdermal estrogen					

Alora
  Climara
  Estraderm
  Vivelle
	Estradiol	0.05–0.1
		0.025 (Climara)
				No indication
				Prevention
				Prevention
				Prevention
					Patches applied once or twice a week depending on manufacturer

Transdermal estradiol/ progesterone					
Combi Patch	Estradiol and norethindrone	0.62 or 81 and 2.7–4.8		No indication for osteoporosis	Patch applied twice a week
Prempro Premphase	Conjugated equine estrogens/ MPA	0.625/2.5 or 5 0.625/5		Prevention Prevention	If excessive bleeding, may consider increasing MPA dose to 5 mg
Femhrt 1/5	Ethinyl estradiol Norethindrone	0.005/1		Prevention	
Progestins Prometrium	Micronized progesterone	100 (daily dose) 200 (cyclic dose)		No indication for osteoporosis	Does not attenuate lipid effects of estrogen

Provera
  Cycrin
  Amen
	MPA	5 or 10 (cyclic dose)
		2.5 (daily dose)
				No indication for osteoporosis	

Aygestin	Norethindrone	2.5–10		No indication for osteoporosis	

FDA, U.S. Food and Drug Administration; MPA, medroxyprogesterone acetate.
From Brown EF, Evans RM, Cole HM, Coble YE (ed): Managing Osteoporosis: Part 3, AMA Continuing Medical Education Program. Chicago, AMA Press, 2000.

- Bone mineral loss in young female athletes with athletic amenhorea of greater than 6 months' duration resembles that seen after menopause.

Resistance Training for Osteoporosis

The other component of an exercise prescription for osteoporosis, resistance training, should involve all major muscle groups so that it will affect the bones of the upper body as well as the legs. Movements should be slow and controlled, with loads set to induce desired muscle fatigue after 10 to 15 repetitions. Good form is critical (utilize trainer or coach initially). Start slowly with a gradual increase in exercise. Following is a list of recommended exercises and the muscle groups that they affect.

Resistance Training Exercises
- Hip extension—gluteal, hamstring, and low back.
- Lumbar extension—low back (**avoid lumbar flexion**).
- Leg press—gluteal, quadriceps, and hamstring.
- Pullover—latissimus dorsi, shoulders, trapezius, and abdominals.
- Torso arm or rowing—latissimus dorsi, shoulders, and biceps.

- Arm cross—chest and shoulders.
- Chest press—chest, shoulders, and triceps.

Ideally, such exercise should initially be supervised and done on machines in a fitness center. Perform resistance exercises every third day.

Patient Education Handout on Exercise

Exercise is important throughout life to build and maintain strong bones and muscles. Bones are similar to muscles in that they respond to exercise by becoming stronger and denser. Just as muscles get flabby if you do not use them, bones lose density if they are not used. People who are bedridden often have low bone density because they cannot get up and move about.

Two types of exercise that are best for bone health are **weight-bearing** and **resistance exercises.** Weight-bearing means that your feet and legs are bearing your weight. Jogging, walking, stair climbing, and dancing are examples of weight-bearing.

Much of the information from this section was derived from the American Medical Association's continuing medical education program, Managing Osteoporosis—Part 3.

Additional resources for osteoporosis patient information include:

- **National Osteoporosis Foundation (NOF)**
  1232 22nd Street NW
  Washington, DC 20037–1292
  202-223-2226
  http://www.nof.org
- **National Institutes of Health**
  Osteoporosis and Related Bone Diseases—National Resource Center
  1232 22nd Street NW
  Washington, DC 20037–1292
  800-624-BONE
  http://www.osteo.org
- **American Academy of Orthopedic Surgeons**
  6300 North River Road
  Rosemont, Ill 60018–4262
  800-346-AAOS
  http://www.aaos.org
- **American College of Rheumatology**
  1800 Century Place, Suite 250
  Atlanta, GA 30345
  404-633-3777
  http://www.rheumatology.com ■

Bibliography

Hamstring Injuries in Athletes

Almekinders LC: Anti-inflammatory treatment of muscular injuries in sports. Sports Med 15:139–145, 1993.

Burkett LN: Investigation into hamstring strains: the case of the hybrid muscle. J Sports Med 3:228–231, 1976.

Burkett LN: Causative factors in hamstring strains. Med Sci Sports 2:39–42, 1970.

Clanton TO, Coupe KJ: JAAOS hamstring strains in athletes: diagnosis and treatment. J Am Acad Orthop Surg 6:237–248, 1998.

Grace TG: Muscle imbalance and extremity injury: a perplexing relationship. Sports Med 2:77–82, 1985.

Heiser TM, Weber J, Sullivan G, et al: Prophylaxis and management of hamstring muscle injuries in intercollegiate football players. Am J Sports Med 12:368–370, 1984.

Jarvinen JJ, Lehto MU: The effects of early mobilization and immobilization on the healing process following muscle injuries. Sports Med 15(2):78–89, 1993.

Kujala UM, Orava S: Ischial apophysis injuries in athletes. Sports Med 16:290–294, 1993.

Liemohn W: Factors related to hamstring strains. J Sports Med 18:71–76, 1978.

Orava S, Kujala UM: Rupture of the ischial origin of the hamstring muscles. Am J Sports Med 23:702–705, 1995.

Safran MR, Garret WE Jr, Seaber AV, et al: The role of warmup in muscular injury prevention. Am J Sports Med 16:123–129, 1988.

Sallay PI, Friedman RL, Coogan PG, Garrett WE: Hamstring muscle injuries among water skiers: functional outcome and prevention. Am J Sports Med 24:130–136, 1996.

Stafford MG, Grana WA: Hamstring quadriceps ratios in college football players: a high-velocity evaluation. Am J Sports Med 12:209–211, 1984.

Worrell TW: Factors associated with hamstring injuries: an approach to treatment and preventative measures. Sports Med 17:338–345, 1994.

Zarins B, Ciullo JV: Acute muscle and tendon injuries in athletes. Clin Sports Med 2:167–182, 1983.

Groin and Hip Pain

Anderson K, Strickland SM, Warren R: Hip and groin injuries in athletes. Am J Sports Med 29(4):521–530.

Lacroix VJ: A complete approach to groin pain. Physician Sports Med 28(1):32–37, 2000.

Swain R, Snodgrass S: Managing groin pain, even when the cause is not obvious. Physician Sports Med 23(1):54–62, 1995.

Quadriceps Strains and Contusions

Aronen JG, Chronister RD: Quadriceps contusions: hastening the return to play. Physician Sports Med 20(7):130–136, 1992.

Aronen JG, Chronister RD, Ove PN, et al: Quadriceps contusions: minimizing the length of time before return to full athletic activities with early mobilization in 120° of knee flexion. Read before the 16th annual meeting of the American Orthopaedic Society for Sports Medicine, Sun Valley, Idaho, July 16–17, 1990.

Brewer BJ: Mechanism of injury to the musculotendinous unit. Instr Course Lect 17:354–358, 1960.

Garrett WE Jr: Strains and sprains in athletes. Postgrad Med 73:200–209, 1983.

Garrett WE Jr, Safran MR, Seaber AV, et al: Biomechanical comparison of stimulated and nonstimulated skeletal muscle pulled to failure. Am J Sports Med 15:448–454, 1987.

Jackson DW, Feagin JA: Quadriceps contusions in young athletes: relation of severity of injury to treatment and prognosis. J Bone Joint Surg 55A:95–105, 1973.

Kaeding CC, Sanka WA, Fisher RA: Quadriceps strains and contusions: decisions that promote rapid recovery. Physician Sports Med 23(1):59, 1995.

Klafs CE, Arnheim DD: Modern Principles of Athletic Training: The Science of Sports Injury Prevention and Management, 4th ed. St. Louis, Mosby, 1977, pp. 370–372.

Martinez SF, Steingard MA, Steingard PM: Thigh compartment syndrome: a limb-threatening emergency. Physician Sports Med 21(3):94–104, 1993.

Novak PJ, Bach BR Jr, Schwartz JC: Diagnosing acute thigh compartment syndrome. Physician Sports Med 20(11):100–107, 1992.

Ryan JB, Wheeler JH, Hopkinson WJ, et al: Quadriceps contusions: West Point update. Am J Sports Med 19(3):299–304, 1991.

Winternitz WA Jr, Metheny JA, Wear LC: Acute compartment syndrome of the thigh in sports-related injuries not associated with femoral fractures. Am J Sports Med 20(4):476–477, 1992.

Zarins B, Ciullo JV: Acute muscle and tendon injuries in athletes. Clin Sports Med 2(1):167–182, 1983.

Aquatic Therapy for the Injured Athlete

American College of Sports Medicine: Guidelines for Graded Exercise Testing and Exercise Prescription. Philadelphia, Lee & Febiger, 1986.

Aquajogger Handbook: the New Wave in Fitness. Eugene, Oregon, Excel Sports Science Inc, 1998.

Aquatic Fitness Professional Manual. Nokomis, Fl, Aquatic Exercise Association, 1998.

Arnheim D: Modern Principles of Athletic Training. St. Louis, St. Louis Mirror/Mosby College, 1985.

Bates A, Hanson N: Aquatic Exercise Therapy. Philadelphia, WB Saunders, 1996.

Becker B, Cole A (eds): Comprehensive Aquatic Therapy. Newton, Mass, Butterworth-Heinemann, 1997.

Borg GV: Psychophysical basis of perceived exertion. Med Sci Sports Exerc 14:377–387, 1982.

Brennan D, Wilder R: Aquarunning: an instructor's manual. Houston, Houston International Running Center, 1990.

Bushman B, Flynn MG, Andres FF: Effect of 4 weeks of deep water run training on running performance. Med Sci Sports Exerc 29(5):694–699, 1997.

Coyle EF, Martin WH, Sinacor DR, et al: Time course of loss adaptations after stopping prolonged intense endurance training. J Appl Physiol 57:1857–1864, 1984.

Eyestone E, Fellingham G, Fisher G: Effect of water running and cycling on maximal oxygen consumption and 2-mile run performance. Am J Sports Med 21:41–44, 1993.

Hickson R, Foster C, Pollock M, et al: Reduced training intensities and loss of aerobic power, endurance, and cardiac growth. J Appl Physiol 58:492–499, 1985.

Huey L, Forester R: The Complete Waterpower Workout Book. New York, Random House, 1993.

HYDRO-FIT News: Special Report: Wave Run Field Rest Study, Summer 1996.

Quinn T, Sedory D, Fisher B: Psychological effects of deep-water running following a land-based training program. Res Q Exerc Sport 64:386–389, 1994.

Ritchie S, Hopkins W: The intensity of exercise in deepwater running. Am J Sports Med 12:27–29, 1991.

Samuelson C: Aquatic one-on-one Rehab with athletes. AKWA Lett April/May 2000, p. 36.

Thein JW, Brody LT: Aquatic-based rehabilitation and training for the elite athlete. J Orthop Sports Phys Ther 27:1, 32–42, 1998 (recommended reading).

Town G, Bradley S: Maximal metabolic responses of deep and shallow water running in trained runners. Med Sci Sports Exerc 23:238–241, 1991.

Wilder RP, Brennan DK: Techniques in aqua running. In Becker B, Cole A (eds): Comprehensive Aquatic Therapy. Boston, Butterworth-Heinemann, 1997, pp. 123–134.

Wilder RP, Brennan DK: Aqua running for athletic rehabilitation. In Buschbacher LP, Braddom R (eds): State of the Art Reviews in Physical Medicine and Rehabilitation: Sports Med in press, 1993a.

Wilder RP, Brennan DK: Physiologic responses to deep water running in athletes. Sports Med 16(6):374–380, 1993a.

Wilder RP, Brennan DK, Schotte D: A standard measure for exercise prescription for aqua running. Am J Sports Med 21:45–48, 1993b.

Running Injuries

Fadale PD, Wiggins ME: Corticosteroid injections: their use and abuse. J Am Acad Orthop Surg 2:133–140, 1994.

James SL: Running injuries of the knee. Instr Course Lect 47:82, 1998.

James SL, Bates BT, Osternig LR: Injuries to runners. Am J Sports Med 6:40–50, 1978.

Leadbetter WB: Cell-matrix response in tendon injury. Clin Sports Med 11:533–578, 1992.

Nigg BM, Nurse MA, Stefanyshyn DJ: Shoe inserts and orthotics for sport and physical activities. Med Sci Sports Exerc Suppl 31:S421–S428, 1999.

Novachek TF: Running injuries: a biomechanical approach. Instr Course Lect 47:397–406, 1998.

Novachek TF, Trost JP: Running: injury mechanisms and training strategies. Instructional Videotape. St. Paul, Minn, Gillette Children's Specialty Healthcare Foundation, 1997.

Scott SH, Winter DA: Internal forces of chronic running injury sites. Med Sci Sports Exerc 22:357–369, 1990.

Concussions: Return to Play

Cantu RC: Guidelines for return to sports after cerebral concussion. Phys Sports Med 14(10):75–83, 1986.

Cantu RC: Second Impact Syndrome: immediate management. Phys Sports Med 20(9):55–66, 1992

Cantu RC: Head injuries in sport. Br J Sports Med 30:289–296, 1996.

Colorado Medical Society Sports Medicine Committee: Guidelines for the Management of Concussions in Sports. Denver, Colorado Medical Society, 1991.

Kelly JP, Nichols JS, Filley CM, et al: Concussion in sports: guidelines for the prevention of catastrophic outcome. JAMA 266(20):2867–2869, 1991.

Kelly JP, Rosenberg J: Practice parameter: the management of concussion in sport (summary statement). Neurology 48(3):581–585, 1997.

Nelson WE, Jane JA, Gieck JH: Minor head injury in sports: a new system of classification and management. Phys Sports Med 12(3):103–107, 1984.

Roberts WO: Who plays? Who sits? Managing concussions on the sidelines. Phys Sports Med 20(6):66–69, 1992.

Roos, R: Guidelines for managing concussion in sports: a persistent headache. Phys Sports Med 24(10):67–74, 1996.

Saunders RL, Harbaugh RE: The second impact in catastrophic contact: sports head trauma. JAMA 252(4):538–539, 1984.

Torg JS: Athletic Injuries to the Head, Neck and Face. Philadelphia, Lea and Febiger, 1982.

Wildberger JE, Maroon JC: Head injuries in athletes. Clin Sports Med 8(1):1–9, 1989.

Osteoporosis

Brown EF, Evans RM, Cole HM, Coble YE (ed): Managing Osteoporosis: Part 3, AMA Continuing Medical Education Program. Chicago, AMA Press, 2000.

Lanyon LE: Using functional loading to influence bone mass and architecture: objectives, mechanisms, and relationship with estrogen of the mechanically adaptive process in bone. Bone 18(Suppl 1):37S–43S, 1996.

Munnings F: Osteoporosis: what is the role of exercise? Phys and Sports Med 20(6):127, 1992.

Shimegi S, Yanagita M, Okano H, et al: Physical exercise increases bone mineral density in postmenopausal women. Endocrine J 41(1):49–56, 1994.

Chapter 8
Reflex Sympathetic Dystrophy

Harris Gellman, MD, and Andrew D. Markiewitz, MD

Causalgia was recognized as early as the Civil War, when it was described by Mitchell (1864). Other names for the condition have included Sudeck's atrophy and shoulder-hand syndrome. The term **reflex sympathetic dystrophy** (RSD; also reflex sympathetic dystrophy syndrome [RSDS]) was introduced by Evans in 1946. Most recently, the designation **complex regional pain syndrome** (CRPS) has been used in an attempt to more accurately describe the syndrome. CRPS is divided into two types: type I, which is not linked to a specific process (RSD), and type II, which is related to a known nerve injury (causalgia). *RSD is defined as a pain state maintained by sympathetic efferent activation, by circulating catecholamines, or by neurochemical action.*

CRPS Type I (RSD)

- Type I is a syndrome that develops after an initiating noxious event.
- Spontaneous pain or allodynia/hyperalgesia occurs, is not limited to the territory of a single peripheral nerve, and is disproportionate to the inciting event.
- There is or has been evidence of edema, skin blood flow abnormality, or abnormal sudomotor activity in the region of the pain since the inciting event.
- This diagnosis is excluded by the existence of conditions that would otherwise account for the degree of pain and dysfunction.

CRPS Type II (Causalgia)

- Type II is a syndrome that develops after a nerve injury.
- Spontaneous pain or allodynia/hyperalgesia occurs and is not necessarily limited to the territory of the injured nerve.
- There is or has been evidence of edema, skin blood flow, abnormality, or abnormal sudomotor activity in the region of the pain since the inciting event.
- This diagnosis is excluded by the existence of conditions that would otherwise account for the degree of pain and dysfunction.

Pathophysiology

Normally, sympathetic stimulation secondary to injury results in vasoconstriction, which decreases blood loss and swelling. Sympathetic tone then decreases after injury, allowing increased blood flow. In the abnormal situation (RSD), inappropriate continuation of sympathetic activity results in edema, with capillary collapse, and ischemia, causing continued pain (positive feedback loop).

Epidemiology

Women are affected with RSD three times as often as men. Because there seems to be an increased risk of the condition in family members of RSD patients, a possible genetic predisposition has been suggested, especially in patients who are resistant to therapy.

The most common history given by the RSD patient is a trivial or minor initial injury accompanied by disproportionate pain persisting long after healing. A common predisposing factor for type I CRPS (RSD) includes Colles' fractures: 25% of patients with Colles' fractures displayed RSD features (Atkins et al, 1989), and 26% of patients had residual features of RSD even as late as 10 years after fracture (Field et al, 1992). Field and coworkers reported that an elevated intracast pressure, indicative of a tight cast and swelling, correlated with a 60% likelihood of developing symptoms of RSD. Bickerstaff and Kanis (1994) found that 50% of their patients with RSD who had residual symptoms 1 year after Colles' fractures also had one of the following: severe fractures or fractures that required manipulation, involvement of the ulnar styloid, or primary casting.

Nerve trauma is causative factor in type II CRPS (causalgia). Richards (1967) reported that of 461 patients with causalgia, 83% had injuries that involved the median or tibial nerves, 53% had more than one nerve affected, and 88% had injuries proximal to the elbow or

knee. Partial nerve injuries tended to produce atypical patterns.

Compression neuropathy at any level can be complicated by RSD (CRPS type II). Grundberg and Reagan (1991) found that of 22 patients with resistant RSD, 7 had nerve compression at other levels; 5 had cubital tunnel syndrome, 1 had compression of the ulnar nerve at Guyton canal, and 1 had a herniated cervical disc. Injury to the infrapatellar branch of the saphenous nerve during knee arthroscopy has also been reported to lead to the development of CRPS II.

Symptoms and Signs

Whatever terminology is used, RSD, RSDS, or CRPS, **the predominant symptom is pain out of proportion to the initial injury.** The pain is usually a constant, persistent aching or burning that is exacerbated by emotional factors. *Swelling, stiffness, and discoloration are initial signs. Secondary signs include bony demineralization, pseudomotor changes, trophic changes, temperature changes, and palmar fibrosis.*

Primary Signs

- Severe hyperalgesia: poorly localized, progressing to a diffuse distribution that does not fit a dermatomal distribution.
- Edema: spreads proximally, changes from soft to hard (brawny) edema with time.
- Stiffness: rapid onset following swelling if swelling is not treated early **(it is very important to initiate physical therapy as quickly as possible);** fibrous ankylosis of joint with time.

Secondary Signs

- Osteopenia.
- Sudomotor or vasomotor changes (mottling, discoloration).
- Temperature changes (cold sensitivity).
- Trophic changes.
- Palmar fibrosis.
- Hyperhydrosis (sweating).
- Skin changes.
- Loss of skin creases.
- Loss of hair.
- Decreased moisture (late).
- Dystonic posture of affected limb.

Associated Findings

- Tremor.
- Weakness, muscle wasting (atrophy).
- Dystonia.

Diagnostic Criteria

- It typically follows an initially innocuous event (e.g., ankle sprain).
- Spontaneous pain, allodynia, and/or hyperesthesia exist beyond the territory of a single peripheral nerve and are disproportionate to the inciting event.
- There is, or has been, evidence of edema, skin blood flow changes, or abnormalities in the pseudomotor activity in that region since the inciting event.
- The existence of any conditions that could otherwise account for the amount of pain and dysfunction present has been excluded.

Special Patient Categories

Patients who are neurologically impaired because of *spinal cord injury* are at risk for the development of RSD. The prevalence of RSD in paraplegic, quadriplegic, and hemiplegic patients is approximately 10%. Braus and colleagues (1994) found symptoms of RSD in 27% of hemiplegic patients with shoulder symptoms and identified as risk factors shoulder subluxation, marked upper extremity weakness, and visual field defects. No correlation of whether the lesion is complete or incomplete has been found between the development of RSD and the level of spinal cord injury.

RSD occurs in approximately 12% of patients with *traumatic brain injuries* and may be difficult to diagnosis because of their inability to vocalize or localize the pain. The only sign may be a withdrawal from pain. The involved extremities may be warmer and more swollen than normal, and the skin may be mottled and glossy. Joint stiffness is not as indicative of RSD in these patients because it may occur regardless of the presence or absence of RSD. Gellman and associates (1997) reported more frequent associated upper extremity injuries in patients with RSD, especially in those with spasticity or patterned motion.

In patients with *strokes,* RSD has been reported to develop in 12 to 25%. *Bone scanning may help identify patients at risk for the development of RSD.* Weiss and coworkers (1993) prospectively studied the value of *three-phase bone scanning* in predicting which patients may develop RSD after stroke. Of 22 patients who had three-phase bone scanning after stroke, 16 scans were considered consistent with RSD; 5 extremities were symptomatic at the time of bone scanning. Of 11 asymptomatic patients with positive scans, 7 subsequently developed RSD. No patient with a negative scan developed RSD.

RSD in *children* has essentially the same presentation as that in adults. It is more frequent in girls than in boys, and the lower extremities are affected more often than the upper extremities. The prognosis for recovery or improvement is better in children than in adults, but children can develop limb-length discrepancies because of altered blood flow and trophic changes.

Diagnosis

Relief of pain or modification of signs after sympathetic block is virtually diagnostic of RSD. Failure of symptoms to improve after block indicates a sympathetically independent source of pain.

The most reliable imaging modality for the diagnosis of RSD is three-phase bone scanning. Periarticular or diffuse mottled demineralization is evident earlier on three-phase bone scanning than on conventional radiographs.

Three-phase Bone Scanning for Diagnosis

- Phase I: angiogram
- Phase II: blood pool
- Phase III: delayed 3 to 4 hours after injection

For a scan to be considered diagnostic of RSD, the delayed phase must show diffusely increased activity in the involved joints with periarticular accentuation in the delayed phase. MacKinnon and Holder (1984) found the delayed bone-uptake phase of the three-phase bone scan to have a **96% sensitivity** and a **98% specificity** in detecting RSD. Werner and coworkers (1989) found a 50% sensitivity and 92% specificity, both of which increased if scanning was done in the first 6 months or in older patients (older than 50 years). A positive bone scan alone, however, does not necessarily correlate with the vascular autonomic dysfunction seen in RSD. Pollock and colleagues (1993) found that vasomotor response patterns to cold stress testing were the same whether or not a patient had a positive bone scan. O'Donoghue and associates (1993) found that marked asymmetry may be seen in all three phases of bone scanning in asymptomatic people as well as those with RSD, especially in the early two phases.

The examiner must order a three-phase bone scan rather than a two-phase standard bone scan when evaluating for possible RSD.

Radiographs often show periarticular or diffuse mottled osteoporosis, but calcium content must be decreased by 30 to 50% to be visible on plain radiographs. Patchy demineralization is nonspecific for RSD; it has been reported to be present in 30 to 80% of patients. Disuse osteopenia may confuse the radiograph in patients with muscle paralysis, and spasticity may limit osteoporosis development.

Thermography to compare the resting blood flow and muscle temperature in the affected extremity with those in the normal extremity may be helpful to confirm the diagnosis of RSD in some patients but is not absolute. Blood flow and muscle temperature measurements after treatment may be helpful to evaluate patient response. Depending on the timing of the test, an increase in temperature of 1°C or more in the affected limb is considered an abnormal result.

Stages of RSD

These stages do not necessarily occur sequentially.

1. **Stage I (Traumatic Phase)**
   a. Onset: at the time of initial injury or within several weeks
   b. Increase in edema
      i. Soft and localized
      ii. Spreads to periarticular tissue, resulting in increasing stiffness
   c. Hyperhidrosis
   d. May see fine tremor (3 to 6 Hz)
   e. Skin
      i. Cool, pale, cyanotic, mottled
      ii. May show erythema and warmth secondary to an increase in superficial blood flow
   f. Increased hair and nail growth
   g. Pain
      i. Increased by movement and weight-bearing
      ii. Voluntary disuse to minimize discomfort
      iii. Increases in severity over time
      iv. Diffuse
   h. Osteopenia on x-rays within 4 to 8 weeks after onset of pain
   i. Duration: 3 to 6 months
2. **Stage II (Dystrophic Phase)**
   a. Onset: 3 to 6 months after onset of pain
   b. Pain becomes more diffuse, increases in severity
   c. Edema changes from soft to brawny edema (creases disappear)
   d. Warmth followed by cyanosis
   e. Trophic changes
      i. Hair loss
      ii. Nails brittle, cracked, grooved
      iii. Glossy skin
      iv. Decreased moisture
   f. Joint range of motion (ROM) decreased, increased stiffness
   g. Muscle weakness or atrophy
   h. Less responsive to sympathetic blockade
   i. Radiographs: osteopenia
   j. Duration: 3 to 6 months
3. **Stage III (Atrophic Phase)**
   a. Onset: 6 to 12 months after injury
   b. Pain
      i. Intractable; although it may decrease
      ii. Proximal spread
      iii. Worsens with motion

   c. Joints
      i. Decreased ROM or lack of functional motion
      ii. Rigid (fibrous ankylosis)
      iii. Flexor tendon contraction
      iv. Joint subluxation
      v. Potentially ankylosed
   d. Skin
      i. Marked trophic changes owing to decreased blood flow
      ii. Cool, pale, dry, glossy
      iii. Subcutaneous fat atrophy (fingers narrow)
   e. Muscle atrophy
   f. Radiographs
      i. Diffuse
      ii. Disuse osteoporosis or osteopenia
   g. Duration: years or permanent

Treatment

Initial treatment should focus on the initiating cause of pain if possible. The goal of treatment is interruption of the continuous feedback loop. A multidisciplinary approach is essential.

Early diagnosis is the best treatment. Poplawski and coworkers (1983), in a review of 126 patients, found that the most important factor in predicting response to treatment was an interval of less than 6 months between onset of symptoms and initiation of therapy.

Delayed diagnosis may result in prolonged rehabilitation and the physical changes secondary to established RSD. A result may be RSD that is more refractory to treatment.

During the **acute postinjury period, treatment** may include nonsteroidal anti-inflammatory drugs (NSAIDs), analgesics, corticosteroid therapy (pulsed), and physical or occupational therapy.

Physical or Occupational Therapy

The primary role of physical and occupational therapy in the early stages of RSD is to help decrease pain and prevent the development of stiffness. Therapy alone may be successful in mild cases. It is important to **use early aggressive physical therapy and encourage motion.** Omer and Thomas (1971) reported that 20% of patients with causalgia were treated successfully with therapy that included elevation, traction, splinting, and conditioning.

Principles of Physical Therapy
- Minimize painful passive motion.
- Home exercise program is important.

- Motor re-education and strengthening as motion permits.
- Mobilize other areas of the extremities to prevent other joints from stiffening and becoming painful (e.g., patients with RSD involving the hand should have attention paid to their elbow and shoulder to avoid stiffness).
- Inappropriate use of physical or occupational therapy may worsen symptoms.
- Heat or ice packs may be used but avoid extreme temperatures.

Active and active-assisted motion (not passive motion) are essential.

- "Stress-loading" program of Watson and Carlson (1987)
  - Traction plus compressive exercises.
  - Improved pain scores.
  - Ninety-five percent improved motion, 84% returned to work, and 88% decreased pain.
- Antiedema measures
  - Elevation of extremity.
  - Place the hand in a position of function.
  - A dependent extremity may have increased edema.
- Massage.
- Compression garments.
- Splinting
  - Used to prevent contractures.
  - Dynamic splints may be necessary in stages II/III disease for stiffness.

Oral Medications

Several drugs have shown promise in the treatment of patients with RSD. For patients who have primarily sympathetically mediated pain, **alpha-adrenegic blockers** seem to be the most effective. The most important effect of alpha-adrenergic blockers is as a vasoconstrictor in the skin and subcutaneous tissue. The blockade allows vessel expansion and increases sodium and water excretion.

Phenoxybenzamine (Dibenzyline) has been found to be an effective blocking agent with few side effects. The *starting dose* of 10 mg/day is maintained for 2 days. If the patient complains of blurred vision, dizziness, lightheadedness, or postural hypotension, the medication is stopped. Postural hypotension is a contraindication to further use of the medication. If no side effects are evident, the dosage should be maintained until symptoms decrease. Increases in dosage can be made every 5 days with monitoring. Complete relief may require dosages as high as 80 mg/day in split doses. Treatment usually lasts 6 weeks.

Phentolamine (Regitine) is another effective alpha-blocking agent, but it is contraindicated in patients with cardiac and asthmatic conditions.

Clonidine (Catapres) stimulates alpha-adrenoreceptors in the brain, decreasing sympathetic outflow. It can be used as a transdermal patch (maximum 0.1-mg patch) to diminish hyperesthesia in the affected limb. The patch is applied to a hairless area, and each patch is good for 7 days at each site; the site should be changed at each application. Clonidine patches have been shown to be effective only in patients who have had relief with sympathetic blocks. Side effects include dry mouth, drowsiness, headache, skin sensitization or contact dermatitis, and rebound hypertension. Clonidine should not be used in patients with hypertension medications unless coordinated with the patient's internist. It should also not be used in patients who have arrhythmia, coronary insufficiencies, cardiac pathologies, or renal failure.

The **beta-blocking medication** propranolol (Inderal) has been shown to be effective in the relief of pain, hyperalgesia and hyperpathia, and it produces less orthostatic hypotension than alpha-blockers. This drug is contraindicated in patients with cardiac problems, asthma, or history of bronchospasm. Recommended dosage is 40 mg every 4 hours to a maximum of 240 mg/day; a 10-mg dose three to four times a day can be used as adjunctive treatment.

Guanethidine is a **postganglionic adrenergic inhibitor** that blocks norepinephrine release, thus modulating the effect of sympathetic nervous system on its target organs. Side effects include depression (loss of appetite, despondency), impotence, orthostatic hypotension, diarrhea, decreased cardiac output, and increased airway resistance. Recommended dosage is 20 to 30 mg/day for 8 weeks. It is contraindicated in patients with asthma.

Mood-modifying drugs have been reported to help reduce the pain and complaints in patients with RSD when used as adjunctive drug therapy. **Amitriptyline (Elavil)** can be used at a dosage starting at 25 mg at bedtime and raised in increments of 25 mg weekly up to 200 mg as needed. This medication decreases anxiety (antidepressants), aids in improving sleep patterns, and helps treat depression. Other mood-modifying agents that have been used in the treatment of patients with RSD include chlorpromazine (Thorazine), trifluoperazine (Stelazine), chlordiazepoxide (Librium), and diazepam (Valium).

Calcium channel blockers have been used in the treatment of RSD because of their ability of reverse vasomotor instability. These drugs induce peripheral vasodilatation without affecting peripheral sympathetic nerve action. They also inhibit movement of calcium ions into cells, thus inhibiting excitation-contraction coupling and producing relaxation of arterial smooth muscle and thereby vasodilatation. Because they have no effect on venous smooth muscles, the risk of orthostatic hypotension is decreased. The antagonistic effects of norepinephrine on smooth muscle interrupts the pain cycle. **Nifedipine** (10 mg three times a day) has been reported to be moderately successful in the treatment of Raynaud's phenomena. The dosage is increased weekly to a maximum of 30 mg three times a day and is maintained for 3 weeks. When pain relief plateaus, the dosage is tapered off. Some patients can be successfully weaned without recurrence. Prough and colleagues (1985) reported that of 13 patients with RSD, 7 had complete relief, 2 had partial relief, and 3 stopped treatment owing to side effects.

NSAIDs are frequently used in the treatment of patients with RSD because they are thought to inhibit pain and decrease swelling and edema. However, **Wilder and associates (1992) reported that 60% of the 70 patients in their series showed no effect from NSAID treatment.** If NSAIDs are used, we prefer **indomethacin** (25 mg PO tid).

The use of **corticosteroids** in the treatment of RSD is controversial. Generally, they are more effective early in the disease course and have been reported to decrease edema and pain. They are less effective in established RSD. Christensen and coworkers (1982) reported that 63% of patients had a good response, but this required dosages of up to 100 mg/day. Good results also have been reported with 60 to 80 mg of prednisone for 2 to 4 days, decreased by 10 to 20 mg every 2 to 4 days until a 40-mg level is reached, followed by a rapid taper to 5 mg, which is maintained for several weeks. The mechanism of action of the corticosteroids is unclear, although the stabilizing effect on basement membranes may reduce capillary permeability and decrease plasma extravasation associated with early RSD. Complications of steroids include weight gain, moon facies, and dyspepsia.

Calcitonin, which modulates osteoclast activity, has been reported to improve motion and decrease pain when administered in a dosage of 100 units/day by nasal spray; however, the effects may not be maintained.

Sympathetic Blocks

Sympathetic blocks can be both diagnostic and therapeutic. Pain relief may last beyond the duration of the block and even be curative. They should be used early if other modalities are ineffective. Blocks can be repeated until the pain is controlled, up to a maximum of 8 to 12 blocks (2 to 3 blocks/wk); a second series may be necessary. If block results are equivocal, a control block with normal saline solution can be done to define the degree of contribution above this level. If relief decreases after repeated blocks, surgical treatment may be considered, and early sympathectomy may prevent the occurrence of irreversible trophic changes and fixed pain patterns. If blocks are ineffective, however, surgical sympathectomy is not indicated.

Stellate ganglion blocks
- Between the C7 and the T1 levels.
- One percent lidocaine or 0.25% bupivacaine (Marcaine).
- Direct anterior approach.
- Easily performed.
- Low complication rate.
- Can be used in a continuous fashion.
- Can be done before surgical procedures on involved extremities (continue into postoperative period).
- Clues to an appropriate block
  - Profound Horner's syndrome.
  - Warming and drying of the hand.
  - Relief of pain.
  - Increased blood flow.
- Complications
  - Minor
    Dizziness.
    Ringing in the ears.
    Blacking out.
    Pain at the site of injection.
    Block of recurrent laryngeal, vagus, or phrenic nerves.
  - Major
    Toxic reaction resulting in respiratory and cardiovascular collapse.
    Total spinal anesthesia.
    Pneumothorax.
    Cerebral air embolism.
- Results
  - Eighty percent pain relief from one or more blocks (Kleinert et al, 1973).
  - Pain relief and improved motion in "most" of 29 patients with continuous blockade and physical therapy (Linson et al, 1983).

Lumbar Block
- More difficult.
- Requires three needles placed approximately 5 cm lateral to the midline opposite the transverse processes of L1, L2, L3, and L4 and directed deeper to place anesthetic along the anterior lateral border of the lumbar vertebra.
- Medication: 10 ml of 1% lidocaine to each needle.
- Signs of successful block: warming and drying of extremity, pain relief.
- Complications
  - Minor
    Paralysis of lumbar nerves.
    Epidural blockade.

- Major
    - Severe systemic toxic reaction.
    - Respiratory and cardiovascular collapse.
    - Seizures.
    - Total spinal anesthesia.

Comparison of treatment based on onset of intervention showed that 70% of the patients improved if treated within 6 months versus only 50% of the patients treated when symptoms had lasted 6 to 12 months. Recognition and initiation of treatment is paramount.

Bier Blocks

- Improvement in ROM and pain relief when combined with reserpine, guanethidine (Hannington-Kiff), or bretylium (Hord) and prednisolone (corticosteroid) followed by joint manipulation.
- Additional medication may prolong duration of pain relief.
- Blocks can be repeated every 48 to 72 hours.
- Blocks are stopped if the patient's response plateaus.
- Motion improved in 46 to 81% after blocks, with patients reporting an 80% reduction in pain.
- Complications
    - Orthostatic hypertension.
    - Dizziness.
    - Somnolence.
    - Nausea.
    - Vomiting.

The use of sympathetic blockade in combination with physical therapy leads to an improvement in 80% of patients.

Chemical Sympathectomy

- Useful if blocks have produced temporary or transient relief.
- Done with 6% aqueous phenol or 50% alcohol.
- May produce sympathetic interruption for weeks to months.
- Use in older or poor-risk patients.

Surgical Sympathectomy

Surgical sympathectomy is useful in patients with only transient relief from sympathetic blocks and in younger patients or patients in good physical condition. It is traditionally done through the posterior approach of Smithwick (1940). Using an open approach, Olcott and colleagues (1991) reported 74% excellent, 17% good, and 9% poor results at 14 months follow-up. Atkins (1954) recommended a transaxillary approach, which has the advantage of providing excellent exposure and direct access to the proximal thoracic chain from T1 to T4. Endo-

scopic surgical sympathectomy has also been described. Complications include increased morbidity because of the required thoracotomy (may be less with endoscopic approach), risk of injury to the peripheral nerves, and pneumothorax.

Biofeedback

Biofeedback may be successful in decreasing pain, and *psychotherapy* may be helpful because long-standing, chronic RSD patients suffer emotional and psychological disturbances owing to duration of pain and disability. Intense psychological support and encouragement are needed, and depression should be treated if present. If severe pathology exists, counseling and medical therapy also need to be instituted.

Alternative Treatment Modalities

Stilz and coworkers (1997) showed *transcutaneous nerve stimulation* to be successful in children, and this modality may be second-line therapy for children. Kesler and associates (1988) reported that 90% of their patients improved with transcutaneous nerve stimulation, and 70% had complete relief after 2 months of treatment.

Electrical stimulation may be considered another second-line therapy in children. Shealy and Maurer (1974) reported complete relief of chronic pain in 25% of patients and partial relief in 60%. *However, physical therapy and oral medications are first-line treatments for children.*

Electroacupuncture, using low-frequency simulation (<10 Hz) for 20 minutes was reported by Chan and Chow (1981) to produce pain relief in 90% of patients. Hill and colleagues (1991) reported improvement in vasodilatation, temperature increases, and erythema. The action of electroacupunture has been theorized to be, at least in part, due to the release of endorphins in the central nervous system. An alternative explanation may be due to large-fiber transmission during acupuncture "closing the gate," thus decreasing pain. Changes in neurovascular responses secondary to central neurochemistry changes may produce lasting changes.

Amputation

Amputation may be considered for persistent pain or if recurrence of pain is common. Many patients are satisfied with the results of amputation despite persistent pain. Dielissen and coworkers (1995) found that 26 of 28 (93%) patients still had pain in the limb after amputation. Most patients are unable to wear a prosthesis after amputation because of pain, and *amputation is not typically recommended.*

Recommended Treatment for Acute RSD Presentation (Fig. 8–1)

Early Diagnosis

Mobilize joints as much as possible.

NSAIDs if not contraindicated.

Analgesics as needed.

Methylprednisolone (Medrol Dosepak).

Amitriptyline (25 mg at bedtime to start).

Elevation and ice.

Physical, occupational therapy.

Follow closely.

Consider alternative modalities (e.g., acupuncture).

Early Follow-up

If improving, continue intervention.

If no improvement, try **two stellate ganglion blocks** and continue methylprednisolone.

Repeat blocks as necessary (if patient responds).

Figure 8–1. Algorithm displaying our management of patients with a post-traumatic or postoperative *acute* pattern of reflex sympathetic dystrophy (RSD) complaints. NSAIDs, nonsteroidal anti-inflammatory drugs; OT, occupational therapy; PT, physical therapy.

Recommended Treatment for Chronic RSD Presentation (Fig. 8-2)

Entertain the diagnosis.

Determine etiology of pain source.

NSAIDs, amitriptyline, and therapy.

Methylprednisolone.

Early trial of sympathetic blocks.

May need to gently manipulate if stiff (under Bier block anesthesia).

Patients with no response to blocks may have other etiology.

Algorithm II. Late presentation of RSD

RSD concerns: pain, swelling, color changes

Yes — Proceed to Algorithm I ← New onset — No → **Established Pain Pattern** With skin changes, finger/wrist stiffness

Yes

No

- Intensive OT or physical therapy
- NSAIDs / analgesics
- Amitriptyline (Elavil)
- Methylprednisolone (Medrol Dosepak) x 2

Improvement — No → Trial of sympathetic blockade

Yes

- Continue present course
- OT three times a week until resolution

Responds to blocks

Yes —
- Full series of 12 stellate blocks (three times a week/4 wks)
- Amitriptyline (Elavil) — for sleep irregularity
- NSAIDs
- Intensive OT
- TENS
- Contrast baths
- Analgesics

No

- Investigate for alternate etiology
- May be nonsympathetically mediated pain
- Refer to pain center for chronic care

- Continue OT
- NSAID therapy ← Yes — Improvement — No → (to Investigate box)

Limited by stiffness

- Manipulate under Bier blocks
- Alternate Bier blocks with stellate blocks
- Consider second set of blocks

Figure 8-2. Algorithm displaying our management of patients with an *established* or *chronic* pattern consistent with RSD. TENS, transcutaneous electrical nerve stimulation.

Prognosis

The prognosis for patients with RSD is better with early diagnosis and treatment, and best if the diagnosis is made and treatment begun in less than 6 months. The prognosis is generally better in children than adults. The primary treatment principle is to treat RSD aggressively early.

Bibliography

Atkins HJB: Sympathectomy by axillary approach. Lancet 1:538, 1954.

Atkins RM, Duckworth T, Kanis JA: Algodystrophy following Colles' fracture. J Hand Surg 14B:161–164, 1989.

Bickerstaff DR, Kanis JA: Algodystrophy: an under-recognized complication of minor trauma. Br J Rheumatol 33:240–248, 1994.

Blanchard EB: The use of temperature biofeedback in the treatment of chronic pain due to causalgia. Biofeedback Self-Regul 4:183, 1979.

Braus DF, Krauss JK, Strobel J: The shoulder-hand syndrome after stroke: a prospective clinical trial. Ann Neurol 36:728–733, 1994.

Chan CS, Chow SP: Electroacupuncture in the treatment of post-traumatic sympathetic dystrophy (Sudeck's atrophy). Br J Anaesth 53:899–901, 1981.

Christensen K, Jensen EM, Noer I: The reflex sympathetic dystrophy syndrome: response to treatment with systemic corticosteroids. Acta Chir Scand 148:653–655, 1982.

Dielissen PW, Claassen ATPM, Veldman PHJM, et al: Amputation for reflex sympathetic dystrophy. J Bone Joint Surg 77B:270–273, 1995.

Evans JA: Reflex sympathetic dystrophy. Surg Gynec Obstet 82:36–43, 1946.

Field J, Protheroe DL, Atkins RM: Algodystrophy after Colles fractures is associated with secondary tightness of casts. J Bone Joint Surg 76B:901–905, 1994.

Field J, Warwick D, Bannister GC: Features of algodystrophy ten years after Colles fracture. J Hand Surg 17B:318–320, 1992.

Gellman H, Collins E: Complex regional pain syndrome in the upper extremity. (In press).

Gellman H, Eckert RR, Botte MJ, et al: Reflex sympathetic dystrophy in cervical spinal cord injury patients. Clin Orthop 233:126–131, 1988.

Gellman H, Nichols D: Upper extremity reflex sympathetic dystrophy. J Am Acad Orthop Surg 5(6):313–322, 1997.

Grundberg AB, Reagan DS: Compression syndromes in reflex sympathetic dystrophy. J Hand Surg 16A:731–736, 1991.

Hannington-Kiff JG: Pharmacological target blocks in hand surgery and rehabilitation. J Hand Surg 9B:29–36, 1984.

Hill SD, Lin MS, Chandler PJ Jr: Reflex sympathetic dystrophy and electroacupuncture. Tex Med 87:76–81, 1991.

Hobelmann CF Jr, Dellon AL: Use of prolonged sympathetic blockade as an adjunct to surgery in the patient with sympathetic maintained pain. Microsurgery 10:151–153, 1989.

Hord AH, Rooks MD, Stephens BO, et al: Intravenous regional bretylium and lidocaine for treatment of reflex sympathetic dystrophy: a randomized, double-blind study. Anesth Analg 74:818–821, 1992.

Jadad AR, Carrol D, Glynn CJ, et al: Intravenous regional sympathetic blockade for pain relief in reflex sympathetic dystrophy: a systematic review and a randomized, double-blind crossover study. J Pain Symptom Manage 10:13–20, 1995.

Kesler RW, Saulsbury FT, Miller LT, et al: Reflex sympathetic dystrophy in children: treatment with transcutaneous electric nerve stimulation. Pediatrics 82:728–732, 1988.

Kleinert HE, Cole NM, Wayne L, et al: Post-traumatic sympathetic dystrophy. Orthop Clin North Am 4:917–927, 1973.

Linson MA, Leffert R, Todd DP: The treatment of upper extremity reflex sympathetic dystrophy with prolonged continuous stellate ganglion blockade. J Hand Surg 8A:153–159, 1983.

MacKinnon SE, Holder LE: The use of three-phase radionuclide bone scanning in the diagnosis of reflex sympathetic dystrophy. J Hand Surg 9A:556, 1984.

Mitchell SW, Morehouse GR, Keen WW: Gunshot Wounds and Injuries of Nerves. New York, JB Lippincott, 1864

O'Donoghue JP, Powe JE, Mattar AG, et al: Three-phase bones scintigraphy. Asymmetric patterns in the upper extremities of asymptomatic normals and reflex sympathetic dystrophy patients. Clin Nucl Med 18(10): 829–836, 1993.

Olcott C IV, Eltherington LG, Wilcosky BR, et al: Reflex sympathetic dystrophy: the surgeon's role in management. J Vasc Surg 14:488–495, 1991.

Omer G, Thomas S: Treatment of causalgia: a review of cases at Brooke General Hospital. Tex Med 67:93, 1971.

Pollock FE Jr, Koman LA, Smith BP, Poehling GG: Patterns of microvascular response associated with reflex sympathetic dystrophy of the hand and wrist. J Hand Surg [Am] 19(5):884–886, 1994.

Poplawski ZJ, Wiley AM, Murray JF: Post-traumatic dystrophy of the extremities: a clinical review and trial of treatment. J Bone Joint Surg 65A:642–655, 1983.

Prough DS, McLeskey CH, Poehling GG, et al: Efficacy of oral nifedipine in the treatment of reflex sympathetic dystrophy. Anesthesiology 62:796–799, 1985.

Richards RL: Causalgia: a centennial review. Arch Neurol 16:339–350, 1967.

Rush PJ, Wilmot D, Saunders N, et al: Severe reflex neurovascular dystrophy in childhood. Arthritis Rheum 28:952–956, 1985.

Shealy CN, Maurer D: Transcutaneous nerve stimulation for control of pain. Surg Neurol 2:45, 1974.

Smithwick RH: The rationale and technique of sympathectomy for the relief of vascular spasm of the extremity. N Engl J Med 222:699, 1940.

Stilz RJ, Carron H, Sanders DB: Case history number 96. Reflex sympathetic dystrophy in a 6 year old: successful treatment by transcutaneous nerve stimulation. Anaesth Analg 56:438–441, 1997.

Sylvest J, Jensen EM, Siggaard-Anderson J, et al: Reflex dystrophy: resting blood flow and muscle temperatures as diagnostic criteria. Scand J Rehabil Med 9:25–29, 1977.

Watson HK, Carlson L: Treatment of reflex sympathetic dystrophy of the hand with an active "stress loading" program. J Hand Surg 12A:779–785, 1987.

Weiss L, Alfano A, Bardfeld P, et al: Prognostic value of triple phase bone scanning for reflex sympathetic dystrophy in hemiplegia. Arch Phys Med Rehabil 74:716–719, 1993.

Werner R, Davidoff G, Jackson MD, et al: Factors affecting the sensitivity and specificity of the three-phase tech-

netium bone scan in the diagnosis of reflex sympathetic dystrophy syndrome in the upper extremity. J Hand Surg 14A:520–523, 1989.

Wilder RT, Berde CB, Wolohan M, et al: Reflex sympathetic dystrophy in children: clinical characteristics and follow-up of seventy patients. J Bone Joint Surg 74A:910–919, 1992.

Chapter 9
Low Back Injuries

S. Brent Brotzman, MD

The accurate, objective study of **low back pain** (LBP), its natural history, and its effective treatment is difficult because of the multiple factors involved. This includes the favorable natural history and spontaneous resolution of most LBP regardless of treatment, the presence of secondary and monetary gain for LBP in Western societies, and the methodological problems in setting up studies.

The incidence of low back disability appears to have dramatically increased in Western society since about 1970. Waddell (1998) concluded, however, that this is not indicative of an increase in the prevalence of LBP but rather of an increase in work loss, sick certification, compensation, and long-term disability awards.

Among industrialized nations, the United States has the highest rate of spinal surgery—five times that of Great Britain, for example (Taylor 1994). Studies examining the outcome of operative and non-operative treatment of back pain have not shown a distinct advantage for surgery. In Weber's (1983) prospective study of 280 patients with herniated nucleus pulposis diagnosed by myelography, the surgical group demonstrated a more rapid recovery than the non-operative treatment group. At four years, however, the outcomes were roughly equivalent, and at ten years there were no appreciable differences in outcome.

Definitions and Common Terms

Acute Mechanical Low Back Pain

The pain is "mechanical"—that is, it **varies with physical activity** (e.g., prolonged sitting, bending forward) and with time. This pain is located in the lumbosacral region, buttocks, and thighs, with no radiation to foot or toes.

Sciatica (Nerve Root Pain)

The term *nerve root pain* is preferable to the use of "sciatica" because it more accurately describes the pathologic origin. Nerve root pain may arise from disc herniation, spinal stenosis, or postoperative scarring. Nerve root pain radiates down one leg in a dermatomal pattern.

The leg pain (unilateral) is described by the patient as worse than the back pain. Numbness and paresthesia (if present) are found in the same nerve root distribution. Straight-leg raise (SLR) testing reproduces the leg pain. Motor, sensory, or reflex changes are classically limited to a single nerve root.

Thus, the term "sciatica," or nerve root pain, is used to describe leg pain that predominates in the distribution of a lumbosacral nerve root, with or without neurologic deficit.

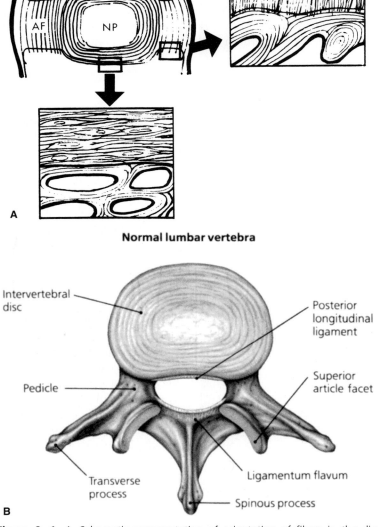

Normal lumbar vertebra

Figure 9–1. *A,* Schematic representation of orientation of fibers in the disc and end plate. AF, annulus fibrosis; NP, nucleus pulposis; CP, cartilaginous plate. *B,* The normal lumbar spine. (*A,* From Canale TE. Campbell's Operative Orthopaedics, 9th ed. St. Louis, Mosby, 1998, p 3018; *B,* from Garfin SR: Acquired spinal stenosis: making the diagnosis in the elderly. J Musculoskel Med 1(1):63, 1987. Artist: C. Boyter.)

Disc Herniation

Disc herniation describes the protrusion of the gelatinous material of the disc (nucleus pulposus) through the annulus fibrosis (Figs. 9–1 and 9–2).

Several studies have shown ***gradual resorption and disappearance of herniated discs on serial MRIs*** without surgical intervention. The larger disc herniations were found to have had more resorption. This favorable

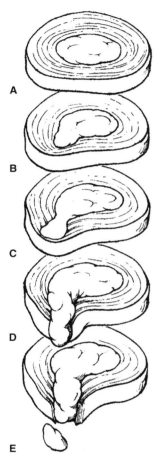

Figure 9–2. *A–E, A,* Normal. *B,* Initial distention of the annulus occurs with posterior displacement of the nucleus, causing protrusion of the intervertebral disk. *C,* Subsequent radial tear of the annulus allows the nucleus to completely protrude posteriorly through the annulus and rest underneath the longitudinal ligament. Shown here is a contained disk herniation (prolapse). *D,* Subsequent protrusion through the posterior longitudinal ligament results in an extruded or uncontained disk herniation. *E,* Finally, a piece of the nucleus separates and migrates to form a sequestered herniation. *F,* On an axial CT image from a CT discogram, a posterior annular tear is identified (*white arrow*). There is *no* herniated nucleus pulposus (HNP). Contrast extends posteriorly into the outer annular fibers and is contained by the posterior annular/posterior longitudinal ligament complex. *G,* At the time of discography, the patient experienced concordant back pain when the L5–S1 disc level was injected and the posterior annular fissure filled with contrast. There was no pain when the normal L3–4 and L4–5 disc levels were injected. (*A–E,* From Gill K: Percutaneous lumbar diskectomy. J Am Acad Orthop Surg 1(1):33–40, 1993; *F* and *G,* Reproduced with permission, from Herzog RG: The radiologic evaluation of lumbar degenerative disk disease and spinal stenosis in patients with back or radicular symptoms. In Eilert RE (ed): Instructional Course Lectures, vol 41. Rosemont, Ill. American Academy of Orthopaedic Surgeons, 1992.)

natural history shows why up to 50% of patients with confirmed, painful herniated discs recover **without surgery** within 1 to 6 months.

Incidence of Low Back Pain

Mechanical LBP is very common, affecting between 70 and 85% of American adults at some point during their lives. An estimated 1.3 billion days a year are lost from work in the United States because of LBP. Back pain complaints are second only to upper respiratory conditions as a cause of work absenteeism. Back pain is also the most common cause of disability in patients younger than 40 years.

In 90% of patients, LBP resolves within 6 weeks (self-limited). In another 5% of patients, the pain resolves by 12 weeks after initiation. Less than 1% of back pain is due to "serious" spinal disease (e.g., tumor, infection). Less than 1% of back pain stems from inflammatory disease (rheumatologic work-up and treatment required). Less than 5% of back pain is true nerve root pain. Most patients with LBP have one or more of four symptoms:

1. Back pain.
2. Leg pain.
3. Neurologic symptoms.
4. Spinal deformity.

False-positive Radiographic Studies in Low Back Pain Evaluation

Diagnostic triage of back pain should be based primarily on an **accurate, focused clinical assessment** (history and physical examination) rather than the growing trend of cursory examination and overreliance on imaging techniques. Asymptomatic patients with no back pain have been found to have a high incidence of "positive" MRI or CT findings. **Jensen and coworkers (1994) found that 64% of asymptomatic individuals who underwent an MRI had "abnormal"-appearing lumbar discs at some level.** Overreliance on the "shotgun approach" of diagnosis with a cursory examination and "knee-reflex" MRI imaging will often obtain an incorrect diagnosis.

Because of the high incidence of false-positive results on MRI (e.g., MRI reading a right-sided L2–3 disc "herniation" in a patient with mechanical LBP only), the physician must correctly correlate the clinical symptoms (right leg L5 sensory and motor changes) with the MRI findings (right herniated disc at the L4–5 level).

"Abnormalities" seen on MRI or CT scan (e.g., age-related disc changes) often are *not* the origin for the patient's back pain (i.e., these tests are **highly sensitive,** but not specific). The crucial part of accurate diagnosis is the physician's clinical findings and their correlation with imaging findings.

We recommend that the primary care physician allow the "back specialist" to order the MRI, CT, or myelogram because different radiologic studies are employed for different suspected clinical diagnosis (e.g., spinal stenosis versus disc space infection versus herniated disc).

Risk Factors Previously Associated with the Development of Low Back Pain

Almost all of us (70 to 85%) will develop LBP at some point. For this reason, it is inappropriate for physicians to tell patients that LBP results from being obese, inactive, or other factors.

Gordon Waddell's recommended text (1998) critically reviews the *poor methodology and science* behind studies that have described risks for LBP including:

- Heavy manual labor.
- Repetitive lifting and twisting.
- Postural stress.
- Whole body vibration.
- Monotonous work.
- Lack of personal control at work.
- Low job satisfaction.
- Poor physical fitness.
- Poor or inadequate trunk strength.
- Smoking.

Waddell, after critical review of these studies, reached several interesting conclusions.

- Most people get back pain; heredity, gender, and body build make little difference.
- It is good general health advice to stop smoking, avoid or correct obesity, and get physically fit. These may possibly help reduce the likelihood of developing new episodes of back pain.
- **Waddell asserts that "social class" is probably the strongest personal predictor of incurring back trouble.** This is in part related to heavy manual labor and in part to "social disadvantage."

"Social class" in Waddell's discussion reflects *occupation* (manual rather than clerical labor) and social disadvantage (e.g., poor medical care). The prevalence of back pain appears to be slightly higher in those patients who perform more manual types of labor. It is unclear which particular aspect of work, social disadvantage (e.g., poor medical care), lifestyle, attitudes, or behavior influences this "social class" finding.

Back pain does have a **greater impact** on people in heavy manual labor jobs. They are more likely to stay off work and stay off longer than "clerical" laborers. This may be a reflection of the *effect* of their back pain (i.e., patient cannot lift the heavy loads required at work) or may reflect the *medical advice* given to them by their physicians (stay off work because of the possibility of aggravating the back pain with resumption of heavy labor).

The examiner should evaluate and rule out potential emergent causes of LBP during history and physical examination. Careful history and review of systems may detect nonmusculoskeletal origin of LBP. **Our approach to the work-up of LBP is to first rule out emergent or nonmusculoskeletal causes of LBP.** Once this is done, the appropriate examinations and tests are performed to confirm or rule out mechanical, nerve root, tumor, infectious, traumatic, systemic, or inflammatory etiology.

Classification of Low Back Pain Syndromes

Mechanical or Activity-related Causes

Segmental and discal degeneration

Myofascial or soft tissue injury/disorder/strain

Disc herniation with possible radiculopathy

Spinal instability with possible spondylolisthesis or fracture

Vertebral body fracture

Spinal canal or lateral recess stenosis

Arachnoiditis, including postoperative scarring

Spondylosis

Facet syndrome

Degenerative joint disease of spine

Systemic Disorders

Primary or metastatic neoplasm, including myeloma

Osseous, discal, or epidural infection

Inflammatory spondyloarthropathy

Metabolic bone disease, including osteoporosis

Vascular disorders such as atherosclerosis or vasculitis

Neurologic Syndromes

Myelopathy from intrinsic or extrinsic processes

Lumbosacral plexopathy, especially from diabetes

Neuropathy, including inflammatory demyelinating type (e.g., Guillain-Barré)

Mononeuropathy, including causalgia

Myopathy, including myositis and metabolic causes

Referred Pain or Psychogenic Etiology

Gastrointestinal disorders

Genitourinary disorders, including nephrolithiasis, prostatitis, and pyelonephritis

Gynecologic disorders, including ectopic pregnancy and pelvic inflammatory disease

Abdominal aortic aneurysm

Hip pathology

Psychosocial causes

Compensable injury

Somatoform pain disorder

Psychiatric syndromes, including delusional pain

Drug seeking

Abusive relationships

Seeking disability or out-of-work status

Modified from Wheeler AH: Low back pain and sciatica. Am Fam Physician 52(5):1333, 1341, 1995.

Red Flags: Indicate Probable Serious Spinal Pathology Requiring Active Work-up and Evaluation of Back Pain

Red Flags

- Presentation age <20 yr or onset >55 yr (tumor?).
- Violent trauma, e.g. fall from a height, MVA (tumor?).
- Constant, progressive, nonmechanical pain.
- Thoracic pain.
- Previous history
  - Carcinoma.
  - Systemic steroids.
  - Drug abuse, HIV.
- Systemically unwell
  - Weight loss.
- Persisting severe restriction of lumbar flexion.
- Widespread neurologic symptoms.
- Structural deformity.
- Positive studies
  - ESR > 25.
  - Plain x-ray: vertebral collapse or bone destruction.

Cauda Equina Syndrome and/or Widespread Neurologic Disorder

- Difficulty with micturition/**urinary retention.**
- Loss of anal sphincter tone or fecal incontinence.
- **Saddle anesthesia** about the anus, perineum, or genitals (numb).
- Widespread (>one nerve root) or **progressive motor weakness in the legs or gait disturbance.**
- Sensory level.

Inflammatory Disorders (Ankylosing Spondylitis and Related Disorders)

- Gradual onset before age 40 yr.
- Marked morning stiffness.
- Persisting limitation of spinal movements in all directions.
- Peripheral joint involvement.
- Iritis, skin rashes (psoriasis), colitis, urethral discharge.

MVA, motor vehicle accident.
From Waddell G: The Back Pain Revolution. New York, Churchill Livingstone, 1998.

Emergent Etiologies of Low Back Pain

Cauda Equina Syndrome

Emergent surgical decompression required.
Only entity affecting the lumbar spine that requires emergent operative intervention.
Low incidence (<1%).
Usual cause is extrinsic pressure on the cauda equina by massive central herniated nucleus pulposus (HNP).
Other possible causes include:

- Epidural abscess.
- Epidural hematoma.
- Trauma.
- Epidural tumor.

Signs and symptoms include:

- **Urinary retention**
  - May exhibit overflow incontinence.
  - "Increased frequency."
- **Saddle anesthesia**
  - Numbness in the distribution of the saddle (perineum, anus, genitals).
- **Bilateral sensory or motor deficits.**
- Lumbar spine pain.

Requires emergent surgical intervention.

Ruptured Abdominal Aortic Aneurysm

- Pulsatile abdominal mass may or may not be palpable (50% of cases).
- Diminished pulses in the lower extremities.
- Unstable hemodynamically.
- Usually older than 50 yr.
- Requires *immediate* vascular surgery consultation and dramatic cardiovascular rescue/stabilization.

Fracture of Lumbar Spine

- High-velocity trauma (e.g., motor vehicle accident) is the typical mechanism.
- Requires immobilization and workup by orthopaedic surgeon/neurosurgery trauma team and appropriate short-term and long-term spine stabilization.
- See a spinal fracture text for further review.

Epidural Abscess

- Symptoms usually progress within a week.
- **Spinal pain with fever.**
- Nerve root pain.
- Weakness.
- Paralysis.
- Central nervous system signs.
- Sepsis.

was still **off work (no return to work) after 6 months.** They found the best predictors, *in order of decreasing accuracy,* were

1. Job characteristics: work history, occupation, job satisfaction, satisfaction with policies and benefits.
2. Patient beliefs about whether back pain was compensable, party at fault, and legal involvement (social factors).
3. Past hospitalization for back pain.
4. Educational level.

Workplace and social factors were by far the most powerful influences on chronicity (84% accurate in predicting who will be chronically disabled). These were more predictive than type of injury, health behavior, or other factors.

Risk Factors for Chronicity of Low Back Pain

- Previous history of LBP
- Significant work loss (due to LBP) in past year
- **Low job satisfaction**
- **Adversarial medicolegal proceedings**
- Radiating leg pain
- Reduced SLR (positive test)
- Signs of nerve root involvement
- Reduced trunk muscle strength and endurance
- Poor physical fitness
- Self-rated poor health
- Heavy smoking
- Psychological distress and depressive symptoms
- Disproportionate illness behavior
- Personal problems—alcohol, marital, financial

Low educational attainment and heavy physical occupation slightly increase the risk of LBP and chronicity but *markedly increase the difficulty of rehabilitation and job retraining.*

Evaluation of Patients with Low Back Pain

A thorough history and examination allows an accurate working diagnosis to be made in 90% of patients with LBP.

Be wary of **constant pain** unrelated to activity or position, nocturnal pain, pain refractory to treatment, or concomitant constitutional symptoms (Table 9–1).

History should also include questioning of nonmusculoskeletal symptoms (e.g., colic symptoms, penile discharge) (Table 9–2).

Predictors of Return-to-Work Status of Patients with Back Pain (Chronicity)

Cats-Barril and Frymoyer (1991) followed 250 patients to evaluate which of numerous factors best predicted who

Table 9–1

Red Flags for Potentially Serious Low Back Pain Conditions (Requiring Further Work-up)

Possible Fracture	Possible Tumor or Infection	Possible Cauda Equina Syndrome (Immediate Emergent Treatment Required)
From medical history:		
Major trauma, such as motor vehicle accident or fall from height	Age older than 50 yr or younger than 20 yr	Saddle anesthesia (numbness) in the area that patient usually rests on (perineum)
	History of cancer	
Minor trauma or even strenuous lifting (in older or potentially osteoporotic patient)	Constitutional symptoms, such as recent fever or chills or unexplained weight loss	Recent onset of bladder dysfunction, such as **urinary retention,** increased frequency, or **overflow incontinence**
	Risk factors for spinal infection: recent bacterial infection (e.g., urinary tract infection); IV drug abuse; or immune suppression from steroids, transplant, or HIV)	Severe or progressive neurologic deficit in the lower extremity
	Pain that worsens when supine: severe night-time pain or pain unrelenting	
From physical examination		Unexpected laxity of the anal sphincter
Back tenderness, possible neurosymptoms	Possible elevated temperature	Perianal/perineal sensory loss
		Major motor weakness: quadriceps (knee extension weakness); ankle plantarflexors, evertors, and dorsiflexors (foot drop)

From Waddell G: The Back Pain Revolution. New York, Churchill Livingstone, 1998.

General History[*]

1. Demographic information
   a. Age
      i. Younger—often discogenic pain.
      ii. Older—stenosis, osseous, lateral disc herniation.
   b. Gender
      i. Male—discogenic, ankylosing spondylitis, Reiter's syndrome more common.
      ii. Female—osteoporosis, fibromyalgia.
   c. Occupation
      i. Specific physical duties—possible increased incidence of back injury with repetitive lifting, twisting, vibration.
      ii. Emotional, work-related stresses—if significant, monitor for nonorganic component to pain.
      iii. Lack of job satisfaction—high correlation with time off work.
      iv. Last date patient worked—the longer the interval off work, the lower the likelihood of return to work.
      v. Feasibility of finding "light" or "clerical" duty at work—we have had much more success with rapid return to work having our patients sit at a desk 8 hours a day (often in a very boring setting), rather than having them stay at home.
      vi. Time left to retirement.
2. Recreational sports

History of Present Illness

1. **Onset of pain**
   a. When did episode begin?
   b. How did pain begin?
      i. Spontaneously
         (a) Sudden onset.
         (b) Gradual onset.
      ii. Traumatically
         (a) Motor vehicle, work-related, nonlegal setting.
         (b) Mechanism—flexion, extension, twist, lift, fall, sneeze, cough, strain, other.
   c. Motor vehicle accidents
      i. Types of cars involved.
      ii. Direction of impact.
      iii. Extent of vehicle damage—however, significant injury can occur with minor damage to vehicle.
      iv. Seat belt used? Lap belt versus shoulder harness—flexion injuries with lap belts, torsional injuries with harness.
      v. Loss of consciousness.
      vi. Did head hit windshield, or did chest hit steering wheel?

*Modified from Cole AJ, Herring SA: The Low Back Pain Handbook. Philadelphia, Hanley & Belfus/Mosby, 1997.

Table 9-2

Conditions That May Mimic Musculoskeletal or Mechanical Back Pain

Vascular

Abdominal aortic aneurysm	Age older than 50 yr Abdominal and back pain Pulsatile abdominal mass

Gynecologic

Endometriosis	Woman of reproductive age Cyclic pelvic and back pain
Pelvic inflammatory disease	Young, sexually active woman Systemically ill (fever, chills) Vaginal discharge or dysuria
Ectopic pregnancy	Missed period Abdominal pain and/or pelvic pain Positive pregnancy test

Genitourinary

Prostatitis	Men older than 30 yr Dysuria Low back and perineal pain
Nephrolithiasis	Flank and groin pain, often colicky in nature Hematuria
Pyelonephritis	Costovertebral angle tenderness—unilateral Fever, dysuria

Gastrointentinal

Pancreatitis or carcinoma	Abdominal pain radiating to back Systemic signs (fever, nausea, vomiting, weight loss) Elevated serum amylase, steatorrhea (fat in stool)
Penetrating or perforated duodenal ulcer	Abdominal pain radiating to back

Rhematologic

Fibromyalgia	Young to middle-aged woman Widespread pain Multiple tender points Disrupted sleep, fatigue Normal radiographs and laboratory values
Polymyalgia rheumatica	Age older than 50–60 yr Hip or shoulder girdle pain and stiffness Elevated ESR Dramatic response to low-dose prednisone
Seronegative spondylo-arthropathies (ankylosing spondylitis, Reiter's syndrome, psoriatic)	Younger male (ankylosing spondylitis, Reiter's syndrome) Lower lumbosacral pain Morning stiffness ("gel") Improvement with activity Radiographic sacroiliitis, may have positive HLA-B27

Diffuse idiopathic skeletal hyperostosis	Age older than 50–60 yr Thoracolumbar stiffness or pain
(Forrestier's disease)	Flowing anterior vertebral calcification on radiographs
Piriformis syndrome	Buttock and leg pain Pain on resisted hip external rotation and abduction Transgluteal or transrectal tenderness
Scheuerman's kyphosis	Age 12–15 yr Thoracic or thoracolumbar pain Increased fixed thoracic kyphosis Three or more wedged vertebrae with endplate irregularities
Trochanteric bursitis, gluteal fasciitis	Pain or tenderness over greater trochanter
Adult scoliosis	Back pain Uneven shoulders, scapular prominence Paravertebral hump with forward flexion

Metabolic

Osteoporosis	Woman older than 60 yr of age Severe acute thoracic pain (fracture) Severe weight-bearing pelvic pain (fracture) Aching dull thoracic pain, relived in supine position (mechanical) Loss of height, increased thoracic kyphosis
Osteomalacia	Diffuse skeletal pain or tenderness Increased alkaline phosphatase
Paget's disease	Bone pain; low back, pelvis, tibia Increased alkaline phosphatase Characteristic radiographic appearance
Diabetic polyradiculopathy	Older patient (>50 yr) Diffuse leg pain, worse at night Proximal muscle weakness
Malignancy	Age older than 50 yr Back pain unrelieved by positional change, night pain Previous history of malignancy Elevated ESR

vii. Specific location of immediate pain, if any.

viii. Visit to emergency department? Diagnostic and therapeutic measures performed.

d. Work-related injuries
   i. Details of specific injury.
   ii. Litigation pending.
   iii. Compensation for time off work.

e. Sports-related injuries
   i. Sports involving torsion (e.g., golf, racquet sports, baseball)—higher incidence of discogenic pain.
   ii. Sports involving repetitive hyperextension (e.g., gymnastics, dance, crew)—greater loading of posterior elements (e.g., spondolysis, facet syndrome).
   iii. Details of specific injury.

2. **Time course of pain**
   a. Intensity of pain—use of **visual analog pain scale** may be helpful
      i. Overall improvement or worsening overall: quantitate with visual analog pain scale or have patient assign a numerical or percent value to pain.
      ii. Response to specific treatment.
   b. Recurrences: frequency and duration.

3. **Location of pain**
   a. **Pain diagram** is helpful (have patient draw on pain diagram)
      i. Structural lesions.
      ii. Possibility of functional component.
   b. Ask about area of most intense pain—back versus leg: right, left, or bilateral?
      i. Primarily back pain—think of annular tear, facet syndrome, local muscular pathology, bony lesion.
      ii. Primarily distal lower extremity pain—think of lateral or extruded herniated nucleus pulposis (HNP), stenosis, nerve lesion.
   c. How has location changed over time and in response to specific treatments?

4. **Relationship of pain to daily routine**
   a. What positions increase the pain?
      i. Prone—pain is increased with facet pain, lateral HNP, systemic process.
      ii. Sitting—increased with annular tear, paramedian HNP.
      iii. Standing—increased with central stenosis, facet syndrome, lateral HNP.
   b. Is there pain on arising from a seat? A positive answer is typical of discogenic pain.
   c. How does walking affect the pain?
      i. How far can the patient walk? Is the distance variable (lumbar stenosis) or constant (vascular claudication)?
      ii. Is there more pain with uphill or downhill walking?
         (a) Patients with spinal stenosis or facet pain have less pain while walking uphill because the lumbar spine is flexed, which increases foraminal and central canal space.
         (b) Discogenic symptoms decrease while walking downhill because the lumbar spine is extended and discs are unloaded.
      iii. Is it more comfortable to walk holding a wagon or carriage or in a flexed posture? A positive answer is typical of stenosis.
   d. How is the pain affected by time of day?
      i. Is the patient awakened from sleep? Consider a systemic process if so.
      ii. Is there morning stiffness? Of what duration? Discogenic patients are stiff for 20 to 30 minutes, whereas rheumatic patients may be stiff for 2 hours.
      iii. Does the pain increase or decrease as the day progresses? The response helps guide treatment.
   e. Is pain intensified by coughing, sneezing, laughing, or Valsalva maneuver? In which location?
      i. Suggests disc disease or, rarely, an intraspinal tumor.
      ii. Reproduction of distal pain strongly supports discogenic pain.
   f. What activities is the patient unable to perform?
   g. Do any positions or maneuvers relieve the pain or other symptoms?

5. **Associated neurologic symptoms**
   a. Location of anesthesia, hypoesthesia, hyperesthesia, paresthesias
      i. Regional.
      ii. Dermatomal.
      iii. Sclerotomal.
      iv. Nonphysiologic.
   b. Does the patient note weakness?
      i. Differentiate inability to perform a task owing to pain from actual weakness.
      ii. Has the patient noted a dragging foot, buckling knee, difficulty with stairs or curbs? Suggestive of myotomal, plexus, cord, or nonphysiologic process.
   c. Has the patient noted bladder, bowel, or sexual dysfunction? If so, consider cauda equina syndrome.
   d. Does the patient have associated upper extremity, central nervous system, or brain stem symptoms?

6. **Diagnostic studies**
   a. Patient should be requested to bring in all images and reports.
   b. Patient should report the results of unavailable studies.

7. **Response to prior treatments**—ask for specifics (answer helps guide treatment)
   a. Bedrest—may be of limited benefit in stenosis.
   b. Medications
      i. Benefits.
      ii. Side effects.
   c. Modalities
      i. Superficial heating and cooling.
      ii. Electric stimulation.
      iii. Ultrasound.
      iv. Transcutaneous electrical nerve stimulation (TENS).
   d. Manual or mechanical therapy
      i. Centralization techniques—passive and active extension, shift correction.
         Positive response suggests discogenic pain.
      ii. Traction.
      iii. Stretching.
      iv. Mobilization.
         (a) Relief with specific facet mobilization suggests facet disease.
         (b) Mobilization may also treat other causes of pain (e.g., segmental dysfunction).
      v. Manipulation may treat facet pain and other sources of lumbar spine pain.
      vi. Rapid response to facet manipulation suggests a facet syndrome.
   e. Exercises
      i. Flexibility.
      ii. Strengthening and stabilization.
      iii. Aerobic conditioning.
   f. Education in proper body mechanics.
   g. Corset or bracing.
   h. Biofeedback.
   i. Soft tissue injections
      i. Trigger points.
      ii. Tendon.
      iii. Ligament.
   j. Spinal injections
      i. Anesthetic phase relief or steroid phase relief.
      ii. Fluoroscopy and/or contrast used?
   k. Percutaneous rhizolysis.
   l. Acupuncture.
   m. Surgery
      i. Specific procedure and date performed.
      ii. Immediate change in symptoms and/or signs.
      iii. Long-term change in symptoms and/or signs.
      iv. Complications.

Medical History

1. **Prior and current medical conditions**
   a. Diabetes.
   b. Hypertension.
   c. Cardiac disease.
   d. Cancer.
   e. Infections.
   f. Rheumatologic diseases.
   g. Gastrointestinal disorders (tolerance for nonsteroidal anti-inflammatory drugs [NSAID] use).
2. **Present medications** and drug allergies.
3. **Operations, injuries, and previous hospitalizations,** with names, addresses, phone numbers of all practitioners involved in patient's care.
4. **Review of systems,** asked selectively
   a. Constitutional symptoms
      i. Weight loss.
      ii. Loss of appetite.
      iii. Fever or night sweats.
      iv. Chills.
      v. Fatigue.
      vi. Night pain.
   b. Integument—rheumatologic disorders (e.g., rashes, psoriasis).
   c. Lymph nodes
      i. Malignancy.
      ii. Infection.
   d. Hematopoietic system
      i. Anemia.
      ii. Bleeding.
   e. Endocrine system—symptoms suggestive of
      i. Diabetes.
      ii. Thyroid dysfunction.
   f. Eyes
      i. Visual loss.
      ii. Inflammation.
   g. Mouth
      i. Pain.
      ii. Ulcerations.
   h. Bones, joints, muscles
      i. Pathologic fractures.
      ii. Peripheral or cervicothoracic joint symptoms.
      iii. Muscle pain or weakness.
   i. Breasts
      i. Pain.
      ii. Lumps.
      iii. Discharge.
   j. Respiratory system
      i. Pain.
      ii. Shortness of breath.
      iii. Cough.
   k. Cardiovascular system
      i. Chest pain.
      ii. Palpitations.
      iii. Orthopnea.

    iv. Dyspnea on exertion.
     v. Intermittent claudication.
    vi. Distal skin lesions.
   vii. Edema.
 l. Gastrointestinal system
     i. Dysphagia.
    ii. Nausea.
   iii. Vomiting.
   iv. Hematemesis.
     v. Jaundice.
   vi. Change in bowel habits.
  vii. Bowel incontinence.
m. Genitourinary system
     i. Urologic
      (a) Nocturia.
      (b) Dysuria.
      (c) Hematuria.
      (d) Pyuria.
      (e) Urinary frequency.
      (f) Retention.
      (g) Incontinence.
    ii. Gynecologic
      (a) Number of full-term pregnancies.
      (b) Last menstrual period (currently pregnant?).
      (c) Are menses regular or irregular?
      (d) Date and results of last pelvic examination and Papanicolaou smear.
      (e) Back or lower extremity pain associated with menses.
 n. Nervous system
     i. Cranial nerves.
    ii. Movement disorders.
   iii. Coordination.
   iv. Convulsions.
     v. Mental status.

Family History

1. Familial conditions.
2. Family members with chronic pain syndromes and/or spine pain.
3. Family members on disability.

Social History

1. Open-ended: "Tell me about your family."
2. Marital status—impact of condition on relationship and vice versa.
3. Children—impact of condition on relationship and vice versa.
4. Substance abuse history
  a. Alcohol intake.
  b. Smoking history.
  c. Illicit drug usage.

5. Social and economic status
  a. Extent of education.
  b. Special financial problems.

Physical Examination of the Lower Back

Several excellent texts on spinal examination are available, including Hoppenfield's *Physical Examination of the Spine and Extremities* (1976), Hoppenfield's *Orthopaedic Neurology* (1988), and Reider's *The Orthopaedic Physical Examination* (1999). Some general guidelines should be followed in the examination of a patient with back pain.

Observation and/or Palpation

- Skin (lipomas, hair over spine—spina bifida) (café-au-lait spots, skintags, neurofibromass for neurofibromatosis).
- Pelvic obliquity or leg-length discrepancy.
- List.
- Scoliosis or kyphosis or lordosis.
- Lumbar lordosis.
- Step-off deformity or flat back syndrome (spondylolisthesis).
- Posture.
- Posterior elements tenderness—facet joints, spinous processes, transverse processes.
- Paraspinous muscles (spasm).
- Iliac crest (traumatic hip pointer or meralgia paresthetica—the latter will have a numb anterior thigh, tender neuroma of the lateral femoral cutaneous nerve at the iliac crest).
- Sacroiliac (SI) joints
- Sciatic notch.
- Palpation for local tenderness in all areas of referred pain including:
  - Groin.
  - Hamstring.
  - Abdomen.
  - Greater trochanter(s) of the hip(s).

Gait

- Heel-walking (tests ankle dorsiflexors → L4 innervated tibialis anterior).
- Toe walking (tests gastrocnemius → L5–S1 disc).
- Antalgic gait or stride length or posture during ambulation.
- Extended hip and flexed knee noted during gait (patients with nerve root irritation will attempt to decrease tension on sciatic nerve by walking with extended hip and flexed knee).

A

B

Transverse section through sacroiliac joint

Ilium

Anterior sacroiliac ligament

Sacrum

Articular cartilage

Interosseous ligaments

Posterior sacroiliac ligament

Sacrotuberous ligament

C

D

Posterior view

Posterior sacroiliac ligament

Sacrospinous ligament

Sacrotuberous ligament

E

Figure 9–3. *A–E,* **SI joint examination maneuvers** designed to provoke pain or detect aberrant motion include the **Patrick test** (*A*), in which the patient lies supine, the ipsilateral leg is flexed at 90 degrees, and an extension force is applied with the hip positioned in flexion, abduction, and external rotation; the **Yeoman test** (*B*), performed with the patient lying prone and the ipsilateral leg placed in 20 degrees of extension and externally rotated; and the **Gaenslen maneuver** (*C*), in which the patient lies supine with the ipsilateral leg hanging off the examination table and the hyperextension force is applied to the hip. A test is considered positive if the patient experiences unilateral back or gluteal pain during the application of these maneuvers. *D* and *E,* Relationship of various components of the SI ligament. The posterior ligament is palpable because it has no muscular coverage. *D,* Transverse section through the SI joint. *E,* Posterior view. (*A–C,* From Slipman CW, Patel RK, Whyte WS, Lenrow DA: Diagnosing and managing sacroiliac pain. J Musculoskel Med 18:325-332, 2001. Artist: C. Boyter.) *D* and *E,* from Mooney V: Understanding, examining for, and treating sacroiliac pain. J Musculoskel Med 10[7]:37–49, 1993. Artist: C. Boyter.)

Table 9-3

Measuring Motor Testing—0–5 Scale

Score	Interpretation
5/5	Normal strength against resistance through full ROM
4/5	Decreased strength against resistance through full ROM
3/5	No resistance through full ROM against gravity
2/5	Decreased ROM without gravity
1/5	Markedly decreased ROM without gravity
0/5	No contraction palpable

ROM, range of motion.

Range of Motion of Lower Back and Hip Joints

- Lumbar flexion (note pain or restricted motion).
- Lumbar extension (pain or restricted motion often indicates posterior element pathology, such as spondylo- or facet syndrome).
- Lateral bending (pain or restricted motion).
- Rotation of spine (pain or restricted motion).

- Hip FABER examination (*flexion*, *abduction*, *external rotation* of hip) (known as Patrick test) (Fig. 9–3A).
- Decreased flexibility of hamstrings and hip flexors (e.g., possible spondylolisthesis).

Muscle Strength (Table 9–3)

- Standing
  - Trendelenburg gait (weak hip abductors).
  - Toe walking (gastrocsoleus—L5–S1 disc).
  - Hip extension (gluteus).
  - Heel-walking (anterior tibial muscle).
  - Toe extension (extensor hallucis longus).
- Sitting
  - Hip flexion (iliapsoas).
  - Knee extension (quadriceps).
  - Knee flexion.
  - Hip abduction.
  - Hip adduction.

Tendon Reflexes, Pathologic Reflexes

- Patellar tendon (L4).
- Achilles tendon (S1).

Figure 9–4. Dermatomal distribution of the sciatic nerve encompasses areas served by the L4, L5, S1, S2, and S3 nerve roots. Involvement of the L4 nerve root causes pain that radiates into the region of the medial leg and foot and the anterior knee. L5 nerve root symptoms present as pain over the lateral lower leg, the dorsum of the foot, and the first dorsal webspace. S1 nerve root pain usually occurs over the sole, heel, and lateral aspect of the foot. S2 nerve root pain occurs over the dorsal toes and posterior medial lower and upper leg, and S3 pain occurs in the medial portion of the buttocks. (From Hoppenfield S: Orthopaedic Neurology: A Diagnostic Guide to Neurologic Levels. Philadelphia, JB Lippincott, 1977.)

Figure 9–5. Straight leg raises (SLR).

Figure 9–6. Lasègue test.

- Beevor sign (rectus abdominus innervation test).
- Babinski reflex (pathologic).
- Ankle clonus (pathologic).

Sensory Testing
- Dermatomal distributions (Fig. 9–4).

Nerve Tension Signs
- SLR (Fig. 9–5).
- Lasègue test (Fig. 9–6).
- Crossed SLR test (Fig. 9–7).
- Bowstring sign (Fig. 9–8).
- Slump test (Fig. 9–9).
- Femoral nerve stretch test (Fig. 9–10).

Nerve Tension Tests

Straight-Leg Raises Test (see Fig. 9–5)
- SLR stretches the L5 and S1 nerve roots. Therefore, an abnormal SLR suggests pathology of the L5 or S1 nerve root. The **sciatic nerve** runs down the posterior thigh and is formed by L4, L5, S1, S2, and S3 nerve roots.
- This test is done with the patient lying comfortably flat. The leg is slowly elevated with the knee in full extension (straight). In normal patients, some hamstring tightness will be felt at 80 to 90 degrees of hip flexion.
- In the presence of sciatica or nerve root irritation, the patient complains of shooting pain

Figure 9–7. Positive crossed SLR test: back pain on the involved side induced by SLR in the uninvolved leg. (From Hoppenfield S: Physical Examination of the Spine and Extremities. Norwalk, Conn, Appleton-Century-Crofts, 1976. Reprinted by permission of Pearson Education, Inc., Upper Saddle River, N.J.)

Figure 9-8. Bowstring leg.

Figure 9-10. Femoral nerve stretch test.

radiating down the posterior thigh, often into the lower leg.

Lasègue Test (see Fig. 9-6)
- This test is an adjunct to the SLR. When the patient complains of reproduction of sciatic pain with an SLR, the examiner passively dorsiflexes the foot of the leg being raised. If this dorsiflexion worsens the sciatica, the Lasègue test is positive.

Crossed Straight-Leg Raises Test (see Fig. 9-7)
- The examiner performs an SLR test on the leg **opposite to that with the sciatica.** If this is positive (e.g., an uninvolved left leg SLR produces the right-sided sciatica), the result is **very sensitive and specific** for a **herniated L5-S1 or L4-5 lumbar disc.**

Bowstring Sign (see Fig. 9-8)
- The examiner starts the test by performing an SLR test until the radicular pain is produced. The knee is then flexed to 90 degrees, typically relieving the patient's symptoms. The examiner then places pressure with the fingers over the posterior aspect of the sciatic nerve in the popliteal fossa. If this reproduces the pain, sciatica is confirmed.

Slump Test (see Fig. 9-9)
- This is a variant of the SLR test and Lasègue test, designed to place tension across the sciatic nerve roots.
- The patient, initially sitting erect, is encouraged to slump forward and then fully forward flex the cervical spine.
- At the same time, the patient performs an SLR.
- The patient then dorsiflexes this same foot (duplicating the Lasègue sign). Repeat for each leg. Reproduction of the radicular pain during these maneuvers is very suggestive of sciatic nerve root tension.

Femoral Nerve Stretch Test (see Fig. 9-10)
- The femoral nerve stretch test is designed to compress the L2, L3, or L4 nerve roots. Compression of these upper lumbar roots is not common.
- The patient is positioned prone on the table with the knee flexed to at least 90 degrees. The examiner then passively extends the hip by lifting the thigh off the examination table. A positive test reproduces the

Figure 9-9. Slump test.

patient's radicular pain in the anterior thigh, rather than a mild feeling of tightness.

Rectal Examination (Sphincter Tone)

Five signs that suggest *nonorganic* pathology (Waddell signs)

1. Superficial or nonanatomic tenderness to palpation
   - Patient reports disproportionate pain to extremely light touch, or tenderness that does correlate with anatomic structures.
2. Simulation sign
   - Axial compression of the head or rotational simulation maneuver (similar to a standing logroll with no true rotation of the affected area) elicits "pain" despite no actual provocation.
3. Distraction sign
   - The same test (e.g., SLR supine versus sitting [Fig. 9–11]) performed on the "distracted" patient does not cause pain, unlike when performed on the patient initially and was "very painful."
4. Regional sensory or motor disturbance
   - A nonanatomic distribution of abnormal sensation (e.g., the entire leg) is reported rather than an anatomic, dermatomal distribution of pain or numbness.
5. Overreaction
   - Patient verbally or physically reacts in an inappropriate, theatrical manner to light touch or gentle examination.

Other Important Areas That Should Be Examined Simultaneously

- Hip(s) (internal and external rotation testing of the hip to rule out intra-articular arthritic involvement)—pain produced on internal or external rotation of the hip is more indicative of intra-articular hip pathology rather than back origin.
- SI joints (FABER maneuver and palpation of the SI joints to rule out sacroiliitis).
- Abdominal examination (e.g., rule out gallbladder, aortic aneurysm).
- Pulses of lower extremities (rule out vascular claudication).
- Sacrum (fracture, tumor).
- Coccyx (rule out coccydynia).
- Lymph nodes (rule out lymphadenopathy associated with sexually transmitted diseases [STDs], infection, tumor).
- Genitalia or meatus or vaginal discharge (STDs).

Figures 9–12 to 9–14 and Tables 9–4 and 9–5 illustrate lumbar disc levels, neurologic levels, and associated motor, sensory, and reflex findings.

We also employ the single-leg hyperextension test (**stork test,** Fig. 9–15) to evaluate for possible spondylolysis in children performing repetitive spine flexion and extension.

Figure 9–12. L4 neurologic level. (From Hoppenfield S: Physical Examination of the Spine and Extremities. Norwalk, Conn, Appleton-Century-Crofts, 1976. Reprinted by permission of Pearson Education, Inc., Upper Saddle River, N.J.)

Figure 9–11. Distraction sign.

L5
NEUROLOGIC LEVEL

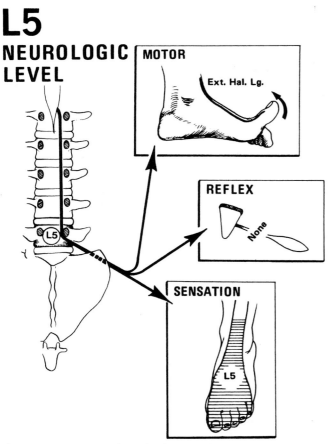

Figure 9–13. L5 neurologic level. Ext. Hal. Lg., extensor hallucis longus. (From Hoppenfield S: Physical Examination of the Spine and Extremities. Norwalk, Conn, Appleton-Century-Crofts, 1976. Reprinted by permission of Pearson Education, Inc., Upper Saddle River, N.J.)

S1
NEUROLOGIC LEVEL

Figure 9–14. S1 neurologic level. Peroneus l. + b., peroneus longus and brevis. (From Hoppenfield S: Physical Examination of the Spine and Extremities. Norwalk, Conn, Appleton-Century-Crofts, 1976. Reprinted by permission of Pearson Education, Inc., Upper Saddle River, N.J.)

Table 9–4

Motor Root Testing in Sciatica/Nerve Root Irritation

Nerve Root	Dermatome	Motor Testing	Comments
L4 (disc level L 3–4).	Inner calf to medial portion of foot (first two toes).	**Tibialis anterior,** tibialis posterior, quadriceps femoris, gluteus medius, gluteus minimus, tensor fascia latae.	Nerve root function best evaluated by testing the strength of the tibialis anterior muscle, which controls **dorsiflexion** and **inversion** of the foot.
L5 (disc level L 4–5).	Dorsum of foot (lateral side of lower leg).	Tibialis anterior, **extensor hallucis longus,** gluteus maximus, hamstring, extensor digitorum longus.	To evaluate L5, test the strength of the extensor hallucis longus (EHL) muscle; it is easier to assess resistance to great toe extension across the metatarsophalangeal joint; a somewhat less sensitive indicator of L5 nerve root function is the strength of the gluteus maximus and long and short toe extensor muscles. Heel-walking tests this nerve root.
S1 (disc level L 5–S1).	Sole, heel, and lateral edge of foot.	**Gastrocnemius,** gluteus maximus, hamstring, foot muscles, peroneus longus, peroneus brevis	The function of the S1 root is most easily evaluated by testing the strength of the gastrocsoleus and plantar flexion muscles. Toe-walking tests this nerve root.
S2.	Posterior medial lower and upper leg.	Flexor digitorum longus, hallucis longus, foot muscle.	Any deformity of the forefoot or toes raises the possibility of a neurologic problem involving S2.
S3.	Medial portion of buttocks.	Helps supply intrinsic muscles of foot.	—

Adapted from Borenstein DG, Wiesel SW, Boden SD: Low Back Pain: Medical Diagnosis and Comprehensive Management, 2nd ed. Philadelphia, WB Saunders, 1995.

Table 9-5

Clinical Features of Lumbar Disc Herniation

Findings	L3–4 Disc, L4 Nerve Root	L4–5 Disc, L5 Nerve Root	L5–S1 Disc, S1 Nerve Root
Pain	Low back, hip, posterolaeral thigh, across patella, anteromedial aspect of leg.	Sacroiliac region, hip, posterolateral thigh, anterolateral leg.	Sacroiliac region, hip, postero-lateral thigh/leg.
Numbness	Anteromedial thigh and knee.	Lateral leg, first webspace.	Back of calf, lateral heel, foot, toe.
Weakness	Knee extension.	Dorsiflexion of great toe (EHL).	Plantar flexion of foot and great toe.
Atrophy	Quadriceps.	Minimal anterior calf.	Gastrocnemius and soleus.
Reflexes	Knee jerk diminished.	None of diagnostic significance.	Ankle jerk diminished or absent.

From Boden SD, Weisel SW, Laws ER, et al: The Aging Spine: Essentials of Pathiophysiology, Diagnosis, and Treatment, 4th ed. Philadelphia, WB Saunders, 1997.

Figure 9–15. To assess localized spondylolysis pain, a single-leg-hyperextension "stork test" is performed. The patient stands on one leg and hyperextends the spine. Reproduction of the patient's pain complaint indicates a diagnosis of spondylolysis until proved otherwise. (From Congeni J: Evaluation spondylolysis in adolescent athletes. J Musculoskel Med 17:123–129, 2000.)

Imaging for Low Back Pain

Plain Films (Fig. 9–16)

The Agency for Health Care Policy and Research guidelines for plain films for LBP:

- Plain films are not recommended for routine evaluation of patients with acute LBP within the first month of symptoms **unless a red flag (see p. 559) is noted on clinical examination.**
- Plain films of the lumbar spine are recommended for ruling out fractures in patients with acute low back problems when any of the following **red flags** are present:
  - Recent significant trauma (all age groups).
  - Recent mild trauma (patients older than 50 yr).
  - History of prolonged steroid use.
  - History of osteoporosis.
  - Patients older than 70 yr.
- Plain x-rays in combination with a **CBC** and **ESR** are useful in ruling out tumor or infection in patients with low back problems when any of the following red flags are present:
  - Prior cancer history or recent infection.
  - Fever over 100°F.
  - IV drug abuse.
  - Prolonged steroid use.
  - LBP with rest.
  - Unexplained weight loss.
- In the presence of red flags (especially for tumor or infection), the use of bone scan, CT, or MRI is clinically indicated even if plain films are negative (Fig. 9–17). The authors recommend letting the back specialist order these imaging studies.
- The routine use of oblique views on the plain lumbar radiographs is not recommended **for adults.**
- A bone scan is recommended in nonpregnant patients to evaluate acute low back problems when spinal tumor, infection, or occult fracture is suspected from red flags on medical history, physical examination, corroborative laboratory tests, or plain x-ray findings. **Bone scans are contraindicated during pregnancy.**
- *Note:* We also recommend obtaining plain films of the lumbar spine in workman's compensation and/or litigation cases, on legal (physician protection) rather than medical grounds.

Text continued on p. 584

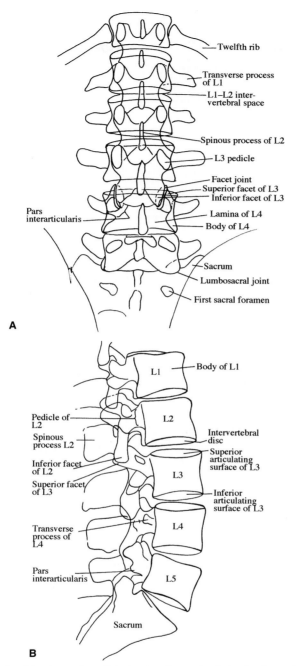

Figure 9–16. *A,* AP radiograph of lumbar spine. *B,* Lateral radiograph of the lumbar spine. (*A* and *B,* From Cole AJ, Herring SA: The Low Back Pain Handbook. Philadelphia, Hanley & Belfus/Mosby, 1997.)

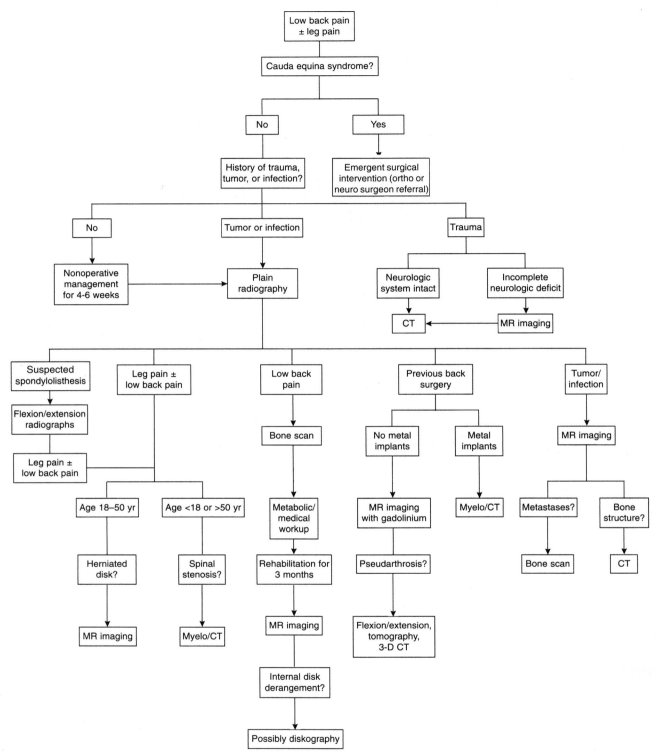

Figure 9–17. Algorithm for utilization of imaging modalities in the evaluation of patients with lumbar spine disorders. Myelo/CT, myelography and CT; 3-D CT, three-dimensional CT. (From Boden SD, Wiesel SW: Lumbar spine imaging: Role in clinical decision making. © 1996 American Academy of Orthopaedic Surgeons. Reprinted from the Journal of the American Academy of Orthopaedic Surgeons, Vol 4[5], p. 238–248, with permission.)

Overview of Management Guidelines for Acute Low Back Pain

Initial Consultation

Diagnostic Triage (Table 9–6 and Figs 9–18 to 9–24)

- Simple backache.
- Nerve root pain (sciatica, radiculopathy).
- Serious spinal pathology >> urgent referral.

Early Management Strategy

Aims:

- Symptomatic relief of pain.
- Prevent disability.

Treatment

- **Prescribe simple analgesia, NSAIDs if not contraindicated**
  - Avoid narcotics if possible and *never more than 2 wk.*
- **Arrange physical therapy if symptoms last more than a few days**
  - Active exercise and physical activity (modifies pain mechanisms, speeds recovery).
- **Advise bedrest *only* if essential: 1–3 days**
  - Prolonged bedrest is harmful.
- **Encourage early (not arduous) activity (e.g., avoid heavy lifting, stooping, bending)**
  - Inactivity is harmful.
  - Activity reduces pain.
  - Physical fitness is beneficial.
- **Practice psychosocial management; this is fundamental**
  - Promote positive attitudes to activity and work.
  - Address concomitant distress and depression.

- **Prescribe absence from work only if unavoidable: early return to work (clerical or light duty)**
  - Prolonged sickness absence makes returning patient to work increasingly difficult.

Biopsychosocial Assessment at 6 Weeks

- Review diagnostic triage.
- ESR, CBC, and x-ray lumbosacral spine if specifically indicated.
- Psychosocial and vocational assessment.

Active Rehabilitation Program

- Incremental aerobic exercise and fitness program of physical conditioning.
- Behavioral medicine principles.
- Work in close liaison with the workplace.

Secondary Referral

- Second opinion.
- Rehabilitation.
- Vocational assessment and guidance.
- Surgery.
- Pain management.

Final outcome measure: maintained productive activity; reduced work loss.

Table 9–6

Symptom Control Methods

RECOMMENDED

Nonprescription analgesics
Acetaminophen (safest)
NSAIDs (aspirin[1], Ibuprofen[1])

Prescribed pharmaceutical methods	Prescribed physical methods	
Nonspecific low back symptoms and/or sciatica	Nonspecific low back symptoms	Sciatica
Prescription NSAIDs[1]	Manipulation/therapy (in place of medication or a shorter trial if combined with NSAIDs)	

OPTIONS

Nonspecific low back symptoms and/or sciatica	Nonspecific low back symptoms	Sciatica
Muscle relaxants [2,3,4]	Physical agents and modalities[2] (heat or cold modalities for home programs only)	Manipulation/therapy (in place of medication or a shorter trial if combined with NSAIDs)
Opioids[3]	Shoe insoles[2]	Physical agents and modalities (heat or cold modalities for home programs only).
		Few days' rest[4]
		Shoe insoles[2]

[1]Aspirin and other NSAIDs are not recommended for use in combination with one another due to the risk of GI complications.
[2]Equivocal efficacy.
[3]Significant potential for producing drowsiness and debilitation; potential for dependency.
[4]Short course (few days only) for severe symptoms.
From Waddell G: The Back Pain Revolution. New York, Churchill Livingstone, 1998.

Modified from Waddell G: The Back Pain Revolution. New York, Churchill Livingstone, 1998.

continued

Overview of Management Guidelines for Acute Low Back Pain *(Continued)*

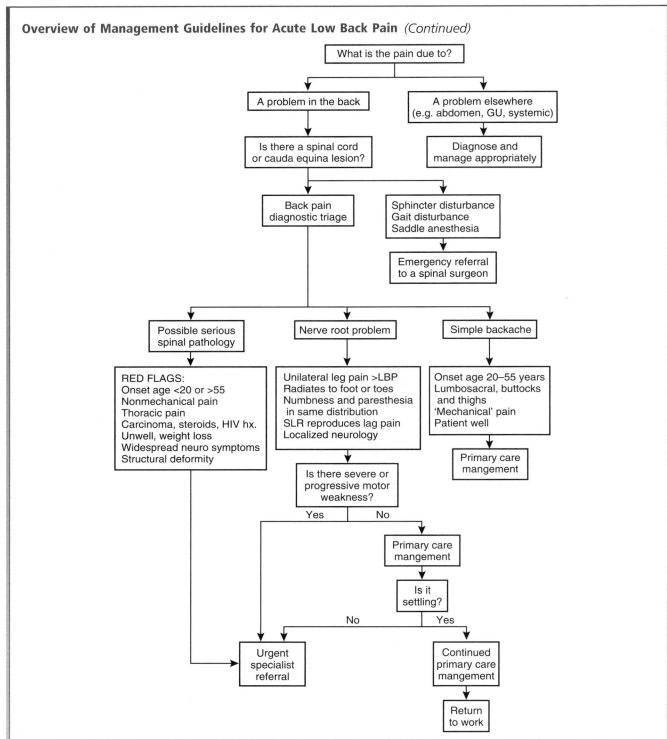

Figure 9–18. Diagnostic triage of back pain. GU, genitourinary; LBP, low back pain; SLR, straight-leg raises; SXS, symptoms. (From Waddell G: The Back Pain Revolution. New York, Churchill Livingstone, 1998.)

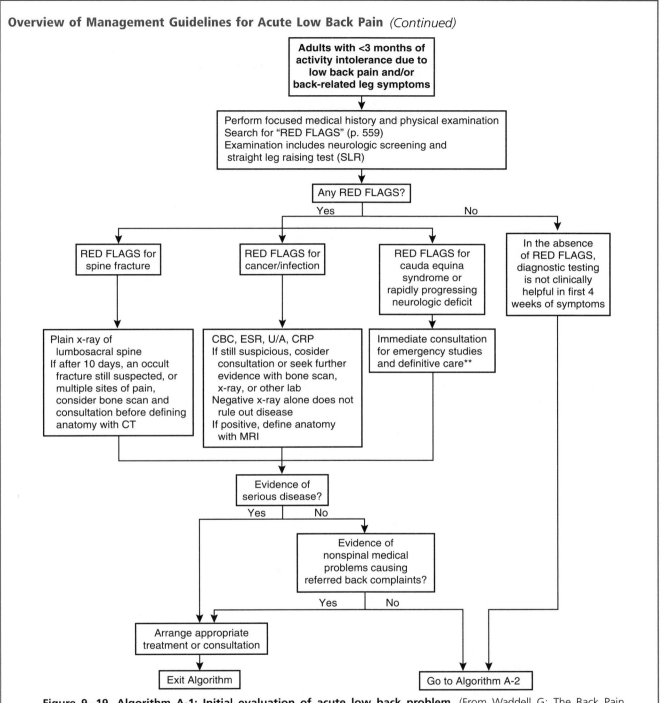

Figure 9–19. Algorithm A-1: Initial evaluation of acute low back problem. (From Waddell G: The Back Pain Revolution. New York, Churchill Livingstone, 1998.)

continued

Overview of Management Guidelines for Acute Low Back Pain *(Continued)*

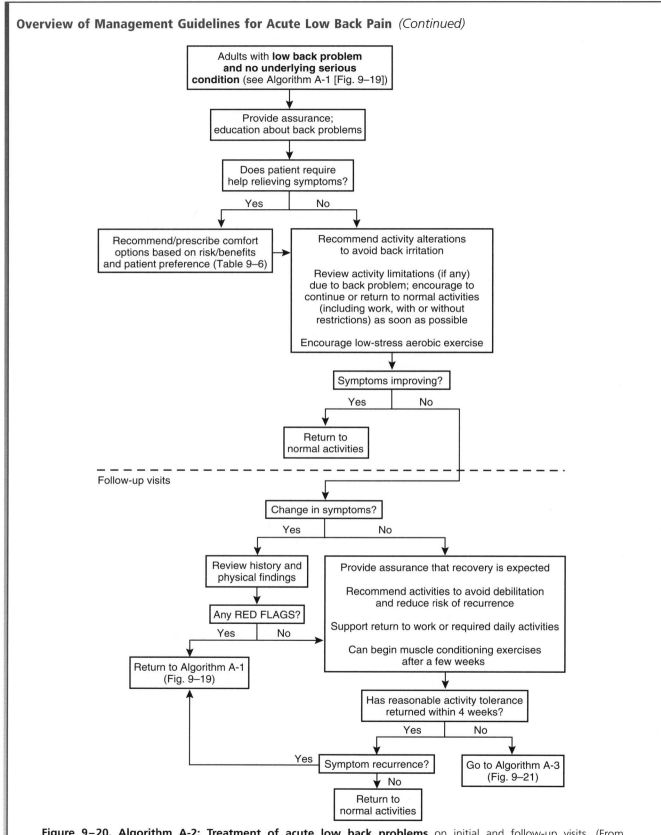

Figure 9–20. Algorithm A-2: Treatment of acute low back problems on initial and follow-up visits. (From Waddell G: The Back Pain Revolution. New York, Churchill Livingstone, 1998.)

Overview of Management Guidelines for Acute Low Back Pain *(Continued)*

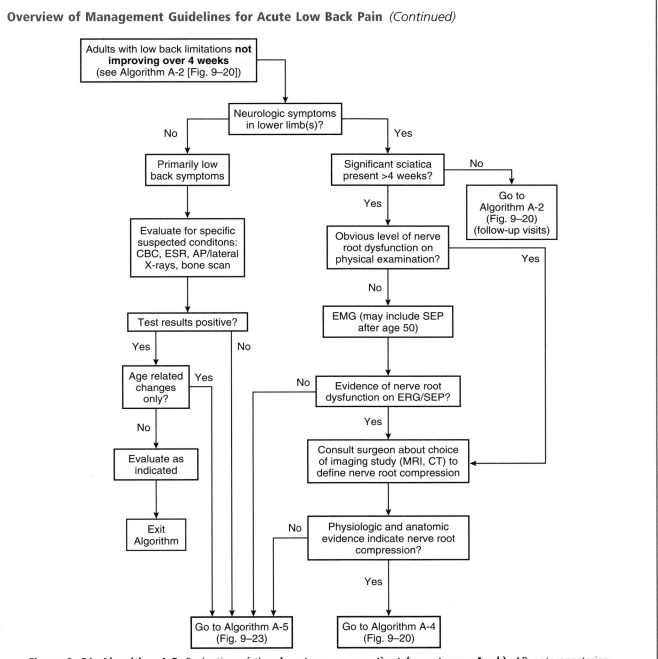

Figure 9–21. Algorithm A-3: Evaluation of the **slow-to-recover patient (symptoms >4 wk).** AP, anteroposterior; EMG, electromyography; SEP, sensory/evoked potentials. (From Waddell G: The Back Pain Revolution. New York, Churchill Livingstone, 1998.)

continued

Overview of Management Guidelines for Acute Low Back Pain *(Continued)*

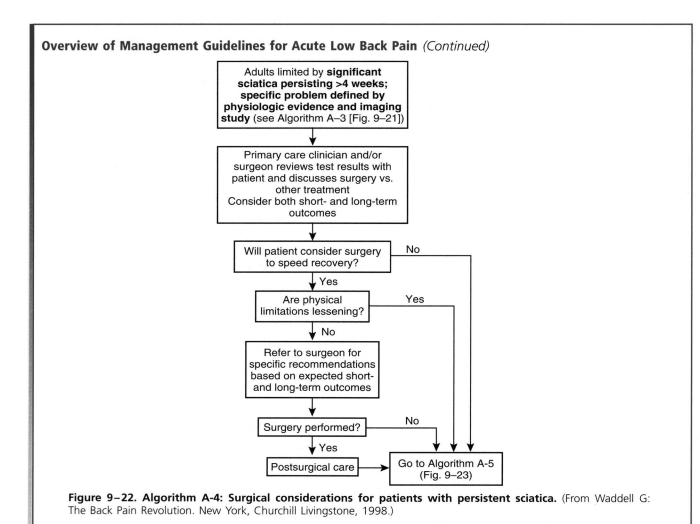

Figure 9–22. Algorithm A-4: Surgical considerations for patients with persistent sciatica. (From Waddell G: The Back Pain Revolution. New York, Churchill Livingstone, 1998.)

Overview of Management Guidelines for Acute Low Back Pain *(Continued)*

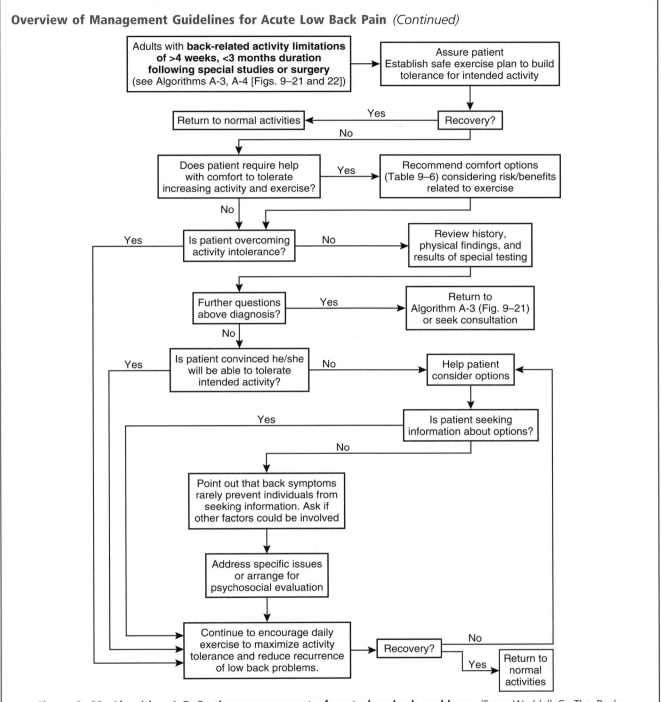

Figure 9–23. Algorithm A-5: Further management of acute low back problems. (From Waddell G: The Back Pain Revolution. New York, Churchill Livingstone, 1998.)

continued

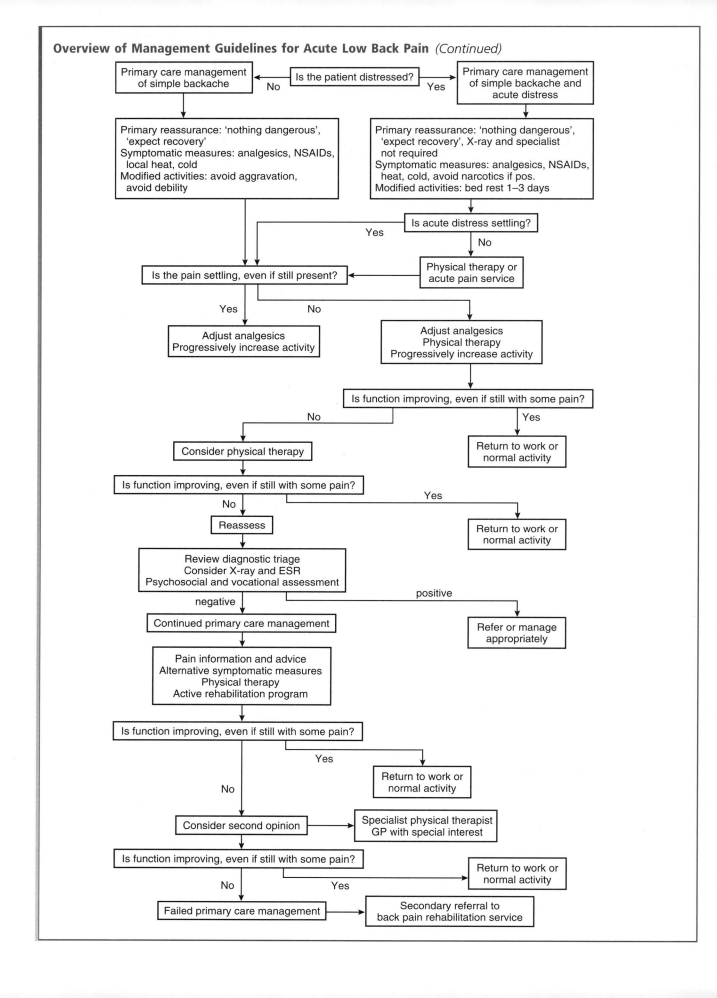

Overview of Management Guidelines for Acute Low Back Pain (*Continued*)

Summary of Management Options for Acute Low Back Pain Based on the Evidence Available in Current Literature

Waddell

At least moderate research **evidence for improvement** *in clinical outcomes.*

- Advise to stay active and continue usual activities.
- NSAIDs.
- Physical therapy in the first 4–6 wk only.

At least moderate research **evidence of no improvement** *in clinical outcomes.*

- Bedrest for more than 2 days.
- TENS.
- Traction.
- Specific back exercises.
- Education pamphlets about low back symptoms.

At least moderate research evidence of **potential harm** *from the following treatments which should* **not** *be used for an episode of acute LBP.*

- Use of narcotics or diazepam (especially for more than 2 wk).

- Bedrest with traction.
- Manipulation under general anesthesia.
- Plaster jacket.

Insufficient research evidence for any improvement in clinical outcomes.

- Conditioning exercises for the trunk muscles.
- Aerobic conditioning.
- Epidural steroid injections.
- Workplace back schools.
- Acupuncture.
- Shoe lifts.
- Corsets.
- Biofeedback.
- Physical modalities (includes ice, heat, shortwave diathermy, massage, ultrasound).

Bedrest Recommendations for the Treatment of Low Back Pain

Royal College of General Practice Guidelines

Conclusions

- For acute or recurrent LBP with or without referred leg pain, **bedrest for 2–7 days is worse than placebo or ordinary activity.** It is not as effective as the alternative treatments to which it has been compared for relief of pain, rate of recovery, return to daily activities, and days lost from work.
- Prolonged bedrest may lead to debilitation, chronic disability, and increasing difficulty in rehabilitation.
- Advice to continue ordinary activity can give equivalent or faster symptomatic recovery from the acute attack, and lead to less chronic disability and less time off work than "traditional" medical treatment with analgesics as required, advice to rest, and let pain be your guide for return to normal activity.
- Graded reactivation over a short period of days or a few weeks, combined with behavioral management of pain, makes little difference to the rate of initial recovery of pain and disability, but leads to less chronic disability and work loss.
- Advice to return to normal work within a planned short time may lead to shorter periods of work loss and less time off work.

Recommendations

- Do not recommend or use bedrest as a treatment for simple back pain.
- Some patients may be confined to bed for a few days as a consequence of their pain but this should not be considered a treatment.
- Advise patients to stay as active as possible and to continue normal daily activities.
- Advise patients to increase their physical activities progressively over a few days or weeks.
- If a patient is working, then advice to stay at work or return to work as soon as possible is probably beneficial.

From RCGP 1996 Clinical Guidelines for the Management of Acute Low Back Pain. London, Royal College of General Physicians, 1996.

Figure 9–24. Algorithm B-2: Primary care management of the simple backache. GP, general practitioner; NSAIDs, nonsteroidal anti-inflammatory drugs; (From Waddell G: The Back Pain Revolution. New York, Churchill Livingstone, 1998.)

Clinical Pearls for Low Back Pain

Disc Herniation

Over 95% of lumbar disc herniation occurs at the L4–5 level (L5 signs) or L5–S1 level (S1 signs). **Seventy-five percent of lumbar herniated discs spontaneously resolve within 6 months.** Leg pain and paresthesias are more symptomatic than the back pain. Only 5 to 10% of patients with persistent sciatica require surgery. Patients with a documented symptomatic herniated lumbar disc treated with surgery have a 10-times-higher risk of developing subsequent disc herniation compared with the general public.

Acute disc herniation is usually characterized by sudden onset of low back discomfort and radicular pain into the leg.

Facet Joint (Posterior Element) Pain

Fifteen to 40% of chronic LBP is due to facet joint pain. The facet joints of the spine are the interfaces where the posterior elements of one spinal segment contact the posterior elements of the next. Like other synovial joints, they can become inflamed. With **lumbar facet syndrome,** pain is typically aggravated by lumbar extension (which compresses the posteriorly located joint) and is relieved by lumbar flexion (which separates the joint surfaces). The diagnosis is clinical (no specific imaging or examination studies) and is one of exclusion. Pain often occurs acutely with extension and rotation of the lumbar spine. The pain usually presents as nonradiating lumbar spine pain (at times radiating to the buttock, rare to radiate below the knee). Approximately 80% of patients with facet syndrome have evidence of prior disc disease. Facet syndrome has no localizing neurologic symptoms associated with its presentation. Sudden attacks of LBP is more suggestive of facet joint involvement. Steadily increasing pain is more common with disc lesions.

A dramatic response to facet manipulation suggests facet syndrome clinically. **Contrast-enhanced facet injections that give relief during the anesthetic phase are diagnostic for facet syndrome.**

Spondylolysis, Spondylolisthesis, and Pars Interarticularis Injuries

Definitions

- **Pars interarticularis**—the area between the superior and the inferior articulating processes of the vertebra,

that is, the point at which the articulating process approaches the pedicle (Fig. 9–25A).
- **Spondylolysis**—the lytic line that crosses the pars interarticularis. Eventually, slippage of the vertebra may occur (spondylolisthesis) (see Fig. 9–25B and C).
- **Spondylolisthesis**—the **resultant forward slippage** of the involved vertebra on the vertebra directly below it (see Fig. 9–25D).

Spondylolysis occurs most commonly in young children who perform repetitive flexion and extension of the spine (e.g., gymnasts). SPECT scanning often confirms a stress fracture of the pars interarticularis (spodylolysis).

Spondylolysis

- Best defined as **a stress fracture of the pars interarticularis.**
- Hereditary predisposition.
- Often a history of repetitive flexion-extension of the spine (e.g., back-walkovers in gymnasts).
- Symptoms usually include low back and occasionally posterior buttock and thigh pain with no neurologic deficit.
- Single-photon emission computed tomography (SPECT) scan shows area of involvement.
- A single-leg hyperextension "stork test" (see Fig. 9–15) is performed to assess localized spondylolysis pain. The patient stands on one leg with the other foot resting on the weight-bearing knee. The patient then hyperextends the lower back. Reproduction of the patient's lower back pain indicates a diagnosis of spondylolysis until proven otherwise.

Spondylolisthesis

- **"Slip" of one vertebra on another.**
- Restricted range of motion of the low back. *This is a very important finding in evaluating children.*
- Sacral prominence with a palpable "step-off."
- Lumbar lordosis is lost (lumbosacral kyphosis).
- Tight hamstrings.
- 75% have low back pain.
- Often back spasms.
- "Heart-shaped" buttocks.
- Slip visualized on standing "spot" lateral.
- Goals of treatment are pain relief, arrest of slip progression, and minimizing deformity.
- Treatment alternatives include serial observation, lumbar stabilization exercises, stretching, spica cast, fusion in situ, laminectomy with fusion, and reduction with fusion.

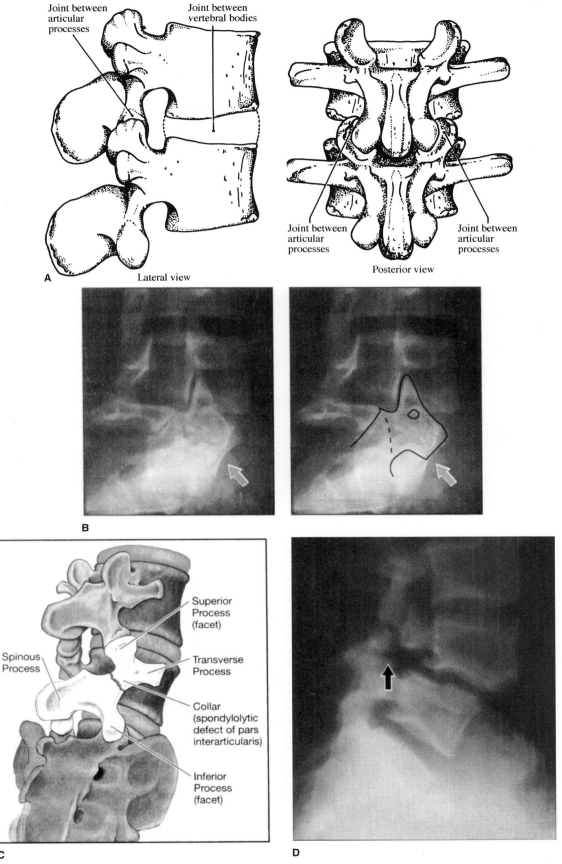

Figure 9–25. *A,* Lateral (*left*) and posterior (*right*) views. *B,* Spondylolysis of the pars interarticularis at L5 is shown on this oblique x-ray of a 17-year-old male's lumbar spine without (*left*) and with (*right*) the "Scottie dog" outlined. *C,* Spondylolytic defects of the pars interarticularis are evident on oblique x-rays as collars on a "Scottie dog." *D,* Spondylolisthesis (slip) at L4–5 (*arrow*) is shown in this lateral x-ray of the lumbar spine of a 30-year-old patient. (*A,* From Cole AJ, Herring SA: The Low Back Pain Handbook. Philadelphia, Hanley & Belfus/Mosby, 1997; *B–D,* from Micheli LS, Couzens GS: How I manage low back pain in athletes. Physician Sports Med 21[3]:182–194, 1993.)

Degenerative Lumbar Spinal Stenosis

Spinal stenosis classically presents with **neurogenic claudication**

- Pain exacerbated by standing or walking.
- Pain radiates into buttocks and lower extremities.
- Pain relieved by forward lumbar flexion.

The presentation is usually a slowly progressive increase in back and radicular symptoms that occur with **walking variable distance.** You must **rule out vascular claudication.**

- Patients with **vascular** claudication usually have a history of smoking, diabetes mellitus, or hyperlipidemia (Table 9–7) and diminished or absent pulses. In **Leriche syndrome,** the patient presents with buttock vascular claudication and impotence owing to aortoiliac occlusive disease.

Degenerative lumbar stenosis is a common cause of disabling back pain in patients over 50. The general **incidence** of degenerative lumbar spinal stenosis ranges from 1.8% to 8% (DeVilliers and Booysen 1976). Lumbar stenosis is caused by reduction of the space available for

Table 9–7

Differentiating Claudication—Vascular versus Neurogenic Characteristics

Vascular Claudication	Neurogenic Claudication
Distribution	
Calf or, less often, buttock	Buttock, thigh, calf or entire leg
Symptoms	
Cramping pain	Cramping pain, numbness, weakness
Triggers	
Exercise in any posture	Walking, running, prolonged standing
Alleviating factors	
Standing or sitting	**Bending forward, sitting, or lying down**
Distance	
Claudication distance fixed	Claudication distance variable
Activities	
Walk uphill has pain	No pain walking uphill
Pain with bicycle ride	No pain riding bicycle
Physical findings	
Pulse diminished or absent	Pulse usually normal
Loss of hair, shiny skin at distal extremities	No loss of hair or skin changes
Spinal movement limitation uncommon	Spinal movement limitation common

Modified from Herkowitz HN: Spinal Stenosis: Clinical Examination. In Eilert RE (ed): Instruct Course Lectures. Rosemont, Ill, AAOS, 1992.

nerve elements due to filling of the spinal canal with hypertrophic tissue. The process begins with degeneration of facet joints and intervertebral disks, resulting in narrowing of the neural foramina and spinal canal. Associated **spinal instability** (defined as more than 3 mm of motion between vertebrae on dynamic lateral radiographs) or a congenitally narrowed spinal canal may exacerbate the stenosis.

Arnoldi et al (1976) classified lumbar stenosis as congenital, acquired, or combined. The term **central stenosis** is used when compression of the dural sac is the main component. **Lateral stenosis** refers to compression of the nerve root in the lateral recess, in the neural foramen, or lateral to the neural foramen (Kirkaldy 1978).

Three types of spinal canals have been described: **round, ovoid, and trefoil.** Trefoil canals have the smallest cross-sectional area and are associated with the highest incidence of symptomatic lumbar stenosis (Bolender et al 1985).

The most common pathophysiology noted is that as the nerve roots of the lumbar spine traverse the lateral recesses, they are encroached on by hypertrophic facet joints, infolded ligamentum flavum, and a bulging annulus fibrosis. The degenerative stenosing process may also be accompanied by the development of segmental spinal instability. We recommend employing preoperative prone and supine lumbar radiographs to evaluate for possible segmental instability. Documented segmental instability on dynamic views is an indication for concomitant intertransverse bone grafting with the decompression.

Clinical Presentation of Spinal Stenosis

Most patients at initial presentation have a long-standing history of lumbar back pain with progression of lower-extremity pain (neurogenic claudication complex). Amundsen et al (1995) reported that the most common symptoms in lumbar spinal stenosis were back pain (95% prevalence) neurogenic claudication (91%), leg pain (71%), and weakness (31%). In 70% of their patients the back pain and leg pain were equally distributed.

There are usually few associated physical findings with spinal stenosis. Amundsen et al (1995) reported sensory changes in 51% of patients, reflex changes in 47%, lumbar tenderness in 40%, reduced spinal mobility in 36%, positive straight-leg raising in 24%, and weakness in 23%. **Post-exercise examination** (e.g., stair-climbing or walking) may reveal greater motor weakness than a static exam.

The key to correctly diagnosing degenerative lumbar spinal stenosis is to recognize the classic neurogenic claudication history. Patients with neurogenic claudication classically complain of pain, weakness, numbness, tingling, or cramping in 1 or both legs. These symptoms occur with walking or standing; **sitting or leaning forward alleviates at least some of the symptoms.** Cycling, which involves forward flexion, is also usually tolerated by patients with lumbar stenosis.

Differential Diagnosis

It is also essential, given the paucity of physical findings, to rule out other conditions that may present with low back and/or lower extremity symptoms.

Patients with **vascular claudication** will have diminished pulses, evidence of peripheral vascular disease, and **relief with rest rather than forward flexion. Other conditions** that should be considered include *peripheral neuropathy*, which presents as dysesthesias and paresthesias rather than activity and position-related changes, and *arthritis of the hip*, which often presents with buttocks pain but should exhibit hip irritability on internal rotation and abduction. Conditions such as *aortic aneurysm, knee arthritis, pelvic or sacral pathology, cervical myelopathy, amyotrophic lateral schlerosis, demyelinating disease, depression, or retroperitoneal tumors* should be ruled out.

Diagnostic Modalities

Plain lumbar spine films are employed to exclude tumor, fracture, infection, etc. In patients with signs and symptoms consistent with spinal stenosis, MRI or post myelographic CT scans are needed to confirm neural element compression. On myelogram, nerve root entrapment in the lateral recess or central canal stenosis is demonstrated by the level of cutoff of contrast material. Herno et al (1994) found that myelographic evidence of complete cutoff of contrast material (severe stenosis) correlated with a better surgical outcome. Riew et al (1998) concluded that **post-myelographic CT is superior to MRI** as a single study for the preoperative planning of decompression for lumbar spinal stenosis. Electrophysiologic studies are rarely useful in the evaluation of lumbar stenosis.

Natural history of Non-operative Treatment

Johnsson et al (1992) studied the progression of symptoms over a 4 year period in 32 patients with lumbar stenosis who refused or were not medically cleared for surgery. 70% of patients were unchanged at 4-year follow-up. Of the remaining 30%, half were better, half worse. The results of the prospective Maine Lumbar Spine Study part 3 (Atlas et al 1996) demonstrated superior outcomes at 1 year for operative treatment of symptomatic lumbar stenosis compared with non-operative treatment. The operative patients maintained their superior status at 3 years.

Non-operative Treatment of Lumbar Stenosis

We recommend use of the algorithm employed by Hilibrand and Rand (1999) (Fig. 9–26) for the non-operative treatment of degenerative lumbar spinal stenosis.

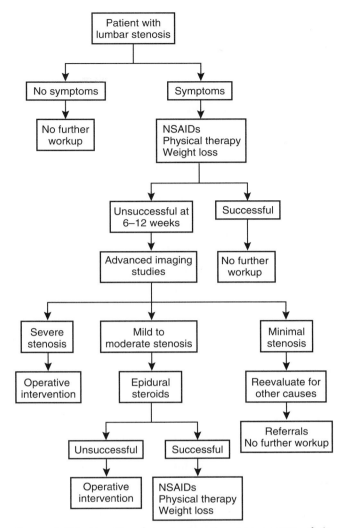

Figure 9–26. Algorithm for non-operative management of degenerative lumbar stenosis. (From Hilibrand AS, Rand N: Degenerative lumbar stenosis: diagnosis and management. J Am Acad Ortho Surg 7:239–248, 1999.)

NSAIDS are part of the initial management unless contraindicated. Physical therapy is employed using a modification of the standard low-back exercise program. Postural exercises **in flexion** are combined with pelvic stabilization and aerobic conditioning. Bicycle exercise is recommended because the slight forward flexion is typically well-tolerated by these patients. A back brace fashioned in slight forward flexion may also be useful, but long-term brace wear may eventually lead to truncal deconditioning.

Epidural steroid injection (ESI) is commonly used to treat patients with lumbar stenosis. Cuckler et al (1985) performed a prospective, randomized, double-blind study of epidural steroids in patients with lumbar radicular symptoms, half of whom had a diagnosis of lumbar spinal stenosis. In the spinal stenosis patients, there was no statistical difference in symptom improvement between the ESI and placebo injections at 24 hours and at 1 year. However, a similar study by Dilke et al (1973) demonstrated a statistically significant (p <0.05) improvement in short-term pain and functional measures.

Hilibrand and Rand (1999) reserve the use of epidural steroid injections for mild to moderate stenosis and major medical co-morbidities for whom physical therapy and other medical treatments have not helped.

Operative Treatment (Fig 9–27)

Success rates for surgical treatment of lumbar stenosis have ranged from 57% to 85% (Spengler 1987; Hilibrand 1999). A thorough work-up is recommended to identify any associated degenerative pathologic changes—such as spondylosisthesis, segmental instability, or scoliosis—that might require concomitant **stabilization** in addition to decompression.

Piriformis Syndrome (Pseudosciatica)

This syndrome results from compression or inflammation of the sciatic nerve as it courses under or through the piriformis muscle in the buttock. The patient presents with pseudosciatica—buttock and leg pain. They have tenderness on piriformis muscle palpation. Fifty percent of patients have LBP; 23% have dyspareunia. To distinguish piriformis syndrome from **lumbar radiculopathy,** perform a nerve tension test (positive in the latter). To distinguish piriformis syndrome from sacroiliitis, review pelvic radiographs. Sclerosis or irregularity of SI joints should be evident in sacroiliitis (Table 9–8).

Physical Therapy Approaches in Low Back Pain—Overview of Extension-Flexion Bias

In patients with LBP and concomitant radiating leg pain, McKenzie (1981) has described a clinical phenomenon known as "centralization." During McKenzie's procedure, a change in pain location from peripheral (or distal) to a more proximal (or central) location is desired during the mechanical assessment and manipulative evaluation.

Determination of the initial movement pattern to be used by the therapist is based on presumed pathology (e.g., discogenic versus posterior element pain), pain pattern, and successful *pain centralization.* Again, this underscores the importance of thorough evaluation that allows the physician to accurately categorize the malady being sent to the therapist for treatment as discogenic, posterior facet joint, or something else.

Extension Bias

As a very generalized guideline, the **extension bias** (see later) is most commonly used with discogenic pathology; symptoms decrease with repetitive extension on motion pattern testing and pain **centralizes** with extension.

- Extension exercises may **reduce intradiscal pressure,** allowing anterior migration of the nucleus pulposus away from the area of pathologic compression (Figs. 9–28 and 9–29).
- Extension exercises may actually **increase symptoms** in patients with large central disc herniation, foraminal stenosis, or foraminal herniation.

Figure 9–27. Algorithm for operative management of degenerative lumbar stenosis. (From Hilibrand AS, Rand N: Degenerative lumbar stenosis: diagnosis and management. J Am Acad Ortho Surg 7:239–248, 1999.)

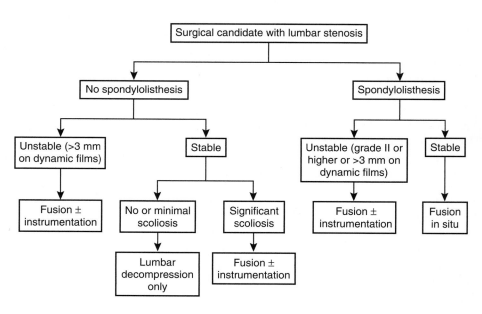

Table 9-8

Common Findings in Conditions of the Lumbar Spine—Summary

Herniated Lumbar Disc (Herniated Nucleus Pulposus)

Reproduction or exacerbation of sciatic symptoms with **nerve tension tests** (SLR, Lasègue test, slump test, bowstring sign).

Reproduction of sciatica with flexion of the lumbar spine.

Reproduction of sciatica with crossed SLR test (highly specific).

Sciatic notch tenderness.

Lumbar muscle spasm or list away from the involved nerve root (variable).

Neurologic deficit in the distribution of the involved nerve root (variable).

Exacerbation of pain by Valsalva (e.g., sneeze, cough, or defecation).

MRI correlates with side (R or L) and neurologic level noted on examination.

Spinal Stenosis

Neurogenic claudication—cramping leg and back pain or numbness increased with walking variable distance and relieved by forward bending, sitting, or lying. Usually bilateral legs and does not follow dermatomal pattern.

Loss of normal lumbar lordosis.

Hallmark is symptom severity change with position change.

Passive spine extension reproduces leg symptoms.

Usually a paucity of neurologic findings such as reflex changes, motor or sensory deficits.

Motor or sensory deficit variable (e.g., depression or loss of ankle jerks, muscle wasting of thighs, calves, and ankle dorsiflexors).

Nerve tension signs are usually absent.

Radiographic evidence of facet hypertrophy, disc narrowing, interlaminar space narrowing.

Lumbar Spondylolysis

Best described as stress fracture of the pars interarticularis.

Lumbar tenderness at the level of involvement (variable).

Decreased lumbar lordosis (variable).

Repetitive hyperextension injury.

SPECT scan and bone scan positive.

Pain aggravated by extension, relieved by flexion.

Hamstring tightness with SLR test and passive ROM testing.

Pain exacerbated by hyperextension of the lumbar spine (passive extension, active extension, **single-leg extension test**) (frequent).

May have signs of associated spondylolisthesis, if present.

Lumbar Fracture

History or trauma (may be minor trauma in osteoporotic patient).

Tenderness at the level of injury.

Localized swelling and hematoma or ecchymosis.

Possible lower motor neuron deficit owing to injury to the cauda equina or the nerve roots (variable).

Possible upper motor neuron deficit if the lesion is above the level of the cauda equina.

Mechanical Low Back Pain

Paraspinous muscle tenderness.

Paraspinous muscle spasm (variable).

Symptoms exacerbated by forward flexion relieved with rest.

List to one side (variable).

Normal neurologic examination, **pain confined locally to low back.**

Annular Tears

Back pain greater than leg pain.

Nerve tension signs present on examination but negative radiographic evidence of nerve impingement.

Discography is diagnostic.

Pain worsened by Valsalva maneuver, coughing, leaning, or sitting forward.

CT and myelogram negative for herniated disc.

Facet Joint Arthropathy

Pain on spine extension and ipsilateral side bending.

Localized unilateral point tenderness posteriorly over facet joint.

Pain well blocked by facet joint injection of lidocaine and/or steroid.

Infection

Elevated sed rate (ESR), WBC count may be normal.

May have positive blood culture or tuberculin test.

Radiographs may show vertebral end-plate erosion, decreased intervertebral disc height. May exhibit bony erosion or reactive bone formation.

Gallium citrate or Indium-labeled leukocyte imaging may be positive.

Malignancy

Increased sed rate (ESR), possible anemia.

Blastic or bony erosions on radiographs.

Prostate-specific antigen (PSA) or alkaline phosphatase level may be elevated.

CT scan localizes cortical lesions earlier than radiographs.

MRI for soft tissue tumor (spinal cord).

Bone scan useful for early demonstration of blastic lesions.

Cauda Equina Syndrome (Emergent)

Unable to void or stand.

Bilateral leg pain and severe back pain.

Saddle distribution anesthesia (numbness) about the anus and perineum.

Widespread or progressive profound motor or sensory loss in lower extremities.

Loss of anal sphincter tone, fecal incontinence.

Table 9-8 *(Continued)*

Common Findings in Conditions of the Lumbar Spine—Summary

Spondylolisthesis	**Discitis**
Hamstring tightness.	Usually ages 1 to 18.
Reversal of lumbar lordosis.	Abrupt onset of severe back pain.
Palpable step-off often.	Fever, malaise, and irritability.
Slip noted on lateral radiographs.	Elevated erythrocyte sedimentation rate (ESR) and C-reactive protein level.
Bilateral pars defects (usually at L5 on S1).	
Inflammatory Spine Disorders	**Sacroiliac Joint (SIJ) dysfunction**
Gradual onset before age 40.	SIJ tenderness to palpation, often a positive FABER test (see Fig. 9–3).
Marked morning stiffness.	Lumbosacral pain with radiation to buttocks, groin, or thigh.
Peripheral joint involvement.	Often schlerosis or irregularity of the SI joints on x-rays.
May have iritis (eye), rash, or urethral discharge (Reiter's).	Confirmation by fluoroscopic SIJ injection.

Modified from Reider B: The Orthopaedic Physical Examination. Philadelphia, WB Saunders, 1999.

- Cardiovascular fitness may then be initiated with an exercise that employs a neutral to extension bias in these patients to avoid aggravation of the patient's back pain during aerobic exercise (e.g., use of aquatic stabilization training or cross-country ski machine).

Flexion Bias

Flexion bias is most commonly used in patients with **posterior spine element (e.g., facet) pain.** In these patients, symptoms decrease with repetitive flexion on motion pattern testing and pain centralizes with flexion.

- Flexion exercises (see later) may act to reduce facet joint compression and provide stretch to lumbar musculature, ligaments, and myofascial structures.
- **Flexion** actually increases intradiscal pressure and **exacerbates discogenic symptoms.**
- Cardiovascular exercises in patients with posterior spine element pain may be initiated with stationary bicycling in slight lumbar flexion or aquatic stabilization exercises in slight lumbar flexion. These activities place the spine in a neutral to flexion bias.

Exercise Programs for Low Back Pain

Several exercise programs have been developed for acute LBP. These include those designed by McKenzie (mainly extension exercises) (1981), Williams (1937), Aston (1999), Heller (1991), and Feldenkrais (Lake 1985), and other lumbar stabilization programs, stretching regimens, and aerobic conditioning programs.

McKenzie Technique

The McKenzie technique is one of the most popular of the many conservative spine care programs. It is a method of diagnosis and treatment based on movement patterns of the spine (Fig. 9–30). For any spinal condition, certain movements aggravate the pain and other movements relieve the pain. Because the McKenzie method works best for acute back pain that responds to lumbar extension, mobilization, and exercises, the technique has been erroneously labeled an extension exercise program. McKenzie, in fact, advocates position and movement patterns, flexion or extension, that best relieve the patient's symptoms.

McKenzie's method is complex and much has been written explaining its theoretical basis. In *The Lumbar Spine: Mechanical Diagnosis and Therapy* (1981), McKenzie classifies LBP based on spinal movement patterns, positions, and pain responses, and describes a *postural syndrome, derangement, and dysfunction.* Each classification has a specific treatment that includes education and some form of postural correction. A basic explanation of the method is as follows.

Some stages of the lumbar degenerative cascade create symptoms because of pathoanatomic abnormalities, which can be positively altered by spinal positioning. This hypothesis has led to several forms of spinal manipulation, including chiropractic and osteopathy.

The McKenzie technique is a more passive form of spinal manipulation in which the patient produces the motion, position, and forces that improve the condition. Examples of pathoanatomic alterations include a tear in the annulus and acute facet arthritis. Repeated lumbar extension may reduce edema and nuclear migration in an annular tear or may realign a facet joint in such a way as to reduce inflammation and painful stimuli. Through trial and error, the position and exercise program that best relieve the patient's symptoms can be found (see Fig. 9–30).

Cyclic range of motion exercises (usually in passive extension) are the cornerstone of the McKenzie program. These repetitive exercises "centralize" pain, and certain postures prevent end-range stress. Lumbar flexion exercises may be added later, when the patient has full spinal range of motion.

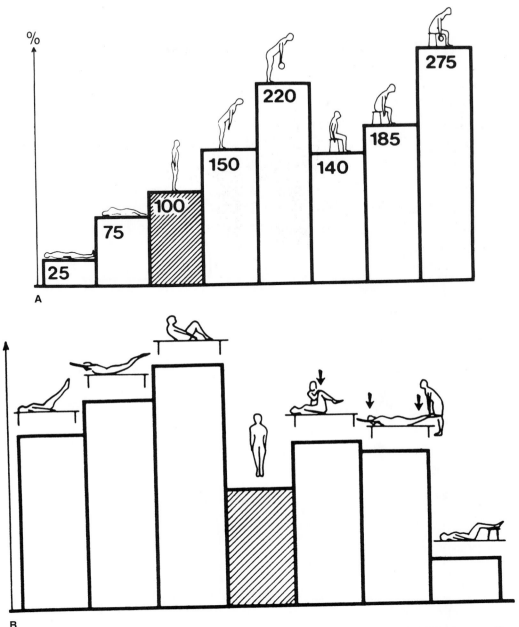

Figure 9-28. *A,* Relative change in the pressure (or load) in the third lumbar disc in various positions in living subjects. *B,* Relative change in the pressure (or load) in the third lumbar disc during various muscle strengthening exercises in living subjects. (*A* and *B,* From Nachemson AL: The lumbar spine, an orthopaedic challenge. Spine 1:59–71, 1976.)

Sagittal view

Axial view

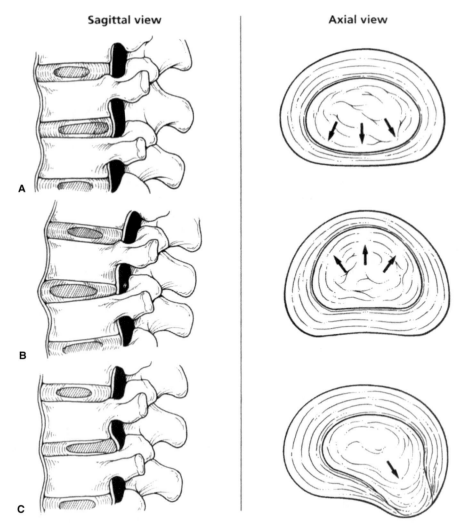

Figure 9–29. Forces applied during asymmetrical compression loading of the disc cause migration of the nucleus pulposus away from the load. They also create a vertical tension on the annulus, opposite the load. *A*, During anterior compression associated with our flexed lifestyles, these stresses are focused on the posterior annulus, frequently causing pain. *B*, In patients with a directional preference for extension, the posterior compression that occurs with extension loading may reverse the direction of these stresses, alleviating those lifestyle-related stresses on this posterior nucleo-annular complex. Pain then centralizes or abolishes. *C*, If the anterior asymmetrical loading forces create a sufficient pressure gradient across the disc to displace nuclear content significantly against the opposite annulus, a herniation could develop, as shown in this example of posterolateral herniation. (*A–C*, From Donelson RG: Mechanical assessment of low back pain. J Musculoskel Med 15[5]: 28–39, 1998. Artist: C. Boyter.)

Treatment is based on evaluation of pain location and maneuvers that change the pain location from referred to centralized (Fig. 9–31). Once identified, the direction of exercise and movement (such as extension) is used for treatment. **Centralization,** as McKenzie use the term, refers to a rapid change in perceived location of pain from a distal or peripheral location to a proximal or central one. Donelson and colleagues (1990) reported centralization of asymmetrical or radiating pain in 87% of patients during the first 48 hours of care.

For a movement to eventually centralize pain, it must be performed **repetitively,** because the initial movement often aggravates or intensifies the pain. Centralization also occurs more rapidly if the initial movements are performed passively to end-range. Centralization most frequently occurs as a result of extension movement, occasionally from lateral movements, and only rarely with flexion.

McKenzie reported that 98% of patients with symptoms for less than 4 weeks who experienced centralization

Figure 9–30. During a McKenzie assessment, the patient is tested sequentially with self-performed, repeated end-range movements. Tests are done with the patient standing (if symptoms allow) and recumbent, first in flexion, then in extension (*A–D*). When end-range flexion and extension testing reveals no centralizing direction, testing progresses to include bilateral side-gliding (*E* and *F*; also performed with the patient standing and recumbent) and supine flexion-rotation (*G*). In an end-range side-glide test, the examiner may hold the patient's shoulders still while the patient moves the pelvis to the side (*E*). In side-gliding (*F*) and flexion-rotation (*G*), the examiner may also apply end-range overpressure for testing.

Once the proper end-range direction of beneficial movement is identified, the clinician can then apply a passive assist to the test movement, frequently including an end-range mobilization. Progress and clinical recovery occasionally require an end-range manipulation in that specific direction. This is needed only to initiate or facilitate the centralizing/abolishing process.

To ensure a safe examination and to maximize the information obtained, the number of repetitions performed during the assessment is dictated by the symptom response. The assessment continues in a follow-up the next day that provides additional opportunity to assess the accuracy, reliability, and consistency of the initial assessment findings.

If a directional preference is identified, the beneficial end-range test movements become the patient's therapeutic home exercise program. At the same time, the patient temporarily avoids positions, activities, and exercises performed in a direction that exacerbates symptoms. (*A–G*, From Donelson RG: Mechanical assessment of low back pain. J Musculoskel Med 15[5]:28–39, 1998. Artist: C. Boyter.)

Figure 9–31. Centralization is a rapid change of pain with maneuvers that result in peripheral or distal pain becoming more centralized (desirable). The converse (peripheralization of the pain) is not sought or desired. (From Donelson RG: Mechanical assessment of low back pain. J Musculoskel Med 15[5]:28–39, 1998. Artist: C. Boyter.)

during their initial assessment had excellent or good results; 77% of patients with subacute symptoms (4 to 12 weeks) had excellent or good results if their pain centralized initially. The critical clinician should always bear in mind the self-limited course typical for patients with low back pain (e.g., a 90% resolution rate at 6 weeks).

The **advantage** of this program is that it gives patients an understanding of their condition and responsibility for maintaining proper alignment and function. **Disadvantages** are that the program requires active, willing participation of the patient, who must have the ability to centralize the pain; better results are obtained for patients with acute pain than for those with chronic pain, and the very complex regimen requires a therapist trained in McKenzie's techniques to obtain the best results.

Each movement is taken to its end-range repetitively as long as distal pain continues to diminish. McKenzie stresses the importance of taking the movements to the end-range permitted by the patient to accurately observe changes in the pain pattern. If distal symptoms worsen, that specific movement is discontinued. Pain locations from these maneuvers are carefully observed and recorded.

Based on the clinical response to centralization, the patient is taught to perform home spinal exercises in that direction of movement (usually extension). For example, for a patient with acute pain, the **self-care exercise program** may include prone extension for a few seconds at a time, with sets of 10 repetitions performed every hour or two. The patient is also taught modified resting positions (for sitting, standing, and lying) and work postures that will maintain centralization and avoid peripheralization.

Most patients have centralization of pain in the first 2 days or sooner. Again, treatment outcomes in "centralizers" are typically good.

McKenzie classified lumbar movements that have the potential to centralize symptoms into extension, flexion, lateral bending, rotation, and side-gliding (combination of lateral bending and rotation). These may be used individually or in combination to diminish the peripheral pain. Gravity-elimination (prone) versus gravity-assisted (standing) symptom reduction further increases the number of lumbar movement combinations that the therapist must understand and possibly use in an effort to centralize symptoms. The result is that more than 40 different exercise regimens are available, and application of the appropriate regimen may require complex customization.

Williams Flexion Exercises (Fig. 9–37)

The goals of this isometric flexion regimen, developed in the 1930s, are to (1) widen the intervertebral foramina and facet joint to reduce nerve compression, (2)

Rehabilitation Protocol
Acute Low Back Pain
McKenzie

McKenzie recommends implementation of this protocol by a therapist with specialized training in the McKenzie method to ensure proper recognition and correct implementation of treatment in response to the patient's clinical relief derived from specific maneuvers. To determine which exercises produce centralization, the physical therapist tests the patient with a *standardized series of lumbar movements, such as flexion, extension (Fig. 9–32), lateral bending, rotation, and side-gliding* (a combination of lateral bending and rotation). Once the therapist identifies the movement (usually extension or lateral bending) that decreases peripheral symptoms, the patient is taught to perform an individualized exercise program in that direction of movement. The movement is performed repetitively to the passive end-range. Maneuvers that "peripheralize" or exacerbate symptoms are discontinued.

Repeat End-Range Movements While Standing

- Back-bending (extension) (Fig. 9–33):
  The patient stands upright with feet slightly apart (A). Place the hands on the small of the back with fingers pointing backward. Bend backward (from the waist) as

Figure 9–33. Extension in a standing posture.

Figure 9–32. Passive extension using a table.

far as possible, using the hands as a fulcrum (B). Keep the knees straight. Hold this position for 1–2 sec, then return to the starting position. This exercise incorporates the effect of gravity because it is performed in an upright position.
- Side-gliding (Fig. 9–34).
- Forward-bending (lumbar flexion).

Recumbent End-Range Movements

- Passive extension while prone (Fig. 9–35):
  In this exercise, the patient lies face down, with hands positioned under the shoulder (A), then pushes up by slowly extending the elbows (B) while keeping the

Rehabilitation Protocol
Acute Low Back Pain *(Continued)*
McKenzie

Figure 9–34. Side-gliding.

pelvis, hips, and legs relaxed (this allows the back to sag). Maintain this position for 1–2 sec, then slowly lower the upper body to the floor. This exercise eliminates the loading effects of gravity because it is performed prone.

- Knees-to-chest while supine (Fig. 9–36):
  The patient lies supine, with knees flexed and feet flat on the floor or bed (A). Place the hands around the knees (B) and slowly pull both knees up toward the chest as far as possible (C). This position is maintained for 1–2 sec, then slowly lower the feet back to the starting position. The patient must not raise the head while performing this exercise or straighten the legs while lowering them.

- Prone lateral shifting of hips off midline (patients with unilateral symptoms):
  The patient lies face down, arms at side (A), moves hips away from the side of pain, and maintains this position for a few seconds (B). With the hips off center, place the elbows under the shoulders and lean on the forearms (C and D); relax in this position for 3 or 4 min. The patient can then perform the maneuver "extension while lying prone," keeping the hips off center.

- Flexion while sitting:
  The patient sits on the edge of a steady chair or stool, with legs apart and hands resting on knees (A). Bend forward from the waist to touch the floor with the hands. Hold this position for 1–2 sec and then slowly return to upright. Once able to bend forward comfortably, the patient can hold onto the ankles and pull farther down (B).

A

Figure 9–35. *A* and *B,* Passive extension while prone.

continued

Rehabilitation Protocol
Acute Low Back Pain *(Continued)*
McKenzie

B

Figure 9–35. *Continued*

A

B

C

Figure 9–36. A–C, Knees to chest while supine.

Figure 9–37. Williams' postural exercises.

stretch hip flexors and back extensors, (3) strengthen abdominal and gluteal muscles, and (4) reduce "posterior fixation" of the lumbosacral junction. *A concern with this method is that certain flexion maneuvers increase intradiscal pressure, possibly aggravating herniated or bulging discs. According to Nachemson (1981), Williams' first exercise increases intradiscal pressure to 210% over that in a standing posture (see Fig. 9–35). Three of the six exercises increase intradiscal pressure, and these three are contraindicated for patients with acute herniated disc.*

Lumbar Stabilization Programs

There is no evidence that early return to activity increases the likelihood of back pain recurrences. On the contrary, physically fit individuals have fewer and shorter attacks of LBP and are more tolerant of pain. With a better understanding of spinal biomechanics, specific activities, and positions that increase loads on the spine, reinjury can be avoided. Numerous studies have shown that patients with LBP can perform selected activities almost normally without increasing pain. Body mechanics that avoid painful positions are called cautious or preventive body mechanics. Body mechanics that attempt to overcome the condition with muscular effort and knowledge of body positions have led to the field of stabilization training.

Back schools, which gained prominence in the 1970s, gave education and training in cautious or preventive body mechanics for routine daily activities, but they did not provide techniques for heavy laborers or for high-performance athletes, who require dynamic, ballistic body mechanics for high-level activities. Practitioners with backgrounds in martial arts or sports training and some therapists with European influences in training developed stabilization training primarily for these patients.

The basic premise of stabilization training is that an individual with back pain (considered an unstable condition) can be taught to stabilize the painful pathologic condition through muscular development and movement patterns that allow painless return to a higher-than-normal level of functional activities. Stabilization training incorporates almost all aspects of conservative treatment: education, body mechanics, manual therapy, the McKenzie technique, Williams' exercises, yoga, martial arts, work hardening, and functional restoration. The techniques of stabilization training have been extensively demonstrated in many texts and videotapes, and the techniques are used by many therapists who treat high performance athletes with back problems.

The main goal of the lumbar stabilization program is to build musculature that stabilizes the torso, with cocontraction of abdominal muscles to provide a corseting effect on the lumbar spine. This concept is centered on the assumption that an injured lumbar motion segment may create a weak link in the kinetic chain, with subsequent predisposition to reinjury. This program is used in conjunction with other methods aimed at controlling acute pain (such as NSAIDs). Emphasis is on positioning the spine in a nonpainful orientation, termed the *neutral spine.* Stretching and range of motion exercises are then completed daily in this configuration. Supervision by an appropriately oriented trainer is advised.

The *second phase* of treatment consists of active joint mobilization methods, including extension exercises in prone and standing positions, and alternating midrange flexion extension in a four-point stance. Simple curl-ups for abdominal muscle strengthening is progressed to dynamic abdominal raising. This includes "dead bug" exercises, using alternate arm and leg movements while supine. Diagonal curl-ups and incline board work are performed.

Progression to aerobic exercise, exercise with a ball, and weight training may be added (see box later). The program endpoint is determined by *maximal functional improvement*, the point beyond which no further improvement in function will result from additional exercise.

Exercise Training in the Lumbar Stabilization Program

Soft Tissue Flexibility

- Hamstring musculotendinous unit.
- Quadriceps musculotendinous unit.
- Iliopsoas musculotendinous unit.
- Gastrocnemius-soleus musculotendinous unit.
- External and internal hip rotators.

Joint Mobility

- Lumbar spine segmental mobility
  - Extension.
  - Flexion (unloaded).
- Hip range of motion.
- Thoracic segmental mobility.

Stabilization Program

- Finding neutral position
  - Standing.
  - Sitting.
  - Jumping.
  - Prone.
- Prone gluteal squeezes
  - With arm raises.
  - With alternate arm raises.
  - With leg raises.
  - With alternate leg raises.
  - With arm and leg raises.
  - With alternate arm and leg raises.
- Supine pelvic bracing.
- Bridging progression
  - Basic position.
  - One leg raised with ankle weights.
  - Stepping.
  - Balance on gym ball.
- Quadruped
  - With alternating arm and leg movements.
- Kneeling stabilization
  - Double knee.
  - Single knee.
  - Lunges, with and without weight.
- Wall-slide quadriceps strengthening.
- Position transition with postural control
  - Abdominal program
    - Curl-ups.
    - Dead bug, supported and unsupported.
    - Diagonal curl-ups.
    - Diagonal curl-ups on incline board.
    - Straight-leg lowering.
  - Gym program
    - Latissimus pull-downs.
    - Angled-leg press.
    - Lunges.
    - Hyperextension bench.
    - General upper body weight exercises.
  - Aerobic program
    - Progressive walking.
    - Swimming.
    - Stationary bicycling.
    - Cross-country ski machine.
    - Running—initially supervised on a treadmill.

From Frymoyer JW: The Adult Spine: Principles and Practice, New York. Raven, 1991.

Bibliography

Amundsen T, Weber H, Lilleas F, Nordal HJ, Abdelnoor M, Magnaes B: Lumbar spinal stenosis: clinical and radiologic features. Spine 20:1178–1186, 1995.

Armstrong J: Lumbar Disk Lesions, 1st ed. London, E & R Livingstone, 1958.

Arnoldi CC, Brodsky AE, Cauchoix J, et al: Lumbar spinal stenosis and nerve root entrapment syndromes: definition and classification. Clin Orthop 115:4–5, 1976.

Aston J: Aston Postural Assessment Workbook: Skills for Observing and Evaluation Body Patterns. Sacramento, Calif, Psychological Corp., March 1999.

Atlas SJ, Deyo RA, Keller RD, et al: The Maine Lumbar Spine Study, Part III: 1 year outcomes of surgical and non-surgical management of lumbar spinal stenosis. Spine 21:1787–1795, 1996.

Basmajian JV: Acute back pain and spasm: a controlled multicenter trial of combined analgesic and antispasm agents. Spine 14:438, 1989.

Boden SD, Wiesel SW: Lumbar spine imaging: role in clinical decision making. J Am Acad Orthop Surg 4(5):238, 1996.

Bogduk N, Twomey LT: Clinical Anatomy of the Lumbar Spine, 2nd ed. Melbourne, Australia, Churchill Livingstone, 1991.

Bolender NF, Schonstrom NS, Spengler DM: Role of computed tomography and myelography in the diagnosis of central spinal stenosis. J Bone Joint Surg Am 67:240–246, 1985.

Borenstein DG, Wiesel SW, Boden SD: Low Back Pain: Medical Diagnosis and Comprehensive Management, 2nd ed. Philadelphia, WB Saunders, 1995.

Brown MD, Seltzer DG: Perioperative care in lumbar spine surgery. Orthop Clin North Am 22:353, 1991.

Cats-Baril WL, Frymoyer JW: Identifying patients at risk of becoming disabled because of low-back pain: the Vermont Rehabilitation Engineering predictive model. Spine 16(6):605–607, 1991.

Cherkin D, Deyo R, Berg A: Evaluation of a physician education intervention to improve primary care for low-back pain. II. Impact on patients. Spine 16:2273, 1991.

Cole AJ, Herring SA: The Low Back Pain Handbook: A Practical Guide for the Primary Care Clinician. St. Louis, Hanley & Belfus/Mosby, 1997.

Cuckler JM, Bernini PA, Wiesel SW, Booth RE Jr, Rothman RH, Pickens GT: The use of epidural steroids in the treatment of lumbar radicular pain: a prospective, randomized, double-blind study. J Bone Joint Surg Am 67:63–66, 1985.

DeVilliers PD, Booysen EL: Fibrous spinal stenosis: a report on 850 myelograms with a water-soluble contrast medium. Clin Orthop 115:140–144, 1976.

Deyo RA: Nonoperative treatment of low back disorders. In Frymoyer JW (ed): The Adult Spine: Principles and Practice. New York, Raven, 1991.

Deyo RA, Diehl AK: Psychosocial predictors of disability in patients with low back pain. J Rheumatol 15:1557, 1988.

Deyo RA, Diehl AK, Rosenthal M: How many days of bedrest for acute low back pain? N Engl J Med 315:1064, 1986.

Dilke TFW, Burry HC, Grahame R: Extradural corticosteroid injection in the management of lumbar nerve root compression. BMJ 2:635–637, 1973.

Dimaggio A, Mooney V: The McKenzie program: exercise effective against back pain. J Musculoskel Med Dec; 4(12):63, 1987a.

Dimaggio A, Mooney V: Conservative care for low back pain: what works? J Musculoskel Med Sep; 63(9):27, 1987b.

Dolan P: Commonly adopted postures and their effects on the lumbar spine. Spine 13:197, 1988.

Donelson R, Silva G, Murphy K: The centralization phenomenon: its usefulness in evaluating and treating referred pain. Spine 15:211, 1990.

Forrsell M: The back school. Spine 6:104, 1981.

Frymoyer JW: Predicting disability from low back pain. Clin Orthop 279:102, 1992.

Frymoyer JW, Nachemson A: Natural history of low back disorders. In Frymoyer JW (ed): The Adult Spine: Principles and Practice, New York, Raven, 1991.

Gilbert JR, Taylor DW, Hildebrand A: Clinical trial of common treatments for low back pain in family practice. BMJ 291:791, 1985.

Gopal A: Evaluation and management of acute low back pain. J Musculoskel Med 19:278–283, 2002.

Greenough H, Fraser R: The effects of compensation on recovery from low back surgery. Spine 14:947, 1989.

Hart D, Stobbe T, Jaraiedi M: Effect of lumbar posture on lifting. Spine 12:138, 1987.

Heller JL: Bodywise. Berkeley, Calif, Wingbow Press, May 1991.

Herno A, Airaksinen O, Saari T, Meittinen H: The predictive value of preoperative myelography in lumbar spinal stenosis. Spine 19:1335–1338, 1994.

Hilibrand AS, Rand N: Degenerative lumbar stenosis: diagnosis and management. J Am Acad Ortho Surg 7:239–248, 1999.

Hoppenfield S: Orthopaedic Neurology. Philadelphia, JB Lippincott, 1988.

Hoppenfield S: Physical Examination of the Spine and Extremities. Norwalk, Conn, Appleton-Century-Crofts, 1976.

Jensen MC, Brant-Zawadski MN, Obucowski N, et al: Magnetic resonance imaging of the lumbar spine in people without back pain. N Engl J Med. Jul 14; 331(2):69–73, 1994.

Johnsson KE, Rosen I, Uden A: The natural course of lumbar spinal stenosis. Clin Orthop 279:82–86, 1992.

Kellett K, Kellett D, Nordholm L: Effects of an exercise program on sick leave due to back pain. Phys Ther 71:283, 1991.

Kelsey JL, Githens PB, White AA 3rd: An epidemiologic study of lifting and twisting on the job and risk for acute prolapsed lumbar intervertebral disk. J Orthop Res 2:61, 1984.

Kirkaldy-Willis WH, Wedge JH, Yong-Hing K, Reilly J: Pathology and pathogenesis of lumbar spondylosis and stenosis. Spine 3:319–328, 1978.

Kjalil T, Alexander AH, Turocy RH: Stretching in the rehabilitation of low-back pain patients. Spine 17:311, 1992.

Kopp JR, Alexander AH, Turocy RH: The use of lumbar extension in patients with acute herniated nucleus pulposus. Clin Orthop 202:211, 1986.

Lake B: Acute back pain: treatment by application of Feldenkrais principles. Aust Family Physician Nov; 14(11):1175–8, 1985.

Liang M, Komaroff M: Roentgenograms in primary care patients with acute low back pain: a cost effectiveness analysis. Arch Intern Med 142:1108, 1982.

Lindstrom I, Ohlund C, Eek C: Mobility, strength, and fitness after a graded activity program for patients with subacute low back pain: a randomized prospective clinical study with a behavioral therapy approach. Spine 17:641, 1992.

Maigne JY, Rime B, Deligne B: Computed tomographic follow-up study of forty-eight cases of nonoperatively treated lumbar intervertebral disk herniation. Spine 17:1071, 1992.

McKenzie RA: The Lumbar Spine: Mechanical Diagnosis and Therapy. Waikanae, New Zealand, Spinal, 1981.

Micheli LJ, Couzens GS: How I manage low back pain in athletes. Phys Sports Med 21:43, 1993.

Nachemson AL: Newest knowledge of low back pain. Clin Orthop 279:8, 1992.

Nachemson AL: Advances in low back pain. Clin Orthop 200:266, 1985.

Nachemson AL: Disc pressure measurements. Spine 6:93, 1981.

Patel AT, Ogle AA: Diagnosis and management of acute low back pain. Am Fam Physician 61(6):1779–86, 1789–90. Review.

Polatin P: The functional restoration approach to chronic low back pain. J Musculoskel Med 7(17):53, 1990.

Reider B: The Orthopaedic Physical Examination. Philadelphia, WB Saunders, 1999.

Riew KD, Hilibrand AS, Bridwell KH, et al: MR- versus CT-myelography: surgical decision-making for lumbar stenosis. In: Proceedings of the 13th Annual Meeting of the North American Spine Society. Rosemont, Ill, North American Spine Society, 1998, pp 117–118.

Robison R: The new back school prescription: stabilization training, part I. Spine State Art Rev 5:341, 1991.

Saal J: The new back school prescription: stabilization training, part II. Spine State Art Rev 5:357, 1991.

Shah J, Hampson W, Jayson M: The distribution of surface strain in the cadaveric lumbar spine. J Bone Joint Surg 60B:246, 1978.

Spengler DM, Bigos SJ, Martin NA: Back injuries in industry: a retrospective study, overview, and cost analysis. Spine 11:241, 1986.

Syms J: Stabilization training can help your back patients gain control. Back Pain Mon 8:101, 1990.

Taylor VM, Deyo RA, Cherkin DC, Krueter W: Low back pain hospitalization: recent U.S. trends and regional variations. Spine 19:1207–12, 1994.

Waddell G: The Back Pain Revolution. New York, Churchill Livingstone, 1998.

Waddell G: A new clinical model for treatment of low back pain. Spine 12:632, 1987.

Waddell G, Somerville D, Henderson L, Newton M: Objective clinical evaluation of physical impairment in chronic low back pain. Spine 17:617, 1992.

Weber H: Lumbar disc herniation. A controlled, prospective study of ten years of observation. Spine 8:131–140, 1983.

Wheeler AH: Diagnosis and management of low back pain and sciatica. Am Fam Physician 52(5):1333, 1347, 1995.

White A, Mattmiller A, White L: Back School and Other Conservative Approaches to Low Back Pain, St. Louis, Mosby–Year Book, 1983.

Wiltse LL: Etiology of spondylolisthesis. J Bone Joint Surg 44A:539, 1962.

Williams PC: The Lumbosacral Spine, Emphasizing Conservative Management. New York, McGraw-Hill, 1965.

Suggested Reading List

Cole AJ, Herring SA: The Low Back Pain Handbook: A Practical Guide for the Primary Care Clinician. St. Louis, Hanley & Belfus/Mosby, 1997.

Hoppenfield S: Orthopaedic Neurology. Philadelphia, JB Lippincott, 1988.

Waddell G: The Back Pain Revolution. New York, Churchill Livingstone, 1998.

Chapter 10
Common Terms, Modalities, and Techniques Employed in Rehabilitation of Orthopaedic Injuries

Anna Williams, PT, MS

Kinematics

Kinematics refers to the science of the motion of bodies in space (Smith et al, 1996). The motion may include the movement of a single point on the body, the position of several segments, the position of a single joint, or motions that occur between adjacent joint surfaces. Kinematics can be further subdivided into two categories: osteokinematics and arthrokinematics.

Osteokinematics refers to the movement between bones. Several terms are associated with osteokinematics. *Mechanical axis* is a line drawn through the moving bone at the starting position of a movement, which passes through the center of the opposing joint surface and is perpendicular to it. *Spin* is the movement of a bone about the mechanical axis (Fig. 10–1A). *Pure swing* is the movement of a bone in which an end of the mechanical axis traces the path of a chord with respect to the ovoid formed by the opposing joint surface (see Fig. 10–1B). *Impure swing* refers to the movement in which the mechanical axis follows the path of an arc with respect to the opposing ovoid surface.

Conjunct rotation is an impure swing accompanied by an element of spin. It may also refer to the rotation that may occur with a succession of swings (Fig. 10–2).

Arthrokinematics refers to the movement between the joint surfaces (Fig. 10–3). Again, several definitions are associated with the types of movements occurring between joint surfaces. *Roll* is the movement in which points at intervals on the moving joint surface contact points at the same intervals on the opposing

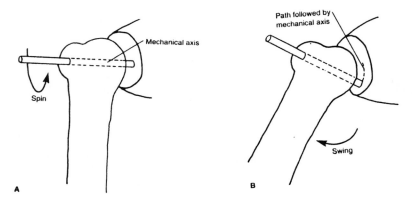

Figure 10–1. Movements such as spin *(A)* and swing *(B)* help to define osteokinematic movements by use of the mechanical axis.

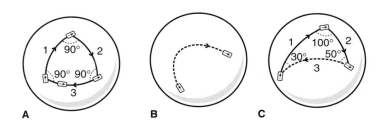

Figure 10–2. Conjunct rotation occurring with a succession of pure swings with return to the starting position *(A)*, with a single impure swing *(B)*, and with a completed cycle of pure and impure swings *(C)*.

surfaces. *Slide* occurs when a single contact point on the moving surface contacts various points on the opposing surface.

When normal arthrokinematic movement is not present, dislocation or impingement may occur as seen in Fig. 10–4, in which normal arthrokinematic movement is absent, resulting in impingement (A) and dislocation (B).

An important rule applies when discussing arthrokinematics and osteokinematics, the *concave-convex rule*. If a concave surface moves on a stationary convex surface, the roll and slide movements must occur in the same direction. When a convex surface moves on a stationary concave surface, the roll and slide movements must occur in opposite directions. This concept can be applied to the restoration of restricted joint motion. However, this rule does not apply to all joints. The concave-convex rule cannot be applied to plane joints, movements for which the axis of rotation passes through the articulating surfaces, and movements of joints in which the concave side of the joint forms a deep socket.

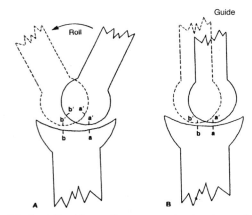

Figure 10–3. Arthrokinematic movements showing roll *(A)* and glide *(B)*. The letters indicate points on the opposing joint surfaces that come in contact with one another. Points a' and b' are on the moving surface; points a and b are on the stationary joint surface. Note that during roll *(A)*, points a and b contact various points on the opposing, moving joint surface; during glide *(B)*, points a and b contact only one point on the moving surface.

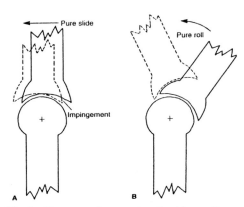

Figure 10–4. Absence of normal arthrokinematic movement, resulting in impingement *(A)* and dislocation *(B)*.

Kinematic Chains

After analyzing individual joints, look at several joints together. A combination of several joints using successive movements constitutes a kinematic chain. Kinematic chains can be referred to as either closed or open (Fig. 10–5). An *open kinematic chain* refers to the distal segment of the chain being able to move in space. Conversely, a *closed kinematic chain*'s distal segment (foot) is fixed and movement occurs at the proximal segment (knee) (Table 10–1).

Closed-packed and Open-packed Positions

In a joint, the ovoid surfaces match perfectly in only one position of the joint. That one position is referred to as the *closed-packed position*. In this position, (1) the maximal area of surface contact occurs, (2) attachments of the ligaments are farthest apart and under tension, (3) capsular structures are taut, and (4) the joint is mechanically compressed and difficult to distract. All other positions of the joint are referred to as the *open-packed position*. Here, the ligaments as well as the capsular structures are slack. The joints may also be distracted several millimeters, allowing accessory motions of spin, roll, and slide as well as decreasing joint friction. Table 10–2 lists the closed-packed position for the joints.

Terminology for Muscle Contractions

Isometric

A muscle contraction that produces force without a measurable change in the joint angle is considered an *isometric contraction*. Isometric contractions can also be referred to as *static* or *holding contractions*. Resistance can be applied either manually or mechanically by having a patient push against an immovable object or holding against a heavy load (Figs. 10–6 and 10–7). The length of a muscle at the time of contraction directly affects the amount of tension that can be produced at a specific point in the range of motion (ROM). However, when muscle length is varied, electromyography (EMG) activity changes. Less EMG activity is seen as a muscle is lengthened with greater tension, while greater EMG activity is seen as a muscle is lengthened with decreased tension.

Isotonic

An **isotonic muscle contraction** causes a joint to move through some ROM. The resistance, whether manual or mechanical, remains constant while the muscle length is continuously changing. Two types of isotonic muscle contractions need to be addressed. A **concentric con-**

A　　　　　　　　　　**B**

Figure 10–5. *A,* Closed kinematic chain. *B,* Open kinematic chain. Open-chain exercises are performed with the distal end of the limb terminating freely in space. Exercising against minimal resistance provided by a length of tubing, as shown here, improves shoulder muscle strength. (*B,* From Richards DB, Kibler B: Sports-related rehabilitation: an overview of concepts. J Musculoskel Med 14[8]:44–63, 1997.)

Table 10-1

Open- versus Closed-chain Exercises

Open-chain Exercises	Closed-chain Exercises	Open-chain Exercises	Closed-chain Exercises
Characteristics	**Characteristics**	Knee ROM exercises.	Hip machine for uninvolved leg.
Distal segment is free.	Distal segment is not free.	Terminal knee extension.	
No weight-bearing.	PWB.	Stationary bicycle.	Sitting with knee flexed, performing towel slides.
Motion is only distal to axis of motion.	Motion is both distal and proximal to axis of motion.	PNF.	***Partial Weight-bearing Closed-chain Exercises***
		Isokinetic exercise equipment.	PWB minisquats.
Muscle contraction is primarily concentric.	Muscle contraction includes concentric, eccentric, isometric, and isotonic.		PWB wall sits.
			PWB lunges.
Movements are usually isolated.	Movements are functional. Can emphasize one muscle group, but entire kinetic chain works together.		Proprioception emphasis using BAPS board.
			Allow PWB ambulation when patient is 50% weight-bearing.
Load is artificial.	Loads are physiologic and through entire kinetic chain.		***Full Weight-bearing Closed-chain Exercises***
Velocity is predetermined.	Velocity is variable.		Wall sits.
Stabilization is often artificial (straps and belts).	Stabilization is a product of normal postural mechanisms.		Minisquats with or without resistance.
			Lunges.
Motion is usually in one cardinal plane.	Motion takes place in all planes.		Proprioception with BAPS board or Fitter treadmill (retro walking and forward walking).
Proprioceptive carry-over to functional activities is questionable.	Significant proprioceptive carry-over to functional activities exists.		Stair machines (forward and reverse stance).
Exercises are often limited by equipment.	Exercises are limited only by imagination.		NordicTrack ski machines.
Exercise Examples	**Exercise Examples**		Agility drills.
Isometrics.	***Non–weight-bearing Closed-chain Exercises***		Step-ups.
Straight leg raises.			Sliding lunges.

BAPS, Biomechanical Ankle Platform System; PNF, proprioceptive neuromuscular facilitation; PWB, partial weight-bearing; ROM, range of motion.

Table 10-2

Close-packed Position of Joints*

Joint	Close-packed Position	Joint	Close-packed Position
Acromioclavicular	Shoulder abducted to 30 degrees	Metacarpophalangeal (thumb)	Maximal opposition
Ankle	Maximal dorsiflexion		
Elbow (radiohumeral)	Elbow flexed 90 degrees, 5 degrees of supination	MTP (toes)	Maximal extension of MTP joints
		Midtarsal (foot)	Maximal supination
Elbow (ulnohumeral)	Maximal elbow extension	Radiocarpal	Maximal extension and maximal ulnar deviation
Facet (spine)	Maximal extension		
Glenohumeral	Maximal shoulder abduction and lateral rotation	Radioulnar (distal)	5 degrees of supination
		Radioulnar (proximal)	5 degrees of supination
Hip	Maximal extension of the hip and maximal medial rotation of the hip	Sternoclavicular	Maximal shoulder elevation
		Subtalar	Maximal supination
IP (fingers)	Maximal extension of IP joints	Tarsometatarsal	Maximal supination
IP (toes)	Maximal extension of IP joints	Temporomandibular	Teeth clenched
Metacarpophalangeal (fingers)	Maximal flexion	Tibiofemoral	Maximal extension and maximal lateral rotation

*In alphabetical order.

IP, interphalangeal; MTP, metatarsophalangeal.

Figure 10–6. Two basic forms of exercise are used in programs to develop muscle strength and endurance: isometric and isotonic. **Isometric** exercise is also known as static exercise because, as one pushes or pulls against a fixed object, the muscle's length remains unchanged and there is no movement.

Isotonic exercise occurs as the muscle shortens (concentric contractions) and lengthens (eccentric contractions) with movement, for example, as one lifts a barbell. Isotonic exercise is dynamic and can entail the full range of motion.

Some weight machines allow athletes to train isokinetically. This method is somewhat similar to isotonic exercise, except that the machine matches the force supplied by the athlete. (From Beckham-Burnett S, Grang WA: Safe and effective weight training for fitness and sport. J Musculoskel Med 4[11]:26–36, 1987.)

traction (Fig. 10–8) causes a shortening of the muscle fibers. The force generated by the muscle fibers is greater than the resistance encountered. Concentric contractions produce acceleration of a body segment. One example of a concentric contraction is performing a biceps curl with light resistance throughout the entire elbow ROM.

An *eccentric contraction* is produced when the resistance encountered is greater than the force produced by the muscle fibers (Fig. 10–9). The muscle fibers lengthen under the resistance. Eccentric contractions produce a deceleration of a body segment as well as provide shock absorption for various activities. However, with eccentric contractions against heavy resistance, there is a potential for excessive stress on the cardiovascular system and these contractions may be contraindicated with some patients. An example of an eccentric contraction is lowering a heavier weight in a controlled manner.

Figure 10–7. During isometric exercise, the muscle contracts without changing length. In this example, the patient is forcefully attempting horizontal abduction against immovable resistance. (From Richards DB, Kibler B: Sports-related rehabilitation: an overview of concepts. J Musculoskel Med 14[8]:44–63, 1997.)

Figure 10–8. In a concentric contraction, muscle shortens against resistance. (From Athletic Training and Sports Medicine. Park Ridge, Ill, American Academy of Orthopaedic Surgeons, 1991.)

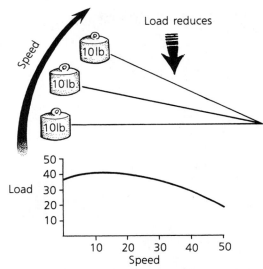

Figure 10–10. Effect of increased speed on muscle load with accelerations at end of range of motion. (From Athletic Training and Sports Medicine. Park Ridge, Ill, American Academy of Orthopaedic Surgeons, 1991.)

Isokinetic

An **isokinetic contraction** is a muscle contraction that occurs at a constant rate of speed. Because the velocity of limb movement allowed is constant, the resistance the muscle fibers encounter will vary. Isokinetic contractions of the muscle may be performed concentrically or eccentrically. Various forms of equipment are used to aid in the production of isokinetic contractions (Fig. 10–10). Different speeds can be set on such equipment and still allow for maximal muscle force production throughout the ROM. A therapist may also reproduce an isokinetic contraction by applying manual accommodating resistance throughout the ROM while controlling the speed of the movement.

Terminology for Muscle Activity

Agonist and Antagonist

The principle muscle or muscle group that produces a joint motion or maintains posture is referred to as an **agonist.** The agonist, or prime mover, contracts to produce an eccentric, concentric, or isometric contraction. An **antagonist** is a muscle or group of muscles that demonstrates the opposite anatomic action of the agonist. The antagonistic muscle passively elongates or shortens to permit motion.

The agonistic and antagonistic muscles vary depending on body position and the effect of gravity on the limb producing the movement. A prime example is elbow flexion with the triceps and biceps brachialis in a variety of positions (Fig. 10–11).

Synergist

The action of the **synergist** is to contract at the same time as the agonist. The synergist contraction may be identical to the agonist, or it may prevent an unwanted action of the agonist acting isometrically. When the agonist contracts, it has the capability to move both the distal and the proximal attachments with the force produced. The synergists automatically contract to fixate that segment at which movement is not meant to occur. The pronator teres is one example of a synergistic muscle. During resisted elbow flexion, the pronator teres inhibits supination caused by the biceps.

Slowly lowering

Figure 10–9. In an eccentric contraction, muscle lengthens against resistance. (From Athletic Training and Sports Medicine. Park Ridge, Ill, American Academy of Orthopaedic Surgeons, 1991.)

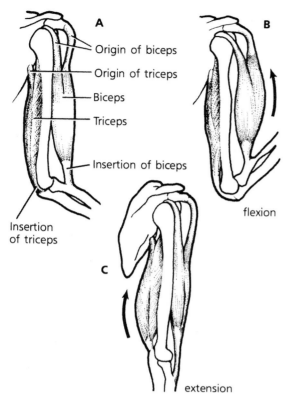

Figure 10–11. *A,* Mechanism of joint motion powered by two opposing muscles. *B,* Biceps contraction flexes the elbow. *C,* Triceps contraction extends the elbow. (*A–C,* From Athletic Training and Sports Medicine. Park Ridge, Ill, American Academy of Orthopaedic Surgeons, 1991.)

Passive Insufficiency

Muscles that are elongated over two or more joints simultaneously may not allow further movement of the agonist at a given point. This phenomenon is referred to as *passive insufficiency.* An example of passive insufficiency is seen in the hamstrings. The hamstrings cross two joints, the hip and knee. When the knee is flexed, the hip can flex to 125 degrees. However, when the knee is extended, the hip can flex to only 60 to 80 degrees, depending on the length of the muscle.

Active Insufficiency

When a muscle attempts to contract with its attachments in close proximity, the force produced is weakened. This is *active insufficiency.* In the body, many muscles cross more than one joint. Length tension relationships must remain favorable to produce desired movements. The body is designed to accommodate such movements. An example of active insufficiency is seen in grip strength. Maximum grip strength is achieved with the wrist slightly extended. As the wrist becomes increasingly flexed, the

Figure 10–12. Tenodesis. Fingers close on wrist extension *(A)* and open on wrist flexion *(B).*

grip strength diminishes. Such diminished grip strength is the result of active insufficiency of the long finger flexors and passive insufficiency of the long finger extensors.

Tenodesis

Tenodesis is the movement of joints caused by passive tension when the muscle is elongated over two or more joints. A prime demonstration of tenodesis is seen when the wrist is flexed and extended. As the wrist flexes, the extensor digitorum causes the fingers to extend passively owing to the increase in tension. Conversely, as the wrist extends, the fingers passively flex because of the increased tension of the flexor digitorum profundus and superficialis muscle (Fig. 10–12).

Therapeutic Techniques Used in Rehabilitation

There are a number of therapeutic techniques in the rehabilitation of a patient. Only a few are discussed to provide the basis of an awareness when speaking to other healthcare providers participating in the patient's rehabilitation.

Proprioceptive Neuromuscular Facilitation

Proprioceptive neuromuscular facilitation (PNF) is a method of increasing the response of the neuromuscular system through the stimulation of the propriocepters (Fig. 10–13). The goal of PNF treatment is to improve and normalize dysfunctional joint movement. In developing the PNF technique, the greatest emphasis was placed on the application of maximal resistance throughout the ROM, using many combinations of patterns and the

Figure 10–13. Proprioceptive neuromuscular facilitation (PNF) exercises are combined movement patterns that use specific sensory input from a therapist to help the patient perform a particular activity. In these exercises, the patient is instructed to retract and depress *(A)* or protract and elevate *(B)* the shoulder while the therapist provides resistance. (*A* and *B*, Andrews JR, Harrelson GL, Wilk KE (eds): Physical Rehabilitation of the Injured Athlete, 2nd ed. Philadelphia, WB Saunders, 1998.)

employment of postural and righting reflexes. The mass movement patterns of facilitation are spiral and diagonal in character and closely resemble the movements used in sports and in work activities. The spiral and diagonal characters are in keeping with the spiral and rotatory characteristics of the skeletal system of bones and joints and the ligamentous structure.

There are **two diagonals of motion** for each of the major parts of the body. Each diagonal is made of two patterns that are antagonistic to each other. A major component of flexion or extension makes up each pattern. There are two flexion and two extension patterns for each part. These major components are always combined with two other components; whether abduction-adduction, external rotation-supination-inversion, or internal rotation-pronation-eversion (Table 10–3).

Many uses exist for PNF in rehabilitation of a patient. The therapist must know in what position to place the patient, proper handling techniques, which pattern to use, which muscle contraction pattern to use, and so on. It is too detailed to discuss for the purposes of this text.

Massage Techniques

Deep Friction Massage

Deep transverse friction massage restores mobility to muscles in the same way a manipulation frees a joint (Tappan, 1988). Deep friction massage (DFM) has a dual effect when performed properly: traumatic hyperemia and movement. Traumatic hyperemia diminishes pain with the enhanced blood supply. With decreased pain, the patient may be able to move the painful structure more freely. DFM also frees adhesions when performed transversely; therefore, it may be performed on muscular, ligamentous, and tendinous lesions. The friction thins out the scar tissue which holds the structure abnormally adherent. However, DFM is not a tolerable method for all patients and should be limited in treatment time.

Myofascial Release

Fascia is a tough connective tissue that has an elastic component, a collagenous or plastic component, and a matrix or ground substance, which under normal condi-

Table 10–3

Patterns of the Diagonals along with Their Acronyms

Head and Neck and Upper Trunk			Lower Trunk		
Pattern	Acronym	Upper Extremities*	Pattern	Acronym	Lower Extremities*
Flexion with rotation to right	D fl, R	D1 ex, R; D2 ex, L	Flexion with rotation to left	D fl, L	D2 fl, L; D1 fl, R
Extension with rotation to left	D ex, L	D2 fl, L; D1 fl, R	Extension with rotation to right	D ex, R	D1 ex, R; D2 ex, L
Flexion with rotation to left	D fl, L	D1 ex, L; D2 ex, R	Flexion with rotation to right	D fl, R	D2 fl, R; D1 fl, L
Extension with rotation to right	D ex, R	D2 fl, R; D1 fl, L	Extension with rotation to left	D ex, L	D1 ex, L; D2 ex, R
Rotation to left	Ro, L	D1 ex, L; D1 fl, R	Rotation to left	Ro, L	D1 ex, L; D1 fl, R
Rotation to right	Ro, R	D1 ex, R; D1 fl, L	Rotation to right	Ro, R	D1 ex, R; D1 fl, L

Note: Bilateral asymmetrical (BA) combinations for reinforcement of diagonal patterns of upper trunk require contact between upper extremities. Forearm and wrist of leading arm are grasped by hand of following arm.

Rotation patterns of upper trunk are reinforced by bilateral reciprocal D1 patterns. Rotation patterns of lower trunk are reinforced by BA patterns of lower extremities (supine position).

Reinforcement of lower trunk by BA combinations of lower extremities requires contact between the extremities.

D, diagonal; ex, extension; fl, flexion; L, left; R, right; Ro, rotation.

After Vose DE: Proprioceptive neuromuscular facilitation. Am I Phys Med 46:846–848. 1967.

tions, is a gelatin-like substance. Cross-restrictions can occur for any number of reasons within the fascia. Myofascial release (MFR), a hands-on technique that applies prolonged light pressure with specific directions into the fascia system, may be used as an adjunct to almost any treatment prescribed for the patient.

Modalities Used in Rehabilitation

Moist Heat

One of the most common heating agents used in rehabilitation are hot packs. Hot packs transfer their heat energy to the body by conduction. Superficial heat usually produces temperature elevation in the underlying tissues to a depth of up to 1 cm. Adipose tissue acts as an insulating layer, which decreases the depth of heat. Commercial hot packs are canvas, usually filled with a hydrophilic substance, that are immersed in 170°F (77°C) water in a thermostatically controlled heater. The packs can retain heat up to 30 minutes. With superficial heat, local metabolism is increased and local vasodilation with hyperemia occurs. Initial vasoconstriction is produced in deep tissue layers, followed by vasodilation. Hot packs also promote muscle relaxation as well as sedation of sensory nerve endings.

Indications
- Subacute or chronic traumatic and inflammatory conditions.
- Preheating before electrical stimulation.

Contraindications
- Acute inflammatory conditions.
- If fever already noted.
- Possible metastases of malignancies.
- Areas of active bleeding.
- Cardiac insufficiency.
- Patients who have received x-ray therapy to the tissue.
- Peripheral vascular disease.

Paraffin

Paraffin is another form of delivering heat, especially to difficult areas such as the distal extremities. A paraffin bath is a container holding a mixture of paraffin (approximately 5 pounds) and mineral oil (approximately 1 pint). The temperature of the melted wax is maintained at 125 to 127°F (52–53°C). Because of the low specific heat, sometimes a higher temperature can be tolerated in the paraffin than in a water mixture. Aside from the heating abilities, paraffin and oil also help soften the skin.

Indications
- Chronic arthritis of the hands or feet.
- Subacute and chronic traumatic and inflammatory conditions.

Contraindications
- Open wounds or infected skin lesion.
- In acute inflammatory joint pathologies, intracapsular heating may promote accelerated destruction of articular cartilage.

Ultrasound

Ultrasound is a deep heating agent commonly used in rehabilitation (Table 10–4). Deep heating agents are capable of causing increased temperatures in tissues up to 3 to 5 cm deep. Ultrasound is a form of acoustic rather than electromagnetic energy. Two common frequencies of the ultrasound are used in rehabilitation: 1 MHz to penetrate deeper tissue and 3 MHz to penetrate more superficial tissue. The ultrasound can use either a pulsed wave, in which the intensity is periodically interrupted and the average intensity of the output over time is reduced, or a continuous wave, in which the intensity remains constant and the energy is produced 100% of the time.

Ultrasound provides increased extensibility of collagen fibers, decreased joint stiffness, decreased muscle spasm, modulation of pain, increased blood flow, and a mild inflammatory response. Two key procedures for the application of ultrasound are to use a gel/lotion medium and to use the applicator in a continuous motion.

Indications

- Soft tissue shortening (joint contractures, scarring).
- Subacute and chronic inflammation.
- Muscle spasms, trigger areas, muscle guarding, neuroma.

Contraindications

- Insufficient arterial circulation.
- Active bleeding.
- Ultrasound over the eyes causes cavitation in the fluid compartments.
- Pregnancy.
- Do not sonate over the spinal cord following a laminectomy because of possible cavitation of the cerebrospinal fluid.
- Infection.
- Do not sonate over the carotid sinuses owing to possible disturbances of the normal pacing of the heart or stimulation of baroreceptors.

Cryotherapy

Cold is used just as heat is in rehabilitation of injuries. Cryotherapy is often used for pain relief, fever reduction, control of bleeding, prevention or reduction of edema from trauma and inflammation, decrease in muscle spasms, and reduction of spasticity. As a general rule of thumb, cold is usually applied during the first 24 to 48 hours following an injury. Applying cold first usually results in decreased fluid filtration into the tissue interstitium, decreased inflammation and pain, and a decrease in the metabolic rate. Cold can be applied by many different techniques, including ice packs, cold whirlpool, ice whirlpool, ice massage, contrast baths, and vasocoolant sprays.

Indications

- Early acute injury or inflammation.
- Muscle spasm.
- Spasticity.
- Fever reduction.
- Edema.
- Emergency care for burns (Athlete Training and Sports Medicine, 1988; Downer, 1988).
- Limited ROM secondary to pain.

Contraindications

- Angina pectoris or cardiac dysfunction.
- Open wounds older than 48 to 72 hours.
- Arterial insufficiency.
- Decreased skin sensation or hypersensitivity.
- Regenerating peripheral nerves.

Electrical Stimulation

Electrical stimulation is another modality commonly used in the rehabilitation of injuries.

Indications

- Reeducate muscles.
- Prevent muscle atrophy.
- Improve muscle contraction.
- Strengthen muscles.
- Stimulate contraction of denervated muscle.
- Stimulate nerve regeneration.
- Decrease muscle spasm and/or muscle guarding.
- Promote wound healing.
- Promote fracture healing.
- Promote ligament and tendon healing.
- Stimulate fibroblasts and osteoblasts.
- Improve circulation.

Contraindications

- Malignancies.
- Infection.
- Pacemakers.
- Pregnancies.

Transcutaneous Electrical Nerve Stimulation

The transcutaneous electrical nerve stimulation (TENS) unit is designed to help control pain of dysfunction as well as reflexogenic and autonomic physiologic responses to nocioception. Various modes can be of benefit to the patient.

Convential Mode

The conventional mode of TENS relieves pain through a proposed spinal cord gating mechanism. It is designed to provide a comfortable tingling sensation at a submotor

Table 10–4

Summary of Research Relating to Ultrasound—Various Settings and Uses for Ultrasound

Application	Authors	Spatial-averaged Temporal Peak		Mode	Regimen	Outcome
		Frequency	**Intensity**			
Soft Tissue Lesions						
Acute injuries			*	P	*	
Sports injuries	Patrick (1978)	*				
Minor fractures			0.5–2.0	P	5 times/wk	Significant improvement
Recent occupational soft tissue injuries	Middlemast and Chatterjee (1978)	1.5				
Subacute			2.0–4.0	*	Up to 5 min daily × 3 then alternate days	Success with acute only
Acute subacromial bursitis	Bearzy (1953)	1.0	0.8–3.0	*	5–10 min × 12	Improvement
Bursitis shoulder	Newman et al (1958)	1.0	1.2–1.3	CW	6 min 3 times/wk × 4	No significant difference
Painful shoulder	Downing and Weinstein (1986)	1.0	0.5	CW	3–5 min × 10	Improvement
Subacromial bursitis	Munting (1978)	1.5	2.0	*	3 times/wk × 3	0.89 MHz more successful
Chronic arthritis	Griffin et al (1978)	0.89/1.0	1.0–2.5	CW	5 min × 8–10	Decreased pain
Plantar fasciitis	Clarke and Stenner (1976)	0.75/1.5	1.05–2.5	CW	5 min × 10	Size unchanged; pain decreased
Rheumatoid nodules		3.0				
Phonophoresis Arthritis	Griffin et al (1967)	1.0	1.5 max	CW	1 time/wk × 9 max	Successful
Epicondylitis or bursitis	Kleinkort and Wood (1975)	1.0	2.0 max	CW	6–9 min	Improvement
Wounds						
Episiotomies	Fieldhouse (1979)	*	0.5–0.8	*	5 min 3 times/wk × 6	Improvement
Episiotomies and surgical wounds	Ferguson (1981)	1.0	0.5	P1:5	3 times daily × 2–4	Improvement
Episiotomies	McLaren (1984)	*	0.5	*	5 min	Improvement
Scars Contracture after hip fixation	Lehmann et al (1981)	*	1.0–2.5	*	5 min daily up to 3 wk	Significant improvement
			1.0–2.0	*	6–8 min, alternate days	Improvement
Hand scars	Bierman (1954)	1.0	0.25–0.75	CW	4–10 min 1 time/wk	Improvement
Dupuytren's contracture	Markham et al (1980)	1.0/3.0	*	*		
Pain						
Low back pain						
Nerve root pain	Patrick (1978)	*	1.0–1.5	P	5 min daily × 10 max	Improvement
Prolapsed intervertebral disc	Nwuga (1983)	*	1.0–2.0	*	10 min 3 times/wk × 4	Significant improvement

*No specific setting for that field.
CW, continuous wave; P, pulsed.
From Prentice WE: Therapeutic Modalities in Sports Medicine, 4th ed. Boston, WCB/McGraw-Hill, 1999.

Table 10-5

Suggested Approaches for Various Treatment Goals Using High-voltage Pulsed Galvanic Stimulation

Goal of Treatment	Rationale	Intensity	Frequency	Polarity Active Electrode	Interval (Intrapulse) (μsec)	Modulation	Active Electrode Site	Treatment Time	Frequency of Treatment
Reduce pain	Stimulate large sensory afferents	Comfortable sensory level only	>50 pps	− to depolarize large sensory afferents	100 for comfort	Continuous	Motor points Acupuncture points Site of pain Myotome Dermatome	30 min or more	prn
Reduce edema (from vessel disruption)	Fluid shift through altered concentration gradient	Sensory level only	High as possible	− to repel proteins	100	Continuous	Cathode over pocket of edema Anode proximal	30–45 min	qd–bid
	Muscle pumping	Sufficient for comfortable contraction	30–40 pps	− to depolarize alpha motoneuron	5	Surged at 1:4 or 1:5 duty cycle	Over muscles that surround venous drainage for injured part	30 min	qd–bid
Wound healing Infected	Destroy bacteria	Sensory level only; wound bed should turn light pink	High as possible	−	100	Continuous	Wound	2 hr	Up to qid
Clean	Unclear, presumably to attract fibroblasts	Sensory only; wound bed should be light pink	High as possible	− days 1–4 + days 1–4	100	Continuous	Wound	45 min–2 hr	bid

Goal	Amplitude	Frequency	Pulse duration	Pulses per burst	Waveform modulation	Electrode placement	Treatment time	Frequency
Muscle exercise to decrease atrophy or increase strength	Strong muscle contraction; high as tolerated	50 pps	— To depolarize alpha motoneuron	5	Surged using duty cycle of 1:5	Over motor points of muscles to be stimulated	10 contractions (10 min)	qd
Muscle exercise for endurance	Comfortable muscle contraction	Minimal tetanic (40 pps)	— to depolarize alpha motoneuron	5	Surged at a comfortable rate	Over motor points of muscles to be stimulated	Progressive length	Build to several sessions per day
Muscle reeducation	Comfortable muscle contraction	Tetanic (30 pps)	—	5	Surged or manually interrupted	Over motor points of muscles to be stimulated	20–30 min	qd
Improve peripheral circulation	Comfortable muscle contraction (10–30% of maximal)	Tetanic (30 pps)	—	5	Surged	Muscles in the area that need increased circulation	10–20 min	qd–bid
Reduce muscle guarding	As strong a muscle contraction as tolerated	Tetanic (30–50 pps)	—	100	Surged	Over muscles that need to be relaxed	10–20 min	qd

level. This mode's parameter ranges include: pulse widths of 50 to 125 and pulse rates of 50 to 100 pulses/p sec, as well as a submotor amplitude that produces either a paraesthesia or a tingling sensation.

This mode may be used on both acute and chronic conditions with relatively fast results in pain modulation. The actual treatment time varies depending on the patient and the condition. However, with the convential mode, adaptation to the stimulus is common. A continuous modification to the pulse width and pulse rate may be necessary to maintain the perceived paresthesia by the patient.

Low-frequency Mode

Low-frequency mode TENS is often referred to as "acupuncture-like" TENS. The purpose of this mode is to provide another means of producing an analgesic response. Low-frequency mode is designed to recruit a variety of deep afferent nerves to produce central inhibitory affects through the endogenous opiates. The parameter ranges for low frequency include: pulse widths of 200 to 500 μsec, pulse rates of 1 to 5 pulses/sec, and an amplitude strong enough to elicit a local muscle contraction in segmentally related myotomes (Hayes, 1993).

Low frequency has several advantages, in that the after effects are longer lasting. Also, the patient's adaptation to the stimulus is minimal. However, some patients may find this uncomfortable and limiting during the actual treatment. Low-frequency mode can be used on both acute and chronic conditions, but the treatments are usually limited to 60-minute sessions once a day.

Burst Mode

The burst mode of TENS is very similar to the low-frequency mode in its mechanism of action and clinical response. Burst mode uses both high- and low-frequency impulses. Each burst pulses at approximately 70 to 100 pulses/sec; pulse width ranges from 200 to 500 μsec, burst rates are 1 to 5 bursts/sec, and the amplitude is strong enough to elicit a local muscle contraction.

As with the low-frequency mode, the burst mode may be used on acute or chronic painful conditions. The lasting effects of the burst mode appear to last longer following the treatment, but the patient may perceive the treatment as uncomfortable.

Brief Intense Mode

Brief intense mode TENS tends to create an almost immediate electroanalgesia when the machine is turned on. This mode is based on the idea that conduction along A-delta and C-fibers is decreased, creating a selective blockage of pain transmission. Parameter ranges include pulse widths at 250 μsec, frequency at 110 pulses/sec, and an amplitude tolerable for maximum paraesthesia.

This mode can be used for both acute and chronic conditions. Brief intense mode is ideal for an extremely acute condition based on the concept of blocking the pain-carrying nerve fibers. It is also used in conjunction with deep friction massage to alleviate the discomfort of the massage technique. Brief intense mode TENS treatment should be limited to 15 minutes because the mechanism of action is theoretically maintaining a conduction block of nerve membrane. However, the treatment can be performed several times a day.

Modulation Mode

Modulation mode TENS operates under the same principles as the conventional mode TENS. The modulation mode is designed to reduce the nerve or perceptual adaptation to the stimulation that often occurs when the stimuli is constant (Wolf, 1989). Pulse width, pulse frequency, and amplitude in the modulation are more cyclically modulated throughout the treatment. Parameters may be modulated individually or in combination.

Treatments can be performed on acute or chronic conditions for any length of time, depending on patient comfort. The effects tend to coincide with the conventional mode TENS.

High-voltage Pulsed Galvanic Stimulation

High-voltage pulsed galvanic stimulation (HVPGS) has an electromotive force of up to 500 volts versus low-voltage units that usually do not exceed 150 volts. Higher voltages bypass the skin's impedance, allowing use of lower voltage current amplitudes in treating patients.

HVPGS consists of paired, unidirectional impulses that rise instantaneously and decay exponentially. The phase duration at the base of each member of a pair is 50 to 100 μsec.

The parameters of HVPGS are appropriate to selectively stimulate large afferent neurons. This causes pain relief through the spinal gating mechanism. Pain may also be relieved through relief of muscle guarding. HVPGS can stimulate a muscle contraction, which in turn, can promote blood flow and produce relaxation. Owing to the possible polar effects of HVPGS, accelerated tissue healing can also be observed. Cathodal stimulation has been shown to be bacteriocidal, whereas anodal stimulation may promote fibroblastic activity. HVPGS can also produce intermittent muscle contractions, which help reduce edema and promote increased blood flow. While reducing edema through creation of muscle contractions, HVPGS will also help decrease muscle atrophy and promote reeducation. Table 10–5 shows several possible indications for HVPGS and suggested ways it may be used to accomplish these goals. Contraindications and precautions are the same as for other modes of electrical stimulation.

Iontophoresis

Iontophoresis is the therapeutic technique that involves introducing ions into the body by means of direct electrical current. Ions are positively or negatively charged and suspended in a solution. These ions move about within the solution depending on the electrically charged current acting on them.

Like charges tend to repel themselves; this is the leading basis for iontophoresis. A positive electrode will drive the positive ions into the body and vice versa for the negative. Low-amperage currents appear to be more effective as a driving force. The recommended current amplitude ranges between 3 to 5 mA. Treatment time will vary between 10 and 20 minutes. The key to iontophoresis is choosing the appropriate ion.

Ions Recommended for Use by the Athletic Trainer

Positive Ions

Antibiotics: Gentamycin sulfate (+), 8 mg/ml, for suppurative ear chondritis.

Calcium (+): from calcium chloride, 2% aqueous solution, believed to stabilize the irritability threshold in either direction, as dictated by the physiologic needs of the tissues. Effective with spasmodic conditions, tics, and "snapping fingers" (joints).

Copper (+): from a 2% aqueous solution of copper sulfate crystals; fungicide, astringent, useful with intranasal conditions (e.g., allergic rhinitis ["hay fever"], sinusitis), and also dermatophytosis ("athlete's foot").

Dexamethasone (+): from Decadron, used for treating musculoskeletal inflammatory conditions.

Hyaluronidase (+): from Wydase, crystals in aqueous solution as directed; for localized edema.

Lidocaine (+): from Xylocaine, 5% ointment, anesthetic/analgesic, especially with acute inflammatory conditions (e.g., bursitis, tendinitis, tic doloreux, and TMJ pain).

Lithium (+): from lithium chloride or carbonate, 2% aqueous solution, effective as an exchange ion with gouty tophi and hyperuricemia.*

Magnesium (+): from magnesium sulfate ("Epsom salts"), 2% aqueous solution, an excellent muscle relaxant, good vasodilator, and mild analgesic.

Mecholyl (+): familiar derivative of acetylcholine, 0.25% ointment, is a powerful vasodilator, good muscle relaxant, and analgesic. Used with discogenic low back radiculopathies and reflex sympathetic dystrophy.

Priscoline (+): from benzazoline hydrochloride, 2% aqueous solution, reported effective with indolent ulcers.

Zinc (+): from zinc oxide ointment 20%, a trace element necessary for healing, especially effective with open lesions and ulcerations.

Negative Ions

Acetate (−): from acetic acid, 2% aqueous solution; dramatically effective as a sclerolytic[‡] exchange ion with calcific deposits.[†]

Chlorine (−): from sodium chloride, 2% aqueous solution, good sclerolytic agent. Useful with scar tissue, keloids, and burns.

Citrate (−): from potassium citrate, 2% aqueous solution, reported effective in rheumatoid arthritis.

Iodine (−): from "Iodex" ointment, 4.7%, an excellent sclerolytic agent, as well as bacteriocidal, fair vasodilator. Also used successfully with adhesive capsulitis ("frozen shoulder"), scars, etc.

Salicylate (−): from "Iodex with methyl salicylate," 4.8% ointment, a general decongestant, sclerolytic, and anti-inflammatory agent. If desired without the iodine, may be obtained from Myoflex ointment (trolamine salicylate 10%) or a 2% aqueous solution of sodium salicylate powder. Used successfully with frozen shoulder, scar tissue, warts, and other adhesive or edematous conditions.

Either

Ringer's solution (±): with alternating polarity for open decubitus lesions.

Tap water (±): usually administered with alternating polarity and sometimes with glycopyrronium bromide in hyperhidrosis.

*The lithium ion replaces the weaker sodium ion in the insoluble sodium urate tophus, converting it to soluble lithium urate.
†The acetate radical replaces the carbonate radical in the insoluble calcium carbonate calcific deposit, converting it to soluble calcium acetate.
‡Sclerolytic: breakdown of calcium build-up or other (hard) deposits.
TMJ, temporomandibular joint.
From Kahn J: Non-steroid iontophoresis. *Clin Manage Phys Ther* 7(1):14–15, 1987.

Possible Indications (Iontophoresis)

- Inflammation.
- Analgesia.
- Muscle spasm.
- Ischemia.
- Edema.
- Calcium deposits.
- Scar tissue.
- Hyperhydrosis.
- Fungi.

- Open skin lesions.
- Herpes.
- Allergic rhinitis.
- Gout.
- Burns.
- Reflex sympathetic dystrophy.

Contraindications

- Skin sensitivity reactions.
- Sensitivity to salicylates.
- Gastritis or active stomach ulcer (hydrocortisone).
- Asthma (mecholyl).
- Sensitivity to metals (zinc, copper, magnesium).
- Sensitivity to seafood (iodine).

Bibliography

Andersson SA: Pain control by sensory stimulation. In Bonica JJ, Liebeskind J, Albe-Fessard DG (eds): Advances in Pain Research and Therapy, vol 3. New York, Raven, 1979, pp. 569–585.

Bearzy JH: Clinical applications of ultrasonic energy in the treatment of acute and chronic subacromial bursitis. Arch Phys Med Rehabil 34:288, 1953.

Bierman W: Ultrasound in the treatment of scars. Arch Phys Med Rehabil 35:209, 1954.

Clark GR, Stenner L: Use of therapeutic ultrasound. Physiotherapy 62(6):85–190, 1976.

Downer AH: Thermal Agents in Rehabilitation, 4th ed. Springfield, Ill, Charles C Thomas, 1988.

Downing DS, Weinstein A: Ultrasound therapy of subacromial bursitis. Phys Ther 66:194, 1986 (abstract).

Ferguson JN: Ultrasound in the treatment of surgical wounds. Physiotherapy 67:12, 1981.

Fieldhouse C: Ultrasound for relief of pain episiotomy scars. Physiotherapy 65:217, 1979.

Griffin JE, Echternach JL, Price RE: Patients treated with ultrasonic driven hydrocortisone and ultrasound alone. Phys Ther 47:594–601, 1967.

Griffin JE, Karsalis TC: Physical Agents for Physical Therapists. Springfield, Ill, Charles C Thomas, 1978.

Hargreaves K, Dionne R: Evaluating endogenous mediators of pain and analgesia in clinical studies. In Max MB, Portenoy RK, Laska EM (eds): Advances in Pain Research and Therapy, vol 18. New York, Raven, 1991, pp. 579–598.

Hayes KW: Manual for Physical Agents, 4th ed. Norwalk, Conn, Appleton & Lange, 1993.

Hertling D, Kessler RM: Management of Common Musculoskeletal Disorders: Physical Therapy Principles and Methods, 3rd ed. Philadelphia, JB Lippincott, 1996.

Hunter-Griffin LY: Athletic Training and Sports Medicine, 2nd ed. Park Ridge, Ill, American Academy of Orthopaedic Surgeons, 1991.

Kisner C, Colby LA: Therapeutic Exercise Foundations and Technique, 2nd ed. Philadelphia, FA Davis, 1990.

Kleinkort IA, Wood F: Phonophoresis with 1 percent versus 10 percent hydrocortisone. Phys Ther 55:1320, 1975.

Lehmann JF: Clinical evaluation of a new approach in the treatment of contracture associated with hip fracture after internal fixation. Arch Phys Med Rehabil 42:95, 1981.

Loubert PV: A qualitative biomechanical analysis of the concave-convex rule. In Proceedings, 5th International Conference of the International Federation of Orthopaedic Manipulative Therapists, Vail, Colo, 1992, pp. 255–256.

MacConaill MA, Basmajian JV: Muscles and Movements: A Basis for Human Kinesiology. Baltimore, Williams & Wilkins, 1969.

Manheimer C, Carlsson C: The analgesic effect of transcutaneous electrical nerve stimulation (TENS) in patients with rheumatoid arthritis: a comparative study of different pulse patterns. Pain 6:329–334, 1979.

Markham DE, Wood MR: Ultrasound for Dopytren's contracture. Physiotherapy 66(2):55–58, 1980.

McLaren J: Randomized controlled trial of ultrasound therapy for the damaged perineum. Clinical Phys Physiol Meas 5:40, 1984 (abstract).

Middlemast S, Chaterjee DS: Comparison of ultrasound and thermotherapy for soft tissue injuries. Physiotherapy 64:331, 1978.

Munting E: Ultrasonic therapy for painful shoulders. Physiotherapy 64:180, 1978.

Newman MK, Kill M, Frampton G: Effects of ultrasound alone and combined with hydrocortisone injections by needle or hydrospray. Am J Phys Med 37:206, 1958.

Nwuga VCB: Ultrasound in treatment of back pain resulting from prolapsed intervertebral disc. Arch Phys Med Rehabil 64:88, 1983.

O'Sullivan SB, Schmitz TJ: Physical Rehabilitation Assessment and Treatment, 3rd ed. Philadelphia, FA Davis, 1994.

Patrick MK: Applications of pulsed therapeutic ultrasound. Physiotherapy 64(4):103–104, 1978.

Prentice WE: Therapeutic Modalities in Sports Medicine, 4th ed. Boston, WCB/McGraw-Hill, 1999.

Rothstein JM, Roy SH, Wolf S: The Rehabilitation Specialist's Handbook, 2nd ed. Philadelphia, FA Davis, 1998.

Sjolund BH, Eriksson M, Loesser J: Transcutaneous and implanted electric stimulation of peripheral nerves. In Bonica JJ (ed): Philadelphia, Lee & Febiger; 1990, pp. 1852–1861.

Smith S, Weiss E, Lehmkuhl LD: Brunnstrom's Clinical Kinesiology, 5th ed. Philadelphia, FA Davis, 1996.

Somers MF: Spinal Cord Injury Functional Rehabilitation. Norwalk, Conn, Appleton & Lange, 1992.

Tappan FM: Healing Massage Techniques: Holistic, Classic, and Emerging Methods, 2nd ed. Norwalk, Conn, Appleton & Lange, 1988.

Thurman BF, Christian EL: Response of a serious circulatory lesion to electrical stimulation. Phys Ther 51:1107–1110, 1971.

Tomberlin JP, Saunders HD: Evaluation, Treatment and Prevention of Musculoskeletal Disorders, vol 2—Extremities, 3rd ed. Philadelphia, WB Saunders, 1994.

Voss DE, Ionta MK, Myers BJ: Propioceptive Neuromuscular Facilitation Patterns and Techniques, 3rd ed. Philadelphia, Harper & Row, 1985.

Wolf CF: Segmental afferent fibre–induced analgesia: In Wall P, Melzack R (eds): Textbook of Pain. New York, Churchill Livingstone, 1989, pp. 884–896.

Yaksh TL: Neurologic mechanisms of pain. In Cousins MJ, Bridenbaugh PO (eds): Neural Blockage in Clinical Anesthesia and Management of Pain. Philadelphia, JB Lippincott; 1988, pp. 791–844.

Glossary

abduction: movement of a body part *away from the midline*.

adduction: the limb distal to the joint is moved *toward the midline*.

Adson test: provocative test for thoracic outlet syndrome, in which the physician tries to eliminate or diminish the patient's radial pulse by abducting and extending the shoulder while rotating the neck.

annulus fibrosis: fibrocartilage circumferential portion of an intervertebral disc.

antalgic gait: gait abnormality caused by increased pain in the involved limb during stance.

anterior: front.

anterior drawer of the ankle: test for anterior talofibular ligament (ATF) laxity or injury of the ankle.

anterior drawer of the knee: test for anterior laxity of the knee (anterior cruciate ligament) in the 90-degree flexed position; not as sensitive as the Lachman test.

Apley compression test: test to elicit pain associated with a meniscus tear by compressing and rotating the knee while flexed at 90 degrees.

apophysitis: inflammation of the apophysis (e.g., Sever's disease).

apprehension test: test to evaluate possible shoulder subluxation (see Chapter 3, Shoulder Injuries).

arthrofibrosis: stiffening, scarring, and loss of motion of a joint.

arthroscopy: surgical procedure allowing viewing of the interior of a joint through a fiberoptic light source and lenses.

avascular necrosis (AVN): death of the cells (bone) as a result of loss of blood supply.

avulsion fracture: fracture during which a piece of bone is pulled loose at its attachment to a tendon, muscle, or ligament.

Babinski sign: abnormal pathologic plantar reflex in which the toes initially dorsiflex on stroking the plantar surface of the foot.

Baker's cyst: swelling in the popliteal space on the posterior part of the knee (see Chapter 4, Knee Injuries).

Beevor sign: sign of the asymmetrical loss of thoracic nerve root motor function, with deviation of the umbilicus away from the dermatome innervated by the injured root when the patient performs a sit-up.

bilateral: affects both left and right sides.

body mass index (BMI): index of a patient's weight in relation to height, determined by dividing the weight in kilograms by the square of the height in meters.

bowstring sign: reproduction of pain by compressing the sciatic nerve in the popliteal fossa (sciatica).

boxer's fracture: fracture of the neck of the fifth metacarpal.

bunion (hallux valgus): enlarged prominence of the medial aspect of the head of the first metatarsal and lateral deviation of the first toe.

bunionette (tailor's bunionette): enlarged prominence of the lateral aspect of the head of the fifth metatarsal.

callus, callosity: thickened, cornified skin of the foot that reflects areas of greater weight-bearing or excess pressure.

carpal tunnel syndrome: symptoms resulting from constriction of the carpal tunnel with resultant pressure on the median nerve.

cauda equina syndrome: emergent spine condition of lower spinal nerve roots with resultant perineal "saddle" numbness, urinary retention, motor loss, and so on (see Chapter 9, Low Back Injuries).

cavus foot (pes cavus): inflexible high-arch foot with poor shock absorption, rigidity.

chondromalacia patella: pathologic diagnosis (not clinical) of degenerative softening of the undersurface of the patella (articular cartilage).

claw toe: toe deformity with metatarsophalangeal joint hyperextension, proximal interphalangeal joint flexion.

closed-chain exercises: closed-kinetic chain (CKC) refers to any exercise in which the limb is restrained against an immobile object (e.g., the ground). A squatting exercise is an example of a closed-chain exercise.

Colles' fracture: eponym for distal radius fracture with dorsal displacement of the distal fragment.

compartment syndrome: increased tissue pressure within an osseofascial compartment compromising muscles and nerves, resulting in necrosis.

concussion: injury to the brain involving transient impairment of function.

contralateral: opposite side.

continuous passive motion (CPM): CPM machine often utilized after knee surgery to improve articular cartilage nutrition, mobilization, effusion, maintain motion, and so on.

contrecoup (counterblow): injury resulting from a blow on the opposite side of the injury (e.g., brain injury).

contusion (bruise): skin or soft tissue injury resulting from a direct blow, with ecchymosis noted.

crepitance: sensation of grating or crackling produced by two irregular surfaces rubbing together.

cubital tunnel syndrome: ulnar nerve irritation or entrapment at the cubital tunnel (elbow) due to throwing.

delayed union of fracture: lack of fracture union within the expected period of time (usually 6–12 mos).

de Quervain's tenosynovitis: tenosynovitis of the abductor pollicis longus or extensor pollicis brevis, i.e., the first dorsal compartment; positive Finklestein test.

dermatome: segment of skin supplied by a given spinal nerve.

discoid meniscus: round, enlarged meniscus that is congenitally "malformed" found in a small percentage of the population.

displaced fracture: bone is out of normal alignment or "moved," often requiring reduction or surgery.

distal: farther from the "central" trunk than a more proximal body part (e.g., the wrist is more distal to the trunk than the elbow).

dorsal: "top" or dorsum of the foot.

dorsiflexion: extension of the foot or ankle, i.e., movement of the foot upward.

drop-arm test: patient is unable to keep the abducted shoulder from falling to the side, a result of a full-thickness rotator cuff (RTC) tear.

eccentric contraction: muscle is exerting tension but is being *lengthened* by an outside force.

ecchymosis: escape of blood into tissue causing bruising or black and blue marks.

edema: swelling.

epiphyseal fracture: fracture of the growth plate of long bones that occurs in children.

epiphysis: ends of long bones.

eversion: the sole (plantar surface) of the foot is turned to the outside (away from the midline).

extension lag: the joint (usually the knee) can be fully passively extended by the examiner (straightened) but not actively extended.

FABER test (Patrick test): provocative test of the sacroiliac joint by *fl*exion of hip, *ab*duction, and *e*xternal *r*otation of the hip and then pressure on the ipsilateral leg causing sacroiliac joint pain.

femoral anteversion, retroversion: the angle between the femoral neck and a plane defined by the shaft of the femur and the flexion axis of the knee; in anteversion, the femoral neck angles anteriorly, in retroversion, it angles posteriorly.

Finklestein test: provocative test in which the thumb is placed inside a fist and then the wrist is ulnarly deviated, eliciting pain over the first dorsal compartment (radial side) of the wrist.

flexion: bending of a joint.

flexion contracture: condition in which the normal extension (straightening) is prevented by soft tissue contracture.

foot drop: weakness or paralysis of the muscles that dorsiflex the foot.

forefoot: "front" area of the foot, composed of the metatarsals and phalanges.

Gaenslen test: provocative test for sacroiliac joint pain in which the joint is stressed by hyperextending the ipsilateral hip off the side of the examination table.

genu recurvatum: ability to hyperextend the knee beyond the neutral position.

genu valgum: valgus deformity of the knee (knock-knee) in which the kneecaps are close, and the distal legs are farther away from the midline than the kneecaps.

genu varum: angulation of the distal legs toward the midline (bowlegs).

gibbus: sharply angled kyphosis.

girth: circumference.

glove-and-stocking sensory loss: circumferential sensory deficit of the limb distal to a certain point (e.g., ankle) typical of peripheral neuropathy (e.g., diabetic, alcoholic neuropathy).

goniometer: protractor instrument used to measure range of motion of a hinged joint.

grind test: test of carpometacarpal arthritis of the thumb, performed by rotating and compressing the metacarpal bone against the trapezium, attempting to elicit grinding in the arthritis joint.

Haglund's deformity (pump bump): abnormal enlargement of the posterior aspect of the calcaneal tuberosity.

hallux rigidus: reduced extension of the first metatarsophalangeal joint.

hallux valgus (bunion): valgus deformity at the first metatarsophalangeal joint; the toe deviates from the midline.

hard corn (heloma durum): dense keratotic tissue occurs over pressure areas of the toes.

Hawkin test (impingement): test of rotator cuff impingement with the shoulder flexed at 90 degrees and internally rotated.

heel counter: back portion of the shoe that rubs or contacts the Achilles portion of the ankle.

heel spur: misnomer; bony prominence at the plantar aspect of the calcaneal tuberosity, the origin of the short toe flexors; *not* the cause of plantar fasciitis.

hemarthrosis: accumulation of blood in a joint.

hindfoot: the "rear foot," including the calcaneus and talus.

hip pointer: contusion to the crest of the ilium.

Homan test: provocative test for deep vein thrombosis of the calf.

hyaline cartilage (articular cartilage): thin layer of smooth cartilage covering the surfaces of a joint.

hyperesthesia: abnormal increase or hypersensitivity to pain, noxious stimuli, light touch, and so on.

hyperextension: forcing the joint into extension beyond the anatomic position.

iliotibial band: strong lateral portion of the deep fascia of the thigh that is the insertion of the tensor fascia lata.

inversion stress test (ankle): test of the calcaneofibular ligament (CF) of the ankle.

ipsilateral: same side.

isometric: muscle contraction producing no change in length of muscle.

isotonic: muscle contraction that produces movement at a joint.

Jersey finger: flexor digitorum profundus rupture of the finger at the tendon's distal attachment to the distal phalanx.

Jones' fracture: fracture at the diaphyseal-metaphyseal junction of the fifth metatarsal, with a high (50%) nonunion rate.

jumper's knee (patellar tendinitis): patellar tendinitis/inflammation typically found at the inferior pole of the patella.

Lachman test: manipulative test of the knee detecting abnormal anterior laxity indicating an anterior cruciate ligament tear; the most sensitive for anterior cruciate ligament integrity of manipulative tests (versus less sensitive anterior drawer).

Lasègue test: passive dorsiflexion of the patient's ankle after straight-leg raising to increase tension on the lower lumbar nerve roots.

lateral: away from the midline of the body.

leg-length discrepancy (LLD): actual or apparent difference between the length of a patient's two lower limbs.

ligament: band of tissue connecting bone to bone.

Lisfranc joints: tarsometatarsal joints of the foot.

Maisonneuve's fracture: proximal (at the knee) fibular shaft fracture with deltoid ligament injury.

malleolus: projection at the distal end of the tibia and fibula.

mallet finger: extensor communis insertion rupture, with inability to actively extend the distal interphalangeal joint.

malunion: fracture uniting with faulty alignment.

manual muscle testing (MMT): subjective grading of muscle strength by applying resistance against active movements.

march fracture: stress fracture of one of the metatarsals; historically common in soldiers walking long distances (fatigue fractures).

McMurray test: provocative knee test to elicit pain and clicking associated with a torn meniscus.

mechanism of injury: manner in which excess force is applied to the body, causing an injury (e.g., valgus blow to the knee causing medial collateral ligament injury).

metatarsalgia: pain and tenderness under the metatarsal heads.

Mulder click: palpable clicking in the third interspace on testing, compressing the neuroma between the metatarsal heads.

Neer impingement test: sign of rotator cuff impingement, produced by maximal forward flexion of the shoulder.

neurapraxia: damage to nerve with "bruising"; not a complete tear or laceration.

nonunion: failure of a fracture to unite (usually > 6 mos).

Ober test: manipulative test to detect contracture of the iliotibial band.

open-chain exercises: the distal end of the extremity is not fixed, allowing the joint to function independently without necessarily causing motion at another joint. One example would be a seated leg extension.

open fracture: fracture associated with a break in the skin (compound fracture).

Osgood-Schlatter syndrome: palpable bony mass at the epiphysis of the tibial tuberosity in athletic adolescents.

paresthesia: abnormal sensation such as burning or prickling of nerve origin.

patella alta: high-riding patella, caused by a "relatively" long patellar tendon.

patella baja (infra): low-riding patella, caused by a short patellar tendon or scarring down of the patella.

periosteum: dense fibrous membrane surrounding long bones.

pes cavus: abnormally high longitudinal arch.

pes planus: flat foot; absent or low longitudinal arch of the foot.

plantar flexion: downward (plantar) movement of the foot or ankle.

plyometric: concentric muscle action immediately preceded by an eccentric action. A plyometric exercise is a quick, powerful movement using a pre-stretch or counter movement that involves the stretch-shortening cycle (SSC). In a stretch-shortening cycle, the muscle is rapidly stretched and then contracted, which increases the force applied to the muscle. Examples include box drills, jumping jacks, single leg hops, jumping in place, etc.

pronation: rotation of the forearm to a palm-down position.

proprioceptive neuromuscular facilitation (PNF): PNF stretching is a type of flexibility exercise combining muscle contraction and relaxation with passive and partner-assisted stretching.

Q-angle (or quadriceps angle): the angle formed in the frontal plane by two line segments: one from the tibial tubercle to the middle of the patella, and the other from the middle of the patella to the anterior superior iliac spine (ASIS).

range of motion (ROM): the natural distance and direction of a joint. Limited ROM indicates a specific joint or body part that can't be moved through its full or normal ROM.

spondylolisthesis: forward displacement or slippage of one vertebra on another.

spondylolysis: defect in the pars interarticularis.

spondylosis: degenerative changes of the vertebrae that can include bony (osteophyte) formation at the disc spaces.

sulcus sign: appearance of a transverse sulcus (divot) between the humeral head and the acromion when the arm is pulled longitudinally, a sign of inferior laxity or multi-directional instability (MDI) of the shoulder.

Thompson test: manipulative test performed by squeezing the calf and observing for normal plantar flexion. Absence of plantar flexion indicates Achilles tendon rupture.

Tinel sign (formication sign): sign of nerve compression, injury, or regeneration after injury in which tapping over the nerve at the site of involvement produces paresthesias or dysesthesias in the distribution of the nerve.

varus: distal portion of the extremity is more proximal than the middle portion (e.g., genu varum or bow-legged).

volar: palmar surface of the hand.

Waddell nonorganic signs: set of five physical signs indicating nonorganic pathology as responsible for the patient's symptoms: nonanatomic tenderness, simulation sign, distraction sign, regional sensory or motor disturbance, and overreaction (see Chapter 9, Low Back Injuries).

Index

Note: Page numbers followed by f indicate figures; those followed by t indicate tables. Italics indicate protocols.

A

Abdominal aortic aneurysm, low back pain due to, 560, 562t
Abdominal muscle tear, groin pain due to, 498t
Abduction pillow, after total hip replacement, 454
Abductor pollicis longus (APL), in de Quervain's tenosynovitis, 72, 72f, 73
Abrasion arthroplasty, of knee, 351, 352, 353
Abscess
  epidural, 560
  of metatarsal, 421
  plantar foot, 437
AC. See Acromioclavicular (AC).
Acceleration, in throwing, 159f, 160
Acetaminophen (Tylenol), for hip arthritis, 444
Achilles paratenonitis, 406–408, 406f, 409–410, 409f, 410f
Achilles tendinitis
  differential diagnosis of, 405
  findings in, 396t
  rehabilitation for, 409–410, 409f, 410f
Achilles tendinosis, 408–410, 409f, 410f
Achilles tendon
  anatomy of, 405
  runner's stretches for, 398, 400f
Achilles tendon dysfunction, 405–412
  classification of, 406
  diagnosis of, 405–406, 405f
  etiology of, 405
  imaging of, 406
  physical examination for, 405–406, 405f
Achilles tendon rupture
  background of, 410
  rehabilitation after, 411, 412
  signs and symptoms of, 396t, 411
  Thompson squeeze test for, 405, 405f, 411
  treatment of, 411–412
ACL. See Anterior cruciate ligament (ACL).
Acromioclavicular (AC) joint
  anatomy of, 125, 126f, 240, 241f
  arthritis of, 151
  injury to, 240–243, 241f, 248
  lidocaine injection in, 151, 151f

Acromioclavicular (AC) joint (cont.)
  palpation of, 131
  testing of, 142, 144f
  weightlifters osteolysis of, 248
Acromioclavicular (AC) ligament, 126f, 240, 241f
Acromion, bone spurs in, 149–150, 151f
Active compression test, 140–141, 143f
Active flexion and extension exercises, after flexor pollicis longus injury, 9, 9f, 10f
Active insufficiency, 609
Activity modification
  for carpal tunnel syndrome, 38
  for knee arthritis, 461
  for lateral epicondylitis, 106, 107f
Actonel (risedronate), for osteoporosis, 534t, 537t
Adductor group attachment, strain of, 497f
Adductor longus muscle injuries, 494, 494f
  rehabilitation for, 501–503, 501f–503f
Adductor tendinitis, groin pain due to, 498t
Adhesive capsulitis, 227–231
  development of, 227
  diagnosis of, 227–228
  differential diagnosis of, 228t
  history taking for, 130
  physical findings in, 248
  stages of, 227
  treatment of, 228–231, 229f
Adson test, 133, 133f
Aerobic conditioning
  after ACL reconstruction, 279
  with arthritis, 449t
AFO (ankle-foot orthosis), for posterior tibial tendon rupture, 416, 416f
Age, ACL injury and, 277–278
Agility training
  after ACL reconstruction, 278, 279
  after articular cartilage procedures of the knee, 353–354
  after MCL injury, 311, 312
Agonist, 608, 609f
Alcohol consumption, and osteoporosis, 532f
Alendronate (Fosamax), for osteoporosis, 534t–537t
Allografts, for ACL reconstruction, 278

Alora (transdermal estradiol), for osteoporosis, 538t
Alpha-adrenergic blockers, for reflex sympathetic dystrophy, 547
Amen (medroxyprogesterone acetate), for osteoporosis, 538t
American Academy of Orthopedic Surgeons, 539
American College of Rheumatology, 539
American Orthopaedic Foot and Ankle Society (AOFAS), on surgical treatment of plantar fasciitis, 403
Amitriptyline (Elavil), for reflex sympathetic dystrophy, 547
Amnesia, post-traumatic, due to concussion, 528, 529t
Amputated parts, replantation and revascularization of, 45–47
Amputation, for reflex sympathetic dystrophy, 549
Analgesics
  for hip arthritis, 444
  for low back pain, 575, 575t
Anatomic snuffbox, tenderness in, 50, 51f
Aneurysm, abdominal aortic, low back pain due to, 560, 562t
Angiofibroblastic hyperplasia, 104
Angiogram, for reflex sympathetic dystrophy, 545
Ankle
  lateral ligament complex of, 372, 372f
  stability of, 371–372, 372f–373f
Ankle brace
  for ankle sprain, 381, 381f, 387
  for posterior tibial tendon rupture, 416, 416f
Ankle dorsiflexion
  after repair of acute unilateral patellar rupture, 347
  for hallux rigidus, 427, 428f
Ankle instability, lateral, 390–392, 392f
Ankle ligament reconstruction, 391–392, 392f
Ankle pain
  chronic, 391
  due to sprain, 383
Ankle pumps, after total hip replacement, 453